THE MEDICAL WORD BOOK

A spelling and
vocabulary guide
to medical transcription

SHEILA B. SLOANE, C.M.T.

President,
Medi-Type, Incorporated

Second Edition

W. B. SAUNDERS COMPANY
PHILADELPHIA/LONDON/TORONTO/
MEXICO CITY/RIO DE JANEIRO/SYDNEY/TOKYO

W. B. SAUNDERS COMPANY
Harcourt Brace Jovanovich, Inc.

The Curtis Center
Independence Square West
Philadelphia, PA 19106

Library of Congress Cataloging in Publication Data

Sloane, Sheila B.
  The medical word book.

  1. Medicine–Terminology. I. Title. [DNLM:
1. Nomenclature. W 15 S634m]
R123.S57 1982   610'.14   81-40691
ISBN 0-7216-8391-6   AACR2

The Medical Word Book   ISBN 0-7216-8391-6

Last digit is the print number: 15   14   13   12   11   10

To
My Husband

JOHN DUSSEAU

With Love and Appreciation for His
Inspiration and the Example
of His High Ideals

PREFACE TO THE
SECOND EDITION

Not many years ago, patient records within both hospitals and the offices of physicians in private practice were kept informally and somewhat casually. The medical secretary was often too busy to take on the task of record keeping, and not infrequently the doctor's wife would come to the office once or twice a week to bring the patients' records up-to-date. The physician, making rounds at the hospital, would scribble a few notes on patients' charts — notes meaningful enough to him but usually indecipherable to anyone else. Writing good case reports was pretty far down on the list of medical priorities.

Advancement and progress in research, the division of medicine into highly specialized fields, and the needs of clinical investigators have now made strict accuracy and careful detail necessary in medical record keeping. No longer are a few scribbled notes acceptable. Trained transcriptionists turn medical data into readily accessible, vital information.

It is the purpose of this book to provide, for those who deal with medical terminology, a simple method for speedily locating sought-after terms. No attempt has been made to make this a complete listing of medical terms. Such an undertaking would be overwhelming and cumbersome. The attempt here is to give the reader a listing of commonly used uncommon medical terms to ease the burden of searching many books. In this attempt, the special needs of transcribers have guided both the organization and arrangement of the content. Particular emphasis has been given to the need for quick reference and reliance on the spoken word — guides to sure usage to all working in the health sciences.

Organization: The book is divided into three major parts. The first comprises Anatomy Illustrated, a series of color plates showing human structure; General Medical Terms, consisting of words common to all specialties; and General Surgical Terms, dealing with such topics as incisions, dressings, sutures, positions, and anesthetics. A new section is made up of an alphabetical list of medications, including radionuclides and chemotherapeutic agents used in treatment of cancer, with proprietary drugs capitalized. Specific tests and pathogenic organisms are listed in Laboratory Terminology, with Normal Laboratory Values ending this part.

The second part is divided into 15 specialties or organ systems. These are arranged alphabetically so that the desired subject can be readily located by flipping through the pages and noting the section title at the top of each page. In this Second Edition, a new section on Radiology and Nuclear Medicine has been added. Neurosurgical terms have been included in the section on Psychiatry and Neurology, and the vocabulary for endocrinology and oncology has been added to the section on Internal Medicine. All terms having to do with surgical procedures, except operations, now appear in General Surgical Terms. Similarly, medications have been separated from the specialty sections and appear in the new section, Drugs and Chemistry. All told, 11,000 new terms appear in the Second Edition. Supplemental plates have been added to provide an anatomic-physiologic perspective in the specialties.

Through the organization of terms by specialty, the time needed to find a specific word is greatly reduced. The transcriber is also relieved of the responsibility of guessing whether a disease entity, an instrument, or the like is listed in one particular specialty rather than another. If a word applies to several specialties, it is listed in each of the appropriate sections. In this respect, repetition of terms has not been avoided; rather, it has been sought out. For example, "sarcoidosis" appears in Cardiovascular System,

Internal Medicine, Orthopedics, and Respiratory System, thus making it unnecessary to flip pages back and forth between sections to find the proper spelling.

A quick glance at the table of contents for the Second Edition will disclose an altogether new concluding part, Guides to Terminology. This provides detailed listings of such diverse subjects as abbreviations; prefixes and suffixes; plurals; chemical elements; and weights, measures, and conversions. The medical transcriptionist, secretary, nurse, student, or physician will find especially useful the meanings of the Greek and Latin roots that make up the complex terminology of medicine.

Arrangement of Terms: Within each section, words are listed so that the familiar term will lead to the unfamiliar; that is, unfamiliar terms are given subentries under familiar main entries. If, for example, the term "Brown-Buerger cystoscope" is used in a urology report, it is only necessary to turn to the section on Urology to find the proper spelling under "cystoscope."

Phonetic Spellings: Selected entries and combining forms are given in two ways: the correct spelling and, at its own alphabetical place, a phonetic spelling. The latter is given in italics, with a cross-reference to the proper spelling. If, for example, the term "ptosis" is used in an ophthalmology report, the transcriptionist may turn to the Ophthalmology section and look for what sounds like "tosis." At that place, one would find the entry "*tosis. See ptosis.*"

As founder and former owner of a busy medical transcription service for 15 years, I watched the needs of transcriptionists become more apparent daily. My years of observing their requirements and concern were responsible for the original conception of *The Medical Word Book.* Their daily use of the book has resulted in suggestions for hundreds of new terms, almost all of which are incorporated in this Second Edition and for whose compilation I am deeply grateful. As in the original edition, I again owe deepest thanks to the staff of the W. B. Saunders Company for skilled help and guidance in the long process from manuscript to printed page.

It is my hope that these pages will answer the needs and improve the skills of health care personnel and will be useful to all concerned with the correct usage and spelling of our vast medical vocabulary. And, finally, I thank the thousands of users of the First Edition who have made the Second necessary.

SHEILA B. SLOANE

CONTENTS

I GENERAL TERMS

II SYSTEMS AND SPECIALTIES

III GUIDES TO TERMINOLOGY

THE
MEDICAL
WORD
BOOK

ORGANS OF SPECIAL SENSE THE EAR

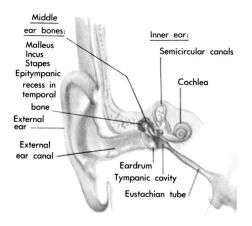

Middle
ear bones:

Malleus
Incus
Stapes
Epitympanic
recess in
temporal
bone

External
ear

External
ear canal

Inner ear:

Semicircular canals

Cochlea

Eardrum
Tympanic cavity
Eustachian tube

THE ORGAN OF HEARING

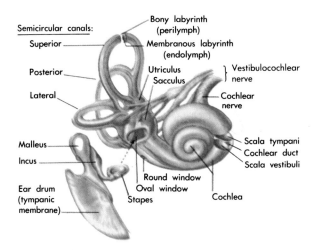

Semicircular canals:

Superior

Posterior

Lateral

Malleus

Incus

Ear drum
(tympanic
membrane)

Bony labyrinth
(perilymph)

Membranous labyrinth
(endolymph)

Utriculus
Sacculus

} Vestibulocochlear
nerve

Cochlear
nerve

Scala tympani
Cochlear duct
Scala vestibuli

Round window
Oval window
Stapes

Cochlea

THE MIDDLE EAR AND INNER EAR

PLATE XII

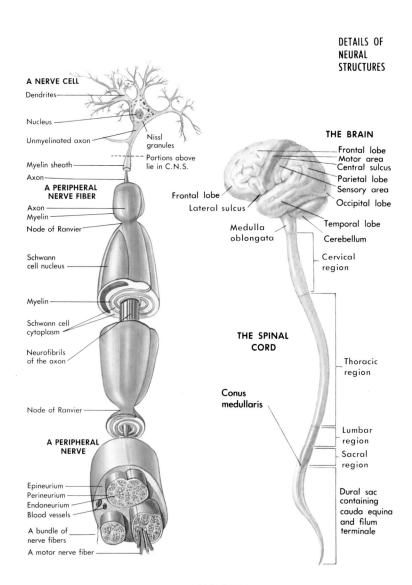

DETAILS OF NEURAL STRUCTURES

A NERVE CELL
Dendrites
Nucleus
Unmyelinated axon
Nissl granules
Portions above lie in C.N.S.
Myelin sheath
Axon

A PERIPHERAL NERVE FIBER
Axon
Myelin
Node of Ranvier
Schwann cell nucleus
Myelin
Schwann cell cytoplasm
Neurofibrils of the axon
Node of Ranvier

A PERIPHERAL NERVE
Epineurium
Perineurium
Endoneurium
Blood vessels
A bundle of nerve fibers
A motor nerve fiber

THE BRAIN
Frontal lobe
Motor area
Central sulcus
Parietal lobe
Sensory area
Occipital lobe
Temporal lobe
Cerebellum
Frontal lobe
Lateral sulcus
Medulla oblongata
Cervical region

THE SPINAL CORD
Thoracic region
Conus medullaris
Lumbar region
Sacral region
Dural sac containing cauda equina and filum terminale

PLATE XI

THE BRAIN AND SPINAL NERVES

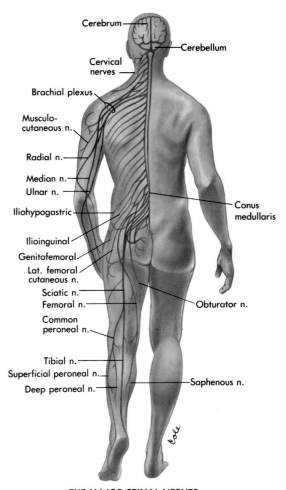

THE MAJOR SPINAL NERVES

Cerebrum

Cerebellum

Cervical nerves

Brachial plexus

Musculo-cutaneous n.

Radial n.

Median n.

Ulnar n.

Iliohypogastric

Ilioinguinal

Genitofemoral

Lat. femoral cutaneous n.

Sciatic n.

Femoral n.

Common peroneal n.

Tibial n.

Superficial peroneal n.

Deep peroneal n.

Conus medullaris

Obturator n.

Saphenous n.

PLATE X

DETAILS OF CIRCULATORY STRUCTURES

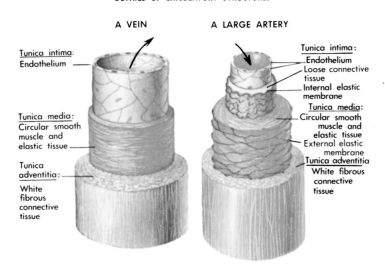

A VEIN

Tunica intima:
Endothelium

Tunica media:
Circular smooth
muscle and
elastic tissue

Tunica
adventitia:

White
fibrous
connective
tissue

A LARGE ARTERY

Tunica intima:
Endothelium
Loose connective
tissue
Internal elastic
membrane

Tunica media:
Circular smooth
muscle and
elastic tissue
External elastic
membrane

Tunica adventitia
White fibrous
connective
tissue

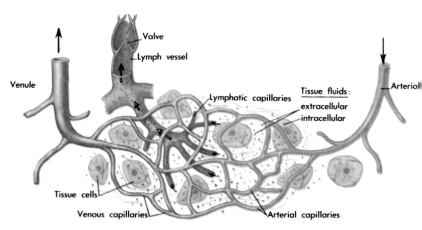

Valve

Lymph vessel

Venule

Lymphatic capillaries

Tissue fluids:
extracellular
intracellular

Arteriole

Tissue cells

Venous capillaries

Arterial capillaries

A CAPILLARY BED

PLATE IX

THE MAJOR BLOOD VESSELS

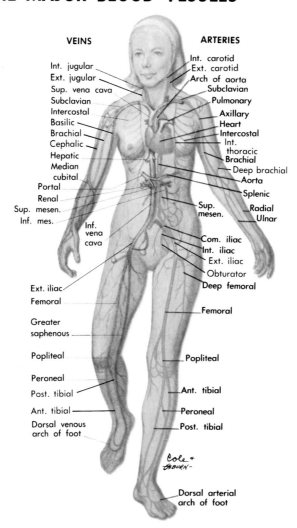

VEINS

Int. jugular
Ext. jugular
Sup. vena cava
Subclavian
Intercostal
Basilic
Brachial
Cephalic
Hepatic
Median
 cubital
Portal
Renal
Sup. mesen.
Inf. mes.
Inf. vena cava
Ext. iliac
Femoral
Greater saphenous
Popliteal
Peroneal
Post. tibial
Ant. tibial
Dorsal venous arch of foot

ARTERIES

Int. carotid
Ext. carotid
Arch of aorta
Subclavian
Pulmonary
Axillary
Heart
Intercostal
Int. thoracic
Brachial
Deep brachial
Aorta
Splenic
Sup. mesen.
Radial
Ulnar
Com. iliac
Int. iliac
Ext. iliac
Obturator
Deep femoral
Femoral
Popliteal
Ant. tibial
Peroneal
Post. tibial
Dorsal arterial arch of foot

Cole & Bourn-

PLATE VIII

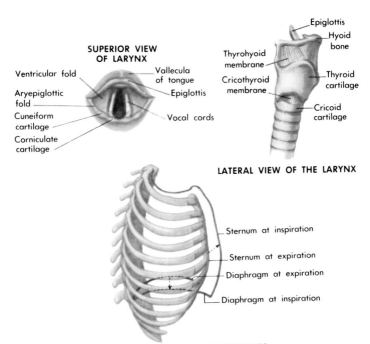

SUPERIOR VIEW OF LARYNX

Ventricular fold
Aryepiglottic fold
Cuneiform cartilage
Corniculate cartilage
Vallecula of tongue
Epiglottis
Vocal cords

Epiglottis
Hyoid bone
Thyrohyoid membrane
Cricothyroid membrane
Thyroid cartilage
Cricoid cartilage

LATERAL VIEW OF THE LARYNX

Sternum at inspiration
Sternum at expiration
Diaphragm at expiration
Diaphragm at inspiration

THORACIC RESPIRATORY MOVEMENTS

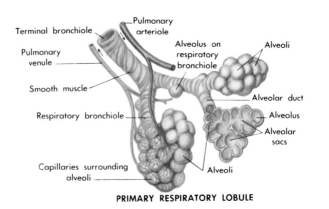

Terminal bronchiole
Pulmonary arteriole
Pulmonary venule
Alveolus on respiratory bronchiole
Alveoli
Smooth muscle
Respiratory bronchiole
Alveolar duct
Alveolus
Alveolar sacs
Capillaries surrounding alveoli
Alveoli

PRIMARY RESPIRATORY LOBULE

PLATE VII

THE ORGANS OF RESPIRATION AND THE HEART

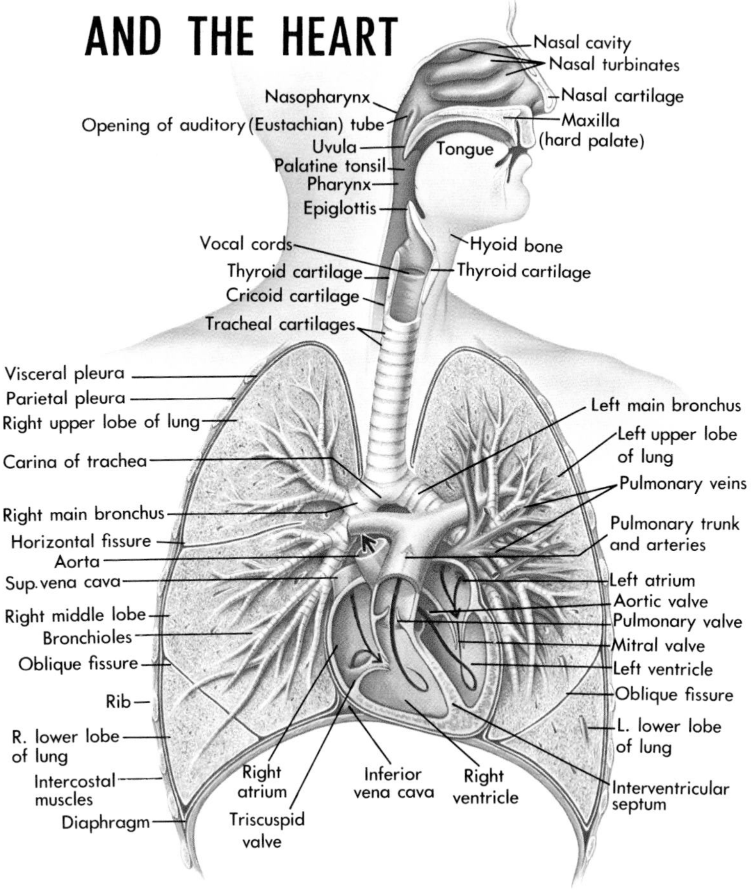

Nasal cavity
Nasal turbinates
Nasal cartilage
Maxilla (hard palate)
Tongue
Nasopharynx
Opening of auditory (Eustachian) tube
Uvula
Palatine tonsil
Pharynx
Epiglottis
Vocal cords
Thyroid cartilage
Cricoid cartilage
Tracheal cartilages
Hyoid bone
Thyroid cartilage
Visceral pleura
Parietal pleura
Right upper lobe of lung
Carina of trachea
Right main bronchus
Horizontal fissure
Aorta
Sup. vena cava
Right middle lobe
Bronchioles
Oblique fissure
Rib
R. lower lobe of lung
Intercostal muscles
Diaphragm
Left main bronchus
Left upper lobe of lung
Pulmonary veins
Pulmonary trunk and arteries
Left atrium
Aortic valve
Pulmonary valve
Mitral valve
Left ventricle
Oblique fissure
L. lower lobe of lung
Interventricular septum
Right atrium
Inferior vena cava
Right ventricle
Triscuspid valve

PLATE VI

SECTION OF STOMACH WALL

Epithelial lining of stomach

Gastric pits

Parietal cells

Gastric glands

Chief cells

Lymph nodule

Smooth muscle: oblique
circular
longitudinal

Submucosa

Blood vessel

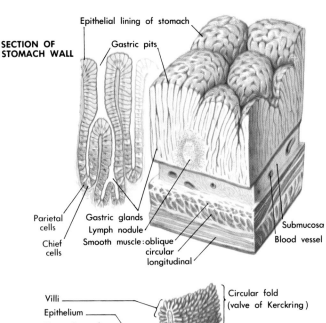

Villi

Epithelium

Mucosal muscle

Blood vessels in submucosa

Smooth muscle
circular
longitudinal

Circular fold (valve of Kerckring)

Lymph follicle

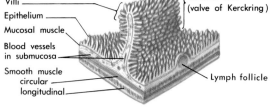

SECTIONS OF SMALL INTESTINE WALL

SECTION OF LARGE INTESTINE (COLON)

Epithelial lining

Openings of glands

Intestinal gland

Submucosal blood vessels

Smooth muscle (circular)

Tenia coli (longitudinal muscle band)

DEMAREST

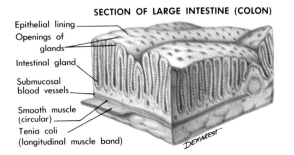

PLATE V

THE ORGANS OF DIGESTION

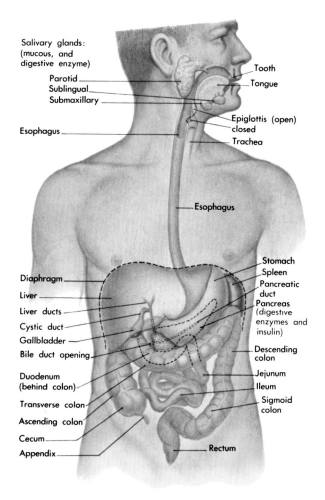

Salivary glands:
(mucous, and
digestive enzyme)

Parotid
Sublingual
Submaxillary

Esophagus

Tooth
Tongue

Epiglottis (open)
closed
Trachea

Esophagus

Diaphragm
Liver
Liver ducts
Cystic duct
Gallbladder
Bile duct opening

Duodenum
(behind colon)

Transverse colon
Ascending colon
Cecum
Appendix

Stomach
Spleen
Pancreatic
duct
Pancreas
(digestive
enzymes and
insulin)

Descending
colon
Jejunum
Ileum
Sigmoid
colon

Rectum

PLATE IV

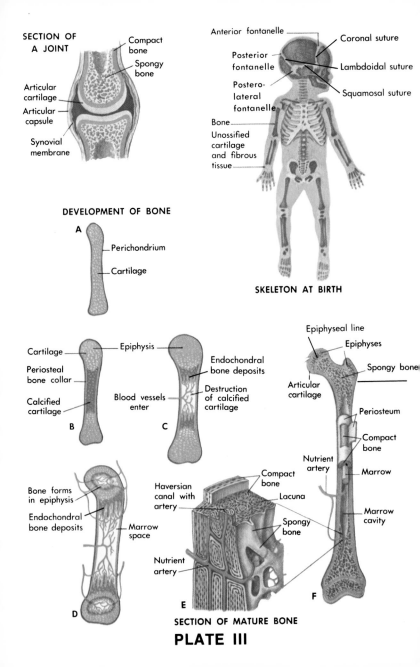

SECTION OF
A JOINT

Compact bone
Spongy bone
Articular cartilage
Articular capsule
Synovial membrane

Anterior fontanelle
Posterior fontanelle
Postero-lateral fontanelle
Bone
Unossified cartilage and fibrous tissue

Coronal suture
Lambdoidal suture
Squamosal suture

SKELETON AT BIRTH

DEVELOPMENT OF BONE

A
Perichondrium
Cartilage

B
Cartilage
Periosteal bone collar
Calcified cartilage
Epiphysis

C
Endochondral bone deposits
Blood vessels enter
Destruction of calcified cartilage

D
Bone forms in epiphysis
Endochondral bone deposits
Marrow space

E
Haversian canal with artery
Nutrient artery
Compact bone
Lacuna
Spongy bone

SECTION OF MATURE BONE

F
Epiphyseal line
Epiphyses
Spongy bone
Articular cartilage
Periosteum
Compact bone
Nutrient artery
Marrow
Marrow cavity

PLATE III

I

GENERAL TERMS

ANATOMY, ILLUSTRATED

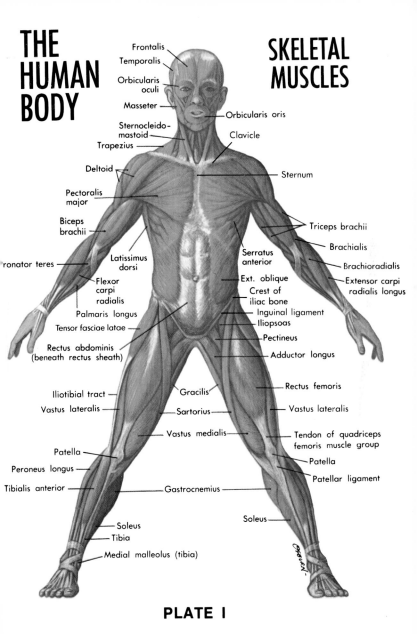

THE HUMAN BODY

SKELETAL MUSCLES

Frontalis
Temporalis
Orbicularis oculi
Masseter
Orbicularis oris
Sternocleido-mastoid
Clavicle
Trapezius
Deltoid
Sternum
Pectoralis major
Biceps brachii
Triceps brachii
Brachialis
Pronator teres
Latissimus dorsi
Serratus anterior
Brachioradialis
Flexor carpi radialis
Ext. oblique
Extensor carpi radialis longus
Crest of iliac bone
Palmaris longus
Inguinal ligament
Tensor fasciae latae
Iliopsoas
Pectineus
Rectus abdominis (beneath rectus sheath)
Adductor longus
Iliotibial tract
Gracilis
Rectus femoris
Vastus lateralis
Sartorius
Vastus lateralis
Vastus medialis
Tendon of quadriceps femoris muscle group
Patella
Patella
Peroneus longus
Patellar ligament
Tibialis anterior
Gastrocnemius
Soleus
Soleus
Tibia
Medial malleolus (tibia)

PLATE I

BONES

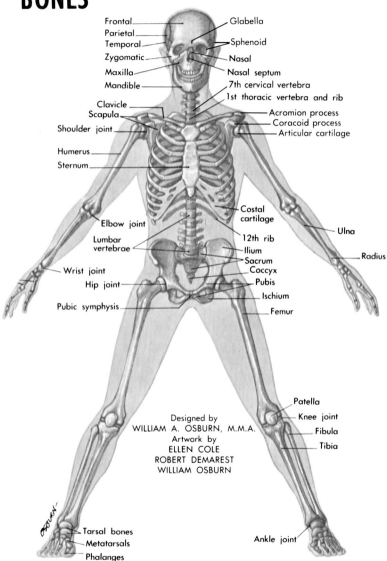

Frontal
Parietal
Temporal
Zygomatic
Maxilla
Mandible
Glabella
Sphenoid
Nasal
Nasal septum
7th cervical vertebra
1st thoracic vertebra and rib
Clavicle
Scapula
Shoulder joint
Humerus
Sternum
Acromion process
Coracoid process
Articular cartilage
Elbow joint
Lumbar vertebrae
Wrist joint
Hip joint
Pubic symphysis
Costal cartilage
12th rib
Ilium
Sacrum
Coccyx
Pubis
Ischium
Femur
Ulna
Radius
Patella
Knee joint
Fibula
Tibia
Tarsal bones
Metatarsals
Phalanges
Ankle joint

Designed by
WILLIAM A. OSBURN, M.M.A.
Artwork by
ELLEN COLE
ROBERT DEMAREST
WILLIAM OSBURN

PLATE II

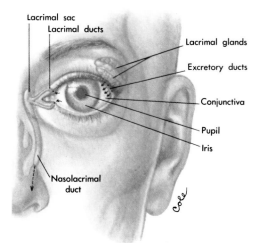

Lacrimal sac
Lacrimal ducts
Lacrimal glands
Excretory ducts
Conjunctiva
Pupil
Iris
Nasolacrimal duct

THE LACRIMAL APPARATUS

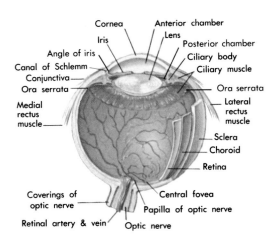

Cornea
Anterior chamber
Iris
Lens
Posterior chamber
Angle of iris
Ciliary body
Canal of Schlemm
Ciliary muscle
Conjunctiva
Ora serrata
Ora serrata
Medial rectus muscle
Lateral rectus muscle
Sclera
Choroid
Retina
Coverings of optic nerve
Central fovea
Papilla of optic nerve
Retinal artery & vein
Optic nerve

HORIZONTAL SECTION OF THE EYE

PLATE XIII

STRUCTURAL DETAILS

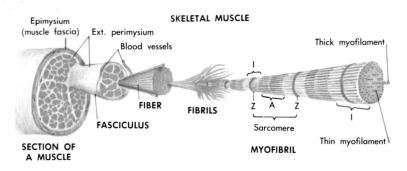

SKELETAL MUSCLE

Epimysium (muscle fascia)
Ext. perimysium
Blood vessels
Thick myofilament
FIBER
FIBRILS
Z A Z
Sarcomere
I
Thin myofilament
FASCICULUS
SECTION OF A MUSCLE
MYOFIBRIL

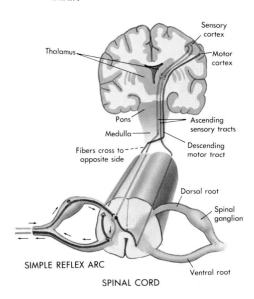

BRAIN

Sensory cortex
Thalamus
Motor cortex
Pons
Ascending sensory tracts
Medulla
Descending motor tract
Fibers cross to opposite side
Dorsal root
Spinal ganglion
SIMPLE REFLEX ARC
Ventral root
SPINAL CORD

PLATE XIV

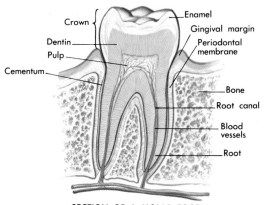

Crown
Enamel
Gingival margin
Dentin
Periodontal membrane
Pulp
Cementum
Bone
Root canal
Blood vessels
Root

SECTION OF A MOLAR TOOTH

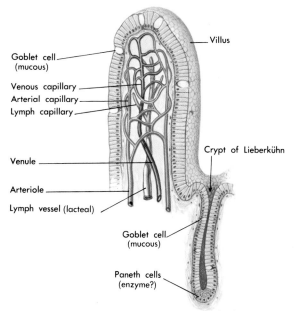

Villus
Goblet cell (mucous)
Venous capillary
Arterial capillary
Lymph capillary
Crypt of Lieberkühn
Venule
Arteriole
Lymph vessel (lacteal)
Goblet cell (mucous)
Paneth cells (enzyme?)
Intestinal gland

SECTIONS OF SMALL INTESTINE WALL

PLATE XV

THE PARANASAL SINUSES

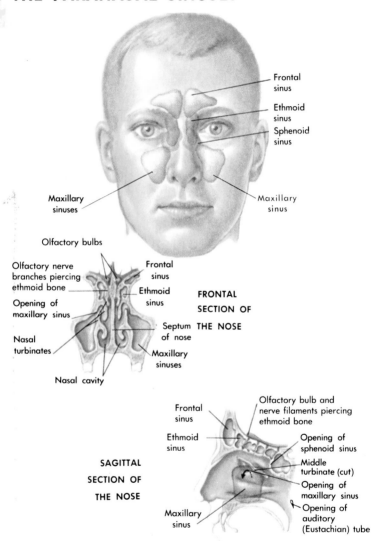

Frontal sinus

Ethmoid sinus

Sphenoid sinus

Maxillary sinus

Maxillary sinuses

Olfactory bulbs

Olfactory nerve branches piercing ethmoid bone

Frontal sinus

Opening of maxillary sinus

Ethmoid sinus

Nasal turbinates

Septum of nose

Nasal cavity

Maxillary sinuses

FRONTAL SECTION OF THE NOSE

SAGITTAL SECTION OF THE NOSE

Frontal sinus

Ethmoid sinus

Maxillary sinus

Olfactory bulb and nerve filaments piercing ethmoid bone

Opening of sphenoid sinus

Middle turbinate (cut)

Opening of maxillary sinus

Opening of auditory (Eustachian) tube

PLATE XVI

THE
MEDICAL
WORDS

GENERAL
MEDICAL TERMS

abacterial
abaissement
abasia
abate
abatement
abdomen
abdominal
abducens
abducent
abduct
abduction
aberrant
aberration
abeyance
abirritant
ablate
ablation
abluent
abnormal
abnormality
abradant
abrasion
abrasive
abscess
absorbent
absorption
a capite ad calcem

acatastasia
acathectic
acathexia
accentuation
accessory
achalasia
ache
acinus
acne
acosmia
acoustic
acquired
acuclosure
acuminate
acute
adduct
adduction
adenitis
adenocarcinoma
adenoma
adenomatous
adenopathy
adhere
adherent
adhesion
adhesive
adhesiveness

adipose
adiposis
aditus
adjunct
adjunctive
adjuvant
ad nauseam
adnerval
adolescence
adolescent
adrenal
adventitia
adventitious
adynamia
adynamic
aerate
aerophagia
afebrile
afferent
afunction
agenesis
agitated
agonal
ailment
akinesia
akinetic
ala
alae
alar
alba
albinism
algogenesia
alimentary
alimentation
allergic
allergy
allotype
alopecia
altricious
alveolus
ambidexterity
ambidextrous

ambient
ambulant
ambulatory
ambustion
amebiasis
amelioration
amnesia
amorphous
ampule
ampulla
ampullae
anabolism
anacatharsis
analgesia
analgesic
analysis
anaphylactic
anasarca
anastomosis
anatomical
anatomy
anemia
anemic
anesthesia
aneurysm
angulus
anhidrosis
anicteric
annectent
annular
annulus
anomalous
anomaly
anorectic
anorexia
anoxemia
anoxia
ansa
antacid
antecedent
ante cibum — before meals
anteflexion

antegrade
anterior
anteroexternal
anterograde
anteroinferior
anterointernal
anterolateral
anteromedian
anteroposterior
anterosuperior
anteroventral
anteversion
anteverted
antexed
anthorisma
antibiotic
antibody
anticholinergic
anticoagulant
antidepressant
antidote
antigen
antihistamine
antipyretic
antisepsis
antiseptic
antitoxin
antitussive
antral
antrum
anus
anxiety
apertura
aperture
apex
aphagia
    a. algera
aphasia
aphasic
apical
apices
aplasia

apnea
apogee
aponeurosis
apposition
approximal
approximate
apyretic
apyrexia
apyrexial
apyrogenetic
apyrogenic
aqueduct
aqueductus
aqueous
arcate
archetype
arciform
arctation
arcual
arcuate
arcuation
arcus
areola
areolar
arrhythmia
arrhythmic
arterial
arteriola
arteriole
arteriosclerosis
artery
arthritis
articulate
articulation
articulo
    a. mortis
artifact
artificial
ascending
ascites
asepsis
aseptic

aspect
    dorsal a.
    ventral a.
asphyxia
asphyxiation
aspirate
aspiration
aspirator
asterixis
asteroid
asthenia
asthenic
asthma
asymmetrical
asymmetry
asymptomatic
asynchronism
ataractic
ataraxia
ataxia
atelectasis
atonic
atonicity
atony
atopic
atopy
atraumatic
atresia
atretic
atrial
atrophy
attenuant
attenuate
attenuation
atypia
atypical
aura
auscultation
autogenesis
autogenous
autopsy
autosomal

autosome
avascular
avulsion
axilla
axillae
axillary
azotemia
azygos
bacteria
ballotable
basal
base line
basilar
belching
benign
bifid
bifurcate
bifurcation
bigeminal
bigeminy
bilateral
bilious
biliousness
bimanual
biochemistry
biochemorphology
biology
biomicroscopy
biophysics
biophysiology
biopsy
bleb
blennogenic
blister
bolus
borborygmus
boss
bosselated
bout
BP — blood pressure
bradycardia
bradykinesia

breadth
brisement
bronchitis
bruise
bruit
bruxism
brwe. See *bruit.*
buccal
bulbar
bulboid
bulbous
bulla
bursa
buttock
cachectic
cachexia
cacoethic
cadaver
caduceus
calcification
calix
calor
calorie
canaliculus
cannula
capillary
capsule
caput
carcinogenesis
carcinoma
cardiomegaly
cardiomyopathy
cardiovascular
carphology
cartilage
cartilaginous
caruncle
catabolism
catamnesis
catharsis
catheter
Caucasian

cauda
caudad
caudae
caudal
caudalis
caudalward
causalgia
cauterization
cautery
cavum
CC — chief complaint
          clinical course
cecal
cellula
cellular
cellulitis
cephalad
cephalalgia
cephalic
cervical
channel
chemotherapy
chorda
chromosome
chronic
cicatrix
circadian
circinate
circulation
circulus
circumferential
circumflex
circumscribed
cirrhosis
claudication
cleft
clinical
clonus
clubbing
clysis
coagulate
coagulation

coalescence
coapt
coarctate
coccygeal
coccyx
coherent
coitus
colic
colicky
collagen
colostomy
coma
comatose
compatible
compensation
competence
complaint
compress
compression
concavity
concentric
concomitant
concrescence
configuration
confluent
congenital
congested
conical
conjugate
consanguinity
conscious
consciousness
conservative
constipated
constipation
constitutional
constriction
consultant
consultation
contagious
contamination
contiguity

contiguous
contour
contractility
contraction
contraindication
contralateral
contusion
convalescence
convalescent
convexity
convoluted
convolution
convulsion
coroner
corpse
corpus
corpuscle
cortex
coryza
cranial
crepitant
crepitation
crepitus
crescent
cribriform
crisis
criterion
critical
croupette
crus
cryoprecipitability
cryoprecipitate
cryotherapy
crypt
cryptogenetic
cul-de-sac
curet
curettage
cutaneous
cyanosis
cyanotic
cyst

debilitate
debility
débouchement
debride
debridement
debris
deceleration
deciduous
decompression
decontamination
decortication
decrement
decrepitate
decrepitation
decrudescence
decrustation
decubation
decubitus
defecation
defervescence
defervescent
deformity
degeneration
deglutition
dehiscence
dehydration
deleterious
delineate
delirious
delirium
delitescence
deltoid
demarcation
demise
demulcent
density
denudation
dermatitis
descending
desiccate
deterioration
detumescence

deviation
dextroposition
diadochokinesia
diadochokinesis
diagnose
diagnosis
    biological d.
    clinical d.
    cytohistologic d.
    cytologic d.
    differential d.
    d. ex juvantibus
    niveau d.
    pathologic d.
    provocative d.
    roentgen d.
    serum d.
diagnostic
diagnostician
dialysis
dialyzed
diameter
diaphoresis
diaphoretic
diaphragm
diarrhea
diastasis
diathermy
diathesis
dichotomy
dietitian
differentiate
differentiation
diffuse
digestion
digestive
digit
digital
dilatation
dilation
dilator
dilution

diminution
dimpling
diplopia
disciform
discoid
discrete
discus
disease
disesthesia
disinfect
disintegration
disorganization
disorientation
disparate
displacement
disposition
disseminated
distad
distal
distalis
distally
distention
distortion
diuresis
diuretic
diurnal
divergent
diverticulum
divulsion
dizziness
donor
dorsal
dorsum
dressing
droplet
duct
ductulus
dysarthria
dysbarism
dyschezia
dyscrasia
dysentery

dysesthesia
dysfunction
dyspepsia
dysphagia
dysphasia
dysplasia
dyspnea
dyspneic
dysponderal
dyspragia
dysrhythmia
dyssymmetry
dystonia
dystonic
dysuria
ebrietas
ebriety
eccentric
ecchymoses
ecchymosis
ecchymotic
eclampsia
écouvillon
écouvillonage
ectad
ectal
ectoentad
ectopic
eczema
edema
edematous
edentulous
efferent
efficacy
efflux
effraction
effusion
egophony
elastica
elective
electrocautery
electrophoresis

electropyrexia
electrotherapy
elicited
elongation
elucidate
emaciated
emanate
embedding
embolism
embryo
embryonic
emesis
emetic
emetocathartic
empiric
en bloc
encapsulated
endemic
endocardium
endocrine
endoplasm
endoscopy
engorged
engorgement
enigmatic
entad
ental
enucleate
enucleation
environment
eparsalgia
epidemic
epigastric
epigastrium
epiphenomenon
epistaxis
epithelial
epithelium
equilibrium
equivocal
erosion
erosive

eructation
eruption
erythema
esophagitis
esophagus
ethanol
etiological
etiology
eucrasia
euphoria
eupnea
euthanasia
euthyroid
evacuation
evanescent
eversion
evert
evisceration
exacerbation
excavation
excise
excoriation
excrescence
excretion
excretory
exenteration
exhaustion
exogenous
exophytic
expiration
expire
exsanguinate
exsanguination
exstrophy
extraocular
extravasation
extremity
extrinsic
extrude
extubate
extubation
exudate

facial
facies
facilitation
Fahrenheit thermometer
fahrma. See words beginning
    pharma-.
falces
falciform
falx
familial
fascia
fascial
fascicle
fasciculation
fasciculus
fatigability
fatigue
FB — foreign body
    fingerbreadth
febrile
fecal
feces
fenestra
fenestrated
fenomenon. See *phenomenon.*
fervescence
fetal
fetid
fetor
fever
FH — family history
fiber
fibra
fibrillation
fibroma
fimbria
fimbriated
fingerbreadth
fissure
fistula
flaccid
flank

flatulence
flatus
flexibility
flexion
flexure
florid
fluctuant
fluctuation
fluoroscope
folium
follicle
folliculus
fontanel, fontanelle
fonticulus
foramen
foramina
forme
    f. fruste
    f. tardive
fornix
fossa
fovea
foveola
fragility
fremitus
frenulum
friable
frontal
fulgurate
fulguration
fulminant
fulminate
fumigation
function
functional
fundus
funduscopy
funiculus
FUO — fever of undetermined
        origin
      fever of unknown
        origin

furuncle
fusiform
gait
ganglion
gangrene
gangrenous
gaseous
gauze
genetic
genitalia
genu
glomerulus
gonorrhea
gracile
gracilis
gradient
gram
granulation
grumous
guaiac
halitosis
haustrum
hemangioma
hematemesis
hematochezia
hematocrit
hematogenous
hematoma
hematopoiesis
hemiparesis
hemiplegia
hemoglobin
hemolysis
hemoptysis
hemorrhage
hemostasis
hepatic
hepatitis
hepatomegaly
hepatorenal
hereditary
heredity

heterogenic
heterotopia
heterotopic
hiatus
hiccup
hidrorrhea
hilus
hirsute
hirsutism
histology
homogeneous
homogenous
homologous
hormone
hospital
H & P — history and physical
HPE — history and physical
            examination
HPI — history of present illness
hyaline
hyalinization
hydration
hydrotherapy
hygiene
hygienic
hygroma
hypalgesia
hypasthenia
hyperemia
hyperesthesia
hyperglycemia
hyperhidrosis
hyperplasia
hyperthermia
hypertonic
hypertonicity
hypertrophy
hyperventilation
hypervolemia
hypochondriac
hypodermic
hypodermoclysis

hypogastric
hypoglycemia
hypoplasia
hypothermal
hypothermia
hypotonia
hypotonic
hypoxia
iatrogenic
icteric
icterus
ictus
idiopathic
idiopathy
idiosyncrasy
illumination
IM — intramuscularly
imbed
imbricated
imbrication
immature
immediate
immobility
immobilization
immune
immunity
immunization
impalpable
impatency
impatent
imperforate
impermeable
impingement
implant
implantation
impressio
in articulo mortis
incarcerated
incidence
incipient
incisura
incompatibility

incompetence
incontinence
incubation
incurable
indigenous
indigestion
indisposition
indolent
induced
indurated
induration
inebriation
inebriety
inert
inertia
in extremis
infantile
infarct
infarction
infection
infectious
inferior
inferolateral
inferomedian
inferoposterior
infestation
infiltrate
infiltration
infirm
infirmity
inflammation
inflammatory
inflation
inflexion
infundibulum
infusion
ingestion
ingravescent
inguinal
inhalation
inherent
inhomogeneous

initial
injection
injury
innominate
inoculate
inoculation
insalubrious
insenescence
insidious
in situ
insomnia
inspiration
inspissated
instillation
insufficiency
insufflation
integration
integument
integumentary
intensity
intensive
intention
intercostal
intermittent
interstitial
intestine
in toto
intoxication
intractable
intramuscular
intrathecal
intravenous
intra vitam
intrinsic
introflexion
introversion
intubate
intubation
intumescence
intumescent
invaginate
inversion

in vivo
involuntary
ipsilateral
irradiation
irreducible
irregular
irregularity
irreversible
irrigation
irritability
irritant
ischemia
isolate
isolateral
isolation
Isolette
isotonia
isotonic
isotope
    radioactive i.
isthmus
IV – intravenous
jactitation
jaundice
jugulation
junction
junctura
juvenile
juxtaposition
kahkekseah. See *cachexia.*
kahkektik. See *cachectic.*
kakoethik. See *cacoethic.*
keloid
keratosis
kilogram
kinetic
kyphosis
labile
labium
lacerated
laceration
lacuna

lamina
laminated
lancinating
laparotomy
laser
lassitude
laterad
lateral
lateralis
latissimus
lavage
lesion
lethal
lethargy
limbus
limen
linear
lipoma
lobe
lobule
lobulus
lobus
longitudinal
lumbar
lumen
lymph
lymphangiogram
lymphatic
lyse
lysis
ma — milliampere
maceration
macula
maim
malabsorption
malacia
malady
malaise
malar
malformation
malfunction
malignancy

malignant
malingerer
malleable
malnutrition
malposition
malpractice
malum
mandible
mandibula
maneuver
manipulation
manual
marasmus
marcid
margin
marginal
margo
marital
marsupialization
masculine
maser
massa
massage
mastication
masticatory
matrix
maxillary
maximum
meatus
medial
medialis
median
medianus
mediastinum
medicable
medicate
medication
medications. See *Drugs and Chemistry* section.
medicinal
medicochirurgic
mediolateral

medius
medulla
medusa
melanemesis
melanoma
melena
melenemesis
melu. See *milieu.*
membrana
membrane
membranous
membrum
mentoanterior
mentoposterior
mentotransverse
mEq — milliequivalent
meridian
meridianus
meridional
mesad
mesal
mesentery
mesiad
mesial
metabolic
metabolism
metamorphosis
metastases
metastasis
metastasize
metastatic
MFB — metallic foreign body
mg — milligram
mgm — milligram
MH — marital history
     medical history
mication
microbiology
microgram
milieu
milliampere
millicurie

milliequivalent
milligram
milliliter
millimeter
millimicrocurie
millimicrogram
millisecond
milliunit
millivolt
mittelschmerz
ml — milliliter
mm — millimeter
mmm — micromillimeter
modality
mongolism
mongoloid
monitor
morbid
morbidity
morcellated
morcellation
moribund
morphology
mortality
motile
motility
msec — millisecond
mucopurulent
mucosa
mucosanguineous
mucus
mummification
mummying
mural
muscle
mutilation
myalgia
myelitis
myelogram
myeloma
myelopathy
myoma

myositis
myxedema
myxoma
nausea
nauseous
nebulization
necropsy
necrosis
neoplasm
neoplastic
nerve
neural
neurasthenia
nexus
niche
nocturia
nocturnal
node
nodular
nodule
nodulus
nodus
nonspecific
normoactive
normocephalic
normotensive
normothermia
normotonia
normotopia
normotrophic
noxious
NPO — nothing by mouth
      (nulla per os)
NTP — normal temperature
      and pressure
nucha
nucleic
nucleoplasm
nucleus
nutrition
N & V — nausea and vomiting
obese

obesity
    exogenous o.
obfuscation
oblique
obliteration
obsolescence
obsolete
obstipation
obstruction
obtund
obturation
obtuse
occipital
occiput
occlusion
occult
oncology
opacity
opaque
OPD — outpatient department
optimum
orbicular
organic
organism
organomegaly
orifice
orthopnea
orthostatic
orthotopic
os
oscillation
oscitation
osculum
osteoid
osteolysis
ostium
P & A — percussion and
      auscultation
pain
    lancinating p.
palliate
palliative

pallor
palpable
palpate
palpation
palpitation
panhidrosis
panhyperemia
panniculus
papilla
papule
paracenesthesia
paracentesis
paradoxical
paralyses
paralysis
paralytic
parenchyma
parenchymal
parenteral
paresis
paresthesia
paries
parietal
pari passu
paroxysm
paroxysmal
patent
pathogen
pathogenesis
pathognomonic
pathologic
pathological
pathology
pathosis
patulous
paucity
PC — after meals (post cibum)
PE — physical examination
peau
    p. d'orange
pectinate
pedal

pedicle
peduncle
peduncular
pedunculated
pelvic
pendulous
percussible
percussion
percutaneous
perfusion
pericardium
periosteum
peripheral
periphery
peritoneal
peritoneum
permeability
permeation
pernicious
per os — by mouth
per primam intentionem
per rectum
perspiration
per tubam
pestilence
petechia
petekeah. See *petechia.*
petrous
PH — past history
pharmaceutical
pharmacist
phenomenon
phthisis
physician
physiologic
physiological
physique
pica
pillion
placebo
plantar
plaque

platelet
plethora
plethoric
pleural
plica
plication
PO — period of onset
po dorahnj. See *peau d'orange.*
polydipsia
polyleptic
polyuria
posterior
posteroinferior
posterolateral
posteromedial
postictal
postmortem
postnatal
postprandial
poudrage
poultice
prandial
preagonal
precursor
premonitory
preponderance
prescription
preventive
primary
procedure
process
prodrome
prodromic
profundus
progeria
prognosis
promontorium
promontory
pronation
prone
prophylactic
prophylaxis

proprioceptive
prostate
prosthesis
prosthetics
prostration
protuberance
provisional
provocative
proximal
proximalis
pruritus
psychic
psychogenic
psychosomatic
ptosis
puberty
pulsatile
pulsion
punctate
punctum
purulent
pustular
pustule
putative
putrescence
putrid
pyelogram
pyemesis
pyemia
pyknic
pyogenesis
pyogenic
pyramid
pyramidal
pyretic
pyrexia
pyrosis
quadrant
qualitative
quantitative
quarantine
quiescent

radial
radialis
radiant
radiate
radiathermy
radiatio
radiation
radical
radioactivity
radioisotope
radiology
radiolucent
radiotherapy
radix
rakoma. See *rhacoma.*
rale
ramification
ramus
raphe
rarefaction
rebound
recapitulation
recidivation
recrudescence
recrudescent
rectus
recumbent
recuperation
recurrence
reducible
redundant
refractory
regimen
regio
regional
regma. See *rhegma.*
regurgitant
regurgitation
rehabilitation
rehydration
reksis. See *rhexis.*
relapse

remedy
remission
remittent
renal
rentgen. See *roentgen.*
resection
reservoir
residual
residue
resilience
resolution
resorption
respiration
respiratory
restitutio
    r. integrum
restitution
restoration
resuscitation
retching
rete
retention
retrograde
retroperitoneal
retroversion
reversion
rhacoma
rhegma
rheumatic
rheumatism
rheumatoid
rhexis
rhonchal
rhonchial
rhonchus
rhythm
rictus
rigidity
    nuchal r.
rigor
    r. mortis
rima

roentgen

rong. See words beginning
   rhonc-.

rongeur

rostrum

rotation

rotexion

rubedo

rubefacient

rubella

rubor

ructus

rudiment

rudimentary

ruga

rugae

rugosity

rumination

rupture

sac

saccular

sacculus

saccus

sacral

sacroiliac

sacrum

sagittal

saliva

salivary

salivation

salubrious

salutary

sanative

sanatorium

sanguine

sanguineous

sarcoma

scalpel

scanning
     radioisotope s.

scanography

scaphoid

sciatica

scirrhous

scirrhus

sclerosing

sclerosis

sclerotic

scyphoid

scythropasmus

sebaceous

seborrhea

secretion

secretory

sedation

sedative

sedentary

seizure

semicomatose

senescence

senile

senility

sensitivity

sensitization

sensorium

sensory

sepsis

septic

septicemia

septulum

sequela

sequelae

serial

serially

seriatim

seropurulent

seropus

serosa

serosanguineous

serous

serpiginous

serrated

sersinat. See *circinate.*

serum

sessile
sexual
sexuality
shivering
shock
    anaphylactic s.
SI — seriously ill
sibling
sign
    vital s's.
Silastic
sinister
sinistrad
sinus
siphon
sithropazmus. See
   scythropasmus.
skeleton
skeletonized
slough
sloughing
sluf. See *slough.*
soluble
somatic
somnolence
spasm
spasmodic
species
specific
specimen
spes
    s. phthisica
spheroid
splenomegaly
spontaneous
sporadic
spurious
stability
stamina
stat — statim (immediately)
status
steatorrhea

steatosis
stellate
stenosis
stenotic
sterile
sterilely
stigma
stigmata
stimulant
stimulation
stimulus
stoma
strangulation
stratum
stria
striae
striated
stricture
stridor
stroma
stupor
stuporous
subacute
subcostal
subcutaneous
subcuticular
sulcus
superficial
superficialis
supernumerary
supination
supine
suppuration
suppurative
susceptible
symbiosis
symmetrical
symphysis
symptom
symptomatic
symptomatology
syncopal

syncope
syndrome
synthesis
tabes
tabescent
tabez. See *tabes.*
tachycardia
tachypnea
tactile
takipneah. See *tachypnea.*
tampon
technique
tegmen
tela
telangiectasis
temperature
tenacious
tenaculum
ter in die
terminal
terminus
tertiary
tessellated
tetralogy
texture
therapeutic
therapist
therapy
thermometer
    centigrade t.
    Fahrenheit t.
thoracic
thoracocentesis
thorax
threshold
throbbing
thyroid
thyromegaly
tinnitus
tisis. See *phthisis.*
tissue
tolerance

tomogram
tonicity
tonus
topical
topography
torpid
torpidity
torpor
torsion
tortuous
torus
tosis. See *ptosis.*
tourniquet
toxemia
toxic
toxicity
trabecula
trachea
tract
tractus
trajector
tranquilizer
transfusion
transillumination
translucent
transmigration
transmissible
transmission
transplantation
transudate
transverse
trauma
traumatic
treatment
tremor
tremulous
trigeminy
trigone
trigonum
trocar
troche
trochlea

truncus
tuba
tubal
tubercle
tuberculum
tuberosity
tubule
tubulus
tumefacient
tumefaction
tumescence
tumid
tumor
tunic
tunica
tunnel
turbid
turbidity
turgescence
turgescent
turgid
turgor
tussive
twinge
twitch
tympanic
tympanitic
uforeah. See *euphoria.*
ukraseah. See *eucrasia.*
ulcerate
ulceration
ultrasonic
ultrasonography
ultrasound
ultraviolet
umbilical
umbilicus
umbo
unciform
unconscious
unction
undernutrition

undifferentiated
undulation
unicentral
unilateral
upnea. See *eupnea.*
uremia
ureter
ureteral
URI — upper respiratory
     infection
urinalysis
urogenital
urticaria
uthahnazeah. See *euthanasia.*
uthiroid. See *euthyroid.*
uvula
vaccinate
vaccine
vacillate
vallecula
valve
variability
variable
variant
vas
vascular
velamen
velamentum
velum
venter
ventral
ventralis
venule
verge
vertebra
vertebrae
vertebral
vertex
vertical
vertigo
vesicle
vesicula

vestibule
vestibulum
vestigial
viable
villus
viral
virile
virulent
virus
viscera
visceral
viscid
viscus
vital
vitality
vitamin
vitium
vitreous
volar
volvulate
vomica

vomit
vomiting
vomitus
    v. cruentus
vortex
vulsella
vulsellum
wakefulness
wart
well-developed
well-nourished
wheal
wheeze
whelk
whorl
wound
xiphoid
zifoid. See *xiphoid.*
zona
zonula
zoster

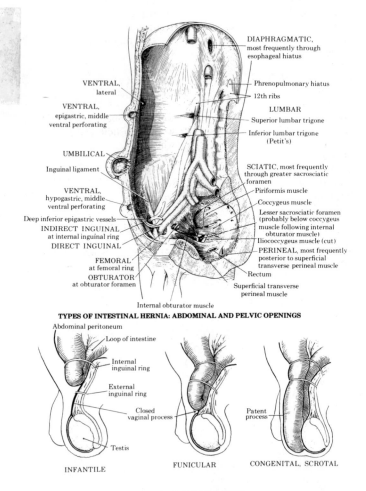

TYPES OF INTESTINAL HERNIA: ABDOMINAL AND PELVIC OPENINGS

DIAPHRAGMATIC, most frequently through esophageal hiatus
Phrenopulmonary hiatus
12th ribs
LUMBAR
Superior lumbar trigone
Inferior lumbar trigone (Petit's)
SCIATIC, most frequently through greater sacrosciatic foramen
Piriformis muscle
Coccygeus muscle
Lesser sacrosciatic foramen (probably below coccygeus muscle following internal obturator muscle)
Iliococcygeus muscle (cut)
PERINEAL, most frequently posterior to superficial transverse perineal muscle
Rectum
Superficial transverse perineal muscle
Internal obturator muscle

VENTRAL, lateral
VENTRAL, epigastric, middle ventral perforating
UMBILICAL
Inguinal ligament
VENTRAL, hypogastric, middle ventral perforating
Deep inferior epigastric vessels
INDIRECT INGUINAL at internal inguinal ring
DIRECT INGUINAL
FEMORAL at femoral ring
OBTURATOR at obturator foramen

Abdominal peritoneum
Loop of intestine
Internal inguinal ring
External inguinal ring
Closed vaginal process
Testis
Patent process

INFANTILE   FUNICULAR   CONGENITAL, SCROTAL

TYPES OF INDIRECT INGUINAL HERNIA

(Courtesy of Dorland's Illustrated Medical Dictionary, 26th ed. Plate XXI. Philadelphia, W. B. Saunders Company, 1981.)

GENERAL
SURGICAL TERMS

Aaron's sign
Abbe's
    operation
    rings
Abbott-Rawson tube
abdomen
abdominal
abdominocentesis
abdominoperineal
abdominoscopy
Abernethy's operation
aberrant
ablation
abrader
abrasion
abscess
    amebic a.
    appendiceal a.
    ischiorectal a.
    mammary a.
    perianal a.
    perirectal a.
    pyogenic a.
    subphrenic a.
absorbable
absorbent
abutment

accessory
Ace bandage
achalasia
    pelvirectal a.
    sphincteral a.
ACMI
    forceps
    gastroscope
    laparoscope
    proctoscope
    telescope
    valve
Acrel's ganglion
ACTH – adrenocorticotropic
            hormone
actinomycosis
acupuncture
Acutrol sutures
Adair's forceps
Adams'
    operation
    position
Adaptic gauze dressing
adenectomy
adenitis
    mesenteric a.
adenocarcinoma

adenofibroma
adenoma
adenomammectomy
adenomatosis
adenomatous
adenomyosis
adenopathy
    axillary a.
adhesion
    attic a's.
adhesiotomy
adhesive
adipectomy
adipocele
adipose
adiposis
adjacent
adnexa
adnexopexy
adrenal
adrenalectomize
adrenalectomy
adrenalorrhaphy
adrenalotomy
Adson's forceps
advancement
adventitia
adventitious
aerate
aeration
aerogram
aerography
Aeroplast dressing
afferent
agenesis
agglutination
Agnew-Verhoff incision
agraffe
akahlazea. See *achalasia.*
Akerlund deformity
akinesia
akinesis

alar
Albert's
    position
    suture
albuginea
Alcon's suture
Alexander's incision
alignment
alimentary
alimentation
Allarton's operation
Allen's
    clamp
    trocar
Allingham's
    operation
    speculum
    ulcer
Allis' forceps
Allis-Ochsner forceps
Allison's suture
allograft
Alm's retractor
alveolar
Americaine anesthetic agent
ampulla
    a. of Vater
amputation
Amussat's operation
Amytal anesthetic agent
anal
anastomosis
    antiperistaltic a.
    Braun's a.
    Clado's a.
    end-to-end a.
    end-to-side a.
    Furniss' a.
    intestinal a.
    isoperistaltic a.
    side-to-end a.
    side-to-side a.

anastomotic
anatomical
anchorage
Andrews' operation
Anectine anesthetic agent
Anestacon anesthetic agent
anesthesia
    absorption a.
    angiospastic a.
    axillary a.
    basal a.
    Bier's local a.
    block a.
    brachial a.
    caudal a.
    chloroform a.
    closed a.
    colonic a.
    compression a.
    conduction a.
    Corning's a.
    electric a.
    endobronchial a.
    endotracheal a.
    epidural a.
    extradural a.
    field block a.
    fractional a.
    general a.
    Gwathmey's oil-ether a.
    high pressure a.
    hyperbaric a.
    hypnosis a.
    hypobaric a.
    hypotensive a.
    hypothermic a.
    infiltration a.
    inhalation a.
    insufflation a.
    intercostal a.
    intramedullary a.
    intranasal a.

anesthesia *(continued)*
    intraoral a.
    intraosseous a.
    intrapulpal a.
    intraspinal a.
    intratracheal a.
    intravenous a.
    intubation a.
    isobaric a.
    Kulenkampff's a.
    local a.
    lumbar epidural a.
    Meltzer's a.
    mixed a.
    nasoendotracheal a.
    nasotracheal intubation a.
    nerve blocking a.
    open a.
    paracervical block a.
    paraneural a.
    parasacral a.
    paravertebral a.
    partial a.
    peridural a.
    perineural a.
    periodontal a.
    permeation a.
    plexus a.
    presacral a.
    pressure a.
    pudendal block a.
    rectal a.
    refrigeration a.
    regional a.
    retrobulbar a.
    sacral a.
    saddle block a.
    semiclosed a.
    semiopen a.
    spinal a.
    splanchnic a.
    stellate block a.

anesthesia *(continued)*
    subarachnoid a.
    surface a.
    surgical a.
    sympathetic block a.
    topical a.
    transsacral a.
    transtracheal a.
    twilight a.
anesthesiologist
anesthesiology
anesthetic
anesthetic agents
    alcohol
    alphaprodine
    Americaine
    amethocaine
    amobarbital
    Amytal
    Anectine
    Anestacon
    anticholinesterase
    Avertin
    benoxinate hydrochloride
    benzocaine
    benzoquinonium chloride
    Blockain
    Brevital
    bupivacaine
      hydrochloride
    butacaine
    butethamine
      hydrochloride
    Butyn
    Carbocaine hydrochloride
    carbon dioxide
    Cetacaine
    chloramine
    chloroform
    chloroprocaine
      hydrochloride
    cinchocaine

anesthetic agents *(continued)*
    Citanest
    cocaine
    cocaine hydrochloride
    curare
    Cyclaine
    cyclomethycaine sulfate
    cyclopentane
    cyclopropane
    decamethonium bromide
    decamethonium iodide
    Demerol
    dibucaine hydrochloride
    diethyl oxide
    Dilaudid
    divinyl ether
    Duranest
    Dyclone
    dyclonine hydrochloride
    edrophonium chloride
    ether
    ether in oil
    ethocaine
    Ethrane
    ethyl chloride
    ethyl ether
    ethyl oxide
    ethyl vinyl ether
    ethylene
    etidocaine hydrochloride
    Evipal
    Fluoromar
    Fluothane
    Forane
    gallamine
    halothane
    helium
    hexobarbital
    hexylcaine hydrochloride
    Holocaine
    Innovar
    ketamine hydrochloride

anesthetic agents *(continued)*
    lidocaine hydrochloride
    lignocaine
    Lorfan
    Marcaine hydrochloride
    meperidine
    mepivacaine
     hydrochloride
    methohexital sodium
    methoxyflurane
    Metycaine hydrochloride
    morphine
    nadbath
    narcotic agents
    narcotic antagonists
    Nembutal
    Nesacaine-CE
    Nisentil
    nitrous oxide
    Novocain
    Nupercaine
     hydrochloride
    Ophthaine
    Oxaine
    oxethazaine
    Penthrane
    pentobarbital
    Pentothal
    Percaine
    piperocaine
     hydrochloride
    Pontocaine
    pramoxine hydrochloride
    prilocaine hydrochloride
    procaine hydrochloride
    proparacaine
     hydrochloride
    propoxycaine
     hydrochloride
    secobarbital
    Seconal
    sodium pentothal

anesthetic agents *(continued)*
    succinyl choline
    Surfacaine
    Tensilon
    tetracaine hydrochloride
    thialbarbitone
    thiamylal sodium
    thiopental sodium
    topical cocaine
    trichloroethylene
    Trilene
    Trimar
    Tronothane
     hydrochloride
    vinyl ether
    vinyl ethyl ether
    Xylocaine with
     epinephrine
anesthetist
anesthetize
aneurysm
aneurysmal
aneurysmectomy
aneurysmoplasty
aneurysmorrhaphy
aneurysmotomy
angiitis
angiopancreatitis
angulation
ankyloproctia
annular
annulorrhaphy
annulus
anoperineal
anoplasty
anorectal
anorectocolonic
anorectum
anoscope
    Bacon's a.
    Bodenheimer's a.
    Boehm's a.

anoscope *(continued)*
>Brinkerhoff's a.
>Buie-Hirschman a.
>Fansler's a.
>Goldbacher's a.
>Hirschman's a.
>Ives' a.
>Muer's a.
>Otis' a.
>Pratt's a.
>Pruitt's a.
>rotating a.
>Sims' a.
>speculum a.
>Welch-Allyn a.

anoscopy
anosigmoidoscopic
anosigmoidoscopy
anospinal
Anson-McVay operation
antecolic
antecubital
anteflexion
anterolateral
anteromedial
anteversion
antimesenteric
antiperistalsis
antiperistaltic
antral
antrum
>pyloric a.
>a. pyloricum
>a. of Willis

anus
apepsia
>achlorhydria a.

aperture
apex
apical
· *aplooshahzh.* See *épluchage.*
aponeurosis

aponeurotic
aponeurotomy
appendalgia
appendectomy
appendekthlipsia
appendical
appendiceal
appendicealgia
appendicectasis
appendicectomy
appendices
appendicism
appendicitis
>acute a
>chronic a.
>a. by contiguity
>fulminating a.
>gangrenous a.
>a. granulosa
>helminthic a.
>a. larvata
>myxoglobulosis a.
>necro-purulent a.
>a. obliterans
>perforating a.
>perforative a.
>stercoral a.
>subperitoneal a.
>suppurative a.
>syncongestive a.
>verminous a.

appendiclausis
appendicocecostomy
appendicocele
appendicoenterostomy
appendicolithiasis
appendicolysis
appendicopathia
appendicopathy
appendicosis
appendicostomy
appendicular

appendiculoradiography
appendix
    auricular a.
    cecal a.
    a. cerebri
    ensiform a.
    vermiform a.
    a. vermiformis
appendolithiasis
appendoroentgenography
appendotome
Appolito's
    operation
    suture
apposition
approximate
approximation
aqueduct
areola
areolae
areolar
areolitis
Argyll-Robertson suture
Arlt's suture
Armsby's operation
arrhythmia
artery
    appendicular a.
    brachial a.
    calcareous a.
    epigastric a.
    femoral a.
    hepatic a.
    intramural a.
    sternocleidomastoid a.
    suprascapular a.
    temporal a.
    thoracoacromial a.
ascites
asepsis
aseptic
Ashford's mamilliplasty

aspirate
aspiration
aspirator
    Thorek's a.
assimilation
asymmetry
asymptomatic
atheromatosis
    a. cutis
athyreosis
atonicity
atony
atraumatic
atresia
atretic
atrial
Atroloc suture
atrophy
augmentation
auricle
auricular
auscultation
autogenous
autograft
autologous
autotransfusion
Auvray's incision
avascular
avascularization
Avertin anesthetic agent
avulsion
aw bissahk. See *en bissac.*
awl
    curved a.
Axenfeld's suture
axilla
axillae
axillary
axis
Babcock's
    clamp
    forceps

Babcock's (*continued*)
    operation
    suture
Backhaus' forceps
Bacon's anoscope
Bainbridge's forceps
Baker's
    cyst
    tube
Bake's dilator
Balfour's
    gastroenterostomy
    retractor
ballooning
ballottement
    abdominal b.
Ball's operation
bandage. See also *dressing*.
    Ace b.
    adhesive b.
    Barton's b.
    circular b.
    compression b.
    cotton elastic b.
    cotton-wool b.
    cravat b.
    crepe b.
    crucial b.
    Curad plastic b.
    demigauntlet b.
    elastic b.
    Elasticon b.
    Elastoplast b.
    Esmarch's b.
    figure-of-eight b.
    fixation b.
    four-tailed b.
    gauntlet b.
    gauze b.
    hammock b.
    immobilizing b.
    Kerlix b.
    Kling b.

bandage *(continued)*
    many-tailed b.
    Marlex b.
    pressure b.
    roller b.
    scultetus b.
    spica b.
    spiral b.
    stockinette b.
    Surgiflex b.
    suspensory b.
    T-bandage
    Thillaye's b.
    Velpeau's b.
    Y-bandage
Band-aid dressing
Bardenheuer's incision
Bard-Parker blades
Barnes'
    dilator
    trocar
Barraquer's suture
Barrett's forceps
Barr's
    hook
    probe
    speculum
Bar's incision
Barth's hernia
Barton's bandage
basal
Bassini's operation
"basting stitch"
    Parker-Kerr b.s.
bath
    sitz b.
Battle-Jalaguier-Kammerer
    incision
Battle's
    incision
    operation
Baynton's operation
Beardsley's clamp

Beatson's operation
Beaver's blades
Beck-Jianu gastrostomy
Beckman's retractor
Beck's gastrostomy scoop
Béclard's
    hernia
    suture
bedsore
Beebe's forceps
Bell's suture
Belmas' operation
Benedict's gastroscope
benign
Berbridge's scissors
Berens'
    retractor
    scoop
Bergman-Israel incision
Bergmann's incision
Berna's retractor
Bernstein's gastroscope
Best's
    clamp
    operation
Bevan's
    forceps
    incision
    operation
Beyea's operation
bezoar
Bier's local anesthesia
Biesenberger's operation
bifrontal
bifurcation
bilateral
biliary
Billroth's
    forceps
    gastroenterostomy I and
        II
    operation
bilobate

bimanual
binder
    Velcro b.
biopsy
    aspiration b.
    excisional b.
    fractional b.
    needle b.
    punch b.
    sponge b.
    surface b.
Bircher's operation
Birkett's hernia
bisection
bistoury
    b. blade
blade
    Bard-Parker b's.
    Beaver's b's.
    bistoury b.
Blake's forceps
Blalock-Hanlon operation
Blalock-Taussig operation
Blanchard's
    cryptotome
    forceps
bleeders
Blockain anesthetic agent
Bloodgood's operation
bloodless
blotchy
Blumer's shelf
Boari's button
Bobb's operation
Bochdalek's foramen
Bodenheimer's anoscope
body
    malpighian b's.
Boehm's
    anoscope
    proctoscope
    sigmoidoscope
boggy

Bogue's operation
bolus
Bonner's position
Bonta's knife
borborygmus
Bose's operation
bosselated
bougie
    acorn-tipped b.
    common duct b.
    olive-tipped b.
    soluble b.
    tunneled b.
    wax-tipped b.
    whistle b.
Bovie unit
bowel
Boyce's position
Boys-Allis forceps
Bozeman's
    position
    suture
Brackin's incision
Bradford's forceps
Braun and Jaboulay
    gastroenterostomy
Braun's anastomosis
Brenner's operation
Brevital anesthetic agent
Bricker's operation
Brinkerhoff's anoscope
Brinton's disease
Brock's incision
Brooks' scissors
Brophy's forceps
Brown-Adson forceps
Brown's forceps
bruit
    b. de clapotement (brwe
      duh klahpotmaw)
Brunner's
    dissector

Brunner's (*continued*)
    forceps
Brunschwig's operation
brwe. See *bruit.*
Bryant's operation
bubo
Buckstein's insufflator
Buerger's disease
Buie-Hirschman
    anoscope
    clamp
Buie's
    clamp
    forceps
    irrigator
    position
    probe
    procedure
    scissors
    sigmoidoscope
    technique
    tube
Buie-Smith
    retractor
    speculum
bunion
bunionectomy
Bunnell's suture
Burnham's scissors
bursa
bursectomy
bursocentesis
bursotomy
Butcher's saw
buttock
button
    Boari's b.
    Chlumsky's b.
    Jaboulay's b.
    Lardennois's b.
    Murphy's b.
    peritoneal b.

button (*continued*)
    polyethylene collar b.
    Villard's b.
Butyn anesthetic agent
Byford's retractor
cadaver
calculus
Caldwell's position
Callisen's operation
Calot's triangle
Camper's fascia
canal
    crural c.
    c. of Nuck
canaliculus
canalization
cannula
    Ingals' c.
    perfusion c.
cannulation
Cantor's tube
capitonnage
capsule
Carbocaine hydrochloride
  anesthetic agent
carbuncle
carcinoma
    basal cell c.
    ductal c.
    infiltrating ductal cell c.
    lobular c.
    metastatic c.
    squamous cell c.
Cargile's membrane
Carmalt's forceps
Carman's tube
Carmody's forceps
carrier
    Deschamps' c.
    Lahey's c.
    Mayo's c.
    Wangensteen's c.

Carter's
    clamp
    splenectomy
cartilage
cartilaginous
caruncle
Casselberry's position
Cassidy-Brophy forceps
catheter
    Foley's c.
    indwelling c.
    Lane's c.
    mushroom c.
    retention c.
    self-retaining c.
    Virden's c.
    Weber's c.
    whistle-tip c.
catheterization
catheterize
cathode
Cattell's
    operation
    tube
cauterization
cautery
cavernous
cavity
    peritoneal c.
cecal
cecectomy
cecocele
cecocolic
cecocolon
cecocoloplicopexy
cecocolostomy
cecofixation
cecoileostomy
cecopexy
cecoplication
cecoptosis
cecorectal

cecorrhaphy
cecosigmoidostomy
cecostomy
cecotomy
cecum
    hepatic c.
    c. mobile
celiac
celiectomy
celiocentesis
celioenterotomy
celiogastrotomy
celioparacentesis
celiopyosis
celiorrhaphy
celioscopy
celiotomy
    ventral c.
Cellolite
cellophane dressing
cellulitus
cellulocutaneous
celluloid
centesis
cephalad
cephalic
Cetacaine anesthetic agent
Chaffin-Pratt tube
Chaput's operation
Chelsea-Eaton speculum
chemosurgery
Cherney's incision
Chernez' incision
Chevalier-Jackson gastroscope
Cheyne's operation
Chiazzi's operation
Chiba needle
Chiene's incision
Child's operation
Childs-Phillips needle
Chlumsky's button
cholangiectasis
cholangioadenoma

cholangiocarcinoma
cholangiocholecystocholedo-
    chectomy
cholangioenterostomy
cholangiogastrostomy
cholangiogram
cholangiography
    operative c.
cholangiohepatitis
cholangiohepatoma
cholangiojejunostomy
    intrahepatic c.
cholangioma
cholangiostomy
cholangiotomy
cholangitis
    c. lenta
cholecyst
cholecystalgia
cholecystatony
cholecystectasia
cholecystectomy
cholecystelectrocoagulectomy
cholecystendysis
cholecystenteric
cholecystenteroanastomosis
cholecystenterorrhaphy
cholecystenterostomy
cholecystgastrostomy
cholecystic
cholecystis
cholecystitis
    c. emphysematosa
    follicular c.
    gaseous c.
    c. glandularis proliferans
cholecystnephrostomy
cholecystocholangiogram
cholecystocolonic
cholecystocolostomy
cholecystocolotomy
cholecystoduodenostomy
cholecystoenterostomy

cholecystogastric
cholecystogastrostomy
cholecystogram
cholecystography
cholecystoileostomy
cholecystojejunostomy
cholecystokinetic
cholecystolithiasis
cholecystolithotripsy
cholecystopathy
cholecystopexy
cholecystoptosis
cholecystopyelostomy
cholecystorrhaphy
cholecystosis
cholecystostomy
cholecystotomy
choledochal
choledochectomy
choledochitis
choledochocele
choledochocholedochorrhaphy
choledochocholedochostomy
choledochoduodenostomy
choledochoenterostomy
choledochogastrostomy
choledochogram
choledochography
choledochohepatostomy
choledochoileostomy
choledochojejunostomy
choledocholith
choledocholithiasis
choledocholithotomy
choledocholithotripsy
choledochoplasty
choledochorrhaphy
choledochoscope
choledochosphincterotomy
choledochostomy
choledochotomy
choledochus

cholelith
cholelithiasis
cholelithotomy
cholelithotripsy
cholelithotrity
cholemesis
cholemia
cholepathia
choleperitoneum
cholescintography
chyle
cicatrectomy
cicatricotomy
cicatrix
cicatrization
circumcision
circumflex
cirsectomy
cirsenchysis
cirsodesis
cirsotome
cirsotomy
cisterna
Citanest anesthetic agent
Clado's anastomosis
Clagett's operation
clamp
      Allen's c.
      Babcock's c.
      Beardsley's c.
      Best's c.
      Buie-Hirschman c.
      Buie's c.
      C. clamp
      Carter's c.
      Cope's c.
      Crile's c.
      Daniel's c.
      DeMartel-Wolfson c.
      Dennis' c.
      Dixon-Thomas-Smith c.
      Doyen's c.

clamp (*continued*)
    Eastman's c.
    Fehland's c.
    Foss' c.
    Friedrich-Petz c.
    Furniss' c.
    Furniss-Clute c.
    Furniss-McClure-Hinton
      c.
    Gant's c.
    Glassman's c.
    Hayes' c.
    Heaney c.
    Herff's c.
    Hunt's c.
    Hurwitz's c.
    Jarvis' c.
    Kapp-Beck c.
    Kelly's c.
    Kocher's c.
    Lahey's c.
    Lane's c.
    Linton's c.
    Lockwood's c.
    MacDonald's c.
    Martel's c.
    Mastin's c.
    Mikulicz's c.
    Moreno's c.
    mosquito c.
    Moynihan's c.
    Nussbaum's c.
    Ochsner's c.
    Parker's c.
    Payr's c.
    Pean's c.
    Pemberton's c.
    Pennington's c.
    Phillips' c.
    Pott's c.
    Rankin's c.
    Ranzewski's c.
    Roosevelt's c.

clamp (*continued*)
    Schoemaker's c.
    Scudder's c.
    Stevenson's c.
    Stone-Holcombe c.
    Stone's c.
    von Petz's c.
    Wangensteen's c.
    Watts' c.
    W. Dean McDonald c.
    Wolfson's c.
    Yellen c.
    Zachary Cope–DeMartel
      c.
claudication
clavicle
clavicular
cleavage
clitoral
clitoridectomy
clitoridotomy
clitoritomy
cloaca
Cloquet's
    fascia
    hernia
    node
    septum
closure
    Smead-Jones c.
clove-hitch
Cloward's retractor
Clute's incision
clysis
coagulate
coagulation
Coakley's suture
coalescence
coapt
coaptation
coarctation
coarctotomy
cobalt

coccyx
Codman's incision
Coffey's incision
colectomy
Cole's retractor
colic
colicky
colitis
Collin's forceps
collodion
colloid
collum
    c. vesicae felleae
colocentesis
coloclysis
colocolostomy
colocutaneous
colofixation
colohepatopexy
coloileal
cololysis
colon
    c. ascendens
    ascending c.
    c. descendens
    descending c.
    irritable c.
    lead-pipe c.
    pelvic c. of Waldeyer
    sigmoid c.
    c. sigmoideum
    thrifty c.
    transverse c.
    c. transversum
colonorrhagia
colonorrhea
colonoscope
colonoscopy
colopexostomy
colopexotomy
colopexy
coloplication

coloproctectomy
coloproctostomy
coloptosis
colorectostomy
colorrhaphy
colosigmoidostomy
colostomy
    ileotransverse c.
    Wangensteen's c.
colotomy
comedocarcinoma
comedomastitis
concretion
condyloma
    c. acuminatum
confluent
Connell's suture
constriction
    duodenopyloric c.
contracture
    Dupuytren's c.
    Volkmann's c.
convolution
Cook's speculum
Cooper's
    hernia
    ligament
    operation
Cope's clamp
cord
    spermatic c.
Corning's anesthesia
Cornish wool dressing
corpora
corpus
cortex
Cotting's operation
cottonoid patty
Courvoisier's
    gallbladder
    incision
Craig's needle

cremaster
cremasteric
cribriform
Crile's
    clamp
    forceps
    retractor
Cripps'
    obturator
    operation
crural
crus
Cruveilhier's ulcer
cryocautery
cryosurgery
cryotherapy
crypt
    c's of Lieberkühn
    Luschka's c's
cryptitis
cryptotome
    Blanchard's c.
cul-de-sac
Curad plastic bandage
curettage
curetted
Curtis' forceps
curvature
    lesser c.
Curvoisier's gastroenterostomy
Cushing's
    forceps
    suture
    ulcer
cutaneous
cuticle
Cyclaine anesthetic agent
cyst
    Baker's c.
    blue dome c.
    branchial c.
    echinococcus c.

cyst (*continued*)
    inclusion c.
    involution c.
    pilonidal c.
    retention c.
    sacrococcygeal c.
    thyroglossal c.
cystauchenotomy
cystduodenostomy
cystectomy
cystic
cysticolithectomy
cysticolithotripsy
cysticorrhaphy
cysticotomy
cystidolaparotomy
cystis
    c. fellea
cystjejunostomy
cystocele
cystocolostomy
cystodiaphanoscopy
cystoduodenostomy
cystogastrostomy
cystojejunostomy
    Roux-en-y c.
cystosarcoma
    c. phylloides
Czerny-Lembert suture
Czerny's
    operation
    suture
dabreedmaw. See *débridement.*
Dacron graft
Dallas' operation
Daniel's clamp
David's speculum
Deaver's
    incision
    retractor
    scissors
DeBakey's scissors

Debove's tube
débride
débridement
decompression
decubitus
defecation
deformity
    Akerlund d.
dehiscence
    wound d.
dehisens. See *dehiscence.*
DeLee's forceps
Delphian node
DeMartel-Wolfson clamp
Demerol anesthetic agent
Denans' operation
Dennis'
    clamp
    forceps
denudation
DePage-Janeway gastrostomy
Depage's position
Dermalene suture
Dermalon suture
descensus
    d. ventriculi
Deschamps' carrier
desiccate
desiccation
Desjardin's
    forceps
    probe
Dexon suture
diaphragm
diaphragmatic
diastalsis
diastasis
    d. recti abdominis
Dieffenbach's operation
dieresis
Dieulafoy's
    erosion

Dieulafoy's *(continued)*
    ulcer
digital
dilation
    digital d.
dilator
    Bakes' d.
    Barnes' d.
    Ferris' d.
    Kron's d.
    Mantz's d.
    Murphy's d.
    Ottenheimer's d.
    Ramstedt's d.
    Wales' d.
    Young's d.
Dilaudid anesthetic agent
dimpling
director
    Larry's d.
    Pratt's d.
discission
discrete
disease. See Medical Specialty
    sections.
dissection
    blunt d.
    radical neck d.
    sharp d.
    supraomohyoid neck d.
dissector
    Brunner's d.
    Kocher's d.
    Wangensteen's d.
disseminated
distention
diverticula
diverticulectomy
diverticulitis
diverticulogram
diverticulopexy
diverticulosis

diverticulum
    Meckel's d.
Dixon-Thomas-Smith clamp
Dowell's operation
Doyen's
    clamp
    forceps
    scissors
drain
    accordion d.
    cigarette d.
    Hemovac d.
    latex d.
    Penrose d.
    polyethylene d.
    polyvinyl d.
    rubber-dam d.
    stab wound d.
    suction d.
    sump d.
    whistle tip d.
dressing. See also *bandage*.
    absorbable d.
    Adaptic gauze d.
    adhesive d.
    Aeroplast d.
    Band-aid d.
    barrel d.
    bolus d.
    brassiere-type d.
    bulky d.
    butterfly d.
    cellophane d.
    cocoon d.
    collar d.
    collodion d.
    compound d.
    compression d.
    Cornish wool d.
    dry pressure d.
    felt d.
    fine mesh d.

dressing (*continued*)
    fluff d.
    fluffy compression d.
    foam rubber d.
    four-tailed d.
    Gelfilm d.
    Gelfoam d.
    Gelocast d.
    impregnated d.
    Lister's d.
    Lubafax d.
    many-tailed d.
    Mersilene d.
    mustache d.
    Nu-gauze d.
    occlusive d.
    paraffin d.
    patch d.
    petrolatum gauze d.
    plastic d.
    pressure d.
    propylene d.
    Raytec d.
    sheepskin d.
    stent d.
    stockinette d.
    Styrofoam d.
    Surgicel gauze d.
    Telfa d.
    tulle gras d.
    Vaseline gauze d.
    Velroc d.
    Vioform d.
    Wangensteen's d.
    Xeroform d.
drugs. See *Drugs and Chemistry* section.
Drummond-Morison operation
duct
    alveolar d.
    biliary d.
    common bile d.

duct (*continued*)
    common hepatic d.
    cystic d.
    efferent d.
    excretory d.
    lactiferous d's.
    mammary d.
    pancreatic d.
    papillary d.
    parotid d.
    prostatic d.
    salivary d.
    d. of Santorini
    semicircular d.
    Stensen's d.
    Wharton's d.
    d. of Wirsung
Dudley's hook
Dudley-Smith speculum
Duhrssen's incision
Duke's trocar
Duncan's position
Dunhill's hemostat
duodenal
duodenectomy
duodenitis
duodenocholangeitis
duodenocholecystostomy
duodenocholedochotomy
duodenocolic
duodenocystostomy
duodenoduodenostomy
duodenoenterostomy
duodenogram
duodenohepatic
duodenoileostomy
duodenojejunostomy
duodenolysis
duodenorrhaphy
duodenoscopy
duodenostomy
duodenotomy

duodenum
Dupuytren's
    contracture
    enterotome
    suture
Duranest anesthetic agent
Duvergier's suture
Dyclone anesthetic agent
dysfunction
dyskinesia
    biliary d.
dysplasia
Earle's probe
Eastman's clamp
ecchymosis
echinococcosis
echinococcotomy
ectocolostomy
ectokelostomy
ectopic
Edebohl's
    incision
    position
edema
edematous
Eder-Chamberlin gastroscope
Eder-Hufford gastroscope
Eder-Palmer gastroscope
Eder's
    gastroscope
    laparoscope
Edward's hook
Ekehorn's operation
Elasticon bandage
Elastoplast bandage
electrocautery
electrocholecystectomy
electrocholecystocausis
electrocoagulation
electrodesiccation
electrogastroenterostomy
electrosurgery

Elliot's position
Elliott's forceps
Ellsner's gastroscope
Elsberg's incision
embolectomy
embolism
embolus
Emerson's stripper
Emmet's suture
en bissac
en bloc
encapsulated
endocholedochal
endoscopy
endothyropexy
engorgement
en masse
enterauxe
enterectasis
enterectomy
enterelcosis
enteritis
enteroanastomosis
enteroapokleisis
enterocele
enterocentesis
enterochirurgia
enterocholecystostomy
enterocholecystotomy
enterocleisis
enteroclysis
enterocolectomy
enterocolitis
enterocolostomy
enteroenterostomy
    Parker-Kerr e.
enteroepiplocele
enterogastritis
enterohepatopexy
enterolith
enterolithiasis
enteropexy
enteroplasty

enteroplexy
enteroptosis
enterorrhaphy
enterostomy
    Witzel's e.
enterotome
    Dupuytren's e.
enterotomy
enucleation
epauxesiectomy
epidermoid
epigastric
epigastrium
epigastrocele
epigastrorrhaphy
epiglottis
epiplocele
epiploectomy
epiploenterocele
epiploic
epiploitis
epiplomerocele
epiplomphalocele
epiploon
epiplopexy
epiploplasty
epiplorrhaphy
epiplosarcomphalocele
epiploscheocele
epithelialization
epithelialize
epithelium
épluchage
eponychium
Equisetene suture
erosion
    Dieulafoy's e.
erythema
erythematous
eschar
Esmarch's
    bandage
    scissors

esofa-. See words beginning
   esopha-.
esogastritis
esophagocardiomyotomy
esophagocologastrostomy
esophagoduodenostomy
esophagoenterostomy
esophagofundopexy
esophagogastrectomy
esophagogastroanastomosis
esophagogastroplasty
esophagogastroscopy
esophagogastrostomy
esophagojejunogastrostomosis
esophagojejunostomy
Ethibond suture
Ethicon suture
Ethiflex suture
Ethilon suture
Ethrane anesthetic agent
euthyroid
evagination
eventration
Evipal anesthetic agent
evisceration
excavation
excision
    wound e.
excoriation
excrement
exenteration
exenteritis
exploratory
exsanguination
exsanguinotransfusion
exteriorize
extirpation
extravasation
extrusion
extubate
exudate

falciform
fanenstel. See *Pfannenstiel.*
Fansler's
    anoscope
    proctoscope
    speculum
Farris' forceps
fascia
    Camper's f.
    Cloquet's f.
    cremaster f.
    cribriform f.
    external oblique f.
    infundibuloform f.
    f. lata femoris
    pectineal f.
    prepubic f.
    Scarpa's f
    f. transversalis
    transverse f.
fascial
fasciaplasty
fascioplasty
fasciorrhaphy
fasciotomy
FB — fingerbreadth
    foreign body
fecal
fecalith
fecopurulent
Federoff's splenectomy
Fehland's clamp
Feilchenfeld's forceps
felon
femoral
femorocele
fenestra
Fenger's probe
feokromositoma. See
   pheochromocytoma.
Ferguson-Coley operation

Ferguson-Moon retractor
Ferguson's
    forceps
    operation
    scissors
    scoop
Fergusson's incision
Ferris'
    dilator
    scoop
Ferris-Smith forceps
fibercolonoscope
fibergastroscope
fiberoptic
fiberscope
    Hirschowitz's f.
fibrin
fibrinopurulent
fibroadenoma
fibroadenosis
fibrocystic
fibroma
fibromatoid
fibromectomy
fibromyoma
fibromyomectomy
fibromyotomy
fibrosis
fimbria
fimbriated
fingerbreadth
Finney's
    operation
    pyloroplasty
fissure
fistula
fistulectomy
fistulization
fistuloenterostomy
fistulotomy
fistulous
fitobezor. See *phytobezoar.*

flap
    cellulocutaneous f.
    island f.
    musculocutaneous f.
    skin f.
    sliding f.
    surgical f.
Flaxedil suture
flebektomee. See *phlebectomy.*
flebitis. See *phlebitis.*
flebo-. See words beginning
    phlebo-.
flegmon. See *phlegmon.*
Flexiton suture
Flexon suture
flexure
    duodenojejunal f.
    hepatic f.
    iliac f.
    sigmoid f.
    splenic f.
fluctuant
fluctuation
Fluoromar anesthetic agent
Fluothane anesthetic agent
Foerster's forceps
Foley's catheter
follicle
    Lieberkühn's f's
follicular
folliculi
    f. lymphatici aggregati
    f. lymphatici aggregati
        appendicis vermiformis
    f. lymphatici gastrici
    f. lymphatici lienales
    f. lymphatici recti
    f. lymphatici solitarii
        intestini crassi
    f. lymphatici solitarii
        intestini tenuis
folliculus

foramen
    f. of Bochdalek
    Morgagni's f.
    f. of Winslow
Forane anesthetic agent
forceps
    ACMI f.
    Adair's f.
    Adson's f.
    Allis' f.
    Allis-Ochsner f.
    Babcock's f.
    Backhaus' f.
    Bainbridge's f.
    Barrett's f.
    Beebe's f.
    Bevan's f.
    Billroth's f.
    Blake's f.
    Blanchard's f.
    Boys-Allis f.
    Bradford's f.
    Brophy's f.
    Brown-Adson f.
    Brown's f.
    Brunner's f.
    Buie's f.
    Carmalt's f.
    Carmody's f.
    Cassidy-Brophy f.
    Collin's f.
    Crile's f.
    Curtis' f.
    Cushing's f.
    DeLee's f.
    Dennis' f.
    Desjardin's f.
    Doyen's f.
    Elliott's f.
    Farris' f.
    Feilchenfeld's f.
    Ferguson's f.
    Ferris-Smith f.
    Foerster's f.
    Foss' f.
    Frankfeldt's f.
    Fulpit's f.
    Glassman-Allis f.
    Glassman's f.
    Gray's f.
    Halsted's f.
    Harrington's f.
    Healy's f.
    Heaney's f.
    Hirschman's f.
    Hoxworth's f.
    Hudson's f.
    Jackson's f.
    Jones' f.
    Judd-Allis f.
    Judd-DeMartel f.
    Kelly's f.
    Kerrison's f.
    Kocher's f.
    Lahey-Pean f.
    Lahey's f.
    Leksell's f.
    Lillie's f.
    Lockwood's f.
    Lovelace's f.
    Lower's f.
    Maier's f.
    Martin's f.
    Mayo-Blake f.
    Mayo-Ochsner f.
    Mayo-Robson f.
    Mayo's f.
    McNealy-Glassman-
        Babcock f.
    McNealy-Glassman-
        Mixter f.
    Mixter's f.
    Moynihan's f.
    New's f.

forceps (*continued*)

    Ochsner-Dixon f.
    Ochsner's f.
    Parker-Kerr f.
    Pean's f.
    Pennington's f.
    Percy's f.
    Porter's f.
    Potts-Smith f.
    Pratt-Smith f.
    Providence f.
    Rankin's f.
    Ratliff-Blake f.
    Rochester-Ewald f.
    Rochester-Mixter f.
    Rochester-Rankin f.
    Rochester's f.
    Roeder's f.
    Russian f.
    Schoenberg's f.
    Schutz's f.
    Scudder's f.
    Semken's f.
    Shallcross' f.
    Singley's f.
    Spencer Wells f.
    Stille's f.
    Stone's f.
    Thoms' f.
    Thorek-Mixter f.
    Virtus' f.
    Walter's f.
    Walther's f.
    Wangensteen's f.
    Weisenbach's f.
    Welch-Allyn f.
    Williams' f.
    Yeomans' f.

Foss'

    clamp
    forceps
    retractor

fossa

    duodenal f.
    epigastric f.
    Hartmann's f.
    ischiorectal f.
    Landzert's f.
    Mohrenheim's f.
    subsigmoid f.

Fowler's

    incision
    position

Fowler-Weir incision

fragmentation

Frankfeldt's

    forceps
    needle
    sigmoidoscope
    snare

Frank's operation

Franz's retractor

Fredet-Ramstedt

    operation
    pyloromyotomy

fren-. See words beginning
    phren-.

frenulum

frenum

Freund's operation

friable

Friedrich-Petz clamp

Frost's suture

FSH — follicle stimulating
    hormone

Fuch's position

fulguration

fulminant

fulminate

Fulpit's forceps

fundus

fundusectomy

funiculopexy

funiculus

Furniss'
    anastomosis
    clamp
    incision
Furniss-Clute clamp
Furniss-McClure-Hinton clamp
furuncle
furunculosis
Gabriel's proctoscope
Gaillard-Arlt suture
galactccele
gallbladder
    Courvoisier's g.
Gallie's
    operation
    transplant
gallstone
Gambee's suture
Gamgee tissue
Gamna nodules
Gandy-Gamna nodules
ganglion
    Acrel's g.
ganglionectomy
ganglionostomy
gangliosympathectomy
gangrene
gangrenous
Gant's clamp
gasserectomy
gastrectomy
    von Haberer-Aguirre g.
gastritis
    cirrhotic g.
    hypertrophic g.
gastrocele
gastrocolic
gastrocolitis
gastrocolostomy
gastrocolotomy
gastrodiaphany
gastroduodenal

gastroduodenoscopy
gastroduodenostomy
gastroenteritis
gastroenteroanastomosis
gastroenterocolostomy
gastroenteroplasty
gastroenterostomy
    Balfour's g.
    Billroth's g. I and II
    Braun and Jaboulay g.
    Curvoisier's g.
    Heineke-Mikulicz g.
    Hofmeister's g.
    Polya's g.
    Roux's g.
    Schoemaker's g.
    von Haberer-Finney g.
    Wölfler's g.
gastroenterotomy
gastroepiploic
gastroesophagostomy
gastrogalvanization
gastrogastrostomy
gastrogavage
gastrohepatic
gastroileitis
gastroileostomy
gastrointestinal
gastrojejunocolic
gastrojejunostomy
gastrolysis
gastromegaly
gastromyotomy
gastronesteostomy
gastropexy
gastroplasty
gastroplication
gastroptosis
gastropylorectomy
gastropyloric
gastrorrhaphy
gastrorrhexis

gastroscope
- ACMI g.
- Benedict's g.
- Bernstein's g.
- Chevalier-Jackson g.
- Eder's g.
- Eder-Chamberlin g.
- Eder-Hufford g.
- Eder-Palmer g.
- Ellsner's g.
- fiberoptic g.
- flexible g.
- Herman-Taylor g.
- Housset-Debray g.
- Janeway's g.
- Kelling's g.
- Schindler's g.
- Wolf-Schindler g.

gastroscopy
gastrosplenic
gastrostomy
- Beck-Jianu g.
- Beck's g.
- DePage-Janeway g.
- Janeway's g.
- Kader's g.
- Marwedel's g.
- Spivack's g.
- Ssabanejew-Frank g.
- Stamm's g.
- Witzel's g.

gastrotome
gastrotomy
Gatellier's incision
gauze
Gelfilm dressing
Gelfoam dressing
Gelocast dressing
Gély's suture
Gersuny's operation
GI — gastrointestinal
Gibbon's hernia

Gibson-Balfour retractor
Gibson's
- incision
- suture

Gill's operation
Gimbernat's ligament
gland
- adrenal g's
- Lieberkühn's g.
- parotid g.
- pineal g.
- pituitary g.
- salivary g.
- sublingual g.
- submaxillary g.
- thyroid g.

Glassman-Allis forceps
Glassman's
- clamp
- forceps

glioma
glossectomy
glossitis
glossoplasty
glossorrhaphy
glossotomy
Goelet's retractor
goiter
- adenomatous g.
- colloid g.
- cystic g.
- exophthalmic g.
- fibrous g.
- nodular g.
- papillomatous g.
- parenchymatous g.
- substernal g.
- toxic g.

Goldbacher's
- anoscope
- needle
- proctoscope

Goldbacher's (*continued*)
    speculum
Gosset's retractor
Gould's suture
Goyrand's hernia
graft
    autogenous g.
    bifurcation g.
    cutis g.
    Dacron g.
    fascial g.
    fiber glass g.
    full-thickness skin g.
    Marlex g.
    split thickness skin g.
    tantalum mesh g.
    Teflon g.
Graham-Roscie operation
granulation
granuloma
granulomatous
Gray's forceps
Greenhow's incision
Green's retractor
Greiling's tube
Gridiron's incision
Grieshaber's retractor
Grondahl-Finney operation
Gruber's hernia
Grynfelt's hernia
guarding
Gudebrod's suture
Guild-Pratt speculum
Gussenbauer's
    operation
    suture
Guyton-Friedenwald suture
Gwathmey's oil-ether
    anesthesia
gynecomastia
Hagedorn's needle
Hahn's operation

hallux
    h. malleus
    h. valgus
    h. varus
Halsted's
    forceps
    hemostat
    incision
    operation
    suture
hamartoma
Handley's
    incision
    operation
Harmon's incision
Harrington-Pemberton
    retractor
Harrington's
    forceps
    retractor
Harris suture
Hartmann's
    fossa
    point
    pouch
haustra coli
haustration
haustrum
Hayes' clamp
healing
    h. by first intention
    h. by granulation
    h. by second intention
    h. by third intention
Healy's forceps
Heaney's
    clamp
    forceps
Heaton's operation
Heerman's incision
Heineke-Mikulicz
    gastroenterostomy

Heineke-Mikulicz (*continued*)
    operation
    pyloroplasty
Heineke's operation
Heller's operation
hemangioma
hemangiosarcoma
hematemesis
hematoma
hemicolectomy
hemicorporectomy
hemigastrectomy
hemihepatectomy
hemipylorectomy
hemisection
hemithyroidectomy
hemoptysis
hemorrhage
hemorrhagic
hemorrhoid
    combined h.
    external h.
    internal h.
    lingual h.
    mixed h.
    mucocutaneous h.
    prolapsed h.
    strangulated h.
    thrombosed h.
hemorrhoidal
hemorrhoidectomy
hemostasis
hemostat
    Dunhill's h.
    Halsted's h.
    Maingot's h.
Hemovac drain
Henke's triangle
Henry's
    incision
    operation
    splenectomy

hepatectomize
hepatectomy
hepatic
hepaticocholangiocholecyst-
    enterostomy
hepaticocholangiojejunostomy
hepaticodochotomy
hepaticoduodenostomy
hepaticoenterostomy
hepaticogastrostomy
hepaticojejunostomy
hepaticolithotomy
hepaticolithotripsy
hepaticostomy
hepaticotomy
hepatitis
hepatobiliary
hepatocele
hepatocholangiocystoduo-
    denostomy
hepatocholangioduodenos-
    tomy
hepatocholangioenterostomy
hepatocholangiogastrostomy
hepatocholangiostomy
hepatocirrhosis
hepatoduodenostomy
hepatoenterostomy
hepatogastric
hepatolithectomy
hepatomegaly
hepatopexy
hepatorrhaphy
hepatosplenomegaly
hepatostomy
hepatotomy
Herff's clamp
Herman-Taylor gastroscope
hernia
    abdominal h.
    acquired h.
    h. adiposa

hernia (*continued*)
  amniotic h.
  Barth's h.
  Béclard's h.
  Birkett's h.
  cecal h.
  Cloquet's h.
  congenital h.
  Cooper's h.
  crural h.
  diaphragmatic h.
  diverticular h.
  duodenojejunal h.
  encysted h.
  epigastric h.
  extrasaccular h.
  femoral h.
  foraminal h.
  funicular h.
  gastroesophageal h.
  Gibbon's h.
  gluteal h.
  Goyrand's h.
  Gruber's h.
  Grynfelt's h.
  Hesselbach's h.
  Hey's h.
  hiatal h.
  hiatus h.
  Holthouse's h.
  incarcerated h.
  incisional h.
  indirect h.
  infantile h.
  inguinal h.
  inguinocrural h.
  inguinofemoral h.
  inguinoproperitoneal h.
  inguinosuperficial h.
  h. in recto
  intermuscular h.
  interparietal h.

hernia (*continued*)
  intersigmoid h.
  interstitial h.
  irreducible h.
  ischiatic h.
  ischiorectal h.
  Krönlein's h.
  Küster's h.
  labial h.
  Laugier's h.
  levator h.
  linea alba h.
  Littre-Richter h.
  Littre's h.
  lumbar h.
  Maydl's h.
  mesenteric h.
  mesocolic h.
  mucosal h.
  oblique h.
  obturator h.
  omental h.
  ovarian h.
  pantaloon h.
  paraduodenal h.
  paraesophageal h.
  paraperitoneal h.
  parasaccular h.
  h. par glissement
  parietal h.
  parumbilical h.
  pectineal h.
  perineal h.
  Petit's h.
  properitoneal h.
  pudendal h.
  pulsion h.
  rectal h.
  reducible h.
  retrocecal h.
  retrograde h.
  retroperitoneal h.

hernia (*continued*)

    Richter's h.
    Riex's h.
    Rokitansky's h.
    sciatic h.
    scrotal h.
    sliding h.
    spigelian h.
    strangulated h.
    subpubic h.
    synovial h.
    thyroidal h.
    tonsillar h.
    Treitz's h.
    tunicary h.
    umbilical h.
    uterine h.
    vaginal h.
    vaginolabial h.
    Velpeau's h.
    ventral h.
    vesical h.
    voluminous h.
    Von Bergmann's h.
    W h.
hernial
herniary
herniated
herniation
hernioappendectomy
hernioenterotomy
hernioid
herniolaparotomy
hernioplasty
herniopuncture
herniorrhaphy
herniotome
herniotomy
Hesselbach's
    hernia
    ligament
    triangle
heteroautoplasty

Heyer-Schulte prosthesis
Hey-Grooves' operation
Hey's hernia
hiatal
hiatopexy
hiatus
hidradenitis
    h. suppurativa
Higgins' incision
Hill-Ferguson retractor
hilum
hilus
Hinckle-James speculum
Hirschman-Martin proctoscope
Hirschman's
    anoscope
    forceps
    proctoscope
Hirschowitz's fiberscope
Hochenegg's operation
Hofmeister's gastroenteros-
    tomy
Hoguet's
    maneuver
    operation
Holocaine anesthetic agent
Holthouse's hernia
homograft
homoplastic
homoplasty
Hood and Kirklin incision
hook
    Barr's h.
    Dudley's h.
    Edwards' h.
    Linton's h.
    Pratt's h.
    Rosser's h.
    Stewart's h.
    Welch-Allyn h.
Hopkins' operation
Horsley's pyloroplasty
Hotchkiss' operation

Housset-Debray gastroscope
Houston's valve
Hoxworth's forceps
Hudson's forceps
Hunt's
    clamp
    operation
Hurwitz's clamp
hydrocele
hydrocelectomy
hydroperitoneum
hydrops
    h. abdominis
hygroma
hyperemic
hyperinsulinism
hyperparathyroidism
hyperpituitarism
hyperplasia
hyperthyroidism
hypertonic
hypertrophic
hypertrophy
hypochondrium
hypocystotomy
hypodermatomy
hypogastric
hypoparathyroidism
hypophysectomy
hypopituitarism
hypoplasia
hypothermia
hypothyroidism
hypotonic
Hyrtl's sphincter
^{131}I — radioactive iodine
I & D — incision and drainage
ileac
ileal
ileectomy
ileitis
    distal i.

ileitis (*continued*)
    regional i.
    terminal i.
ileocecal
ileocecostomy
ileocecum
ileocolic
ileocolitis
ileocolostomy
ileocolotomy
ileocystoplasty
ileoileostomy
ileoproctostomy
ileorectal
ileorectostomy
ileorrhaphy
ileosigmoid
ileosigmoidostomy
ileostomy
    Koch i.
ileotomy
ileotransversostomy
ileum
    terminal i.
ileus
iliocolotomy
iliohypogastric
ilioinguinal
iliolumbocostoabdominal
iliopectineal
iliopubic
imbricated
imbrication
impaction
implant
    Silastic i.
incarcerated
incarceration
incised
incision
    abdominal
    abdomir

incision (*continued*)

    ab externo i.
    Agnew-Verhoeff i.
    alar i.
    Alexander's i.
    angular i.
    aortotomy i.
    arcuate i.
    areolar i.
    arteriotomy i.
    Auvray's i.
    backcut i.
    Bardenheuer's i.
    Bar's i.
    Battle-Jalaguier-
      Kammerer i.
    Battle's i.
    bayonet i.
    Bergman-Israel i.
    Bergmann's i.
    Bevan's i.
    bivalved i.
    Brackin's i.
    Brock's i.
    bur-hole i.
    buttonhole i.
    celiotomy i.
    cervical i.
    Cherney's i.
    Chernez' i.
    Chiene's i.
    circular i.
    circumareolar i.
    circumcisional i.
    circumferential i.
    circumlimbal i.
    circumscribing i.
    Clute's i.
    Codman's i.
    Coffey's i.
    collar i.
    firmatory i.

incision (*continued*)

    conjunctival i.
    corneoscleral i.
    cortical i.
    Courvoisier's i.
    crescent i.
    crosshatch i.
    crucial i.
    cruciate i.
    curved i.
    curvilinear i.
    Deaver's i.
    deltopectoral i.
    dorsolateral i.
    Duhrssen's i.
    dural i.
    Edebohls' i.
    elliptical i.
    Elsberg's i.
    endaural i.
    enterotomy i.
    exploratory i.
    Fergusson's i.
    fishmouth i.
    flank i.
    flexed i.
    Fowler's i.
    Fowler-Weir i.
    Furniss' i.
    Gatellier's i.
    Gibson's i.
    Greenhow's i.
    Gridiron's i.
    guillotine i.
    Halsted's i.
    Handley's i.
    Harmon's i.
    Heerman's i.
    hemitransfixion i.
    Henry's i.
    Higgins' i.
    hockey-stick i.

incision (*continued*)
- Hood and Kirklin i.
- horizontal i.
- inframammary i.
- infraumbilical i.
- inguinal i.
- intercartilaginous i.
- intracapsular i.
- Jackson's i.
- J-shaped i.
- Kammerer's i.
- Kehr's i.
- Kocher's i.
- Küstner's i.
- lamellar i.
- Lamm's i.
- Langenbeck's i.
- lateral flank i.
- lateral rectus i.
- lazy-S i.
- Lempert's i.
- Lilienthal's i.
- limbal i.
- linear i.
- Linton's i.
- longitudinal i.
- Lonquet's i.
- Mackenrodt's i.
- Mason's i.
- Maylard i.
- Mayo-Robson i.
- McArthur's i.
- McBurney's i.
- McLaughlin's i.
- McVay's i.
- meatal i.
- median i.
- Meyer's hockey stick i.
- midline i.
- Mikulicz' i.
- Morison's i.
- muscle splitting i.

incision (*continued*)
- myringotomy i.
- Nagamatsu i.
- oblique i.
- Ollier's i.
- Orr's i.
- paracostal i.
- parainguinal i.
- paramedian i.
- paramuscular i.
- parapatellar i.
- pararectus i.
- parasagittal i.
- parascapular i.
- paraumbilical i.
- paravaginal i.
- Parker's i.
- Pean's i.
- perianal i.
- periareolar i.
- perilimbal i.
- periscapular i.
- peritoneal i.
- Perthes' i.
- Pfannenstiel's i.
- Phemister's i.
- popliteal i.
- postauricular i.
- posterior i.
- posterolateral i.
- proximal i.
- pyelotomy i.
- racquet i.
- radial i.
- rectus muscle splitting i.
- recumbent i.
- relaxing i.
- relief i.
- retroauricular i.
- rim i.
- Risdon's extraoral i.
- Rocky-Davis i.

incision (*continued*)
 Rodman's i.
 Rollet's i.
 Rosen's i.
 Roux-en-Y jejunal loop i.
 saber-cut i.
 salmon backcut i.
 Sanders' i.
 Schobinger's i.
 Schuchardt's i.
 scratch type i.
 semicircular i.
 semiflexed i.
 semilunar i.
 serpentine i.
 Shambaugh's i.
 shelving i.
 shoulder-strap i.
 Simon's i.
 Singleton's i.
 Sloan's i.
 Smith-Peterson i.
 spiral i.
 stab-wound i.
 stellate i.
 sternal splitting i.
 Stewart's i.
 Strombeck's i.
 subcostal i.
 subinguinal i.
 submammary i.
 subtrochanteric i.
 subumbilical i.
 supracervical i.
 suprapubic i.
 supraumbilical i.
 temporal i.
 Thomas-Warren i.
 thoracoabdominal i.
 thoracotomy i.
 Timbrall-Fisher i.
 transection i.

incision (*continued*)
 transmeatal i.
 transrectus i.
 transverse i.
 trap-door i.
 T-shaped i.
 U-shaped i.
 vertical i.
 Vischer's i.
 V-shaped i.
 Warren's i.
 Watson-Jones i.
 Weber-Fergusson i.
 wedge i.
 Whipple's i.
 Wilde's i.
 Willie-Meyer i.
 W-shaped i.
 Y-type i.
 Z-flap i.
 Z-plasty i.
 Z-shaped i.
incisional
incisive
incisura
 i. angularis ventriculi
 i. cardiaca ventriculi
inclusion
incontinence
indurated
induration
infarction
 intestinal i.
infiltration
inflammation
inframamillary
inframammary
infundibula
infundibuliform
infundibulopelvic
infundibulum
Ingals' cannula

inguinal
inguinoabdominal
inguinocrural
inguinolabial
inguinoscrotal
Inlay's operation
Innovar anesthetic agent
inoperable
in situ
instillation
insufflation
insufflator
    Buckstein's i.
    Weber's i.
intercostal
interfemoral
interstitial
intestinal
intestine
intima
intractable
intracystic
intraductal
intubation
intumescence
intussusception
intussusceptum
intussuscipiens
invagination
inversion
inverted
irradiation
irrigator
    Buie's i.
ischioanal
ischiococcygeal
ischiorectal
ischochymia
island
    i's of Langerhans
isograft
Israel's retractor
isthmectomy

isthmus
Ivalon's suture
Ives' anoscope
Jaboulay's
    button
    operation
    pyloroplasty
Jackson's
    forceps
    incision
    retractor
Jacobs-Palmer laparoscope
Jam-Shidi needle
Janeway's
    gastroscope
    gastrostomy
Jarvis' clamp
jaundice
jejunectomy
jejunitis
jejunocecostomy
jejunocolostomy
jejunoileitis
jejunoileostomy
jejunojejunostomy
jejunorrhaphy
jejunostomy
jejunotomy
jejunum
Jelk's operation
Jenckel method
Jobert's suture
Jobst stocking
Johnson's tube
Jones'
    forceps
    position
    scissors
Jonge's position
Jonnesco's operation
Jorgenson's scissors
J-shaped incision
Judd-Allis forceps

Judd-DeMartel forceps
Judd's pyloroplasty
juncture
    saphenofemoral j.
Jutte tube
Kader-Senn operation
Kader's gastrostomy
Kalt's suture
Kammerer's incision
Kapp-Beck clamp
Keeley's stripper
Keel's operation
Keen's operation
Kehr's incision
Keith's needle
Kelling's gastroscope
Kelly's
    clamp
    forceps
    proctoscope
    retractor
    sigmoidoscope
    suture
    tube
keloid
keloplasty
kelotomy
kemo-. See words beginning
   chemo-.
keratosis
Kerlix bandage
Kerrison's
    forceps
    punch
    retractor
    rongeur
kyl. See *chyle.*
Killian-King retractor
King's retractor
Kirby's suture
Kirschner's
    suture

Kirschner's (*continued*)
    wire
Klatskin's needle
Kleenspec sigmoidoscope
Klemme's retractor
Kling bandage
knife
    Bonta's k.
Knowles' scissors
Koch ileostomy
Kocher-Crotti retractor
kocherization
Kocher's
    clamp
    dissector
    forceps
    incision
    operation
    ulcer
koilonychia
kol-. See words beginning
   chol-.
kolangi-. See words beginning
   cholangi-.
kole-. See words beginning
   chole-.
kolo-. See words beginning
   cholo-.
Kondoleon operation
Kraske's
    operation
    position
    retractor
Krönlein's hernia
Kron's
    dilator
    probe
Kulenkampff's anesthesia
Kurten's stripper
Küster's hernia
Küstner's incision
laceration

lacuna
    l. musculorum
    l. vasorum
lacunar
Lahey-Pean forceps
Lahey's
    carrier
    clamp
    forceps
    operation
    retractor
    tenaculum
lamella
lamina
Lamm's incision
Landzert's fossa
Lane's
    catheter
    clamp
    operation
Langenbeck's incision
Langerhans islands
laparectomy
laparocholecystotomy
laparocolostomy
laparocolotomy
laparocystectomy
laparocystidotomy
laparoenterostomy
laparoenterotomy
laparogastroscopy
laparogastrostomy
laparogastrotomy
laparohepatotomy
laparoileotomy
laparomyomectomy
laparorrhaphy
laparoscope
    ACMI l.
    Eder's l.
    Jacobs-Palmer l.
    Lent's l.
laparoscopic

laparoscopy
laparosplenectomy
laparosplenotomy
laparotomaphilia
laparotome
laparotomy
laparotrachelotomy
laparotyphlotomy
Lardennois's button
La Roque's technique
Larry's
    director
    probe
laser
Laugier's hernia
lavage
Law's position
Le Dran's suture
LeFort's suture
leiomyoma
leiomyomata
Leksell's
    forceps
    rongeur
Lembert's suture
Lempert's incision
Lempka's stripper
Lent's laparoscope
lesion
leukonychia
Levin's tube
Lieberkühn's
    crypts
    follicles
    glands
Lieberman's
    proctoscope
    sigmoidoscope
lien
    l. accessorius
    l. mobilis
lienal
lienculus

lienopancreatic
lienorenal
ligament
    arcuate l.
    Cooper's l.
    gastrocolic l.
    gastrohepatic l.
    gastrolienal l.
    gastrophrenic l.
    Gimbernat's l.
    hepatogastric l.
    Hesselbach's l.
    inguinal l.
    lacunar l.
    lienorenal l.
    pancreaticosplenic l.
    pectineal l.
    phrenicocolic l.
    phrenicolienal l.
    phrenicosplenic l.
    Poupart's l.
    splenocolic l.
    splenorenal l.
    l. of Treitz
ligation
    high saphenous vein l.
ligature
    McGraw's elastic l.
Lilienthal's incision
Lillie's forceps
Lincoff's sponge
line
    iliopectineal l.
    median l.
    pectinate l.
    pectineal l.
    Spieghel's l.
linea
    l. alba
    l. semilunaris
linitis
    l. plastica

Linton's
    clamp
    hook
    incision
    operation
    retractor
    tube
lipectomy
lipoma
Lister's
    dressing
    scissors
lithotome
lithotomy
lithotony
lithotresis
Littauer's scissors
Little's retractor
Littre-Richter hernia
Littre's
    hernia
    suture
lobe
    Riedel's l.
lobectomy
lobular
lobule
lobulette
lobulus
Lockwood's
    clamp
    forceps
Löffler's suture
Lonquet's incision
Lord's operation
Loreta's operation
Lorfan anesthetic agent
Lotheissen-McVay technique
Lotheissen's operation
Lovelace's forceps
Lower's forceps
Lubafax dressing

Luer-Korte scoop
lumen
lunula
Luschka's crypts
lymphadenectomy
lymphadenitis
lymphadenopathy
    giant follicular l.
lymphosarcoma
Lynch's operation
lyse
lysis
MacDonald's clamp
Macewen's operation
Mackenrodt's incision
Mackid's operation
Madden technique
Maier's forceps
Maingot's hemostat
Mair's operation
malacotomy
malignant
malpighian bodies
mamilla
mammaplasty
mammary
mammectomy
mammiform
mammilliplasty
    Ashford's m.
mammogram
mammography
mammoplasia
mammoplasty
    augmentation m.
maneuver
    Hoguet's m.
Mann-Williamson ulcer
Manson's schistosomiasis
Mantz's dilator
Marcaine hydrochloride
    anesthetic agent

Marcy's operation
Marlex
    bandage
    graft
    mesh
    suture
marsupialization
Martel's clamp
Martin's
    forceps
    needle
    retractor
    speculum
Marwedel's
    gastrostomy
    operation
Mason's incision
mastadenitis
mastadenoma
mastectomy
masthelcosis
Mastin's clamp
mastitis
mastocarcinoma
mastochondroma
mastodynia
mastogram
mastography
mastoncus
mastopathia
    m. cystica
mastopathy
    cystic m.
mastopexy
mastoplastia
mastoplasty
mastoptosis
mastorrhagia
mastoscirrhus
mastosis
mastostomy
mastotomy

Mathew's speculum
matrix
Maunsell's suture
maxilla
Maydl's
    hernia
    operation
Mayer's position
Maylard incision
Mayo-Blake forceps
Mayo-Collins retractor
Mayo-Harrington scissors
Mayo linen suture
Mayo-Lovelace retractor
Mayo-Noble scissors
Mayo-Ochsner forceps
Mayo-Robson
    forceps
    incision
    operation
    position
    scoop
Mayo-Sims scissors
Mayo's
    carrier
    forceps
    needle
    operation
    probe
    retractor
    scissors
    scoop
    stripper
McArthur's
    incision
    method
    operation
McBurney's
    incision
    operation
    point
W. Dean McDonald clamp
McEvedy's operation

McGraw's elastic ligature
McLaughlin's incision
McNealy-Glassman-Babcock
    forceps
McNealy-Glassman-Mixter
    forceps
McVay's
    incision
    operation
Meckel's diverticulum
mediastinal
mediastinum
medications. See *Drugs and
    Chemistry* section.
Medrafil's wire suture
medulla
medusa
megacolon
megalogastria
Meigs' suture
Meltzer's anesthesia
membrane
    Cargile m.
membranous
Menghini's needle
Mercurio's position
Mermingas' operation
Mersilene
    gauze dressing
    suture
mesenteric
mesenteriopexy
mesenteriorrhaphy
mesenteriplication
mesentery
mesentorrhaphy
mesh
    Marlex m.
    tantalum m.
    Teflon m.
mesoappendicitis
mesoappendix
mesocecum

mesocolon
    ascending m.
    descending m.
    sigmoid m.
    transverse m.
mesocoloplication
mesogastrium
mesorectum
mesosigmoid
mesosigmoidopexy
metastases
metastasis
metastatic
metatarsal
method
    Jenckel m.
    McArthur's m.
    Morison's m.
Metycaine hydrochloride
    anesthetic agent
Metzenbaum's scissors
Meyerding's retractor
Meyer's
    hockey stick incision
    retractor
MFB − metallic foreign body
microgastria
microsurgery
Mikulicz's
    clamp
    incision
    operation
Miles' operation
milium
    colloid m.
Miller-Abbott tube
Miller's scissors
Mixter's forceps
Mohrenheim's fossa
Montague's
    proctoscope
    sigmoidoscope
Moore's scoop

Moreno's clamp
Morgagni's foramen
Morison's
    incision
    method
    pouch
Morton's toe
Moschcowitz's operation
motility
Moynihan's
    clamp
    forceps
    operation
    position
    probe
    scoop
mucocutaneous
    m. hemorrhoid
mucopurulent
mucosa
Mueller-Frazier tube
Mueller-Pool tube
Mueller-Pynchon tube
Mueller-Yankauer tube
Muer's anoscope
multilocular
Murphy's
    button
    dilator
    needle
    retractor
    treatment
muscle
    cremaster m.
    deltoid m.
    external oblique m.
    internal oblique m.
    latissimus dorsi m.
    masseter m.
    pectineus m.
    pectoralis major m.
    pectoralis minor m.
    pyramidalis m.

muscle (*continued*)
    rectococcygeal m.
    rectus m.
    scalene m.
    serratus anterior m.
    serratus magnus m.
    sternohyoid m.
    sternothyroid m.
    subscapularis m.
    transversus m.
Myers' stripper
myoma
myomectomy
myotomy
Nabatoff's stripper
Nachlas' tube
Nagamatsu incision
Narath's operation
narcosis
    Nussbaum's n.
narcotic
navel
necropsy
necropurulent
necrosis
necrotic
needle
    Chiba n.
    Childs-Phillips n.
    Craig's n.
    Frankfeldt's n.
    Goldbacher's n.
    Hagedorn's n.
    Jam-Shidi n.
    Keith's n.
    Klatskin's n.
    Martin's n.
    Mayo's n.
    Menghini's n.
    Murphy's n.
    pop-off n.
    Reverdin's n.
    Rochester's n.

needle (*continued*)
    Silverman's n.
    Vim-Silverman n.
Nembutal anesthetic agent
neoplasm
neoplastic
nerve
    hypogastric n.
    iliohypogastric n.
    ilioinguinal n.
    phrenic n.
Nesacaine-CE anesthetic agent
neurectomy
    gastric n.
Neurolon suture
nevus
    melanocytic n.
    pigmented n.
Newman's proctoscope
New's
    forceps
    scissors
nipple
    invaginated n.
Nisentil anesthetic agent
Noble's position
node
    axillary n's
    cervical lymph n's
    Cloquet's n.
    Delphian n.
nodular
nodule
    Gamna n's
    Gandy-Gamna n's
nonfunctioning
nonperforating
Northbent's scissors
Norwood's snare
Novocain anesthetic agent
NPO — nothing by mouth
    (nulla per os)
Nuck's canal

Nu-gauze dressing
Nupercaine hydrochloride
   anesthetic agent
Nussbaum's
     clamp
     narcosis
Nuttall's operation
O'Beirne's
     sphincter
     tube
Oberst's operation
oblique
     external o.
     internal o.
obliteration
obstruction
     intestinal o.
obturator
     Cripps' o.
occlusion
     enteromesenteric o.
occult
Ochsner-Dixon forceps
Ochsner's
     clamp
     forceps
     scissors
     tube
Oddi's sphincter
Ogilvie's operation
Ollier's incision
omentectomy
omentopexy
omentoplasty
omentorrhaphy
omentosplenopexy
omentotomy
omentum
     gastrocolic o.
     gastrohepatic o.
     gastrosplenic o.
     splenogastric o.

omphalectomy
omphalelcosis
omphalic
omphalitis
omphalocele
onychauxis
onychectomy
onychia
onychomycosis
onychorrhexis
onychotomy
operation
     Abbe's o.
     Abernethy's o.
     Adams' o.
     Allarton's o.
     Allingham's o.
     Amussat's o.
     Andrews' o.
     Anson-McVay o.
     Appolito's o.
     Armsby's o.
     Babcock's o.
     Ball's o.
     Bassini's o.
     Battle's o.
     Baynton's o.
     Beatson's o.
     Belmas' o.
     Best's o.
     Bevans' o.
     Beyea's o.
     Biesenberger's o.
     Billroth's o.
     Bircher's o.
     Blalock-Hanlon o.
     Blalock-Taussig o.
     Bloodgood's o.
     Bobb's o.
     Bogue's o.
     Bose's o.
     Brenner's o.

operation (*continued*)

    Bricker's o.
    Brunschwig's o.
    Bryant's o.
    Callisen's o.
    Cattell's o.
    Chaput's o.
    Cheyne's o.
    Chiazzi's o.
    Child's o.
    Clagett's o.
    Cooper's o.
    Cotting's o.
    Cripps' o.
    Czerny's o.
    Dallas' o.
    Denans' o.
    Dieffenbach's o.
    Dowell's o.
    Drummond-Morison o.
    Ekehorn's o.
    Ferguson-Coley o.
    Ferguson's o.
    Finney's o.
    Frank's o.
    Fredet-Ramstedt o.
    Freund's o.
    Gallie's o.
    Gersuny's o.
    Gill's o.
    Graham-Roscie o.
    Grondahl-Finney o.
    Gussenbauer's o.
    Hahn's o.
    Halsted's o.
    Handley's o.
    Heaton's o.
    Heineke-Mikulicz o.
    Heineke's o.
    Heller's o.
    Henry's o.
    Hey-Grooves o.

operation (*continued*)

    Hochenegg's o.
    Hoguet's o.
    Hopkins' o.
    Hotchkiss' o.
    Hunt's o.
    Inlay's o.
    interval o.
    Jaboulay's o.
    Jelk's o.
    Jonnesco's o.
    Kader-Senn o.
    Keel's o.
    Keen's o.
    Kocher's o.
    Kondoleon o.
    Kraske's o.
    Lahey's o.
    Lane's o.
    Linton's o.
    Lord's o.
    Loreta's o.
    Lotheissen's o.
    Lynch's o.
    Macewen's o.
    Mackid's o.
    Mair's o.
    Marcy's o.
    Marwedel's o.
    Maydl's o.
    Mayo-Robson o.
    Mayo's o.
    McArthur's o.
    McBurney's o.
    McEvedy's o.
    McVay's o.
    Mermingas' o.
    Mikulicz's o.
    Miles' o.
    Moschcowitz's o.
    Moynihan's o.
    Narath's o.

operation (*continued*)
- Nuttall's o.
- Oberst's o.
- Ogilvie's o.
- Pirogoff's o.
- Polya's o.
- Poth's o.
- radical o.
- Ramstedt's o.
- Rehn-Delorme o.
- Rose's o.
- Routier's o.
- Roux-en-Y o.
- Scarpa's o.
- Schede's o.
- Schlatter's o.
- Senn's o.
- Sotteau's o.
- State o.
- subcutaneous o.
- Swenson's o.
- Talma's o.
- Tanner's o.
- Tansini's o.
- Textor's o.
- Thiersch's o.
- Torek's o.
- Travel's o.
- Trendelenburg's o.
- Treves' o.
- Turner's o.
- van Buren's o.
- Vermale's o.
- Verneuil's o.
- Vidal's o.
- Wangensteen's o.
- Warren's o.
- Watson's o.
- Waugh's o.
- Weir's o.
- Whipple's o.
- Whitehead's o.

operation (*continued*)
- Winiwarter's o.
- Wise's o.
- Witzel's o.
- Wölfler's o.
- Wützer's o.
- Wyeth's o.
- Wyllys-Andrews o.
- Zieman's o.
- Zimmerman's o.
- Z-plasty

operable
Ophthaine anesthetic agent
OR — operating room
organomegaly
Orr's incision
os pubis
O'Sullivan-O'Connor retractor
O'Sullivan's retractor
Otis' anoscope
Ottenheimer's dilator
Owen's position
Oxaine anesthetic agent
Oxycel pack
oxygen
- o. therapy

oxygenation
oxygenator
oxyuriasis
Oxyuris
- *O. vermicularis*

Pagenstecher's linen thread
Palfyn's suture
palliate
palliative
palma
- p. manus

palmar
palpation
pampiniform
Pancoast's suture
pancolectomy

pancreas
    aberrant p.
    accessory p.
    p. divisum
    Willis' p.
    Winslow's p.
pancreatectomy
pancreatic
pancreaticoduodenostomy
pancreaticoenterostomy
pancreaticogastrostomy
pancreaticojejunostomy
pancreaticosplenic
pancreatitis
pancreatoduodenectomy
pancreatoduodenostomy
pancreatoenterostomy
pancreatography
pancreatolithectomy
pancreatolithotomy
pancreatotomy
pancreolithotomy
panniculus
panproctocolectomy
Panzer's scissors
papilla
    p. of Vater
papillae
papillary
papillate
papillectomy
papilloma
papillosphincterotomy
paracentesis
    abdominal p.
    p. abdominis
    p. vesicae
parathyroid
parathyroidectomy
Paré's suture
parenchyma
paries

parietal
parietes
Parker-Kerr
    "basting stitch"
    enteroenterostomy
    forceps
    suture
Parker's
    clamp
    incision
    retractor
Parkinson's position
paronychia
parotid
parotidectomy
parotitis
pars
    p. pylorica
    p. superior duodeni
paste
    Unna's p.
patency
patent
patulous
Paul Mixter tube
Payr's clamp
Péan's
    clamp
    forceps
    incision
    position
peau d'orange
pectenotomy
pectineal
pectoral
pectoralis
pedicle
peduncle
pedunculated
pelvis
Pemberton's clamp
pendulous

Pennington's
   clamp
   forceps
   speculum
Penrose drain
Penthrane anesthetic agent
Pentothal anesthetic agent
peptic
Percaine anesthetic agent
percutaneous
Percy's forceps
perforation
perianal
periappendicitis
perigastric
perineal
perineorrhaphy
perineum
periphery
perirectal
peristalsis
peristaltic
peritoneal
peritonealize
peritoneocentesis
peritoneoclysis
peritoneography
peritoneoplasty
peritoneoscope
   Wolf's p.
peritoneoscopy
peritoneotomy
peritoneum
   parietal p.
   visceral p.
peritonitis
peritonization
peritonize
perityphlitis
   p. actinomycotica
periumbilical
per primam intentionem

Perthes' incision
Petit's
   hernia
   suture
Pfannenstiel's incision
phalanx
Phemister's incision
pheochromocytoma
Phillips' clamp
phlebectomy
phlebitis
phlebolith
phlebolithiasis
phleboplasty
phlebosclerosis
phlebothrombosis
phlebotomy
phlegmon
phrenemphraxis
phrenic
phrenicectomized
phrenicectomy
phreniclasis
phrenicoexeresis
phreniconeurectomy
phrenicotomy
phrenicotripsy
phytobezoar
pillar
pilonidal
pinealectomy
pinealoma
Pirogoff's operation
pituitectomy
plantar
platysma
pledget
plexus
   brachial p.
   pampiniform p.
plica
   p. duodenalis

plica (*continued*)
    p. duodenojejunalis
    p. duodenomesocolica
    p. epigastrica
    p. gastropancreatica
    p. ileocecalis
    p. paraduodenalis
    p. umbilicalis
plication
plombage
plug
    p. gastrostomy
po dorahnj. See *peau d'orange.*
point
    Hartmann's p.
    McBurney's p.
pollicization
Polya's
    gastroenterostomy
    operation
Polydek suture
polyethylene
polyp
polypectomy
polypoid
polyposis
    p. gastrica
    p. intestinalis
    p. ventriculi
polypotome
polyunguia
Ponka technique
pons
    p. hepatis
Pontocaine anesthetic agent
Pool's tube
porta
    p. hepatis
    p. lienis
portacaval
portal
    intestinal p.
Porter's forceps

position
    Adams' p.
    Albert's p.
    anatomical p.
    arm-extension p.
    Bonner's p.
    Boyce's p.
    Bozeman's p.
    Buie's p.
    Caldwell's p.
    Casselberry's p.
    coiled p.
    decortical p.
    decubitus p.
    Depage's p.
    dorsal p.
    dorsal elevated p.
    dorsal inertia p.
    dorsal lithotomy p.
    dorsal recumbent p.
    dorsal rigid p.
    dorsodecubitus p.
    dorsolithotomy p.
    dorsorecumbent p.
    dorsosacral p.
    dorsosupine p.
    Duncan's p.
    Edebohls' p.
    Elliot's p.
    emprosthotonos p.
    fetal p.
    Fowler's p.
    frog-legged p.
    Fuch's p.
    genucubital p.
    genufacial p.
    genupectoral p.
    head dependent p.
    hinge p.
    horizontal p.
    hornpipe p.
    jackknife p.
    Jones' p.

position (*continued*)
 Jonge's p.
 kidney p.
 knee-chest p.
 knee-elbow p.
 kneeling-squatting p.
 Kraske's p.
 lateral decubitus p.
 lateral prone p.
 lateral recumbent p.
 Law's p.
 leapfrog p.
 lithotomy p.
 Mayer's p.
 Mayo-Robson p.
 Mercurio's p.
 Moynihan's p.
 neck extension p.
 Noble's p.
 opisthotonos p.
 orthopnea p.
 orthotonos p.
 Owen's p.
 Parkinson's p.
 Péan's p.
 Proetz's p.
 prone p.
 Robson's p.
 Rose's p.
 Samuel's p.
 Schüller's p.
 Scultetus' p.
 semi-Fowler p.
 semiprone p.
 semireclining p.
 shoe-and-stocking p.
 Simon's p.
 Sims' p.
 Stenver's p.
 Stern's p.
 supine p.
 Trendelenburg's p.
 upright p.

position (*continued*)
 Valentine's p.
 Walcher's p.
 Waters-Waldron p.
 Wolfenden's p.
Poth's operation
Pott's
 clamp
 scissors
Potts-Smith forceps
pouch
 Hartmann's p.
 Morison's p.
Poupart's
 ligament
 shelving edge, of P's
  ligament
Pratt-Smith forceps
Pratt's
 anoscope
 director
 hook
 probe
 scissors
 speculum
prepped and draped
probe
 Barr's p.
 Buie's p.
 Desjardin's p.
 Earle's p.
 Fenger's p.
 Kron's p.
 Larry's p.
 Mayo's p.
 Moynihan's p.
 Pratt's p.
 Welch-Allyn p.
procedure
 Buie's p.
procidentia
proctalgia
 p. fugax

proctectasia
proctectomy
procteurynter
proctitis
proctococcypexy
proctocolectomy
proctocolitis
proctocolpoplasty
proctocystoplasty
proctocystotomy
procto-elytroplasty
proctologic
proctology
proctoperineoplasty
proctopexy
proctoplasty
proctoptosis
proctorrhaphy
proctoscope
    ACMI
    Boehm's p.
    Fansler's p.
    Gabriel's p.
    Goldbacher's p.
    Hirschman-Martin p.
    Hirschman's p.
    Kelly's p.
    Lieberman's p.
    Montague's p.
    Newman's p.
    Pruitt's p.
    Strauss' p.
    Turell's p.
    Tuttle's p.
    Vernon-David p.
    Welch-Allyn p.
    Yeomans' p.
proctoscopy
proctosigmoidectomy
proctosigmoiditis
proctosigmoidoscopy
proctostenosis

proctostomy
proctotome
proctotomy
proctovalvotomy
Proetz's position
prolapse
    rectal p.
prolapsus
    p. ani
    p. recti
proliferation
properitoneal
prosthesis
    Heyer-Schulte p.
protrusion
Providence forceps
Pruitt's
    anoscope
    proctoscope
pruritus
    p. ani
pseudocyst
    pancreatic p.
psoas
pubic
pubioplasty
pubiotomy
pubis
pudendal
pudic
pulsatile
punch
    Kerrison's p.
punctate
puncture
    epigastric p.
Purcell's retractor
purulent
pylon
pylorectomy
pyloric
pyloristenosis

pylorodilator
pylorodiosis
pyloroduodenitis
pylorogastrectomy
pyloromyotomy
    Fredet-Ramstedt p.
pyloroplasty
    Finney's p.
    Heineke-Mikulicz p.
    Horsley's
    Jaboulay's p.
    Judd's p.
    Ramstedt's p.
pyloroptosis
pyloroscopy
pylorospasm
pylorostomy
pylorotomy
pylorus
Pynchon's tube
pyocelia
pyramid
    p. of thyroid
pyramidalis
raclage
radioisotope
rafe. See *raphe.*
Ramdohr's suture
Ramstedt's
    dilator
    operation
    pyloroplasty
ramus
Rankin's
    clamp
    forceps
Ranzewski's clamp
ranula
    pancreatic r.
raphe
Ratliff-Blake forceps
Raytec gauze dressing

rectal
rectectomy
rectocele
rectorectostomy
rectoromanoscopy
rectoscopy
rectosigmoid
rectosigmoidectomy
rectostomy
rectovaginal
rectovesical
rectum
redundant
Rehn-Delorme operation
reperitonealize
resection
    gastric r.
retinaculum
retractor
    Alm's r.
    Balfour's r.
    Beckman's r.
    Berens' r.
    Berna's r.
    Buie-Smith r.
    Byford's r.
    Cloward's r.
    Cole's r.
    Crile's r.
    Deaver's r.
    Ferguson-Moon r.
    Foss' r.
    Franz's r.
    Gibson-Balfour r.
    Goelet's r.
    Gosset's r.
    Green's r.
    Grieshaber's r.
    Harrington-Pemberton r.
    Harrington's r.
    Hill-Ferguson r.
    Israel's r.

retractor (*continued*)
    Jackson's r.
    Kelly's r.
    Kerrison's r.
    Killian-King r.
    King's r.
    Klemme's r.
    Kocher-Crotti r.
    Krasky's r.
    Lahey's r.
    Linton's r.
    Little's r.
    Martin's r.
    Mayo-Collins r.
    Mayo-Lovelace r.
    Mayo's r.
    Meyerding's r.
    Meyer's r.
    Murphy's r.
    O'Sullivan's r.
    Parker's r.
    Purcell's r.
    Richardson-Eastman r.
    Richardson's r.
    Rigby's r.
    Rochester-Ferguson r.
    Roux's r.
    Senn's r.
    Sistrunk's r.
    Sloan's r.
    Smith-Buie r.
    Theis' r.
    Volkmann's r.
    Walker's r.
    Walter-Deaver r.
    Webster's r.
    Weinberg's r.
    Weitlaner's r.
    Wolfson's r.
retrocecal
retroflexion
retrograde

retromammary
retroperitoneal
retroversion
Reverdin's needle
Richardson-Eastman retractor
Richardson's
    retractor
    suture
Richter's
    hernia
    suture
Riedel's
    lobe
    struma
Riex's hernia
Rigal's suture
Rigby's retractor
rima
ring
    Abbe's r's
    inguinal r.
Ringer's lactate solution
Risdon's extraoral incision
Ritisch's suture
Rives' splenectomy
Robson's position
Rochester-Ewald forceps
Rochester-Ferguson
    retractor
    scissors
Rochester-Mixter forceps
Rochester-Rankin forceps
Rochester's
    forceps
    needle
Rocky-Davis incision
Rodman's incision
Roeder's forceps
Rokitansky's hernia
Rollet's incision
rongeur
    Kerrison's r.

rongeur (*continued*)
    Leksell's r.
Roosevelt's clamp
Rosen's
    incision
    operation
Rose's position
rosette
Rosser's hook
Routier's operation
Roux-en-Y
    cystojejunostomy
    jejunal loop incision
    operation
Roux's
    gastroenterostomy
    retractor
    sign
Rovsing's sign
RR — Recovery Room
Rubin's tube
ruga
    r. gastrica
rugae
Rumel's tourniquet
rupture
Russian forceps
Ryle's tube
sac
    hernial s.
    serous s.
saccular
sacculation
sacculus
Saenger's suture
Samuel's position
Sanders' incision
sanguineous
Santorini's duct
saphenectomy
saphenofemoral
saphenous
sarcoid

sarcoma
saucerization
saw
    Butcher's s.
scalene
scalenectomy
scalenotomy
scalenus
scalpel
Scarpa's
    fascia
    operation
    sheath
    triangle
Schede's operation
Schindler's gastroscope
schistosomiasis
    intestinal s.
    Manson's s.
Schlange's sign
Schlatter's operation
Schobinger's incision
Schoemaker's
    clamp
    gastroenterostomy
Schoenberg's forceps
Schuchardt's incision
Schüller's position
Schutz's forceps
scirrhous
scirrhus
scissors
    Berbridge's s.
    Brooks' s.
    Buie's s.
    Burnham's s.
    Deaver's s.
    DeBakey's s.
    Doyen's s.
    Esmarch's s.
    Ferguson's s.
    Jones' s.
    Jorgenson's s.

scissors (*continued*)
Knowles' s.
Lister's s.
Littauer's s.
Mayo-Harrington s.
Mayo-Noble s.
Mayo-Sims s.
Mayo's s.
Metzenbaum's s.
Miller's s.
New's s.
Northbent's s.
Ochsner's s.
Panzer's s.
Potts' s.
Pratt's s.
Rochester-Ferguson s.
Shortbent's s.
Sistrunk's s.
Thorek-Feldman s.
Thorek's s.
Vezien's s.
sclerotherapy
sclerosis
gastric s.
scoop
Beck's s.
Berens' s.
Desjardin's s.
Ferguson's s.
Ferris' s.
Luer-Korte s.
Mayo-Robson s.
Mayo's s.
Moore's s.
Moynihan's s.
Scribner's shunt
scrotal
scrotectomy
scrotocele
scrotoplasty
scrotum

Scudder's
clamp
forceps
Scultetus' position
scybalous
scybalum
sebaceous
Seconal anesthetic agent
section
frozen s.
semi-Fowler position
Semken's forceps
Senn's
operation
retractor
sentinel pile
sepsis
septum
Cloquet's s.
crural s.
s. femorale
serosa
serosanguineous
serositis
serous
sessile
sfinkter-. See words beginning
sphincter-.
Shallcross's forceps
Shambaugh's incision
sheath
rectus s.
s. of rectus abdominis
muscle
Scarpa's s.
shelf
Blumer's s.
Shortbent's scissors
shotty nodes
shunt
portacaval s.
postcaval s.

shunt (*continued*)
    Scribner's s.
sibah-. See words beginning
  scyba-.
sigmoid
sigmoidectomy
sigmoiditis
sigmoidopexy
sigmoidoproctostomy
sigmoidorectostomy
sigmoidoscope
    Boehm's s.
    Buie's s.
    disposable s.
    fiberoptic s.
    Frankfeldt's s.
    Kelly's s.
    Kleenspec s.
    Lieberman's s.
    Montague's s.
    Solow's s.
    Turell's s.
    Tuttle's s.
    Vernon-David s.
    Welch-Allyn s.
    Yeomans' s.
sigmoidoscopy
sigmoidosigmoidostomy
sigmoidostomy
sigmoidotomy
sigmoidovesical
sign
    Aaron's s.
    Roux's s.
    Rovsing's s.
    Schlange's s.
    Stokes' s.
    Tansini's s.
    Thomayer's s.
    Toma's s.
    Volkovitsch's s.
    Wachenheim-Reder s.

sign (*continued*)
    Wahl's s.
    Wölfler's s.
    Wolkowitsch's s.
    Wreden's s.
Silastic implant
silicone
Silverman's needle
Simon's
    incision
    position
    suture
Sims'
    anoscope
    position
    speculum
    suture
Singleton's incision
Singley's forceps
sinus
    pilonidal s.
    sacrococcygeal s.
    thyroglossal s.
siphon
Sistrunk's
    retractor
    scissors
situs
    s. inversus viscerum
    s. perversus
    s. solitus
    s. transversus
skeletization
skeletonize
Sloan's
    incision
    retractor
sloughing
sluffing. See *sloughing*.
Smead-Jones closure
Smith-Buie retractor
Smith-Peterson incision

snare
    Frankfeldt's s.
    Norwood's s.
sois. See *psoas.*
Solow's sigmoidoscope
solution
    Ringer's lactate s.
Sotteau's operation
Southey's trocar
speculum
    Allingham's s.
    Barr's s.
    Buie-Smith s.
    Chelsea-Eaton s.
    Cook's s.
    David's s.
    Dudley-Smith s.
    Fansler's s.
    Goldbacher's s.
    Guild-Pratt s.
    Hinckle-James s.
    Martin's s.
    Mathew's s.
    Pennington's s.
    Pratt's s.
    proctoscopic s.
    Sims' s.
    Vernon-David s.
Spencer Wells forceps
sphincter
    Hyrtl's
    O'Beirne's s.
    Oddi's s.
    prepyloric s.
sphincteralgia
sphincterectomy
sphincterismus
sphincteritis
sphincteroplasty
sphincteroscope
sphincteroscopy
sphincterotome

sphincterotomy
    choledochal s.
spicular
spiculated
spicule
spiculum
Spieghel's line
Spivack's gastrostomy
splanchnicectomy
spleen
    accessory s.
splenectomize
splenectomy
    Carter's thoraco-
      abdominal s.
    Federoff's s.
    Henry's s.
    Rives' s.
    subcapsular s.
splenectopia
splenic
splenitis
splenocele
splenocleisis
splenomegaly
splenoncus
splenopexy
splenoportography
splenoptosis
splenorenal
splenorrhagia
splenorrhaphy
splenotomy
splenulus
sponge
    Lincoff's s.
Ssabanejew-Frank gastrostomy
Stamm's gastrostomy
stapler
    TA-30
    TA-55
stasis

State operation
steatorrhea
stenosis
    pyloric s.
stenotic
Stensen's duct
Stenver's position
stent
stercoraceous
sterile
sterilely
sterility
sterilize
Steri-strip
Stern's position
sternal
sternum
Stevenson's clamp
Stewart's
    hook
    incision
Stille's forceps
stocking
    Jobst s.
Stokes' sign
stoma
stomach
    dumping s.
    leather bottle s.
Stone-Holcombe clamp
Stone's
    clamp
    forceps
strangulation
stratum
Strauss' proctoscope
stria
stricture
stripper
    Emerson's s.
    intraluminal s.
    Keeley's s.

stripper (*continued*)
    Kurten's s.
    Lempka's s.
    Mayo's s.
    Myers' s.
    Nabatoff's s.
    Webb's s.
    Wilson's s.
stroma
Strombeck's incision
struma
    Riedel's s.
strumectomy
stump
    invaginated s.
Sturmdorf's suture
subareolar
subcutaneous
submammary
subscapular
sudosist. See pseudocyst.
sulcus
    s. intermedius
superficial
superficialis
supernumerary
supination
supine
suppuration
suppurative
Supramid suture
Surfacaine anesthetic agent
surgical procedures. See
    operation.
Surgical gauze dressing
Surgiflex bandage
Surgilene suture
Surgilon suture
Surgilope suture
suspension
suture
    absorbable s.

suture (*continued*)

    Acutrol s.
    Albert's s.
    Alcon's s.
    Allison's s.
    alternating s.
    anchoring s.
    angle s.
    Appolito's s.
    apposition s.
    Argyll-Robertson s.
    Arlt's s.
    atraumatic s.
    Atroloc s.
    Axenfeld's s.
    Babcock's s.
    back-and-forth s.
    Barraquer's s.
    baseball s.
    Béclard's s.
    Bell's s.
    biparietal s.
    black-braided s.
    black silk s.
    blanket s.
    bolster s.
    Bozeman's s.
    braided s.
    bregmatomastoid s.
    bridle s.
    bunching s.
    Bunnell's s.
    buried s.
    button s.
    cable wire s.
    capitonnage s.
    cardiovascular s.
    catgut s.
    celluloid s.
    chain s.
    chromic catgut s.
    circular s.

suture (*continued*)

    circumcision s.
    clavate s.
    Coakley's s.
    coaptation s.
    cobbler's s.
    collagen s.
    compound s.
    Connell's s.
    continuous s.
    corneoscleral s.
    coronal s.
    Cushing's s.
    cushioning s.
    cutaneous s.
    cuticular s.
    Czerny-Lembert s.
    Czerny's s.
    dacron s.
    dekalon s.
    deknatel s.
    delayed s.
    dentate s.
    dermal s.
    Dermalene s.
    Dermalon s.
    Dexon s.
    double-armed s.
    double-button s.
    dulox s.
    Dupuytren's s.
    Duvergier's s.
    edge-to-edge s.
    elastic s.
    Emmet's s.
    Equisetene s.
    Ethibond s.
    Ethicon s.
    Ethiflex s.
    Ethilon s.
    ethmoideomaxillary s.
    everting s.

suture (*continued*)

- far and near s.
- figure-of-eight s.
- fixation s.
- Flaxedil s.
- Flexiton s.
- Flexon s.
- free ligature s.
- Frost's s.
- furrier's s.
- Gaillard-Arlt s.
- Gambee's s.
- Gély's s.
- Gibson's s.
- Glover's s.
- Gould's s.
- guy s.
- groove s.
- Gudebrod's s.
- Gussenbauer's s.
- gut chromic s.
- Guyton-Friedenwald s.
- Halsted's s.
- Harris s.
- helical s.
- hemostatic s.
- horizontal mattress s.
- horsehair s.
- imbricated s.
- interlocking s.
- intermaxillary s.
- interrupted s.
- intradermal s.
- inverted s.
- Ivalon's s.
- Jobert's s.
- Kalt's s.
- kangaroo tendon s.
- Kelly's s.
- Kirby's s.
- Kirschner's s.
- lace s.
- lambdoid s.

suture (*continued*)

- Le Dran's s.
- LeFort's s.
- Lembert's s.
- ligation s.
- limbal s.
- Littre's s.
- living s.
- locking s.
- lock-stitch s.
- Löffler's s.
- loop s.
- Marlex s.
- mattress s.
- Maunsell's s.
- Mayo-linen s.
- Medrafil's wire s.
- Meigs' s.
- Mersilene s.
- monofilament s.
- multifilament s.
- multistrand s.
- near-and-far s.
- Neurolon s.
- nonabsorbable s.
- noose s.
- nylon monofilament s.
- over-and-over s.
- overlapping s.
- Palfyn's s.
- Pancoast's s.
- Paré's s.
- Parker-Kerr s.
- pericostal s.
- Petit's s.
- pin s.
- plain catgut s.
- plastic s.
- plicating s.
- plication s.
- Polydek s.
- polyester s.
- polyethylene s.

suture (*continued*)

- polyfilament s.
- polypropylene s.
- presection s.
- primary s.
- prolene s.
- pulley s.
- pull-out wire s.
- pursestring s.
- quilled s.
- quilted s.
- Ramdohr's s.
- reinforcing s.
- relaxation s.
- retention s.
- ribbon gut s.
- Richardson's s.
- Richter's s.
- Rigal's s.
- Ritisch's s.
- rubber s.
- running continuous s.
- Saenger's s.
- sagittal s.
- secondary s.
- seminal s.
- seromuscular s.
- seroserosal silk s.
- seroserous s.
- serrated s.
- shotted s.
- silk s.
- silk-braided s.
- silkworm gut s.
- silver wire s.
- Simon's s.
- simple s.
- Sims' s.
- single-armed s.
- sling s.
- spiral s.
- stainless steel s.
- staple s.

suture (*continued*)

- stay s.
- steel mesh s.
- stick-tie s.
- Sturmdorf's s.
- subcuticular s.
- superficial s.
- support s.
- Supramid s.
- surgical s.
- Surgilene s.
- Surgilon s.
- Surgilope s.
- tantalum-wire s.
- Taylor's s.
- tendon s.
- tension s.
- Tevdek s.
- Thermo-flex s.
- Thiersch's s.
- through-and-through s.
- tiger gut s.
- Tom-Jones s.
- tongue-and-groove s.
- traction s.
- transfixing s.
- transfixion s.
- twisted s.
- Tycron s.
- unabsorbable s.
- uninterrupted s.
- Verhoeff's s.
- vertical mattress s.
- Vicryl s.
- Viro-Tec s.
- visceroparietal s.
- whipstitch s.
- white braided s.
- white silk s.
- wire s.
- Wölfler's s.
- Wysler's s.
- Y-s.

suture (*continued*)
  Z-s.
  Zytor's s.
Swenson's operation
sympathectomy
syndrome. See Medical
  Specialty sections.
syngraft
syringe
syringectomy
syringotome
syringotomy
Talma's operation
tamponade
Tanner's operation
Tansini's
  operation
  sign
tantalum mesh
Taylor's suture
T-bandage
technique
  Buie t.
  La Roque's t.
  Lotheissen-McVay t.
  Madden t.
  Ponka t.
  time diffusion t.
  vest-over-pants t.
Teflon
  graft
  mesh
Telfa dressing
tenaculum
  Lahey's t.
tendon
  conjoined t.
tenectomy
tenesmus
tenomyoplasty
tenotomy
Tensilon anesthetic agent
teratoma

testicle
Tevdek suture
Textor's operation
thalamectomy
thalamotomy
Theis' retractor
theleplasty
thelerethism
thelitis
thelorrhagia
thenar eminence
Thermo-flex suture
Thiersch's
  operation
  suture
Thillaye's bandage
Thomas-Warren incision
Thomayer's sign
Thoms' forceps
thoracotomy
Thorek-Feldman scissors
Thorek-Mixter forceps
Thorek's
  aspirator
  scissors
thread
  celluloid t.
  Pagenstecher's linen t.
thrombectomy
thrombophlebitis
thymectomize
thymectomy
thymus
thyroglossal
thyrohyal
thyroid
thyroidea
  t. accessoria
  t. ima
thyroidectomize
thyroidectomy
thyroiditis
thyroidotomy

thyromegaly
thyroparathyroidectomy
thyrotomy
thyrotoxicosis
Timbrall-Fisher incision
tissue
    Gamgee t.
toe
    Morton's t.
toilet
Toma's sign
Tom-Jones suture
Torek's operation
torsion
tortuous
tourniquet
    Rumel's t.
trabeculae
    t. lienis
    t. of spleen
trabecular
tracheostomy
tracheotomy
tract
    alimentary t.
    biliary t.
transduodenal
transection
transfixion
transfusion
transplant
    Gallie t.
transplantation
transposition
transversalis
transversostomy
Travel's operation
treatment
    Murphy's t.
Treitz's
    hernia
    ligament of T.

Trendelenburg's
    operation
    position
Treves' operation
triangle
    Calot's t.
    Henke's t.
    Hesselbach's t.
    Scarpa's t.
trigone
trigonectomy
Trilene anesthetic agent
Trimar anesthetic agent
trocar
    Allen's t.
    Barnes' t.
    Duke's t.
    Ochsner's t.
    Southey's t.
Tronothane hydrochloride
    anesthetic agent
TSH — thyroid stimulating
    hormone
T-shaped incision
T-tube
tube
    Abbott-Rawson t.
    Baker's t.
    Buie's t.
    Cantor t.
    Carman's t.
    Cattell's t.
    Chaffin-Pratt t.
    Debove's t.
    Greiling's t.
    Johnson's t.
    Jutte's t.
    Kelly's t.
    Levin's t.
    Linton's t.
    Miller-Abbott t.
    Mueller-Frazier t.

tube (*continued*)
    Mueller-Pool t.
    Mueller-Pynchon t.
    Mueller-Yankauer t.
    Nachlas' t.
    O'Beirne's t.
    Ochsner's t.
    Paul-Mixter t.
    Pool's t.
    Pynchon's t.
    Rubin's t.
    Ryle's t.
    Wangensteen t.
    Yankauer's t.
tuber
    t. omental
tubercle
    pubic t.
tumor
tunica
    t. abdominalis
    t. adventitia
    t. albuginea
    t. dartos
    t. fibrosa hepatis
    t. fibrosa lienis
    t. mucosa ventriculi
    t. mucosa vesicae felleae
    t. muscularis coli
    t. muscularis intestini
      tenuis
    t. muscularis recti
    t. muscularis ventriculi
    t. serosa
    t. serosa coli
    t. serosa hepatis
    t. serosa intestini tenuis
    t. serosa lienis
    t. serosa peritonei
    t. serosa ventriculi
    t. serosa vesicae felleae
Turell's
    proctoscope

Turell's (*continued*)
    sigmoidoscope
Turner's operation
Tuttle's
    proctoscope
    sigmoidoscope
Tycron suture
ulcer
    Allingham's u.
    Cruveilhier's u.
    Cushing's u.
    decubitus u.
    Dieulafoy's u.
    duodenal u.
    follicular u.
    gastric u.
    gastroduodenal u.
    gastrojejunal u.
    jejunal u.
    Kocher's u.
    Mann-Williamson u.
    marginal u.
    peptic u.
    perforating u.
    stomal u.
ulceration
ultrasonography
ultrasound
umbilectomy
umbilical
umbilicus
unguis
    u. incarnatus
Unna's paste
unit
    Bovie u.
urachus
U-shaped incision
uthiroid. See *euthyroid.*
vagal
vagotomy
vagus
Valentine's position

valve
    Houston's v.
valvula
    v. ileocolica
    v. pylori
van Buren's operation
varicocele
varicose
varicosity
varicotomy
varix
vas deferens
vasa
    v. brevia
vascular
vasectomy
Vaseline gauze dressing
Vater's
    ampulla
    papilla
vein
    azygos v.
    femoral v.
    portal v.
    saphenous v.
Velcro binder
Velpeau's
    bandage
    hernia
Velroc dressing
vena
    v. cava
venesection
venipuncture
venoperitoneostomy
ventral
ventrocystorrhaphy
verge
    anal v.
Verhoeff's suture
Vermale's operation
vermicular

vermiculation
vermiculous
vermiform
vermifugal
Verneuil's operation
Vernon-David
    proctoscope
    sigmoidoscope
    speculum
verruca
    v. acuminata
    v. digitata
    v. filiformis
    v. plana
    v. plantaris
    v. vulgaris
vesicointestinal
vessel
    circumflex v.
    external pudic v.
    hypogastric v.
    iliac v.
    pudendal v.
    pudic v.
vest-over-pants technique
Vezien's scissors
Vicryl suture
Vidal's operation
Vi-drape
Villard's button
villoma
villus
villusectomy
Vim-Silverman needle
Virden's catheter
Vioform dressing
Viro-Tec suture
Virtus' forceps
viscera
visceral
visceroparietal
visceroperitoneal

visceropleural
visceroptosis
viscerosensory
viscerotome
Vischer's incision
viscid
viscidity
viscus
Vitallium
Volkmann's
    contracture
    retractor
Volkovitsch's sign
volvulus
vomica
Von Bergmann's hernia
von Haberer-Aguirre gastrec-
    tomy
von Haberer-Finney gastro-
    enterostomy
von Petz's clamp
V-shaped incision
Wachenheim-Reder sign
Wahl's sign
Walcher's position
Waldeyer's colon
Wales' dilator
Walker's retractor
Walter-Deaver retractor
Walter's forceps
Walther's forceps
Wangensteen's
    carrier
    clamp
    colostomy
    dissector
    dressing
    forceps
    operation
    tube
Warren's
    incision
    operation

wart
    plantar w.
Waters-Waldron position
Watson-Jones incision
Watson's operation
Watts' clamp
Waugh's operation
Webb's stripper
Weber-Fergusson incision
Weber's
    catheter
    insufflator
Webster's retractor
Weinberg's retractor
Weir's operation
Weisenbach's forceps
Weitlaner's retractor
Welch-Allyn
    anoscope
    forceps
    hook
    probe
    proctoscope
    sigmoidoscope
Wharton's duct
W hernia
Whipple's
    incision
    operation
Whitehead's operation
whitlow
    melanotic w.
    thecal w.
Wilde's incision
Williams' forceps
Willie-Meyer incision
Willis'
    antrum
    pancreas
Wilson's stripper
Winiwarter's operation
Winslow's
    foramen

Winslow's (*continued*)
    pancreas
wire
    Kirschner's w.
Wirsung's duct
Wise's operation
Witzel's
    enterostomy
    gastrostomy
    operation
Wolfenden's position
Wölfler's
    gastroenterostomy
    operation
    sign
    suture
Wolf-Schindler gastroscope
Wolfson's
    clamp
    retractor
Wolf's peritoneoscope
Wolkowitsch's sign
Wreden's sign
W-shaped incision
Wützer's operation
Wyeth's operation
Wyllys-Andrews operation

Wysler's suture
Xeroform gauze dressing
xiphoid
Xylocaine with epinephrine
    anesthetic agent
xyster
Yankauer's tube
Y bandage
Yellen clamp
Yeomans'
    forceps
    proctoscope
    sigmoidoscope
Young's dilator
Y-suture
Y-type incision
Zachary Cope-DeMartel clamp
Z-flap incision
Zieman's operation
Zimmerman's operation
zister. See *xyster.*
Z-plasty
    incision
    operation
Z-shaped incision
Z-suture
Zytor's suture

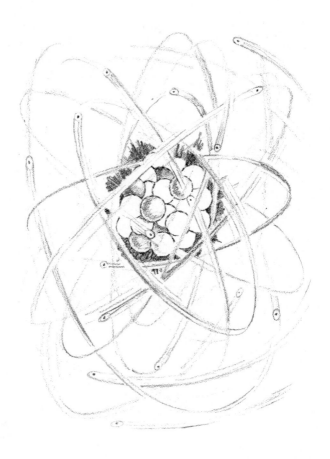

(Courtesy of Graham, B. J., and Thomas, W. N.: An Introduction to Physics for Radiologic Technologists. Philadelphia, W. B. Saunders Company, 1975.)

DRUGS AND CHEMISTRY

Abbokinase
Accelerase
Accurbron
acenocoumarin
acenocoumarol
acetaminophen
acetazolamide
acetic acid
acetohexamide
Acetonide
acetophenazine
acetylcholine chloride
acetylcysteine
acetyldigitoxin
acetylsalicylic acid
Achromycin
    A. V
Achrostatin V
Acidophilus
Acidulin
Aci-Jel jelly
Acnaveen
Acne-Dome
acrisorcin
ACTH — adrenocorticotropic
    hormone

Acthar
Acticort
Actidil
Actifed
actinomycin
    a. D
Actrapid
Acylanid
Adapin
Adipex-P
adrenalin chloride
Adriamycin
adriamycinone
Adroyd
Adrucil
Aerolone
Aeroseb-Dex
Aeroseb-HC
Aerosporin
Afrin
Afrinol
aggregated albumin (human)
aggregated radioiodinated
    (I 131) albumin (human)
    (MAA I 131)
Agoral

A-hydroCort
Akineton
Akrinol
Alba-3
Albamycin
Albatussin
Albuminar-5
albumin microspheres (human)
Albumotope ^{125}I, ^{131}I
    A. L-S
Alconefrin
Aldactazide
Aldactone
Aldoclor
Aldomet
Aldoril
Alerin-TD
Alka-Seltzer
alkavervir
Alkeran
Alkets
allantoin
Allecur
allobarbital
allopurinol
Allpyral
Alpha Chymar
alpha-chymotrypsin
Alphaderm
Alpha Keri
alphaprodine
alseroxylon
AlternaGEL
Aludrine
Aludrox
aluminum acetate
    a. hydroxide
    a. nicotinate
    a. phosphate
Alupent
Alzinox
amantadine hydrochloride

Ambenyl
Ambodryl
Amcill
Amen
Americaine-Otic
Amesec
A-MethaPred
amethocaine
Amicar
amikacin sulfate
Amikin
aminacrine hydrochloride
aminocaproic acid
Amino-Cerv
Aminodur
Aminophyllin
aminophylline
aminosalicylate sodium
aminosalicylic acid
Amipaque
Amitid
amitriptyline hydrochloride
ammonium biphosphate
    a. carbonate
    a. chloride
    a. ichthyosulfonate
    a. mandelate
    a. tartrate
Amnestrogen
amobarbital
amoxapine
amoxicillin
Amoxil
Amphedroxyn
amphetamine
    a. aspartate
    a. saccharate
    a. sulfate
Amphojel
amphotericin B
ampicillin
Amsustain

amyl nitrite
Amytal
Anadrol
Ananase
Anaspaz
Ancef
Android
Anectine
    A. Flo-Pack
Anestacon
Anesthesin
Angio-CONRAY (contrast
   material)
angiotensin
Anhydron
anhydrous
    a. theophylline
anileridine
anisindione
anisotropine methylbromide
Ansolysen Bitartrate
Anspor
A-N stannous aggregated
   albumin
Antabuse
antazoline
Antepar
anthracycline
Anthra-Derm
anthralin
Antifoam A Compound
Antilirium
Antiminth
Antistine
Antivert
Antrenyl
    A. Bromide
Antuitrin "S"
Anturane
APC with codeine
A.P.L.
apomorphine hydrochloride

apothesine
A-Poxide
Apresazide
Apresoline
    A.-Esidrix
Aquacare
AquaMEPHYTON
Aquaphor
Aquaphyllin
Aquatensen
ara-C (cytosine arabinoside)
Aralen
Aramine
Arco-Lase
Arfonad
Argyrol
Aristocort
Aristoderm
Aristospan
Arlidin
Artane
Arthralgen
Asbron G Inlay-Tab
Ascodeen
ascorbic acid
Ascriptin
Asendin
asparaginase
L-asparaginase
aspirin
Atabrine
Atarax
Athemol
Athrombin
Ativan
Atromid-S
atropine
    a. methyl nitrate
    a. sulfate
attapulgite
Attenuvax
^{198}Au (gold)

Auralgan
Aureomycin
Aureotope
Auroloid-198
aurothioglucose
AVC cream
Aveeno bath
Aventyl HCl
Avertin
Avitene
azapetine phosphate
azathioprine
Azene
Azo-Gantanol
Azo-Gantrisin
Azolid
Azo-Mandelamine
Azotrex
Azulfidine
Azulfidine EN-tabs
Bacimycin
Bacitracin
baclofen
Bactrim
BAL in Oil
Balneol
Balnetar
Banthine
Barachlor
Basaljel
basis soap
BCNU — bischloroethylnitro-
            sourea
beclomethasone dipropionate
Beclovent
Belladenal
belladonna
Bellergal
benactyzine hydrochloride
Benadryl
Bendectin
bendroflumethiazide

Benemid
Benisone
Benodaine
benoxinate
Bentyl
Benylin
Benzagel
benzalkonium chloride
benzathine
            penicillin G b.
Benzedrine
benzene hexachloride
benzestrol
benzocaine
benzoic acid
benzonatate
benzothiadiazine
benzoyl peroxide
benzphetamine
benzthiazide
benztropine mesylate
benzyl benzoate
benzylpenicilloyl-polylysine
Betadine
betahistine
Betalin
betamethasone
            b. benzoate
            b. valerate
Betapen-VK
bethanechol chloride
Bicillin
BiCNU
Bilopaque
Bio-Heprin
Biomydrin
Biozyme-C Ointment
biperiden
            b. hydrochloride
            b. lactate
bisacodyl
bischloroethylnitrosourea

bishydroxycoumarin
bismuth subcarbonate
bis-Tropamide
Blefcon
Blenoxane
bleomycin
    b. sulfate
Blephamide
Bonadoxin
Bonine
Bontril PDM
boracic acid
boric acid
Borofax
B & O suppositories
Bradosol
Breokinase
Breonesin
Brethine
bretylium tosylate
Bretylol
Brevicon
Brevital
Bricanyl
Bristamycin
bromelain
bromocriptine
    b. mesylate
bromodiphenhydramine
bromophenol blue
brompheniramine
Brondecon
Bronkaid
Bronkephrine
Bronkodyl
Bronkosol
Bronkotabs
buclizine
Bufferin
Burow's solution
busulfan
butabarbital sodium

butacaine
butadiene
butambem picrate
butaperazine
Butazolidin
    B. Alka
Butesin Picrate
butethamine
Buticaps
Butisol
butorphanol tartrate
Butyn
cade oil
Cafergot
caffeine
Caladryl cream
calamine
Calcidrine syrup
calcifediol
Calciferol
Calcimar
calcitonin-salmon
calcitriol
calcium carbonate
    c. chloride
    c. gluceptate
    c. glycerophosphate
    c. iodide
CaldeCort
Calderol
Caldesene
Calphosan
Cama Inlay-Tab
Camalox
Camoquin
Campho-phenique
camphorated parachlorophenol
Candeptin
Candex
candicidin
Cantharone
Cantil

Capastat Sulfate
Capital
Capitrol
Capla
capreomycin
capreomycin sulfate
Caprokol
captodiame
captopril
carbachol
carbamazepine
carbarsone
carbenicillin disodium
    c. indanyl sodium
carbetapentane citrate
carbidopa
carbinoxamine
Carbocaine Hydrochloride
carbol-fuchsin
carbon dioxide
Carbo-Resin
Carboxin
Carbrital
carbromal
Carcholin
Cardilate
Cardiocreme
Cardioquin
Cardrase
carisoprodol
Carmol HC
carmustine
carphenazine
Cartrax
casanthranol
cascara sagrada
castor oil
Catapres
Cathomycin
Ceclor
Cedilanid
CeeNU

cefaclor
cefadroxil
    c. monohydrate
Cefadyl
cefamandole nafate
cefazolin sodium
cefoxitin sodium
Celestone
Cellothyl
Celontin
Cenadex
Cenalene
Centrax
cephalexin
cephaloridine
cephalothin sodium
cephapirin sodium
cephradine
Cerebro-Nicin
Cerespan
Cerubidine
Cetacaine
Cetaphil
Cetapred
charcoal
Chardonna
Chestamine
Chlo-Amine
chlophedianol hydrochloride
chloral hydrate
Chloramate
chlorambucil
chloramine-T
chloramphenicol
Chloraseptic
chlorcyclizine
chlordantoin
chlordiazepoxide
    hydrochloride
chlorhydroxyquinolin
chlormerodrin
    c. Hg 197

chlormerodrin (*continued*)
    c. Hg 203
chlormezanone
chloroform
Chloromycetin
Chloromyxin
chloroprocaine hydrochloride
Chloroptic-P
chloroquine hydrochloride
chlorothen
chlorothiazide
chlorotrianisene
chlorpheniramine maleate
chlorpromazine
chlorpropamide
chlorprothixene
chlorquinaldol
chlortetracycline
    hydrochloride
chlorthalidone
Chlor-Trimeton
chlorzoxazone
Cho-Free
Choledyl
cholestyramine
choline magnesium
    trisalicylate
Choloxin
Chorex
chorionic gonadotropin
Chromalbin
chromic phosphate P 32
Chromitope Sodium
chromium Cr 51 serum albumin
chrysarobin
chrysazin
Chymar
Chymoral
chymotrypsin
cimetidine
cinnamedrine hydrochloride
Circanol

Circubid
cisplatin
cis-retinoic acid
Citanest
citrate of magnesia
clemizole
Cleocin
clidinium bromide
clindamycin hydrochloride
Clinistix
Clinoril
Clistin
clofibrate
Clomid
clomiphene citrate
clonazepam
clonidine hydrochloride
Clonopin
clorazepate dipotassium
    c. monopotassium
Chlorpactin XCB
clortermine hydrochloride
clotrimazole
cloxacillin sodium
CMF (Cytoxan, methotrexate,
    5-fluorouracil)
C-MOPP (cyclophosphamide,
    vincristine, procarbazine,
    prednisone)
^{57}Co, ^{58}Co, ^{60}Co (cobalt)
cobalt
cocaine
    c. hydrochloride
Codalan
codeine
    c. phosphate
Codimal
Cogentin
Colace
ColBENEMID
colchicine
colistimethate sodium

colistin
collagenase
colloidal sulfur
Collo Kit
Coly-Mycin
Combid
Combipres
Compazine
Conestron
Congespirin
Conjutabs
COP (Cytoxan, Oncovin,
    prednisone)
Copavin
copper oleate
    c. sulfate
Co-Pyronil
Coramine
Cordran
Corgard
Coricidin
Cor-Tar-Quin
Cort-Dome
Cortef
Corticaine
corticotropin
Cortifar
cortisol
cortisone
Cortisporin
Cortogen
Cortone
Cortril
Co-salt
Cosmegen
Cotazym
CoTylenol
Coumadin
Co-Xan
C-Quins
cranberry juice
Cresatin

cromolyn sodium
crotamiton
Cruex
cryptenamine
crystalline warfarin sodium
crystal violet
Crysticillin
Crystodigin
Cuemid
cupric sulfate
Cuprimine
curare
CVP (Cytoxan, vincristine,
    prednisone)
cyanocobalamin Co 57, Co 58,
    Co 60
    radioactive c.
cyclacillin
Cyclaine
Cyclamycin
cyclandelate
Cyclapen-W
cyclizine lactate
cyclobenzaprine hydrochloride
Cyclogyl
Cyclohexane
cyclomethycaine
Cyclomydril
Cyclopar
cyclopentane
cyclopentolate
cyclophosphamide
cyclopropane
cycloserine
Cyclospasmol
cyclothiazide
cycrimine hydrochloride
Cylert
cyproheptadine hydrochloride
Cystospaz
Cytellin
Cytomel

Cytosar-U
cytosine arabinoside
Cytoxan
dacarbazine
Dacriose
Dactil
dactinomycin
Dalmane
danazol
Danex shampoo
Danilone
Danocrine
danthron
Dantrium
dantrolene sodium
dapsone
Daranide
Daraprim
Darbid
Daricon
Daro Tablets
Dartal
Darvocet
Darvon
Datril
daunorubicin hydrochloride
Davoxin
Dayalets
Deaner
deanol acetamidobenzoate
Decadron
Deca-Durabolin
Decholin
Declomycin
Declostatin
Decubitex
dehydrocholic acid
Deladumone
Delalutin
Delatestryl
Delestrogen
Delfen

Delta-Cortef
Deltasone
Deltra
Delvex
demecarium
demeclocycline hydrochloride
Demerol
Demser
Demulen
Dendrid
Depakene
Depen
Depo-Medrol
Depo-Provera
Depo-Testosterone
Deprol
Dermacort
dermatomycin
Dermoplast
DES – diethylstilbestrol
Desenex
deserpidine
Desferal
desipramine hydrochloride
deslanoside
desonide
desoximetasone
desoxycorticosterone acetate
Desoxyn
desoxyribonuclease
Desquam-X
Devegan
dexamethasone
dexbrompheniramine
dexchlorpheniramine maleate
Dexedrine
dexpanthenol
dextroamphetamine
dextromethorphan
    hydrobromide
dextropantothenyl alcohol
dextropropoxyphene

dextrose
dextrothyroxine sodium
Diabinese
Diafen
Dialog
Dialose
diaminodiphenylsulfone
Diamox
diamthazole
Dianabol
diazepam
diazoxide
Dibenzyline
dibucaine hydrochloride
dicarbazine
dichloralphenazone
dichlorphenamide
dicloxacillin
    d. sodium monohydrate
Dicodid
Dicopac
Dicorvin
dicumarol
dicyclomine hydrochloride
Didrex
Didronel
dienestrol
diethylstilbestrol
    d. diphosphate
diflorasone diacetate
Digitaline Nativelle
digitalis
digitoxin
digoxin
dihydrocodeinone bitartrate
dihydrohydroxycodeinone
dihydromorphinone
dihydrotachysterol
dihydroxyaluminum amino-
    acetate
diiodohydroxyquin
Diiodohydroxyquinoline

diisopropyl fluorophosphate
Dilantin
Dilatrate-SR
Dilaudid
Dilor
dimenhydrinate
dimercaprol
Dimetane
Dimetapp
dimethindene maleate
dimethisoquin hydrochloride
Dimethpyrindine
dimethyl sulfoxide
Dimocillin
dioctyl calcium sulfosuccinate
    d. sodium sulfosuccinate
Diodoquin
Diodrast
Dionosil
dioxyline phosphate
diphemanil methylsulfate
diphenhydramine hydro-
    chloride
diphenidol
diphenoxylate hydrochloride
diphenylhydantoin
diphenylpyraline
Diprosone
dipyridamole
Disalcid
Disomer
disopyramide phosphate
dithiazanine iodide
Ditropan
Diucardin
Diupres
Diuretin
Diuril
Diutensin
dobutamine hydrochloride
Dobutrex
docusate sodium

Dolene
Dolonil
Dolophine
Domeboro
domiphen bromide
Donnagel
Donna-sed
Donnatal
Donnazyme
dopamine
Dopram
Dorbane
Doriden
Dorsacaine
doxapram hydrochloride
doxepin hydrochloride
Doxinate
doxorubicin hydrochloride
doxycycline
doxylamine
Dramamine
Drinalfa
Drize
Drolban
dromostanolone propionate
droperidol
DTIC-Dome
Dulcolax
Duofilm
Duoprin
Duosterone
Duotrate
Duphaston
Durabolin
Duracillin
Duragesic
Duranest
Duraquin
Duricef
Duvoid
Dyazide
Dyclone

dyclonine
Dymelor
Dynacaine
Dynapen
dyphylline
Dyrenium
echothiophate
Edecrin
Edrisal
edrophonium chloride
E.E.S.
Efroxine
Efudex
Elase
Elavil
Elixicon
Elixophyllin
Elorine
Elspar
Elutek
emetine
Emetrol
Emivan
Empirin
Empracet
Emprazil
Emulave
E-Mycin
enanthate
Enarax
Endep
Enduron
Enduronyl
Enovid
ephedrine hydrochloride
E-Pilo
epinephrine
    e. bitartrate
epinephryl borate
Epitrate
Eppy
Equagesic

Equanil
ergocalciferol
Ergomar
ergonovine maleate
Ergostat
ergotamine tartrate
Ergotrate
erythrityl tetranitrate
Erythrocin
  E. Lactobionate
  E. Stearate
erythrol tetranitrate
erythromycin
  e. estolate
  e. ethylsuccinate
  e. lactobionate
  e. stearate
eserine
Esgic
Esidrix
Esimil
Eskalith
Estar
Estinyl
Estivin
Estrace
estradiol
  e. valerate
Estradurin
Estratest
estrone
Estrovarin
Estrovis
Estrugenone
Estrusol
Eta-Lent
Etamon
ethacrynic acid
ethambutol hydrochloride
ethamivan
Ethaquin
Ethatab

ethaverine hydrochloride
ethchlorvynol
ethinamate
ethinyl estradiol
ethionamide
ethosuximide
ethotoin
ethoxazene hydrochloride
Ethril
ethyl aminobenzoate
etidronate disodium
Etrafon
eucatropine
eugenol
Eumydrin
Eurax
Euresol
Euthroid
Eutonyl
Eutron
Evex
Excedrin
Exna
Extendryl
Exzit
^{18}F (fluorine)
Factorate
F-Cortef
Fedrazil
Feldman buffer solution
Femogen
fenoprofen calcium
fentanyl
Feosol
Fergon
Fer-In-Sol
Fero-Folic-500
Fero-Grad-500
Fero-Gradumet
ferrous
  f. citrate Fe 59
  f. gluconate

ferrous (*continued*)
 f. sulfate
Festalan
fibrinolysin
Fiorinal
Flagyl
Flavin
flavoxate hydrochloride
Fleet enema
Flexeril
florantyrone
Floraquin
Florinef
Floropryl
floxuridine
Fludrocortisone
fludrocortisone acetate
flumethasone pivalate
fluocinolone acetonide
Fluonid
fluorescein
fluorine
 f. F 18
Fluoritab
Fluoroplex
fluorouracil
 5-f.
fluoxymesterone
fluphenazine hydrochloride
flurandrenolide
flurazepam hydrochloride
flurothyl
folic acid
Folvite
Forhistal
formocresol
Fostex
Fostril
Fototar
frusemide
5-FU — 5-fluorouracil
FUDR — flox uridine

Fulvicin
fumagillin
Fungizone
Furacin
Furadantin
furazolidone
furosemide
Furoxone
furtrethonium
^{67}Ga (gallium)
gallium citrate Ga 67
Gallogen
Gamastan
Gammagee
gamma globulin
Gammar
Gammimune
Gamulin Rh
Gantanol
Gantrisin
Garamycin
Gaviscon
Gaysal
Gelfoam
Gelusil
Gemonil
gentamicin
gentian violet
Geocillin
Geopen
Gerandrest
Gexane
Gifford and Smith buffer
 solution
Gitaligin
gitalin
Glaucon
Glofil-125
glucagon
glucosamine hydrochloride
glutamic acid hydrochloride
Glutest

glutethimide
glycerin
glyceryl guaiacolate
    α-g. guaiacol ether
    g. trinitrate
glycopyrrolate
Gly-Oxide
Glyrol
gold Au 198
    g. sodium thiomalate
gramicidin
Granulex
Grifulvin V
Grisactin
griseofulvin
Gris-PEG
G-strophanthin
Guaianesin
guaifenesin
guanethidine monosulfate
    g. sulfate
Gustase
Gyne-Lotrimin
Gynergen
Gynetone
Hague solution
Haldol
Haldrone
Halog
haloperidol
haloprogin
Halotestin
Halotex
Harmonyl
Hasacode
Hasamal
Hedspa
Hedulin
Hema-Combistix
Hemo-Vite
heparin
Hepathrom

Hep-B-Gammagee
heroin
Herplex
Hesper
hetacillin
Hetrazan
Hexa-Betalin
hexachlorophene
Hexadrol
Hexalet
hexocyclium methylsulfate
hexylresorcinol
Hippuran
Hipputope
Hiprex
Hispril
Histabid
Histachlor
Histadur
Histadyl
Histalog
histamine
        h. diphosphate
        h. phosphate
Histaspan
Histionex
Historal
Histrey
homatropine
Hormonin
Humorsol
Hycodan
Hycomine
Hycotuss
Hydeltrasol
Hydeltra-T.B.A.
Hydergine
hydralazine hydrochloride
Hydrillyn
hydriodic acid
hydrochloric acid
hydrochlorothiazide

hydrocodone bitartrate
hydrocortisone
    h. sodium succinate
    h. valerate
Hydrocortone
HydroDIURIL
hydroflumethiazide
Hydrolose
hydromorphone hydrochloride
Hydromox
Hydropres
hydroxyamphetamine
hydroxychloroquine sulfate
hydroxydaunomycin
14-Hydroxydihydrocodeinone
hydroxymesterone
hydroxyprogesterone
    h. caproate
hydroxyzine hydrochloride
    h. pamoate
Hygroton
Hykinone
hyoscine
hyoscyamine sulfate
Hyperab
Hyper-Tet
Hytone
^{125}I, ^{131}I (iodine)
Iberet-Folic-500
Iberol Filmtab
Ibrin
ibuprofen
ichthammol
Ichthyol
idoxuridine
^{131}I-HSA
Iletin
Ilidar
Ilopan
Ilosone
Ilotycin
    I. Gluceptate

Ilozyme
^{131}I-MAA
Imferon
imipramine
    i. hydrochloride
    i. pamoate
Immu-G
Immuglobin
immune serum globulin
Imodium
Imuran
^{113m}In (indium)
Inapsine
^{113m}In-colloid
Inderal
Inderide
indigo carmine
Indocin
Indoklon
indomethacin
Indon
^{111}In-DTPA
INH (isonicotine hydrazine) −
    isoniazid
Innovar
insulin
Intal
interferon
Intropin
Inversine
iodinated glycerol
    i. I 125 fibrinogen
    i. I 131 aggregated
      albumin (human)
    i. I 125 serum albumin
    i. I 131 serum albumin
      (human)
iodine
    radioactive i.
iodochlorhydroxyquin
iodohippurate sodium I 131
iodoquinol

Iodotope
iopanoic acid
[131]I-ortho-iodohippurate
ipecac
Iprenol
[131]I-rose bengal
Ismelin
isoamyl nitrite
Iso-Bid
isobucaine
isobutylallylbarbituric acid
isocarboxazid
isoetharine hydrochloride
isoflurophate
Isohist
isometheptene
Isomil
isoniazid
isonicotinic acid hydrazide
isopropamide iodide
isopropylarterenol
isoproterenol hydrochloride
  i. sulfate
Isopto Cetapred
Isordil
  I. Tembids
  I. Titradose
isosorbide dinitrate
isothipendyl
isoxsuprine hydrochloride
Isuprel
Ivadantin
Janimine
Jectofer
juniper tar
Kalpec
kanamycin sulfate
Kantrex
Kanulase
Kaochlor
kaolin
Kaon

Kaon-Cl
Kaopectate
Kay Ciel
Kayexalate
KEFF
Keflex
Keflin
Kefzol
Kemadrin
Kenalog
Kenacort
Keralyt
Ketaject
Ketalar
ketamine hydrochloride
khellin
Klaron
Klor
Klorvess
Klotrix
K-Lyte
Koāte
Komed
Komex
Konakion
Kondremul
Konsyl
Konȳne
K-Phos
K-Tabs
Kudrox
Ku-Zyme
Kwell
LāBID
Labstix
Lacril
LactAid
Lactobacillus acidophilus
lanatoside C
Lanoxin
Largon
Larodopa

Larotid
Larylgan
Lasix
Lassar's zinc paste
lauryl sulfoacetate
Ledercillin VK
Lentard
Lente Iletin
Lentopenil
Leritine
Leukeran
levallorphan tartrate
levarterenol bitartrate
levodopa
Levo-Dromoran
Levoid
Levophed
Levoprome
levopropoxyphene napsylate
levorphanol tartrate
Levothroid
levothyroxine sodium
Levsin
Librax
Libritabs
Librium
Lidaform
Lidex
lidocaine
    l. hydrochloride
Lidone
Lidosporin
lignocaine
Limbitrol
lime solution
Lincocin
lincomycin hydrochloride
lindane
Lioresal
liothyronine sodium
liotrix
Lipancreatin

Lipo-Hepin
Lipo-Nicin
Liquaemin Sodium
Liquamar
Liquiprin
Lithane
lithium carbonate
Lithonate
lobeline
Locorten
Loestrin
Lomotil
lomustine
Loniten
Lo/Ovral
loperamide hydrochloride
Lopressor
Lopurin
lorazepam
Lorelco
Lorfan
Loridine
Loroxide
Lotrimin
Lowila Cake
loxapine hydrochloride
    l. succinate
Loxitane
Lufyllin
Lugol's solution
Lullamin
Luminal
Lungaggregate Reagent
Lutrexin
lututrin
lypressin
lysergic acid diethylamide
    (LSD)
Lysodren
Lyteers
MAA Kit
Maalox

Macrodantin
Macroscan-131
Macrotec
mafenide acetate
magaldrate
Magan
Magnesia Magma
magnesium carbonate
 m. citrate
 m. gluconate
 m. oxide
 m. salicylate
 m. sulfate
 m. trisilicate
Mandacon
Mandalay
Mandelamine
mandelic acid
Mandol
mannitol
Mantadil Cream
Marax
Marcaine
Marezine
Marplan
Matropinal
Matulane
Maxidex
Maxiflor
Maxitrol
mazindol
Mebaral
mebutamate
mecamylamine
mechlorethamine hydro-
 chloride
Mecholyl
meclizine hydrochloride
meclofenamate sodium
Meclomen
Mediatric
Medihaler-Iso

Medrol
medroxyprogesterone acetate
medrysone
mefenamic acid
Mefoxin
Megace
megestrol acetate
Mektec 99
Mellaril
melphalan
menadiol sodium diphosphate
menadione
Menest
Menformon
Menic
Menrium
mepacrine
mepenzolate bromide
Mepergan
meperidine hydrochloride
mephenesin
mephentermine
mephenytoin
mephobarbital
mepivacaine hydrochloride
meprobamate
Meprospan
meprylcaine
meralluride
Meratran
merbromin
mercaptomerin sodium
6-mercaptopurine
Mercodinone
Mercuhydrin
Mercurochrome
mercury, ammoniated
Merthiolate
Mesantoin
mescaline
Mesopin
mesoridazine besylate

Mestinon
Mesulphen
metabutethamine
metabutoxycaine
metacresol acetate
Metahydrin
Metamine
Metamucil
Metandren
Metaprel
metaproterenol sulfate
metaraminol bitartrate
Metatensin
methacholine
methacycline hydrochloride
methadone
methallenestril
methaminodiazepoxide
methamphetamine hydro-
    chloride
methandrostenolone
methantheline bromide
methapyrilene
methaqualone
metharbital
methazolamide
methdilazine
Methedrine
methenamine
        m. hippurate
        m. mandelate
Methergine
methicillin sodium
methimazole
methixene hydrochloride
methocarbamol
methohexital sodium
Methorate
methotrexate
methotrimeprazine
methoxamine
methoxsalen

methscopolamine bromide
methsuximide
methyclothiazide
methylcellulose
methyldopa
methyldopate hydrochloride
methylene blue
methylergonovine maleate
methylparaben
methylphenidate hydro-
    chloride
methylphenylethylhydantoin
methylphenylsuccinimide
methylprednisolone
        m. acetate
        m. sodium succinate
Methyl red—bromothymol blue
    reagent
methylrosaniline
methyltestosterone
methylthionine chloride
methyl violet
methyprylon
methysergide maleate
Meticortelone
Meticorten
Metimyd
metoclopramide
metocurine iodide
metolazone
Metopirone
metoprolol tartrate
Metrazol
Metreton
metrizamide
metronidazole
Metubine
Metycaine
metyrapone
metyrosine
Mexate
MicaTin

miconazole
Micrainin
MICRhoGAM
microNEFRIN
Midol
Midrin
Migral
Migralam
milk of magnesia
Milontin
Milpath
Milprem
Miltown
Miltrate
Minipress
Minitec
Minizide
Minocin
minocycline hydrochloride
Minotal
minoxidil
Mintezol
Miochol
Miradon
Mithracin
mithramycin
mitomycin
mitotane
Mixtard
Moban
Mobidin
Modane
Moderil
Modicon
molindone hydrochloride
Monistat
Monocaine
Monodral
Monsel's solution
MOPP (nitrogen mustard,
    Oncovin, prednisone,
    procarbazine)

morphine
    m. hydrochloride
    m. sulfate
Motrin
6-MP — 6-mercaptopurine
MPI Iodine 123
MPI stannous diphosphonate
MTX — methotrexate
Mucilose
Mucomyst
Mudrane
Murine
Mustargen
Mutamycin
Myambutol
Mycelex
Mycifradin
Mycitracin
Mycolog
Mycostatin
Mydriacyl
Mylanta
Myleran
Mylicon
Myochrysine
Myodigin
Myophen
Myotonachol
Mysoline
Mysteclin
Mytrex
Nacton
nadolol
Nafcil
nafcillin sodium
nalbuphine hydrochloride
Naldecon
Nalfon
Nal I 125
nalidixic acid
Nalline
nalorphine

naloxone hydrochloride
nandrolone decanoate
    n. phenpropionate
naphazoline
Naprosyn
naproxen
Naqua
Naquival
Narcan
narcotine
Nardil
Naturetin
Navane
Nebcin
Nectadon
NegGram
Nembutal
Neo-Antergan
Neo-Calglucon
Neo-Cobefrin
Neo-Cortef
Neo-cultol
NeoDECADRON
Neo-Delta-Cortef
Neo-Deltef
Neohetramine
Neo-Hydeltrasol
Neolax
Neolin
Neo-Medrol
neomycin
Neo-Polycin
Neosone
Neosporin
neostigmine methylsulfate
Neo-Synephrine
Neothylline
Nephrox
Neptazane
Nesacaine
Neutrogena

niacin
niacinamide
nialamide
Niamid
Nico-400
Nicobid
Nicolar
Nico-Metrazol
Niconyl
Nico-Span
nicotinamide
nicotinic acid
nicotinyl alcohol
nifedipine
Niferex
nikethamide
Nilstat
Nipride
Nisentil
Nitranitol
Nitrazine
Nitretamin
Nitro-Bid
nitrofurantoin
    n. macrocrystals
    n. sodium
nitrofurazone
nitrogen mustard
nitroglycerin
Nitroglyn
Nitrol Ointment
Nitrong Ointment
Nitrospan
Nitrostat
Noctec
Nolamine
Noludar
Nolvadex
norepinephrine bitartrate
norethindrone
    n. acetate

Norflex
Norgesic
norgestrel
Norinyl
Norisodrine
Norlestrin
Norlutate
Norlutin
Norodin
Norpace
Norpramin
Norquen
nortriptyline hydrochloride
noscapine
Novafed
Novahistine
Novatrin
novobiocin
Novocain
Novrad
Nubain
Nucofed
Numorphan
Nupercainal
Nupercaine
Nutramigen
Nydrazid
nylidrin hydrochloride
Nystaform
nystatin
Obetrol
Ocusert
Ogen
oleic acid I 125
Omnipen
Oncovin
Ophthaine
Ophthalgan
Ophthetic
Ophthochlor
Ophthocort
Optef

Optilets-500
Oracaine
Orasone
Ora-Testryl
Oratrol
Orenzyme
Oretic
Oreticyl
Oreton
Organidin
Orimune
Orinase
Orlex Otic Solution
Ornade
Ornex
orphenadrine citrate
orthoboric acid
Ortho-Novum
Osmitrol
Osmoglyn
Osteolate
Osteoscan
Otrivin
ouabain
Ovcon
Ovral
Ovrette
Ovulen
oxacillin sodium
Oxaine
Oxalid
oxazepam
ox bile extract
oxethazaine
Oxsoralen
oxtriphylline
oxybutynin chloride
oxycodone
Oxydess
oxymetholone
oxymorphone hydrochloride
oxyphenbutazone

oxyphencyclimine hydro-
    chloride
oxyphenonium bromide
oxytetracycline hydrochloride
oxytocin
^{32}P (potassium)
Pabalate
Pabirin
Pagitane
PAM (melphalan) − phenylala-
    nine mustard
Pamelor
Pamine
Pamisyl
Panaquin
Pancrease
pancreatin
pancrelipase
pancuronium bromide
Panheprin
Panitol
Panmycin
PanOxyl
Panteric
panthenol
Pantopon
Pantothenylol
Panwarfin
papaverine hydrochloride
para-aminosalicylic acid
paracetaldehyde
parachlormetaxylenol
Paradione
Paradol
Paraflex
Parafon Forte
paraldehyde
paramethadione
paramethasone acetate
Para-Pas
Parasal
Paredrine

paregoric
pargyline hydrochloride
Parlodel
Parnate
PAS − para-aminosalicylic acid
Pathibamate
Pathilon
Pathocil
Pavabid
Pavakey
Paveril
Pavulon
PBZ Lontabs
PBZ-SR
pectin
Pediacof
Pedialyte
Pediamycin
Pediazole
Peganone
pemoline
Penbritin
penicillamine
penicillin
    p. G benzathine
    p. G procaine
    p. V potassium
Pensyn
pentaerythritol tetranitrate
pentagastrin
pentapiperide methylsulfate
pentapyrrolidinium bitartrate
pentazocine hydrochloride
    p. lactate
penthienate bromide
Pentids
pentobarbital sodium
pentolinium tartrate
Pentritol
pentylenetetrazol
Pen-Vee K
Perandren

Perazil
Perchloracap
Percocet-5
Percodan
Percogesic
Percorten
Pergonal
Periactin
Peri-Colace
Peritrate
Permapen
Permitil
Pernox
perphenazine
Persantine
Persistin
Pertofrane
Pertscan
peruvian balsam
PETN (pentaerythritol tetra-
    nitrate)
Petrogalar
peyote
Pfi-Lith
Phazyme
phenacemide
phenacetin
phenaglycodol
Phenaphen
phenaphthazine
phenazopyridine hydrochlorid
phencyclidine
phendimetrazine tartrate
phenelzine sulfate
Phenergan
Phenetron
phenindamine
phenol red
phenolsulfonphthalein
phenothiazine
phenoxybenzamine hydro-
    chloride

phenprocoumon
phensuximide
phentolamine
Phenurone
phenylalanine mustard
L-phenylalanine mustard
phenylbutazone
phenylephrine hydrochloride
phenylpropanolamine hydro-
    chloride
phenyl salicylate
phenyltoloxamine citrate
phenytoin sodium
pHisoDerm
pHisoHex
pHos-pHaid
Phosphocol P 32
Phospholine Iodide
Phosphotec
Phosphotope
Phrenilin
Phyllocontin
physostigmine salicylate
Physpan
phytonadione
phenindione
pheniramine
phenmetrazine hydrochloride
phenobarbital
phenol
phenolphthalein
picrotoxin
pilocarpine
Pima
pipazethate hydrochloride
pipenzolate bromide
piperacetazine
piperazine estrone sulfate
piperidolate hydrochloride
piperocaine
piperoxan
pipradrol

Piptal
pirbuterol
Pitocin
Pitressin
Pituitrin
pix juniperi
Placidyl
Plaquenil
Platinol
Pnu-Imune
podophyllin
podophyllum resin
Polaramine
poldine methylsulfate
Polycillin
Polycitra
Polycycline
polyestradiol phosphate
Poly-histine
Polymox
polymyxin B
Polysporin
Polytar
polythiazide
Poly-Vi-Flor
Poly-Vi-Sol
POMP (prednisone, Oncovin,
    methotrexate, 6-mercap-
    topurine)
Ponstel
Pontocaine
Potaba
potassium
        p. acetate
        p. *p*-aminobenzoate
        p. chloride
        p. gluconate
        p. iodide
        p. perchlorate
        p. permanganate
        p. phosphate
Povan

Pragmatar
pralidoxime chloride
Pramosone
pramoxine
Prantal
prazepam
prazosin hydrochloride
Prednefrin
prednisolone
        p. tebutate
prednisone
Pregnyl
Prelu-2
Preludin
Premarin
Pre-Mens
Pre-Pen
Pressonex
Primacaine
primaquine phosphate
primidone
Principen
Priscoline
Privine
Pro-Banthine
probenecid
probucol
procainamide hydrochloride
procaine hydrochloride
Procan
procarbazine hydrochloride
prochlorperazine
Procholon
procyclidine hydrochloride
Prodox
Profenil
progesterone
Progestin
Progestoral
Proglicem
Progynon
Proketazine

Proklar
Prolixin
Prolixin Decanoate
Proloid
Proloprim
Proluton
promazine
promethazine hydrochloride
Pronestyl
propantheline bromide
proparacaine hydrochloride
Propion Gel
propoxycaine
propoxyphene hydrochloride
    p. napsylate
propranolol hydrochloride
Propylparaben
propylthiouracil
Prostaphlin
Prostigmin
Protalba
protamine sulfate
Protopam Chloride
protoveratrine A
protriptyline hydrochloride
Provell
Provera
Provest
pseudoephedrine
    p. hydrochloride
    p. sulfate
psyllium hydrophilic mucilloid
    p. seed
Pulmolite
Purinethol
Purodigin
Pyocidin-Otic
pyrantel pamoate
pyrazinamide
Pyribenzamine
Pyridium
pyridostigmine bromide

pyridoxine hydrochloride
pyrilamine
pyrimethamine
Pyrolite
Pyronil
pyrrobutamine
pyrrocaine
pyvinium pamoate
Quaalude
Quadetts
Quadnite
Quadramin
Quadramoid
Quadrinal
Quadsul
Quan-III
Quarzan
Quelicin
Quelidrine
Queltuss
Questran
Quibron
Quide
Quilene
quinacrine
Quinaglute
Quinamm
Quine
quinestrol
quinethazone
Quinidex
quinidine
    q. gluconate
    q. polygalacturonate
    q. sulfate
quinine
    q. sulfate
Quinite
Quinora
Quintess
Quiphile
Quotane

racephedrine
Rachromate-51
Racobalamin[57]
Racobalamin[60]
radioiodinated I 125 serum
    albumin (human)
    r. s. a. (h.) (IHSA I 125,
    I 131)
radioiodine
radionuclide-labeled 125 I
    fibrinogen (human)
Raphetamine
Raudixin
Rau-Sed
Rautensin
Rautina
Rauwiloid
Rauwoldin
rauwolfia serpentina
Rauzide
Ravocaine
Reactrol
Regitine
Regonol
Regroton
Remsed
Renacidin
Renelate
Renese
Renotec (Tc 99m-Iron-
    Ascorbate-DTPA)
Repan
Repoise
rescinnamine
reserpine
Reserpoid
resorcin
resorcinol
Respaire
Restophen
Restrol
retinoic acid

Rezamid
RhoGAM
Rifadin
Rifaldazine
Rifamate
rifampicin
rifampin
rifamycin
Rimactane
Rimifon
Rimso-50
Ringer's lactate
Riopan
RISA-125-H
RISA-131-H
Ritalin
ritodrine hydrochloride
Robalate
Robamox
Robaxin
Robaxisal
Robenogatope
Robicillin VK
Robimycin
Robinul
Robitussin
Rocaltrol
Roma-Nol
Romilar
Rondec-DM
Rondomycin
Roniacol
rose bengal sodium
rotoxamine
Rubratope[57]
Rubratope[60]
Rum-K
Ru-Tuss
salicylazosulfapyridine
salicylic acid
Salpix
Salrin

salsalate
Saluron
Salutensin
Sandril
Sanorex
Sansert
Sarapin
Scarlet Red Ointment
ScintiCheck
scopolamine
^{75}Se (selenium)
Sebizon
Sebucare
Sebulex
Sebutone
secobarbital
Seconal
selenium
    s. sulfide
selenomethionine Se 75
Selsun
Semikon
Semilente Iletin
Semitard
Semoxydrine
Senokot
Septra
Ser-Ap-Es
Serax
Serc
Serenium
Serentil
Serfin
Seromycin
Serpasil
    S.-Apresoline
    S.-Esidrix
Sethotope
Setrol
Sidonna
Sigesic
Silain

Silvadene
silver nitrate
    s. sulfadiazine
Simeco
simethicone
Sine-Aid
Sinemet
Sinequan
Singlet
Singoserp
Sintrom
Sinulin
sitosterols
Slo-Phyllin
Slow-K
sodium acetate
    s. bicarbonate
    s. biphosphate
    s. butabarbital
    s. chloride
    s. chromate Cr 51
    s. ethylmercurithio-
      salicylate
    s. fluoride
    s. hyposulfite
    s. indigotin disulfonate
    s. iodide I 123, I 125,
      I 131
    s. iodohippurate I 131
    s. iothalamate I 125
    s. levothyroxine
    s. nitroprusside
    s. oxychlorosene
    s. para-aminohippurate
    s. pentobarbital
    s. pertechnetate Tc 99m
    s. phosphate P 32
    s. polystyrene sulfonate
    s. rose bengal I 131
    s. salicylate
    s. sulfathiazole
    s. thiosulfate

Softran
Solacen
Solganal
Solu-Cortef
Solu-Medrol
Soma
Somnafac
Somnos
Somophyllin
Sonilyn
Sorbitrate
Sparine
spartejne
Spartocin
Spectrocin
spironolactone
Sporostacin
^{85}Sr, ^{87m}Sr (strontium)
SSKI (supersaturated solution
   of potassium iodine)
Stadol
stanozolol
Staphcillin
Staticin
Statobex
Statrol
Steclin
Stelazine
Stemutrolin
Sterane
stilbestrol
Stilbetin
Stilphostrol
Stoxil
Streptase
streptokinase
streptomycin
streptozocin
Stronscan-85
strontium nitrate Sr 85
strontium Sr 87m
strophanthin

Strotope
Suavitil
Sublimaze
succinylcholine chloride
Sucostrin
Sudafed
Sudan IV
Suladrin
Sulamyd
sulfacetamide sodium
Sulfacet-R
sulfadiazine
Sulfadrin
sulfamethizole
sulfamethoxazole
Sulfamylon
sulfasalazine
sulfathiazole
sulfinpyrazone
sulfisoxazole
     s. diolamine
sulfonamide
sulfosalicylic acid
sulfur
sulindac
Sultrin
Sumycin
Supac
Superinone
Surfacaine
Surfak
Surgicel
Surmontil
Sus-Phrine
Sustaire
Suvren
Symmetrel
Synalar
Synalgos
Synatan
Syncillin
Syncuma

Syndrox
Synemol
Synestrol
Synirin
Synkayvite
Synophylate
Synthroid
Syntocinon
Syntrogel
syrosingopine
Tabron
Tacaryl
TACE
Tagamet
Tagathen
Taka-diastase
Talwin
tamoxifen citrate
Tandearil
TAO — triacetyloleandomycin
    troleandomycin
Tapazole
Taractan
Tavist
^{99m}Tc (technetium)
^{99m}Tc-albumin
^{99m}Tc-albumin microspheres
^{99m}Tc-dimercaptosuccinate
^{99m}Tc-DTPA
^{99m}Tc-glucoheptonate
^{99m}Tc-iron ascorbate
^{99m}Tc-MAA
^{99m}Tc-pertechnetate
^{99m}Tc-phosphate
^{99m}Tc-pyrophosphate
^{99m}Tc-sulfur colloid
Tc 99m sulfur colloid
TechneColl
TechneScan MAA
TechneScan PYP
technetated albumin (human)
    lungaggregate

technetium Tc 99m
    t. Tc 99m aggregated
      albumin
    t. Tc 99m diphosphonate
    t. 99m DTPA
    t. Tc 99m etidronate
      sodium
    t. 99m HSA
    t. Tc 99m medronate
      sodium
    t. Tc 99m pentetate
      sodium
    t. Tc 99m polyphosphate
    t. Tc 99m pyrophosphate
    t. Tc 99m serum albumin
    t. Tc 99m stannous
      pyrophosphate
    t. Tc 99m sulfur colloid
Technetope II
Tedral
Tegopen
Tegretol
Teldrin
Telepaque
Temaril
Tempra
Tensilon
terbutaline sulfate
terpin hydrate
Terra-Cortril
Terramycin
Terrastatin
Teslac
Tessalon
Tes-Tape
Test-Estrin
testolactone
testosterone
    t. cypionate
    t. propionate
Testred
Testryl

Tesuloid
tetracaine hydrochloride
tetrachloroethylene
tetracycline
Tetracyn
tetraethylammonium chloride
tetrahydrozoline hydrochloride
Tetrastatin
Tetrex
Texacort
6-TG — 6-thioguanine
thallous chloride Tl 201
Theelin
Thenfadil
thenyldiamine
Theobid
theobrominal
theobromine
    t. magnesium oleate
Theocalcin
Theoclear L.A.
Theo-Dur
Theolair
Theophyl
theophylline
    t. anhydrous
    t. ethylenediamine
Theovent
Thephorin
Theragran
Theratuss
Theruhistin
thiabendazole
thiamine hydrochloride
thiazide
thiethylperazine
thimerosal
thioguanine
Thiomerin
thiopental
thiopropazate
thioridazine

Thiosulfil
Thio-TEPA
thiothixene
Thiouracil
thiphenamil hydrochloride
thonzylamine
Thorazine
thrombin
Thrombostat
thyroglobulin
Thyrolar
D-thyroxine
L-thyroxine
^{201}Ti (titanium)
Ticar
ticarcillin disodium
Tigan
Timoptic
Tinactin
tincture of opium
Tindal
Tinver
Titralac
^{201}Tl (thallium)
tobramycin
    t. sulfate
tocamphyl
Toclase
Tocosamine
Tofranil
Tolazamide
tolazoline hydrochloride
tolbutamide
Tolectin
Tolinase
tolmetin sodium
tolnaftate
Tolserol
Topicort
Topsyn
Torecan
TP — testosterone propionate

Tral
Trancopal
Transact
transaminase
Tranxene
tranylcypromine sulfate
Trasentine
Travase ointment
Travasol
Trecator
Trest
triacetyloleandomycin
triamcinolone
    t. acetonide
    t. diacetate
    t. hexacetonide
Triaminic
triamterene
Triavil
tribromoethanol
Triburon
trichlormethiazide
triclobisonium
Tricoloid
Tri-Cone
tricyclamol chloride
Tridesilon
tridihexethyl chloride
Tridione
triethylenemelamine (TEM)
trifluoperazine hydrochloride
triflupromazine hydrochloride
trifluridine
trihexyphenidyl hydrochloride
Tri-Immunol
Trilafon
Trilene
Trilisate
trimeprazine tartrate
trimethadione
trimethaphan camsylate

trimethobenzamide hydro-
    chloride
trimethoprim
Trimeton
trimipramine maleate
Trimox
Trimpex
Trinsicon
triolein I 131
    t. (glyceryl trioleate)
    I 131
trioxsalen
tripelennamine citrate
    t. hydrochloride
triprolidine hydrochloride
Trisoralen
Triton WR-1339
Tri-Vi-Sol
Trobicin
Trocinate
Trofan
troleandomycin
trolnitrate
Tronothane Hydrochloride
tropicamide
L-tryptophan
tubocurarine chloride
Tuinal
Tusquelin
Tussar
Tusscapine
Tussend
Tuss-Ornade
Twiston
tybamate
Tylenol
Tylox
tyloxapol
Tympagesic
Tyvid
Tyzine
U-Gencin

Ulo
Ultandren
Ultracef
Ultralente Iletin
Ultran
Ultratard
Ultra-TechneKow
Unguentum Bossi
Unipen
Unitensen
Uracid
Ureaphil
Urecholine
Urex
uricosuric
Urised
Urisedamine
Urispas
Uristix
Uritone
Urobiotic-250
urokinase
Uro-Phosphate
Uroqid-acid
Urostat
Usanol
Uteracon
Uticillin VK
Uticort
Utrasul
Vagilia
Vagisec
Valadol
Valisone
Valium
Vallestril
Valmid
Valpin
valproic acid
Vancocin
vancomycin hydrochloride
vanillic acid diethylamide

Vanobid
Vanocyn
Vanoxide
Vaponefrin
Vapo-N-Iso
Vasocidin
Vasodilan
vasopressin
Vasospan
Vasoxyl
V-Cillin K
Veetids
Velban
Velosef
Velosulin
Veralba
Vergo
Veriloid
Vermox
Versapen
Vesprin
Vibramycin
Vicodin
Vi-Daylin
Vinactane
vinblastine sulfate
vincristine
     v. sulfate
Viocin
Vioform
Viokase
viomycin sulfate
Vio-Thene
Viroptic
Visine
Vistaril
Vistrax
Vita-Metrazol
Vitron-C
Vivactil
Vivonex
Vleminckx' solution

Vontrol
Voranil
Voxin-Pg
Vytone
WANS
warfarin
Westcort cream
white precipitate
Wigraine
WinGel
Winstrol
Wyamine
Wyamycin E
Wycillin
Wydase
Wygesic
Wymox
Wynestron
^{133}Xe (xenon)
Xeneisol Xe 133
xenon Xe 133
    x. Xe 133 V.S.S.
      (Ventilation Study
      System)
Xeroform

Xseb shampoo
Xylocaine
Xylometazoline
^{169}Yb (ytterbium)
ytterbium Yb 169 DTPA
    y. Yb 169 pentetate
      sodium
Yutopar
Zactirin
Zanchol
Zarontin
Zaroxolyn
Zephiran Chloride
Zetar
zinchlorundesal
Zincon
zinc sulfate
Ziradryl
Zolyse
Zomax
zomepirac sodium
Zorprin
zorubicin
Zyloprim
Zypan

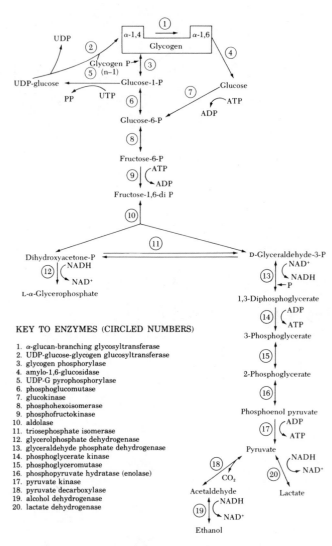

KEY TO ENZYMES (CIRCLED NUMBERS)

1. α-glucan-branching glycosyltransferase
2. UDP-glucose-glycogen glucosyltransferase
3. glycogen phosphorylase
4. amylo-1,6-glucosidase
5. UDP-G pyrophosphorylase
6. phosphoglucomutase
7. glucokinase
8. phosphohexoisomerase
9. phosphofructokinase
10. aldolase
11. triosephosphate isomerase
12. glycerolphosphate dehydrogenase
13. glyceraldehyde phosphate dehydrogenase
14. phosphoglycerate kinase
15. phosphoglyceromutase
16. phosphopyruvate hydratase (enolase)
17. pyruvate kinase
18. pyruvate decarboxylase
19. alcohol dehydrogenase
20. lactate dehydrogenase

EMBDEN-MEYERHOF PATHWAY OF GLUCOSE METABOLISM

(Courtesy of Dorland's Illustrated Medical Dictionary, 26th ed. Plate XLI. Philadelphia, W. B. Saunders Company, 1981.)

LABORATORY TERMINOLOGY
Normal Laboratory Values*

AA – acetic acid
abetalipoproteinemia
ablastin
ABO
- antibodies
- antigens
- compatibility
- incompatibility
- typing

ABO-blood groups (named for agglutinogens)
ABO-Rh typing
Abrams' test
Absidia
absorption
- fat a.
- iron a.

Acanthamoeba
Acanthamoeba/Hartmannella
Acanthocheilonema perstans
acanthocyte
acanthocytosis
Acaridae
acatalasia
Acaulium
ACD – acid, citrate, dextrose
acetaldehyde
acetaminophen
Acetest
Acetobacter
- *A. aceti*
- *A. melanogenus*
- *A. oxydans*
- *A. rancens*
- *A. roseus*
- *A. suboxydans*
- *A. xylinus*

acetone
acetonemia
acetophenetidin
acetylcholinesterase
acetyl-CoA
acetylcoenzyme A
acetylcysteine
Acholeplasma laidlawii
Achorion
achroacyte
achromia

*Normal Laboratory Values section begins on page 206.

Achromobacter
Achromobacteraceae
acid
      acetoacetic a.
      acetylsalicylic a.
      amino a.
      aminolevulinic a.
      argininosuccinic a.
      ascorbic a.
      chloranilic a.
      deoxyribonucleic a.
      diacetic a.
      ethacrynic a.
      folic a.
      formiminoglutamic a.
      glucuronic a.
      glutamic a.
      hippuric a.
      homogentisic a.
      homovanillic a.
      hydrochloric a.
      5-hydroxyindoleacetic a.
      lactic a.
      nalidixic a.
      phenylpyruvic a.
      pyruvic a.
      ribonucleic a.
      teichoic a.
      tricarboxylic a.
      trichloroacetic a.
      uric a.
      valproic a.
      vanillylmandelic a.
      xanthurenic a.
acidemia
acid-fast
acidifiable
acidifier
acidify
acidimetry
acidity
acidocyte

acidocytopenia
acidocytosis
acidogenic
acidophil
acidophilic
acidosis
acid phosphatase
acid-Schiff stain
Acinetobacter
      A. anitratum
      A. calcoacceticus
      A. parapertussis
Acladium
Acremonium
Acrotheca pedrosoi
Acrothesium floccosum
ACTH — adrenocorticotropic
          hormone
ACTH test
actin
Actinobacillus
      A. actinomycetemcom-
          itans
      A. mallei
      A. pseudomallei
actinochemistry
Actinomadura
      A. madurae
actinomyces
Actinomyces
      A. bovis
      A. israelii
Actinomycetaceae
Actinomycetales
actinomycetes
actinomycetic
actinomycin
actinomycosis
actinomycotic
Actinoplanaceae
Actinoplanes
Actinopoda

Actonia
Adamkiewicz's test
Addis count
adenasthenia
adenine
adenosine
    a. deaminase
adenovirus
adenyl
ADH — alcohol dehydrogenase
    antidiuretic hormone
adjuvant
    Freund a.
Adler's test
ADP — adenosine diphosphate
Aedes
    A. aegypti
    A. albopictus
    A. cinereus
    A. flavescens
    A. leucocelaenus
    A. scutellaris pseudo-
      scutellaris
    A. sollicitans
    A. spencerii
    A. taeniorhynchus
Aerobacter
    A. aerogenes
    A. cloacae
aerobe
aerobia
aerobian
aerobic
aerobiotic
aerogenic
aerogenous
Aeromonas
    A. hydrophila
    A. liquefaciens
    A. punctata
    A. salmonicida
AFB — acid-fast bacillus

agammaglobulinemia
    Bruton's a.
    Swiss type a.
Agamodistomum
    A. ophthalmobium
Agamonema
Agamonematodum migrans
A/G ratio test — albumin-
   globulin ratio test
agar
    bile-esculin a.
    bird seed a.
    brain-heart infusion a.
    chocolate a.
    Columbia blood a.
    corn meal a.
    deoxyribonuclease a.
    DNase a.
    Hektoen a.
    inhibitory mold a.
    lysine iron a.
    mycobiotic a.
    MacConkey a.
    Middlebrook's a.
    nitrate a.
    nutrient a.
    phenylethyl alcohol a.
    potato dextrose a.
    rabbit blood a.
    Sabhi a.
    Sabouraud's dextrose a.
    Salmonella-Shigella a.
    Schaedler blood a.
    Simmons' citrate a.
    thistle seed a.
    trichophyton a.
    triple sugar iron a.
    tryptic soy a.
    urea a.
    Wilkins-Chilgren a.
    xylose-lysine-
      deoxycholate a.

Agarbacterium
agent
    adrenergic blocking a.
    alkylating a.
agglutination
    acid a.
    bacteriogenic a.
    cold a.
    H a.
    intravascular a.
    latex a.
    macroscopic a.
    mediate a.
    microscopic a.
    O a.
    platelet a.
    salt a.
    spontaneous a.
    T-a.
    Vi a.
agglutinator
agglutinin
    alpha a.
    anti-Rh a.
    beta a.
    chief a.
    cold a.
    febrile a.
    flagellar a.
    group a.
    H a.
    haupt-a.
    immune a.
    latex a.
    leukocyte a.
    Mg a.
    O a.
    platelet a.
    Rh a.
    somatic a.
    warm a.
agglutinogen

aglobulia
aglobuliosis
aglobulism
aglycemia
aglycogenosis
agranulocyte
agranuloplastic
ahaptoglobinemia
AHF — antihemophilic factor
AHG — antihemophilic
      globulin
      antihuman globulin
AHT — antihyaluronidase
      titer
AIHA — autoimmune hemo-
      lytic anemia
akaryocyte
akoreon. See *Achorion.*
akro-. See words beginning
      achro-.
ALA — aminolevulinic acid
alamecin
alangine
alanine
albumin
    a. A
    acetosoluble a.
    acid a.
    alkali a.
    a. of Bence Jones
    caseiniform a.
    coagulated a.
    derived a.
    hematin a.
    iodinated serum a.
    normal human serum a.
    Patein's a.
    radio-iodinated serum a.
    serum a.
    a. tannate
    triphenyl a.
albuminuria

albumosuria
> Bence Jones a.
> Bradshaw's a.
> enterogenic a.
> pyogenic a.

Alcaligenes
> *A. bookeri*
> *A. bronchosepticus*
> *A. faecalis*
> *A. marshallii*
> *A. metalcaligenes*
> *A. recti*
> *A. viscolactis*

alcohol
ALD — aldolase
Alder-Reilly anomaly
aldolase
aldosterone
aldosteronism
aleukocytosis
Alginobacter
Alginomonas
alkalemia
alkalescence
alkali
alkaline
> a. phosphatase

alkalosis
> compensated a.
> hypokalemic a.
> metabolic a.

allele
allergen
Allescheria
> *A. boydii*

alloantibody
Allodermanyssus
> *A. sanguineus*

allogenic
allotype
alpha$_1$
alpha$_2$

alpha
> a. acid glycoprotein
> a. amino acids
> a. amino nitrogen
> a. amylase
> a. antichymotrypsin
> a. antiplasmin
> a. antitrypsin
> a.-beta variation
> a. cells
> a. chain
> a. fetoglobin
> a. fetoprotein
> a. globulin antibodies
> A-1 globulins
> A-2 globulins
> a-1-4 glucosidase
> deficiency
> a. ketoglutarate
> a. lipoproteins
> a. macroglobulin
> a. melanocytic-
> stimulating hormone
> a. methyldopa
> a. nephthyl acetate
> esterase reaction
> a. particles
> a. protease inhibitor
> a. receptors
> a. seromucoid
> a. thalassemia
> a. trypsin

alphavirus
Alternaria
Amanita
> *A. muscaria*
> *A. pantherina*
> *A. phalloides*
> *A. rubescens*
> *A. verna*

ameba
> coprozoic a.

amebiasis
ameboflagellate
Ames Lab-Tek cryostat
amino
    a. acid
aminoaciduria
aminopeptidase
    leucine a.
aminotransferase
Amoeba
    A. buccalis
    A. cachexica
    A. coli
    A. coli mitis
    A. dentalis
    A. dysenteriae
    A. histolytica
    A. limax
    A. meleagridis
    A. urinae granulata
    A. urogenitalis
    A. verrucosa
amorphous
AMP — adenosine monophos-
      phate
amylase
    pancreatic a.
    salivary a.
    serum a.
    urinary a.
amyloclast
amyloid
amyloidosis
ANA — antinuclear antibodies
anaerobe
    facultative a's
    obligate a's
anaerobia
anaerobian
anaerobiase
anaerobic
anaerogenic

analbuminemia
Anaplasma
Anaplasmataceae
Ancylostoma
    A. braziliense
    A. duodenale
androgen
androstanedione
androstene
anemia
    aplastic a.
    autoimmune hemolytic a.
    Cooley's a.
    hemolytic a.
    hypochromic a.
    leukoerythroblastic a.
    macrocytic a.
    microcytic a.
    normochromic a.
    normocytic a.
    pernicious a.
    sickle cell a.
anergy
aneuploidy
Angiostrongylus
    A. cantonensis
angiotensin I, II, III
angiotensinase
anion
anisocytosis
anisohypercytosis
anisohypocytosis
anisokaryosis
anisoleukocytosis
anomaly
    Alder-Reilly a.
    Pelger-Huët nuclear a.
Anopheles
    A. maculipennis
Anoplura
anoxemia
anoxemic

Anthomyia
    A. canicularis
    A. incisura
    A. manicata
    A. saltatrix
    A. scalaris
Anthomyiidae
    A. Fannia
    A. Hydrotea
    A. Hylemyia
anthrax
antibiotic
    bactericidal a.
    bacteriostatic a.
    broad spectrum a.
    oral a.
antibody
    ABO a's
    alloantin-D a.
    antinuclear a.
    Duffy a's, Fy^a, Fy^b
    Lewis a's, Le^a, Le^b
anticholinesterase
anticoagulant
anticoagulative
anticoagulin
anticolibacillary
anticollagenase
anticolloidoclastic
anti-DNA
antigen
    ABO a's
    erythrocyte a.
    HLA a's
    Kell a's
    Kveim a.
    Rh a.
    Vi a.
antigenic
antigenicity
antigenotherapy
antiglobulin

antihemagglutinin
antihemolysin
antihemolytic
antihemophilic
antiheterolysin
antihyaluronidase
    a. titer
anti-invasin
    a. I
    a. II
anti-isolysin
antilewisite
    British a.
antimicrobial
antinuclear
antistaphylolysin
antistreptococcic
antistreptococcin
antistreptokinase
antistreptolysin
    a. O
aplasmic
aplastic
apoenzyme
apolipoprotein
appliqué form
Apt test
Arachis
    A. hypogaea
Arachnia
    A. propionica
Arachnida
arbovirus
arenavirus
Argas
    A. reflexus
arginine
argininosuccinicaciduria
Argo corn starch test
Arizona
    A. hinshawii
Armanni-Ebstein cell

Arthrographis
    A. langeroni
Arthropoda
arthrospore
arylamine
ASA — acetylsalicylic acid
    argininosuccinic acid
ascariasis
ascaricidal
ascaricide
ascarides
Ascaris
    A. lumbricoides
Aschheim-Zondek test
Ascomycetes
ascorbate
ascospore
ascotrophosome
ascus
ASO titer — antistreptolysin
          O titer
aspartate
aspergillosis
Aspergillus
    A. auricularis
    A. barbae
    A. bouffardi
    A. clavatus
    A. concentricus
    A. flavus
    A. fumigatus
    A. giganteus
    A. glaucus
    A. gliocladium
    A. mucoroides
    A. nidulans
    A. niger
    A. ochraceus
    A. pictor
    A. repens
assay
    ELISA (enzyme-linked
    immunosorbent a.)

assay (*continued*)
    hemagglutination a.
    immunofluorescent a.
    leukotactic a.
AST — aspartate aminotrans-
    ferase
Asterococcus
astrocyte
Atelosaccharomyces
ATP — adenosine triphosphate
ATPase stain
atypia
atypical
Auer's bodies
aurococcus
Australian X disease virus
autoagglutination
autoagglutinin
autoantibody
autoanticomplement
autoantigen
autoantitoxin
autoerythrophagocytosis
autohemolysin
autohemolysis
autoimmune
autoimmunity
autosensitization
aviadenovirus
avipexvirus
AZ test — Aschheim-Zondek
        test
B cells
Babesia
    B. microti
bacilli
    acid-fast b.
Bacillus
    B. acidi lactici
    B. aerogenes capsulatus
    B. aertrycke
    B. alvei
    B. anthracis

Bacillus (continued)
    B. botulinus
    B. brevis
    B. bronchisepticus
    B. cereus
    B. circulans
    B. coli
    B. diphtheriae
    B. dysenteriae
    B. enteritidis
    B. faecalis alcaligenes
    B. influenzae
    B. larvae
    B. leprae
    B. mallei
    B. oedematiens
    B. oedematis maligni
      No. II
    B. pertussis
    B. pestis
    B. pneumoniae
    B. polymyxa
    B. proteus
    B. pseudomallei
    B. pumilus
    B. pyocyaneus
    B. stearothermophilus
    B. subtilis
    B. suipestifer
    B. tetani
    B. tuberculosis
    B. tularense
    B. typhi
    B. typhosus
    B. welchii
    B. whitmori
bacillus
    b. abortivus equinus
    Bang's b.
    Battey bacilli
    Boas-Oppler b.

bacillus (*continued*)
    Bordet-Gengou b.
    Calmette-Guérin b.
    Döderlein's b.
    Ducrey's b.
    Escherich's b.
    Fick's b.
    Flexner-Strong b.
    Flexner's b.
    Friedländer's b.
    Gärtner's b.
    Ghon-Sachs b.
    glanders b.
    Hansen's b.
    Hofmann's b.
    Johne's b.
    Klebs-Löffler b.
    Klein's b.
    Koch-Weeks b.
    Morax-Axenfeld b.
    Morgan's b.
    Newcastle-Manchester b.
    Nocard's b.
    paracolon b.
    Pfeiffer's b.
    Preisz-Nocard b.
    rhinoscleroma b.
    Schmitz's b.
    Schmorl's b.
    Shiga's b.
    smegma b.
    Sonne-Duval b.
    Strong's b.
    swine rotlauf b.
    timothy b.
    tubercle b.
    typhoid b.
    vole b.
    Welch's b.
    Whitmore's b.
bacteremia

bacteria
  gram-negative b.
bacterioagglutinin
bacteriology
bacteriophage
Bacterium
  B. aerogenes
  B. aeruginosum
  B. anitratum
  B. cholerae suis
  B. cloacae
  B. coli
  B. dysenteriae
  B. pestis bubonicae
  B. sonnei
  B. tularense
  B. typhosum
bacteriuria
Bacteroides
  B. corrodens
  B. fragilis
  B. funduliformis
  B. melaninogenicus
bacteroides
Bactometer
Balantidium
  B. coli
bands
Bang's bacillus
Bargen's streptococcus
Barr bodies
Bartonella
  B. bacilliformis
Bartonellaceae
Baso — basophil
basophil
basophilia
basophilic
basophilism
  Cushing's b.
  pituitary b.
Battey bacilli

BEI — butanol extractable
  iodine
Bence Jones
  albumin
  albumosuria
  protein test
  proteinuria
  reaction
Benedict's test
bentonite flocculation test
benzidine
Bessey-Lowry unit
Beta 1, 2, 2A, 2M, 3
Beta-endorphin
Beta-lactamase
Bethesda-Ballerup Citrobacter
BFP — biologic false positive
BFT — bentonite flocculation
  test
Bifidobacterium
  B. eriksonii
bile
bilirubin
bilirubinemia
bioassay
biosynthesis
biuret
Blastocystis
  B. hominis
Blastomyces
  B. brasiliensis
  B. coccidioides
  B. dermatitidis
blastomycin
blastomycosis
bleeding time
  Duke's method b.t.
  Ivy's method b.t.
blood
  cord b.
blood serum
  Löffler's b.s.

blood urea nitrogen
Bloor's test
Bloxam's test
BMR — basal metabolic rate
Boas' test
Boas-Oppler
    bacillus
    lactobacillus
Bodansky unit
Bodo
    B. caudatus
    B. saltans
    B. urinaria
Bodonidae
body
    Auer's b's
    Barr b's
    Cabot's ring b's
    chromatin b's
    Donovan's b's
    Heinz b's
    Heinz-Ehrlich b's
    Howell-Jolly b's
    Howell's b's
    inclusion b's
    Jolly's b's
    ketone b's
    Leishman-Donovan b's
    Mallory's b's
    Maragiliano b.
    Negri b's
    psammoma b.
    Todd's b.
    X chromatin b's
Bombay phenotype
Bonanno's test
bone marrow
Bordet-Gengou bacillus
Bordetella
    B. bronchiseptica
    B. parapertussis
    B. pertussis

Borrelia
    B. anserina
    B. berbera
    B. buccalis
    B. carteri
    B. caucasica
    B. duttonii
    B. hermsii
    B. hispanica
    B. kochii
    B. parkeri
    B. persica
    B. recurrentis
    B. refringens
    B. turicatae
    B. venezuelensis
    B. vincentii
Bowie's stain
Bradshaw's albumosuria
bradykinin
Branhamella
    B. catarrhalis
British antilewisite
bromsulphalein
broth
    brain-heart infusion b.
    hippurate b.
    indole-nitrate b.
    Middlebrook's b.
    Mueller-Hinton b.
    nutrient b.
    selenite b.
    thioglycollate b.
    Todd-Hewitt b.
    Voges-Proskauer b.
Brucella
    B. abortus
    B. bronchiseptica
    B. canis
    B. melitensis
    B. suis
Brucellaceae

brucellosis
Brugia
    B. malayi
    B. microfilariae
Brunhilde virus
Bruton's agammaglobulinemia
BSP — bromsulphalein
BUN — blood urea nitrogen
Bunyamwera virus
Busse's Saccharomyces
Butyribacterium
Bwamba fever virus
C — centigrade
C_{alb} — albumin clearance
C_{am} — amylase clearance
C_{cr} — creatinine clearance
C_{in} — insulin clearance
C_{pah} — para-aminohippurate
        clearance
C_u — urea clearance
Cabot's ring bodies
Cache valley virus
calcium
calcivirus
California virus
Calliphora
    C. vomitoria
Calmette-Guérin bacillus
calorimetry
Calymmatobacterium
    C. granulomatis
Campylobacter
    C. fetus
Candida
    C. albicans
    C. albidus
    C. guilliermondi
    C. krusei
    C. laurentii
    C. luteolus
    C. parakrusei
    C. parapsilosis

Candida (*continued*)
    C. pseudotropicalis
    C. stellatoidea
    C. tropicalis
candidiasis
candidosis
carbon
    c. dioxide
    c. monoxide
carboxyhemoglobin
carboxypeptidase
Cardiobacterium
    C. hominis
cardiolipin
carotene
carotenoid
Carpoglyphus
    C. passularum
carrier
Casoni's intradermal test
cast
    granular c.
    hyaline c.
    waxy c.
Castellanella
    C. castellani
Castellani's test
CAT — computed axial
        tomography
        computerized axial
        tomography
Catalpa
catalysis
cataphylaxis
catecholamine
Catenabacterium
CA virus — croup-associated
        virus
CBC — complete blood count
CEA — carcinoembryonic
        antigen
Celebes' vibrio

cell

    alpha c's
    aneuploid c's
    argentaffin c's
    Armanni-Ebstein c.
    B c's
    band c's
    beta c's
    buffy-coated c's
    burr c.
    chromaffin c's
    crenated c's
    delta c's
    endothelial c's
    ependymal c's
    epithelial c's
    erythroid c's
    Ferrata's c's
    gamma c's
    Gaucher's c.
    H-2^b mouse c's
    HeLa c's
    islet c's
    Kupffer's c's
    Leydig's c's
    lymphoid c's
    mast c's
    mesothelial c's
    metallophil c's
    monosomic c's
    null c's
    packed c's
    plasma c's
    progenitor c's
    reticulum c's
    sickle c.
    stem c's
    T c's
    target c.
    tart c.
    trisomic c's
    Türk's c.

cellular
Cellvibrio
    C. flavescens
    C. fulvus
    C. ochraceus
    C. vulgaris
centrifugation
cephalin
Cephalosporium
    C. granulomatis
Ceph floc — cephalin
        flocculation
cercaria
ceruloplasmin
cestode
cestodiasis
CF — complement fixation
CF antibody titer
Chagas' disease
Charcot-Leyden crystals
Chediak's test
chemoluminescence
chemotactic
chemotaxis
chemstrip
Cheyletiella
    C. parasitovorax
Chikungunya virus
Chilomastix
    C. mesnili
Chlamydia
    C. oculogenitalis
    C. psittaci
    C. trachomatis
Chlamydiaceae
Chlamydobacteriaceae
Chlamydobacteriales
Chlamydophrys
chlamydospore
Chlamydozoaceae
Chlamydozoon
chloride

chloroleukemia
cholecystokinin
Choleraesuis
    C. salmonella
cholesterol
cholinesterase
chorionic gonadotropin
chromatin
chromatography
chromoblastomycosis
chromomycosis
chromosomal
chromosome
    gametic c.
    Philadelphia c.
    X, Y c.
Chrysops
CHS — cholinesterase
chylomicron
chymotrypsin
CI — colloidal iron
    crystalline insulin
circadian
Citrobacter
    Bethesda-Ballerup C.
    C. diversus
    C. freundii
Cladosporium
    C. carrionii
    C. werneckii
clasmatocyte
Clathrochloris
Clathrocystis
clearance
    blood urea c.
    creatinine c.
    urea c.
Clinitest
clonorchiasis
Clonorchis
    C. endemicus
    C. sinensis
clostridia

Clostridium
    C. acetobutylicum
    C. aerofoetidum
    C. agni
    C. bifermentans
    C. botulinum
    C. butylicum
    C. chauvoei
    C. cochlearium
    C. fallax
    C. feseri
    C. haemolyticum
    C. histolyticum
    C. kluyveri
    C. multifermentans
    C. nigrificans
    C. novyi
    C. oedematiens
    C. ovitoxicus
    C. paludis
    C. parabotulinum
    C. parabotulinum equi
    C. pasteurianum
    C. pastorianum
    C. perfringens
    C. ramosum
    C. septicum
    C. sordellii
    C. sporogenes
    C. sticklandii
    C. tertium
    C. tetani
    C. tetanomorphum
    C. thermosaccharolyti-
      cum
    C. tyrosinogenes
    C. welchii
clotting time
clumping
CMV — cytomegalovirus
CO_2 — carbon dioxide
coagulant
coagulase

coagulate
coagulation
coagulin
coagulogram
coccidia
Coccidioides
    C. immitis
coccidioidin
coccidioidomycosis
coccidium
coccobacillus
coccobacteria
coccus
Coe virus
colibacillary
coliform
collagen
collagenase
colloid
colloidal gold
colony
Colorado tick fever virus
Columbia blood agar
compatibility
    ABO c.
complement
    c. activation
    c. fixation
complex
    Ghon c.
ConA — concanavalin A
condenser
conglutination
Congo red
    stain
    test
contagium
    c. animatum
    c. vivum
contaminant
conversion
    Mantoux c.

Cooley's anemia
Coombs' test
    direct
    indirect
coprohematology
Copromastix
    C. prowazeki
Copromonas
    C. subtilis
coproporphyria
coproporphyrin
coproporphyrinogen
Cordylobia
    C. anthropophaga
coronavirus
corpuscle
corticosteroid
cortisol
Cortrosyn
Corynebacteriaceae
Corynebacterium
    C. acnes
    C. belfantii
    C. diphtheriae
    C. enzymicum
    C. equi
    C. hemolyticum
    C. hofmannii
    C. infantisepticum
    C. minutissimum
    C. murisepticum
    C. mycetoides
    C. necrophorum
    C. ovis
    C. parvulum
    C. pseudodiphtheriticum
    C. pseudotuberculosis
    C. pyogenes
    C. renale
    C. tenuis
    C. ulcerans
    C. vaginale

Corynebacterium (*continued*)
    C. xerosis
Coulter counter
count
    Addis c.
    reticulocyte c.
    Schilling blood c.
counter
    Coulter c.
counterimmunoelectrophoresis
Coxiella
    C. burnetii
Coxsackie virus
CPK — creatine phosphokinase
C-reactive protein test
creatinase
creatine
    c. kinase
    c. phosphate
    c. phosphokinase
creatininase
creatinine
crenation
CRF — corticotropin-releasing
        factor
crossmatching
CRP — C-reactive protein
cryocrit
cryofibrinogen
cryogammaglobulin
cryoglobulin
cryoglobulinemia
cryoprecipitate
cryostat
    Ames Lab-Tek c.
cryptococcal
cryptococci
cryptococcosis
Cryptococcus
    C. albidus/albidus
    C. albidus/diffluens
    C. capsulatus

Cryptococcus (*continued*)
    C. epidermidis
    C. gilchristi
    C. histolyticus
    C. hominis
    C. laurentii
    C. luteolus
    C. meningitidis
    C. neoformans
    C. terreus
cryptozoite
crystal
    Charcot-Leyden c's
C & S — culture and sensitivity
CSF — cerebrospinal fluid
Ctenocephalides
Culex
Culicoides
culture
    attenuated c.
    blood c.
    chorioallantoic c.
    direct c.
    flask c.
    hanging-block c.
    hanging-drop c.
    needle c.
    plate c.
    sensitized c.
    shake c.
    slant c.
    smear c.
    stab c.
    stock c.
    streak c.
    stroke c.
    thrust c.
    tissue c.
    tube c.
    type c.
Cushing's basophilism
C virus — Coxsackie virus

cyclase
    adenyl c.
    adenylate c.
cyclic
    c. AMP
    c. GMP
    c. nucleotides
cylindroid
cysticerci
Cysticercus
    C. acanthrotrias
    C. bovis
    C. cellulosae
    C. fasciolaris
    C. ovis
    C. tenuicollis
cysticercus
cystine
cytocentrifugation
cytocentrifuge
cytochemistry
cytofluorography
cytogenetics
cytology
cytolysate
    blood c.
cytolysis
cytomegalovirus
cytoplasm
cytotoxicity
DAGT – direct antiglobulin test
Dale-Laidlaw's clotting time method
dehydrogenase
    isocitric d.
    lactate d. (LDH)
dehydropeptidase
Dematium
Demodex
    D. folliculorum
dengue

Dermacentor
    D. andersoni
    D. occidentalis
    D. variabilis
Dermacentroxenus
Dermanyssus
    D. avium et gallinae
Dermatobia
    D. hominis
dermatomycosis
Dermatophilus
    D. penetrans
Dermatophytin "O"
dermatophytosis
diacetate
Diagnex Blue test
Dialister
    D. pneumosintes
diastase
Dick test
Dicrocoelium
    D. dendriticum
Dientamoeba
    D. fragilis
differential
difilo-. See words beginning *diphyllo-*.
dilution
dilutor
Dimastigamoeba
p-dimethylaminoazobenzene
dimethyl sulfoxide
dinitrochlorobenzene
Dipetalonema
    D. perstans
diphtheroid
diphyllobothriasis
Diphyllobothrium
    D. latum
    D. parvum
    D. taenioides
diplobacillus

diplobacterium
Diplococcus
    D. pneumoniae
diplococcus
    d. of Morax-Axenfeld
    d. of Neisser
    Weichselbaum's d.
Diplogonoporus
    D. brauni
    D. grandis
dipstick
Dipylidium
    D. caninum
Dirofilaria
    D. immitis
    D. tenuis
dis-. See also words beginning
   dys-.
disease
    Chagas' d.
    Gaisböck's d.
    Gaucher's d.
    Osler's d.
    Schottmüller's d.
    Vaquez-Osler d.
    Vaquez's d.
dish
    Petri's d.
Distoma
distomiasis
DIT — diiodotyrosine
DMSO — dimethylsulfoxide
DNA — deoxyribonucleic acid
DNase — deoxyribonuclease
DNase agar
Döderlein's bacillus
Dolichos
    D. biflorus
Donath-Landsteiner test
Donovania
    D. granulomatis
Donovan's bodies

Dracunculus
    D. medinensis
drepanocyte
drepanocytemia
drepanocytic
Drepanospira
drumstick
Ducrey's bacillus
Duffy antibodies, Fy^a, Fy^b
Duke's method bleeding time
duovirus
D-xylose tolerance test
dye
    aniline d.
dyscrasia
    blood d.
    lymphatic d.
dysdiemorrhysis
dysemia
dysentery
    amebic d.
    bacillary d.
    balantidial d.
    bilharzial d.
    catarrhal d.
    ciliary d.
    ciliate d.
    flagellate d.
    Flexner's d.
    fulminant d.
    malarial d.
    protozoal d.
    scorbutic d.
    Sonne d.
    spirillar d.
    sporadic d.
    viral d.
dysgammaglobulinemia
dyskaryosis
eastern equine encephalo-
   myelitis virus
Eberthella

EBV — Epstein-Barr virus
ECBO virus — enteric cyto-
pathogenic bovine orphan
virus
ECDO virus — enteric cytopathogenic dog orphan
virus
ECF — extracellular fluid
ECFA — eosinophil chemo-
tactic factor of
anaphylaxis
ECG — electrocardiogram
echinococcosis
Echinococcus
  E. granulosus
  E. multilocularis
Echinorhynchus
echinosis
Echinostoma
ECHO virus — enteric cyto-
pathogenic human orphan
virus
ECHO 28 virus
ECMO virus — enteric cyto-
pathogenic monkey orphan
virus
E. coli — *Escherichia coli*
ECSO virus — enteric cyto-
pathogenic swine orphan
virus
ectoplasm
EDTA — ethylenediaminotetra-
acetate
Edwardsielleae
Edwardsiella
  E. tarda
EEE virus — eastern equine
encephalomyelitis virus
EEG — electroencephalogram
eelworm
Ehrlich's
  reaction

Ehrlich's (*continued*)
  test
Eikenella
  E. corrodens
EKG — electrocardiogram
ekino-. See words beginning
  echino-.
elastase
electrocardiogram
electrocardiograph
electrochemistry
electroencephalogram
electroimmunoassay
electrolyte
  amphoteric e.
  colloidal e.
  protein e.
  serum e.
electrophoresis
  serum protein e.
ELISA — enzyme-linked
immunosorbent
assay
Ellsworth-Howard test
El Tor's vibrios
eluate
elution
EMC virus — encephalomyo-
carditis virus
Endamoeba
  E. blattae
Endolimax
  E. nana
Endomyces
  E. albicans
  E. capsulatus
  E. epidermatidis
  E. epidermidis
endomycosis
endoplasm
endotheliocyte
endotoxin

Entamoeba
    E. buccalis
    E. buetschlii
    E. coli
    E. gingivalis
    E. hartmanni
    E. histolytica
    E. kartulisi
    E. nana
    E. nipponica
    E. polecki
    E. tetragena
    E. tropicalis
    E. undulans
Enteritidis
    E. salmonella
Enterobacter
    E. aerogenes
    E. agglomerans
    E. alvei
    E. cloacae
    E. hafniae
Enterobacteriaceae
enterobiasis
Enterobius
    E. vermicularis
enterococcus
enteroglucagon
Enteromonas
    E. hominis
enterovirus
enzyme
    serum e.
Eos — eosinophils
eosinopenia
eosinophil
    polymorphonuclear e.
eosinophilia
epidemiology
Epidermophyton
    E. floccosum
    E. inguinale

Epidermophyton (*continued*)
    E. rubrum
epithelium
Epstein-Barr virus
eratirus. See *Eratyrus.*
Eratyrus
erisip-. See words beginning
    erysip-.
erithremea. See *erythremia.*
erithro-. See words beginning
    erythro-.
Erwinieae
Erwinia
    E. amylovora
Erysipelothrix
    E. insidiosa
    E. rhusiopathiae
erythremia
Erythrobacillus
erythroblast
erythroblastoma
erythroblastosis
    e. fetalis
    e. neonatorum
erythrocyte
erythrocythemia
erythrocytophagy
erythrocytosis
    leukemic e.
    e. megalosplenica
erythrogenesis
erythroid
erythrokinetics
erythron
erythroneocytosis
erythropenia
erythrophagocytosis
erythropoiesis
erythropoietin
Escherichia
    E. aerogenes
    E. alkalescens

Escherichia (*continued*)
    E. aurescens
    E. coli
    E. dispar
    E. dispar var. *ceylonensis*
    E. dispar var. *madampensis*
    E. freundii
    E. intermedia
Escherichieae
Escherich's bacillus
esherikea. See *Escherichia.*
esherikiee. See *Escherichieae.*
ESR — erythrocyte sedimentation rate
ester
esterase
estradiol
estrogen
estrus. See *Oestrus.*
ethosuximide
etiocholanolone
Eubacteriales
Eubacterium
    E. alactolyticum
    E. lentum
    E. limosum
Euglena
    E. gracilis
euglobulin
eugonic
eumycotic
Euproctis
    E. chrysorrhoea
Eurotium
    E. malignum
Eusimulium
Eutriatoma
Eutrombicula
    E. alfreddugesi
exfoliative
exocrine

exopeptidase
Exophiala
    E. jeanselmei
    E. mycetoma
    E. werneckii
extracellular
extracorpuscular
exudate
F — Fahrenheit
factor
    coagulation f's, I, II, III, IV, V, VII, VIII, IX, X, XI, XII
    Hageman f.
fago-. See words beginning *phago-.*
FANA — fluorescent antinuclear antibody
faneroplazm. See *phaneroplasm.*
Fannia
    F. canicularis
Fasciola
    F. gigantica
    F. hepatica
Fasciolopsis
    F. buski
FBS — fasting blood sugar
Fehleisen's streptococcus
Fehling's test
fenilketonurea. See *phenylketonuria.*
fenistiks. See *Phenistix.*
feno-. See words beginning *pheno-.*
feo-. See words beginning *pheo-.*
fermentation
    mannitol f.
Ferrata's cells
Ferribacterium
ferritin

ferroflocculation
ferrokinetics
Feulgen test
fibrin
fibrinogen
fibrinogenase
fibrinolysin
    seminal f.
Fick's bacillus
Ficoll-Hypaque technique
fiferz. See *Pfeiffer's.*
Filaria
    F. bancrofti
    F. conjunctivae
    F. hominis oris
    F. juncea
    F. labialis
    F. lentis
    F. lymphatica
    F. palpebralis
    F. philippinensis
filariasis
Filarioidea
fisaloptera. See *Physaloptera.*
Fishberg's concentration test
fixative
    Heidenhain's Susa f.
    Zenker's f.
Flagellata
flagellate
flagellum
flavivirus
Flavobacterium
    F. meningosepticum
flebotomus. See *Phlebotomus.*
Flexner-Strong bacillus
Flexner's
    bacillus
    dysentery
flocculation
    cephalin f.
    Ramon f.

floccule
    toxoid-antitoxin f.
flocculoreaction
flora
fluke
    blood f.
fluorescence
fluorometry
Fonsecaea
    F. compactum
    F. pedrosoi
formalin
forme
    f. fruste
fos-. See words beginning
    phos-.
fractionation
fragility
    erythrocyte f.
    osmotic f.
    red cell f.
Francisella
    F. tularensis
Frei test
Freund adjuvant
Friedländer's
    bacillus
    pneumobacillus
Friedman's test
fructose
FSH — follicle stimulating
    hormone
FTA — fluorescent treponemal
    antibody
FTI — free thyroxine index
function
    liver f.
Fungi Imperfecti
fungus
furosemide
Fusarium
Fusiformis

Fusobacterium
    F. fusiforme
    F. mortiferum
    F. necrophorum
    F. nucleatum
    F. plautivincenti
    F. varium
fusocellular
fusospirillary
fusospirillosis
fusospirochetal
fusospirochetosis
fusotreptococciosis
FVC — forced vital capacity
Gaffkya
    G. tetragena
Gaisböck's disease
galactin
galactose
gallium
gamma A, D, E, G, M
gamma globulin
gamma glutamyl transferase
Gärtner's bacillus
gastrin
Gaucher's
    cell
    disease
GC — gonococcus
    gonorrhea
    granular casts
genestatic
genetic
genotype
geotrichosis
Geotrichum
    G. candidum
Gerhardt's test
GFR — glomerular filtration
    rate
GG — gamma globulin
GGT — gamma glutamyl trans-
    ferase

Ghon complex
Ghon-Sachs bacillus
Giardia
    G. lamblia
Giemsa's stain
GLC — gas-liquid chromato-
    graphy
globulin
    A-1 g's
    A-2 g's
    alpha g's
    beta g's
    gamma g's
    immune serum g.
    g. X
Glossina
glucocorticosteroids
glucose
glucosuria
glutamate
glutaminase
glutamine
glutaraldehyde
glycerolization
glycine
Glyciphagus
    G. buski
    G. domesticus
glycogen
glycoprotein
glycosuria
GMP — guanosine monophos-
    phate
Gomori's stain
gonadotropin
    chorionic g.
Gongylonema
    G. pulchrum
gongylonemiasis
gonococcus
gonorrhea
G6PD — glucose-6-phosphate
    dehydrogenase

GPT — glutamic pyruvic
    transaminase
gram-negative
gram-positive
Gram's stain
Gram-Weigert stain
granulocyte
granulocytosis
Gravindex test
gravity
    specific g.
Gruber-Widal reaction
GTT — glucose tolerance test
guaiac
Guaroa virus
Guthrie test
Gutman unit
Haemonchus
    H. contortus
Haemophilus. See *Hemophilus.*
Haemosporidia
Hageman factor
H agglutination
H agglutinin
half-life
Ham's test
Hanger's test
Hansen's bacillus
haploid
haplophase
haplotype
hapten
    group A h.
haptoglobin, Hp^1 and Hp^2
Harrison's test
Hartmanella
    H. hyalina
Haverhillia multiformis
$H-2^b$ mouse cells
Hb — hemoglobin
HBD — hydroxybutyrate
    dehydrogenase

HCG — human chorionic
    gonadotropin
HCT — hematocrit
HDL — high density lipoprotein
H & E — hematoxylin and eosin
Heidenhain's Susa fixative
Heinz bodies
Heinz-Ehrlich bodies
Hektoen agar
HeLa cells
helminth
helminthic
Helminthosporium
Helophilus
hemadsorption
hemagglutination
hemagglutinin
Hemastix
Hematest
hematocrit
hematocrystallin
hematogen
hematogenesis
hematogenous
hematohyaloid
hematologist
hematology
hematopoiesis
    extramedullary h.
heme
Hemispora stellata
hemizygosity
hemoccult
hemochromogen
hemochromometry
hemocytoblast
hemocytometer
hemoflagellate
hemofilus. See *Haemophilus.*
hemoglobin
hemoglobinemia
hemoglobinometry

hemoglobinuria
hemogram
hemohistioblast
hemolysin
hemolysis
hemolytic
hemolyze
hemonkus. See *Haemonchus.*
hemophil
hemophilia
Hemophilus
    H. aegyptius
    H. aphrophilus
    H. bovis
    H. bronchisepticus
    H. ducreyi
    H. duplex
    H. haemolyticus
    H. hemoglobinophilus
    H. hemolyticus
    H. influenzae
    H. parahaemolyticus
    H. parainfluenzae
    H. parapertussis
    H. paraphrophilus
    H. pertussis
    H. suis
    H. vaginalis
hemophilus
    h. of Koch-Weeks
    h. of Morax-Axenfeld
hemosiderin
hemosiderinuria
hemosiderosis
hemosporidea. See
    Haemosporidia.
hemostasis
Hemostix
hemotherapy
heparin
hepatocellular

hepatogram
hepatotoxicity
Herellea
    H. vaginicola
Hermetia illucens
herpesvirus
Heterodera
    H. marioni
heterophil
Heterophyes
    H. heterophyes
    H. katsuradai
Heterophyes/Metagonimus
heterophyiasis
heterozygous
HF — Hageman factor
HGF — hyperglycemic-glyco-
    genolytic factor
HIAA — hydroxyindoleacetic
    acid
Hicks-Pitney thromboplastin
    generation test
Hinton test
Histalog test
histamine
histiocyte
histiocytosis
histocompatibility
    h. complex
histology
histopathology
Histoplasma
    H. capsulatum
    H. duboisii
histoplasmin
histoplasmosis
HLA — human leukocyte
    antigens
HLDH — heat-stable lactic
    dehydrogenase
Hofmann's bacillus

Hogben test
Homalomyia
homogentisuria
homozygous
hookworm
Hormodendrum
    H. carrionii
    H. compactum
    H. pedrosoi
Howard test
Howell-Jolly bodies
Howell's bodies
HPF — high power field
HPL — human placental
    lactogen
Huebener-Thomsen-
    Friedenreich phenomenon
human chorionic gonadotropin
humoral
hyaline
hyalinization
Hycel-17
Hydatigera
    H. infantis
17-hydroxycorticosteroid
5-hydroxyindoleacetic acid
21-hydroxylase
17-hydroxysteroid
5-hydroxytryptamine
hymenolepiasis
Hymenolepis
    H. diminuta
    H. murina
    H. nana
hyperaldosteronism
hyperbetalipoproteinemia
hyperbilirubinemia
hypercalcemia
hypercalciuria
hypercapnia
hypercholesterolemia
hyperchromasia

hyperchromatism
hyperchromemia
hyperchromia
hypercorticosolism
hypercupremia
hypergammaglobulinemia
hyperglobulinemia
hyperglycemia
hyperimmunoglobulinemia
hyperkalemia
hyperlipemia
hyperlipidemia
hyperlipoproteinemia
hypernatremia
hyperphosphatemia
hyperprolactinemia
hyperthermia
hyperuricemia
hyperviscosity
hypha
hypoalbuminemia
hypobetalipoproteinemia
hypocalcemia
hypocapnia
hypochromasia
hypochromemia
    idiopathic h.
hypochromia
hypochromic
hypochrosis
Hypoderma
    H. bovis
hypogammaglobulinemia
hypoglycemia
hypokalemia
hyponatremia
hypophosphatasia
hypophosphatemia
hypoplastic
hypoproteinemia
hypothermia
hypotransferrinemia

hypovolemia
hypoxemia
IBC — iron-binding capacity
ICD — isocitric dehydrogenase
icteric index
^{131}I uptake test (radioactive
     iodine)
Ig — immunoglobulin
IgA — gamma A
          immunoglobulin
IgD — gamma D
          immunoglobulin
IgE — gamma E
          immunoglobulin
IgG — gamma G
          immunoglobulin
IgM — gamma M
          immunoglobulin
iksodez. See *Ixodes.*
iksodiasis. See *ixodiasis.*
Ilheus virus
immune
immunity
immunization
immunize
immunoassay
immunocatalysis
immunochemistry
immunocompetence
immunocyte
immunodeficiency
immunodiagnostic
immunodiffusion
immunoelectrophoresis
     countercurrent i.
immunoferritin
immunofiltration
immunofixation
immunofluorescence
immunoglobulin
     gamma A i. (IgA)
     gamma D i. (IgD)

immunoglobulin (*continued*)
     gamma E i. (IgE)
     gamma G i. (IgG)
     gamma M i. (IgM)
immunohematology
immunoperoxidase
immunosuppression
incompatibility
     ABO i.
index
     acidophilic i.
     hematopneic i.
     hemolytic i.
     icteric i.
     Krebs' leukocyte i.
     maturation i.
     phagocytic i.
     pyknotic i.
     sedimentation i.
indican
indices
indole
Infusoria
INH — isonicotinic acid
          hydrazide
inhibitor
     inter-alpha-trypsin i.
inoculum
insulin
intracellular
iodameba. See *Iodamoeba.*
Iodamoeba
     I. büetschlii
     I. williamsi
iodine
iontophoresis
iron-binding capacity
irovirus
ISG — immune serum globulin
isochromosome
isoenzyme
isohemagglutination

isohemagglutinin
isoimmunization
isolation
Isoparorchis
  I. trisimilitubis
Isospora
  I. belli
  I. hominis
isosporiasis
isotope
Ivy's method bleeding time
Ixodes
  I. bicornis
  I. cavipalpus
  I. frequens
ixodiasis
Ixodoidea
Japanese B encephalitis virus
jaundice
Jenner-Giemsa stain
JH virus
Johne's bacillus
Jolly's bodies
Jones-Cantarow test
Junin virus
K — potassium
Kahn test
kallikrein
Karmen units
karyocyte
karyotype
Katayama's test
KAU —King-Armstrong units
Kell antigens
ketoacidosis
ketogenic
ketone
ketonemia
ketonuria
ketosis
17-ketosteroid
Ketostix

kilomastiks. See *Chilomastix.*
kimotripsin. See *chymotrypsin.*
kinase
kinetocyte
kinetoplast
King-Armstrong unit
klahmidea. See *Chlamydia.*
klahmideasee. See *Chlamy-*
  diaceae.
klahmido-. See words
  beginning *Chlamydo-.*
Klebs-Löffler bacillus
Klebsiella
  K. friedländeri
  K. ozaenae
  K. pneumoniae
  K. rhinoscleromatis
Klebsielleae
Klein's bacillus
klorid. See *chloride.*
kloro-. See words beginning
  chloro-.
Koch-Weeks
  bacillus
  hemophilus
KOH — potassium hydroxide
koksakee. See *Coxsackie.*
kokseela. See *Coxiella.*
koksidi-. See words beginning
  coccidi-.
kol-. See words beginning
  chol-.
Kolmer's test
koreonik. See *chorionic.*
korinee-. See words beginning
  Coryne-.
Krebs' leukocyte index
kromatin. See *chromatin.*
kromo-. See words beginning
  chromo-.
Kumba virus
Kunkel's test

Kupffer's cells
Kveim antigen
Kyasanur Forest disease virus
label
      radioactive l.
Lactobacillaceae
Lactobacilleae
Lactobacillus
      L. acidophilus
      L. arabinosus
      L. bifidus
      L. bulgaricus
      L. casei
      L. catenaforme
      L. fermentans
      L. fermenti
      L. leichmannii
      L. plantarum
lactobacillus
      l. of Boas-Oppler
Lactobacteriaceae
lactose
Ladendorff's test
Laelaps
Lange's colloidal gold test
Lansing virus
larva
Lassa virus
LD — lymphocyte defined
LDH — lactic dehydrogenase
LE — lupus erythematosus
LE test
lecithin
lecithinase
lectin
Lee-White clotting time
      method
Leishman-Donovan bodies
Leishmania
      L. braziliensis
      L. donovani
      L. infantum

Leishmania (continued)
      L. tropica
      L. tropica mexicana
leishmaniasis
      cutaneous l.
      mucocutaneous l.
      naso-oral l.
      nasopharyngeal l.
      visceral l.
Leishman's stain
lelaps. See *Laelaps.*
Leon virus
leptocyte
leptocytosis
Leptomitus
      L. epidermidis
      L. urophilus
      L. vaginae
Leptospira
      L. australis
      L. autumnalis
      L. biflexa
      L. canicola
      L. grippotyphosa
      L. hebdomidis
      L. hyos
      L. icterohaemorrhagiae
      L. interrogans
      L. pomona
leptospirosis
      l. icterohemorrhagica
Leptothrix
Leptotrichia
      L. buccalis
      L. placoides
Leptotrombidium
      L. akamushi
      L. deliense
lesithin. See *lecithin.*
lesithinas. See *lecithinase.*
leucine
leukapheresis

leukemia
    lymphoblastic l.
    lymphocytic l.
    monocytic l.
    myeloblastic l.
    myelocytic l.
    myelogenous l.
    reticuloendothelial cell l.
leukoagglutinins
leukocyte
leukocytosis
    eosinophilic l.
    lymphocytic l.
leukogram
leukopenia
leukotaxis
level
    barbiturate l.
    ethanol l.
    isoelectric l.
    lead l.
Levinson test
Lewis antibodies, Le[a], Le[b]
Lexosceles
    L. reclusus
Leydig's cells
Lichtheimia corymbifera
likthimea korimbifera. See
    Lichtheimia corymbifera.
Limnatis
    L. granulosa
    L. mysomelas
    L. nilotica
Limulus
    L. polyphemus
lipase
lipid
lipidase
lipocyte
lipoid
liponisus. See *Lyponyssus.*

lipoprotein
liquefaction
Lissoflagellata
Listeria
    L. monocytogenes
Loa
    L. loa
Löffler's blood serum
LPF — low power field
    lymphocytosis-
        promoting factor
lukemea. See *leukemia.*
luko-. See words beginning
    leuko-.
Lunyo virus
lupus
    l. erythematosus
lusin. See *leucine.*
lutein
lymphoblast
lymphoblastomid
lymphoblastosis
lymphocyte
    atypical l.
    plasmacytoid l.
lymphocytopenia
lymphocytosis
    neutrophilic l.
    l. promoting factor
lymphs — lymphocytes
Lyponyssus
lysin
lysine
lysing
lysis
lysokinase
lysolecithin
lysosome
lysozyme
MacConkey agar
macroaleuriospore

macroblast
macrocyte
macrocythemia
    hyperchromatic m.
macrocytic
macroglobulin
macroglobulinemia
    Waldenström's m.
Macromonas
    M. bipunctata
    M. mobilis
macromonocyte
macromyeloblast
macronormoblast
macrophage
macropolycyte
Macrostoma mesnili
Madurella
    M. grisea
maedivirus
magnesium
malabsorption
malaria
malasezeah. See *Malassezia.*
Malassezia
    M. furfur
    M. macfadyani
    M. tropica
mallein
Malleomyces
    M. mallei
    M. pseudomallei
    M. whitmori
Mallory's bodies
Malmejde's test
Mansonella ozzardi
Mantoux
    conversion
    skin test
Maragiliano body
marrow
    bone m.

Masson stain
mastadenovirus
Mastigophora
materia
maturation
Mayaro virus
May-Grünwald-Giemsa stain
MBC – minimal bactericidal
    concentration
MCD – mean cell diameter
    mean corpuscular
    diameter
MCH – mean corpuscular
    hemoglobin
MCHC – mean corpuscular
    hemoglobin con-
    centration
MCV – mean corpuscular
    volume
mean cell diameter
mean corpuscular diameter
mean corpuscular hemoglobin
mean corpuscular hemoglobin
    concentration
mean corpuscular volume
MEG – megakaryocytes
megakaryoblast
megakaryocyte
megaloblast
meiosis
melanin
Melanolestes
    M. picipes
Meloidogyne
Mengo virus
meningococci
meningococcin
meningococcus
meningocyte
meniscocyte
Merulius
    M. lacrimans

mesangial
mesangium
mesobacterium
metachromatic
metagglutinin
metaglobulin
metagonimiasis
Metagonimus
    M. ovatus
    M. yokogawai
metamorphosis
metamyelocyte
metanephrine
metaphase
Methanobacterium
Methanococcus
methemalbumin
methemalbuminemia
methemoglobin
methemoglobinemia
methemoglobinuria
method
    chromolytic
    (dyed-starch) m.
    Dale-Laidlaw's clotting
    time m.
    Lee-White clotting
    time m.
methyl
    m. methacrylate
Metopirone test
Mg agglutinin
Microbacterium
microbiology
microbroth
microchemistry
Micrococcaceae
Micrococcus
    M. pyogenes var. *aureus*
microcyte
microcytic

Microfilaria
    M. bancrofti
    M. streptocerca
microne
microorganism
microphage
microprotein
microscope
microscopic
microscopy
    electron m.
microspherocyte
Microsporon furfur
Microsporum
    M. audouini
    M. canis
    M. felineum
    M. fulvum
    M. furfur
    M. gypseum
    M. lanosum
Middlebrook-Dubos hemag-
    glutination test
Middlebrook's
    agar
    broth
MIF — migration-inhibition
    factor
miksopod. See *myxopod.*
miksosporidea. See
    Myxosporidia.
Mima
    M. polymorpha
minimal bactericidal concentra-
    tion
miosis. See *meiosis.*
mitochondria
mitogen
mitogillin
mitokinetic
mitomalcin

mitoplasm
mitosis
Miyagawanella
    M. illinii
    M. louisianae
    *M. lymphogranulomato-
        sis*
    M. ornithosis
    M. pneumoniae
    M. psittaci
MLC — minimal lethal concen-
        tration
moiety
molality
molar
molarity
Monadina
Monas
Monilia
monilial
moniliasis
Moniliformis
monoblast
monochromator
monoclonal
monocyte
monocytopenia
monocytosis
mononuclear
Monos — monocytes
monosaccharide
monosomic
monosomy G, X
Monosporium
    M. apiospermum
Monotricha
Morax-Axenfeld
    bacillus
    diplococcus
    hemophilus
Moraxella
    M. lacunata

Moraxella (continued)
    M. liquefaciens
morbillivirus
Morgan's bacillus
morococcus
morphology
mosaicism
Mosenthal's test
motile
motility
Motulsky dye reduction test
mouse unit
MU — mouse unit
mucopolysaccharidase
mucopolysaccharide
mucoprotein
Mucor
    M. corymbifer
    M. mucedo
    M. pusillus
    M. racemosus
    M. ramosus
    M. rhizopodiformis
mucormycosis
mucus
Mueller-Hinton broth
muramidase
Murphy-Pattee test
Murray Valley encephalitis
    virus
murtofilum. See
    Myrtophyllum.
mycoagglutinin
mycobacteria
Mycobacteriaceae
mycobacteriosus
Mycobacterium
    M. avium-intracellulare
    M. balnei
    M. berolinenis
    M. bovis
    M. butyricum

Mycobacterium (continued)
    M. chelonei
    M. flavescens
    M. fortuitum
    M. gastri
    M. gordonae
    M. habana
    M. intracellularis
    M. kansasii
    M. leprae
    M. leprae murium
    M. luciflavum
    M. marinum
    M. microti
    M. paratuberculosis
    M. phlei
    M. scrofulaceum
    M. simiae
    M. smegmatis
    M. szulgai
    M. terrea-nonchromo-
      genicum-triviale
    M. tuberculosis
    M. tuberculosis var.
      avium
    M. tuberculosis var.
      bovis
    M. tuberculosis var.
      hominis
    M. ulcerans
    M. xenopi
Mycocandida
Mycococcus
Mycoderma
    M. aceti
    M. dermatitis
    M. immite
mycology
Myconostoc
    M. gregarium
Mycoplana
    M. bullata

Mycoplana (continued)
    M. dimorpha
Mycoplasma
    M. buccale
    M. faucium
    M. fermentans
    M. hominis
    M. orale
    M. pharyngis
    M. pneumoniae
    M. salivarium
Mycoplasmataceae
Mycoplasmatales
mycosis
    m. fungoides
mycotic
myeloblast
myeloclast
myelocyte
myiasis
myoglobin
Myriapoda
Myrtophyllum
    M. hepatis
myxopod
Myxosporidia
myxovirus
NAD — nicotinamide adenine
        dinucleotide
Naegleria
NANA — N-acetylneuraminic
        acid
NBT — nitroblue tetrazolium
Necator
    N. americanus
Negri bodies
Neisseria
    N. caviae
    N. catarrhalis
    N. flava
    N. flavescens
    N. gonorrhoeae

Neisseria (continued)
    N. intracellularis
    N. lactamicus
    N. meningitidis
    N. mucosa
    N. ovis
    N. sicca
    N. subflava
Neisseriaceae
Neisser's diplococcus
Nematoda
nematode
neocyte
neocytosis
nephelometry
neuraminidase
neutropenia
neutrophil
    band n.
neutrophile
    juvenile n.
    mature n.
    polymorphonuclear n.
    segmented n.
neutrophilia
Newcastle disease virus
Newcastle-Manchester bacillus
Nitrobacter
Nitrobacteraceae
Nitrocystis
Nocardia
    N. asteroides
    N. brasiliensis
    N. caviae
    N. madurae
nocardiosis
Nocard's bacillus
norepinephrine
normoblast
    acidophilic n.
    basophilic n.
    intermediate n.

normoblast (*continued*)
    orthochromatophilic n.
    polychromatophilic n.
normoblastosis
normocyte
normocytic
normocytosis
normo-orthocytosis
nosomycosis
NPDL — nodular, poorly
    differentiated
    lymphocytes
NPN — nonprotein nitrogen
NSQ — not sufficient quantity
nucleoprotein
nucleus
numo-. See words beginning
    pneumo-.
O agglutination
O agglutinin
O antistreptolysin
Obermayer's test
Obermeier's spirillum
Obermüller's test
occult blood
Ochromyia
    O. anthropophaga
OCT — ornithine carbamyl
    transferase
Octomitus
    O. hominis
Octomyces
    O. etiennei
Oestrus
    O. hominis
    O. ovis
OHCS — hydroxycortico-
    steroid
Oidiomycetes
oidiomycosis
oligemia
oligocythemia

Onchocherca
    O. caecutiens
    O. volvulus
onchocerciasis
O'nyong-nyong virus
Oospora
opisthorchiasis
Opisthorchis
    O. felineus
    O. noverca
    O. viverrini
orbivirus
organic
organism
    Arizona o.
    Rickett's o.
    Vincent's o.
Oropouche virus
orthopoxvirus
Osler's disease
osmolality
osmometry
osmosis
Ostertag
    streptococcus of O.
Otomyces
    O. hageni
    O. purpureus
otomycosis
    o. aspergillina
ova
ovum
oxalate
oxygen
oxyhemoglobin
oxyhemogram
oxyhemograph
oxysteroid
Oxyuris
    O. incognita
    O. vermicularis
PAH – para-aminohippurate

pancytopenia
Pandy's test
panhematopoietic
panhemocytophthisis
Papanicolaou's
    smear
    stain
    test
papillomavirus
Papovaviridae
papovavirus
Pappenheim's stain
Parachordodes
Paracoccidioides
    P. brasiliensis
paracoccidioidomycosis
Paracolobactrum
    P. aerogenoides
    P. arizonae
    P. coliforme
    P. intermedium
paraffin
Paragonimus
    P. westermani
Paragordius
    P. cintus
    P. tricuspidatus
    P. varius
parahormone
paramyxovirus
Parasaccharomyces
    P. ashfordi
parasite
parasitic
parasitology
parathormone
paratyphi S.C.
paratyphoid A and B
paravirus
Parvobacteriaceae
Parvoviridae
parvovirus

PAS — para-aminosalicylic acid
Pasteurella
    P. haemolytica
    P. multocida
    P. pestis
    P. pseudotuberculosis
    P. tularensis
Patein's albumin
pathogen
Paul-Bunnell-Barrett test
Paul-Bunnell test
PBG — porphobilinogen
PBI — protein-bound iodine
pCO_2 — carbon dioxide
    pressure
PCV — packed cell volume
Pectobacterium
    P. carotovorum
Pediculoides
    P. ventricosus
Pediculus
    P. humanus var. *capitis*
    P. humanus var. *corporis*
    P. inguinalis
    P. pubis
Pelger-Huët nuclear anomaly
pellicle
Penicillium
    P. barbae
    P. bouffardi
    P. minimum
    P. montoyai
    P. notatum
    P. patulum
    P. spinulosum
Pentastoma
    P. constrictum
    P. denticulatum
    P. taenioides
pentastomiasis
Pentatrichomonas
    P. ardin delteili

pentatrichomoniasis
pentolysis
pentosan
pentosazon
pentose
pepsin
peptidase
    leucine amino p.
Peptococcus
    P. asaccharolyticus
    P. magnus
    P. prevotii
Peptostreptococcus
    P. anaerobius
    P. intermedius
    P. micros
pericyte
peroxidase
Petriellidium
Petri's
    dish
    test
Pfeiffer's bacillus
pH — hydrogen ion concen-
    tration
phagocyte
phagocytic
phagocytoblast
phagocytolysis
phagocytosis
phaneroplasm
Phenistix
phenol
    p. liquefactum
    p. red
    p. salicylate
phenolphthalein
phenolsulfonphthalein
phenothiazine
phenomenon
    Huebener-Thomsen-
      Friedenreich p.

phenomenon (*continued*)
    prozone p.
phenotype
    Bombay p.
phenylalanine
phenylketonuria
pheochromocyte
pheochromocytoma
pheresis
Phialophora
    P. jeanselmi
    P. verrucosa
Philadelphia chromosome
Phlebotomus
    P. argentipes
    P. chinensis
    P. intermedius
    P. macedonicum
    P. noguchi
    P. papatasii
    P. sergenti
    P. verrucarum
    P. vexator
phosphatase
    acid p.
    alkaline p.
    serum p.
phosphate
phosphatidylethanolamine
phosphocreatine
phosphofructokinase
phospholipase
phospholipid
phosphorus
phosphorylase
Phthirus
    P. pubis
Phycomycetes
phycomycosis
Physaloptera
    P. caucasica
    P. mordens

phytohemagglutination
Piazza's test
picogram
piedra
Piedraia
    P. hortae
pigment
pinworm
Pityrosporon
    P. orbiculare
    P. ovale
    P. versicolor
PKU — phenylketonuria
plasma
plasmablast
plasmacyte
plasmacytoma
plasmacytosis
plasmagene
plasmahaut
plasmalogen
plasmapheresis
plasmarrhexis
plasmid
plasmin
plasminogen
plasmocyte
Plasmodium
    P. falciparum
    P. malariae
    P. ovale
    P. pleurodyniae
    P. vivax
    P. vivax minuta
plasmodium
    exoerythrocytic p.
platelet
plateletpheresis
pleokaryocyte
pleomorphic
pneumobacillus
    Friedländer's p.

pneumococcal
pneumococcus
Pneumocystis
    P. carinii
pneumovirus
pO_2 — partial pressure of
    oxygen
poikiloblast
poikilocyte
poikilocytosis
polarography
Poly — polymorphonuclear
    leukocyte
polychromasia
polychromatic
polychromatophilia
polychromatosis
polychromemia
polyclonal
polycyte
polycythemia
    p. hypertonica
    myelopathic p.
    p. rubra
    splenomegalic p.
    p. vera
polycytosis
polyemia
    p. aquosa
    p. hyperalbuminosa
    p. polycythaemica
    p. serosa
polymorphocyte
polymorphonuclear
    p. basophil
    p. eosinophil
    p. leukocyte
    p. neutrophil
polynuclear
polyomavirus
polyploid
polyploidy

polyribosome
polysaccharide
polysomaty
polysomy X
Porges-Meier test
Porges-Salomon test
Porocephalus
    P. armillatus
    P. clavatus
    P. constrictus
    P. denticulatus
porphobilinogen
porphyria
porphyrin
postprandial
potassium
potentiometry
Powassan virus
poxvirus
PP — postprandial
PPD — purified protein
    derivative
prealbumin
pregnanediol
pregnanetriol
Preisz-Nocard bacillus
premyeloblast
premyelocyte
proerythroblast
proerythrocyte
profibrinolysin
profile
    liver p.
prolactin
proliferate
proliferation
prolymphocyte
promegaloblast
promoblast
promonocyte
promyelocyte
pronormoblast

Propionibacterium
   P. acnes
proplasmacyte
Proteeae
proteidin
     pyocyanase p.
protein
    C-reactive p.
proteinemia
proteinosis
proteinuria
    Bence Jones p.
proteoclastic
proteolipid
proteolytic
Proteomyces
proteose
proteosuria
Proteus
   P. inconstans
   P. mirabilis
   P. morganii
   P. OX-K
   P. OX-2
   P. OX-19
   P. rettgeri
   P. vulgaris
prothrombin
prothrombinase
prothrombinogen
prothrombinokinase
prothrombinopenia
protoanemonin
Protobacterieae
protocoproporphyria
protoporphyrin
Protozoa
protozoan
protozoon
protozoophage
Providencia
   P. alcalifaciens

Providencia (continued)
   P. stuartii
Prowazekia
prozone
psammoma
PSD — peptone-starch-dextrose
Pseudamphistomum
   truncatum
Pseudomonadaceae
Pseudomonadales
Pseudomonadineae
Pseudomonas
   P. aeruginosa
   P. eisenbergii
   P. fluorescens
   P. fragi
   P. non-liquefaciens
   P. pseudomallei
   P. pyocyanea
   P. syncyanea
   P. viscosa
Pseudomonilia
PSP — phenolsulfonphthalein
PTA — plasma thromboplastin
     antecedent
PTC — plasma thromboplastin
     component
PTT — partial thromboplastin
     time
Pulex
   P. irritans
Pullicidae
pullorin
Pullularia
purpura
    thrombocytopenic p.
pyknosis
pyknotic
pyocyanase
pyogenic
pyrogen
pyroglobulin

QNS – quantity not sufficient
qualitative
quantitative
Quick's test
RA – rheumatoid arthritis
rabdo-. See words beginning
   rhabdo-.
radioassay
radioimmunoassay
radioisotope
radiolabeled
radionuclide
radioreceptor
RAI – radioactive iodine
RAI scan
     uptake
RA latex fixation test
Ramon flocculation
rate
     sedimentation r.
ratio
     myeloid-erythroid r.
RBC – red blood cell
     red blood count
RBC/hpf – red blood cells per
       high power field
RBE – relative biological
      effectiveness
reaction
     Bence Jones r.
     Ehrlich's r.
     glycine-arginine r.
     Gruber-Widal r.
     sigma r.
     Wassermann r.
     Weil-Felix r.
     Widal r.
reagent
     Sickledex r.
renin
renogram
reovirus

reticulin
reticulocyte
reticuloendothelial
Retortamonas
     R. intestinalis
RH – Rhesus (factor)
rhabdocyte
Rhabdomonas
Rh agglutinin
Rh antigen
Rhinocladium
Rhizobiaceae
Rhizobium
Rhizoglyphus
     R. parasiticus
Rhizopoda
Rhizopus
     R. equinus
     R. niger
     R. nigricans
Rhodotorula
     R. rubra
RhoGAM vaccine
RIA – radioimmunoassay
riboflavin
Rickett's organism
Rickettsia
     R. akamushi
     R. akari
     R. australis
     R. burnetii
     R. conorii
     R. diaporica
     R. mooseri
     R. muricola
     R. nipponica
     R. orientalis
     R. pediculi
     R. prowazekii
     R. quintana
     R. rickettsii
     R. sibiricus

Rickettsia (*continued*)
    R. tsutsugamushi
    R. typhi
    R. wolhynica
Rickettsiaceae
rickettsial
rickettsialpox
Rift Valley fever virus
Ringer's solution
rinokladeum. See
    Rhinocladium.
RISA — radioactive serum
    albumin
rizo-. See words beginning
    Rhizo-.
RNA — ribonucleic acid
RNase — ribonuclease
rod-shaped
Romanowsky's stain
roolo. See *rouleau* and
    rouleaux.
Rose's test
Rose-Waaler test
rotavirus
Rothera's test
Rotter's test
rouleau
rouleaux
roundworm
Rourke-Ernstein sedimentation
    rate
Rous test
Rowntree and Geraghty's test
RPF — renal plasma flow
RS virus
rubella
rubivirus
rubrum
Russell unit
Russian spring-summer
    encephalitis virus
Sabhi agar

Sabouraud's dextrose agar
Saccharomyces
    S. albicans
    S. anginae
    S. apiculatus
    Busse's s.
    S. cantliei
    S. capillitii
    S. carlsbergensis
    S. cerevisiae
    S. coprogenus
    S. epidermica
    S. galacticolus
    S. glutinis
    S. lemonnieri
    S. mellis
    S. mycoderma
    S. neoformans
Salmonella
    S. choleraesuis
    S. derby
    S. durazzo
    S. enteritidis
    S. gallinarum
    S. minnesota
    S. montevideo
    S. muenchen
    S. newington
    S. paratyphi A, B, C
    S. pullorum
    S. schottmülleri
    S. sendai
    S. thompson
    S. typhi
    S. typhimurium
    S. typhisuis
    S. typhosa
    S. virginia
Salmonella-Shigella agar
Salmonelleae
Salvia
    S. horminium

Salvia (*continued*)
    S. sclarea
Sappinia diploidea
Saprospira
Sarcina
Sarcocystis
sarcocyte
Sarcodina
Sarcophaga
    S. carnaria
    S. dux
    S. fuscicauda
    S. haemorrhoidalis
    S. nificornis
Sarcoptes
    S. scabiei
scan
    bilirubin s.
    brain s.
    CAT (computed axial
      tomography) s.
    gallium s.
    kidney s.
    krypton s.
    liver s.
    RAI s.
    risa s.
    spleen s.
    technetium s.
SCG — serum chemistry graph
Schaedler blood agar
Schick test
Schilling
    blood count
    test
schistocyte
Schistosoma
    S. haematobium
    S. intercalatum
    S. japonicum
    S. mansoni
schistosome

schistosomiasis
Schizoblastosporion
schizogony
Schmitz's bacillus
Schmorl's bacillus
Schottmüller's disease
schwannoma
Schwann's white substance
scintiphotograph
scolecoid
scolex
Scopulariopsis
    S. americana
    S. aureus
    S. blochi
    S. brevicaulis
    S. cinereus
    S. koningi
    S. minimus
scopulariopsosis
sediment
sedimentation
    erythrocyte s.
sedimentation rate
    Rourke-Ernstein s.r.
    Westergren's s.r.
    Wintrobe's s.r.
    Zeta s.r.
sefalin. See *cephalin.*
sefalosporeum. See
    Cephalosporium.
Seg — segmented (leukocyte)
SEGS — segmented neutro-
      phils
Semliki Forest virus
Sendai virus
sensitivity
septicemia
serine
serkarea. See *cercaria.*
serodiagnosis
serological

serology
serotonin
serotype
serous
Serratia
    S. indica
    S. kiliensis
    S. liquefaciens
    S. marcescens
    S. piscatorum
    S. plymuthica
    S. rubidaea
Serratieae
serum creatinine
sfero-. See words beginning
    with *sphero-.*
SGOT — serum glutamic
            oxaloacetic trans-
            aminase
SGPT — serum glutamic
            pyruvic trans-
            aminase
SH — serum hepatitis
shaletela. See *Cheyletiella.*
Shiga's bacillus
Shigella
    S. alkalescens
    S. ambigua
    S. arabinotarda Type A,
      B
    S. boydii
    S. ceylonensis
    S. dispar
    S. dysenteriae
    S. etousae
    S. flexneri
    S. madampensis
    S. newcastle
    S. paradysenteriae
    S. parashigae
    S. schmitzii
    S. shigae
    S. sonnei

Shigella (*continued*)
    S. wakefield
Shinowara-Jones-Reinhard unit
Sia test
sickle cell
Sickledex reagent
sickling
Siderobacter
sideroblast
Siderocapsa
Siderocapsaceae
Siderococcus
siderocyte
siderophilin
sifasea. See *Syphacia.*
sigmavirus
Simbu virus
Simmons' citrate agar
Sims-Huhner test
Sindbis virus
skisto-. See words beginning
    schisto-.
skizo-. See words beginning
    schizo-.
SMA-12 profile test
smear
    fungi s.
    Papanicolaou's s.
    TB s.
sodium
solution
    formaldehyde s.
    Ringer's s.
somatomedin
somatostatin
Somogyi unit
Sonne-Duval bacillus
Sonne dysentery
sparganosis
sparganum
SPCA — serum prothrombin-
            conversion
            accelerator

spectrometer
spectrophotometry
SPF — specific pathogen free
sp. gr. — specific gravity
spherocyte
spherocytosis
sphingomyelin
sphingosine
Spirillaceae
Spirillum
    S. minor
    Obermeier's S.
Spirochaeta
    S. daxensis
    S. eurystrepta
    S. marina
    S. pallida
    S. plicatilis
    S. stenostrepta
    S. vincenti
spirochete
spirochetemia
spirogram
spirometry
Sporothrix
    S. schenckii
sporotrichosis
Sporozoa
sporozoite
sporozoon
sputum
SSKI — saturated solution of
      potassium iodide
Stab — stabnuclear neutrophil
staf-. See words beginning
   staph-.
stain
    acid-Schiff s.
    alcian blue s.
    ATPase s.
    Bowie's s.

stain (*continued*)
    carbol fuchsin s.
    chlorazol black E. s.
    Congo red s.
    cresyl violet s.
    eosin s.
    Giemsa's s.
    Gomori's s.
    Gram's s.
    Gram-Weigert s.
    hematoxylin-eosin s.
    Jenner-Giemsa s.
    Leishman's s.
    Masson s.
    May-Grünwald-Giemsa s.
    methenamine silver s.
    Papanicolaou's s.
    Pappenheim's s.
    polychrome methylene
      blue s.
    quinacrine s.
    Romanowsky's s.
    Truant's s.
    van Gieson's s.
    Wade-Fite-Faraco s.
    Weigert's s.
    Wright's s.
    Ziehl-Neelsen's s.
staphylocoagulase
staphylococcal
staphylococcemia
staphylococci
Staphylococcus
    S. albus
    S. aureus
    S. citreus
    S. epidermidis
staphylolysin
    α s., alpha s.
    β s., beta s.
    δ s., delta s.

staphylolysin (*continued*)
    ε s., epsilon s.
    γ s., gamma s.
steroid
stippling
    basophilic s.
St. Louis encephalitis virus
Stormer viscosimeter
Streptobacillus
    S. moniliformis
streptococcal
Streptococceae
streptococci
Streptococcus
    S. agalactiae
    S. anginosus
    S. bovis
    S. cremoris
    S. durans
    S. equi
    S. equisimilis
    S. faecalis
    S. faecium
    S. fecalis
    S. hemolyticus
    S. lactis
    S. liquefaciens
    S. MG
    S. mitis
    S. pneumoniae
    S. pyogenes
    S. salivarius
    S. uberis
    S. viridans
    S. zooepidemicus
    S. zymogenes
streptococcus
    alpha s.
    anhemolytic s.
    Bargen's s.
    beta s.
    Fehleisen's s.

streptococcus (*continued*)
    gamma s.
    hemolytic s.
    nonhemolytic s.
    s. of Ostertag
streptolysin O, S
Streptomyces
    S. madurae
    S. pelletieri
    S. somaliensis
Streptothrix
Strong's bacillus
Strongyloides
    S. stercoralis
strongyloidiasis
STS − serologic test for
      syphilis
    standard test for
      syphilis
STU − skin test unit
study
    erythrokinetic s's
    fat absorption s's
subculture
substance
    white s. of Schwann
    zymoplastic s.
Sudan
    S. black
    S. I
    S. II
    S. G. S. III
    S. IV
    S. yellow G
sudo-. See words beginning
    pseudo-.
sulfhemoglobin
sulfmethemoglobin
sulfobromophthalein
Sulkowitch's test
survival
    red blood cell s.

Swiss-type agammaglobulin-
emia
Syphacia
    S. obvelata
T_3 — triiodothyronine
T_4 — thyroxine, levothyroxine,
    tetraiodothyronine
tachogram
Taenia
    T. africana
    T. brunerri
    T. confusa
    T. echinococcus
    T. philippina
    T. saginata
    T. solium
T agglutination
Takata-Ara test
tapeworm
target cell
TAT — tetanus antitoxin
    toxin-antitoxin
    turn around time
TB — tubercle bacillus
    tuberculosis
TBC — tuberculosis
TBG — thyroxine-binding
    globulin
TBI — thyroxine binding index
T cells
technique
    Ficoll-Hypaque t.
    zinc sulfate centrifugal
    flotation t.
tenea. See *Taenia.*
tenosefalidez. See
    Ctenocephalides.
Teschen virus
test
    Abrams' t.
    acetic acid t.
    acetic acid and potassium
    ferrocyanide t.

test (*continued*)
    acetoacetic acid t.
    acetone t.
    acidified serum t.
    acidity reduction t.
    acid-lability t.
    acidosis t.
    acid phosphatase t.
    ACTH t.
    Adamkiewicz's t.
    Adler's t.
    adrenalin t.
    adrenocortical
    inhibition t.
    A/G ratio t.
    agglutination t.
    albumin t.
    adolase t.
    aldosterone t.
    alizarin t.
    alkali t.
    alkali denaturation t.
    alkali tolerance t.
    alkaline phosphatase t.
    alkaloid t.
    alpha amino nitrogen t.
    amylase t.
    antiglobulin t.
    Apt t.
    arginine t.
    Argo corn starch t.
    arylsulfatase t.
    Aschheim-Zondek t.
    ascorbate cyanide t.
    ascorbic acid t.
    automated reagin t.
    AZ t.
    Bence Jones protein t.
    Benedict's t.
    bentonite flocculation t.
    bile acid t.
    bile pigment t.
    bile solubility t.

test (*continued*)

bilirubin t., direct,
    indirect
bilirubin tolerance t.
biuret t.
blood urea nitrogen t.
Bloor's t.
Bloxam's t.
Boas' t.
Bonanno's t.
bromosulfalein t.
butanol extractable
    iodine t.
calcium t.
capillary fragility t.
carbon dioxide combin-
    ing power t.
Casoni's intradermal t.
Castellani's t.
catecholamine t.
cephalin-cholesterol
    flocculation t.
cephalin flocculation t.
cetylpyridium chloride t.
Chediak's t.
cholesterol t.
cholesterol-lecithin
    flocculation t.
cholinesterase t.
chromogenic cephalo-
    sporin t.
coagulation t.
colloidal gold t.
complement-fixation
    (C-F) t.
Congo red t.
Coombs' t., direct,
    indirect
coproporphyrin t.
cortisone-glucose
    tolerance t.
C-reactive protein t.

test (*continued*)

creatine t.
creatinine clearance t.
cyanide-nitroprusside t.
dexamethasone suppres-
    sion t.
dextrose t.
Diagnex Blue t.
Dick t.
dinitrophenylhydrazine t.
direct antiglobulin t.
dithionite t.
Donath-Landsteiner t.
edrophonium chloride t.
Ehrlich's t.
electrophoresis t.
Ellsworth-Howard t.
Fehling's t.
ferric chloride t.
Feulgen t.
fibrinogen t.
Fishberg's concentration
    t.
flocculation t.
fluorescent treponemal
    antibody t.
formol-gel t.
fragility t.
Frei t.
Friedman's t.
frog t.
galactose tolerance t.
Gerhardt's t.
glucagon t.
glucose tolerance t.
glycogen storage t.
Gravindex t.
Guthrie t.
Ham's t.
Hanger's t.
Harrison's t.
hemagglutination t.

test (*continued*)

heterophile antibody t.
Hicks-Pitney thrombo-
plastin generation t.
Hinton t.
hippuric acid t.
Histalog t.
histamine t.
Hogben t.
homogentisic acid t.
Howard t.
17-hydroxycortico-
steroid t.
5-hydroxyindoleacetic
acid t.
^{131}I (radioactive iodine)
uptake t.
icterus index t.
indican t.
indigo-carmine t.
indole t.
insulin clearance t.
insulin tolerance t.
interference t.
iron-binding capacity t.
isoiodeikon t.
isopropanol precipitation
t.
Jones-Cantarow t.
Kahn t.
Katayama's t.
17-ketosteroid t.
Kolmer's t.
Kunkel's t.
lactic acid t.
lactic dehydrogenase t.
lactose tolerance t.
Ladendorff's t.
Lange's colloidal gold t.
latex fixation t.
latex slide agglutination t.
LE t.

test (*continued*)

leucine aminopeptidase t.
Levinson t.
levulose tolerance t.
limulus lysate t.
lipase t.
lipid t.
lymphocyte transfer t.
magnesium t.
malaria film t.
mallein t.
Malmejde's t.
Mantoux skin t.
mastic t.
melanin t.
methylene blue t.
Metopirone t.
Middlebrook-Dubos
hemagglutination t.
monocyte function t.
Mosenthal's t.
Motulsky dye reduction t.
mucoprotein t.
Murphy-Pattee t.
nitrate utilization t.
nitroblue tetrazolium t.
nitroprusside t.
nonprotein nitrogen t.
Obermayer's t.
Obermüller's t.
occult blood t.
osazone t.
osmotic fragility t.
Pandy's t.
Papanicolaou's t.
partial thromboplastin
time t.
Paul-Bunnell t.
Paul-Bunnell-Barrett t.
Petri's t.
phenolphthalein t.
phenolsulfonphthalein t.

test (*continued*)

    phenylketonuria t.
    phosphatase t.
    phospholipid t.
    phosphoric acid t.
    Piazza's t.
    plasma hemoglobin t.
    Porges-Meier t.
    Porges-Salomon t.
    porphobilinogen t.
    porphyrin t.
    potassium t.
    precipitin t.
    prolactin t.
    protein t.
    protein-bound iodine t.
    prothrombin t.
    purine bodies t.
    quantitation t.
    Quick's t.
    RA latex fixation t.
    radioactive iodine t.
    reactone red t.
    resorcinol t.
    rose bengal t.
    Rose's t.
    Rose-Waaler t.
    Rothera's t.
    Rotter's t.
    Rous t.
    Rowntree and Geraghty's t.
    Schick t.
    Schilling t.
    secretin t.
    sedimentation t.
    serology t.
    serum alkaline phosphatase t.
    serum globulin t.
    Sia t.
    sickle cell t.

test (*continued*)

    sickling t.
    silver nitroprusside t.
    Sims-Huhner t.
    SMA-12 profile t.
    sodium t.
    streptozyme t.
    Sulkowitch's t.
    sweat t.
    T-3 uptake t.
    Takata-Ara t.
    tetrazolium t.
    Thayer-Martin t.
    Thorn t.
    thromboplastin generation t.
    thymol turbidity t.
    thyroxine binding index t.
    tine t.
    tolbutamide tolerance t.
    transaminase t. (SGOT - SGPT)
    trypsin t.
    tyrosine t.
    Tzanck t.
    Uffelmann's t.
    urea clearance t.
    urea nitrogen t.
    urease t.
    uric acid t.
    urine acetone t.
    urobilinogen t.
    van den Bergh t.
    vanilmandelic acid t.
    Van Slyke t.
    VDRL t.
    Voges-Proskauer t.
    Volhard's t.
    Wassermann t.
    Watson-Schwartz t.
    wire loop t.
    xylose concentration t.

test (*continued*)
    D-xylose tolerance t.
    zinc flocculation t.
    zinc turbidity t.
Tes-Tape
tetraploidy
TGT — thromboplastin
    generation test
    thromboplastin
    generation time
thalassemia
THAM — trihydroxymethyl-
    aminomethane
Thayer-Martin test
Theiler's virus
theolin
thermogram
thiocyanate
Thorn test
thread
    mucous t's
thrombasthenia
thrombin
thrombocyte
thrombocytopenia
thrombocytopoiesis
thrombocytosis
thrombometer
thromboplastic
thromboplastin
thromboplastinogen
thrombostasis
thrombosthenin
thrombotest
thymidine
thymol turbidity
thyrocalcitonin
thyrotropin
thyroxine
TIBC — total iron-binding
    capacity
timothy bacillus

titer
    agglutination t.
    antihyaluronidase t.
    CF antibody t.
titration
TLC — thin-layer chromato-
    graphy
TNTC — too numerous to
    count
Todd-Hewitt broth
Todd's bodies
Todd units
toluidine
    t. blue O
Torula
    T. capsulatus
    T. histolytica
Torulopsis
    T. glabrata
toxicology
toxin
Toxocara
    T. canis
    T. cati
    T. mystax
toxocariasis
toxoid
toxoid-antitoxoid
Toxoplasma
    T. gondii
    T. pyrogenes
toxoplasmosis
TPI — *Treponema pallidum*
    immobilization
TPTZ — tripyridyltriazine
Trachybdella bistriata
transaminase
transferase
transferrin
Trematoda
    T. *Clonorchis*
    T. *Dicrocoelium*

Trematoda (*continued*)
  T. *Echinostoma*
  T. *Fasciola*
  T. *Fasciolopsis*
  T. *Gastrodiscoides*
  T. *Heterophyes*
  T. *Metagonimus*
  T. *Opisthorchis*
  T. *Paragonimus*
  T. *Schistosoma*
trematode
Treponema
  T. *calligyrum*
  T. *carateum*
  T. *genitalis*
  T. *macrodentium*
  T. *microdentium*
  T. *mucosum*
  T. *pallidum*
  T. *pertenue*
  T. *pintae*
TRF – thyrotropin-releasing
      factor
TRH – thyrotropin-releasing
      hormone
Tricercomonas
Trichinella
  T. *spiralis*
trichinosis
trichomonad
Trichomonas
  T. *buccalis*
  T. *hominis*
  T. *intestinalis*
  T. *pulmonalis*
  T. *tenax*
  T. *vaginalis*
trichomoniasis
Trichophyton
  T. *concentricum*
  T. *epilans*
  T. *ferrugineum*

Trichophyton (*continued*)
  T. *mentagrophytes*
  T. *rosaceum*
  T. *rubrum*
  T. *sabouraudi*
  T. *schoenleini*
  T. *sulfureum*
  T. *tonsurans*
  T. *verrucosum*
  T. *violaceum*
trichophytosis
Trichoptera
Trichosporon
  T. *beigelii*
  T. *cutaneum*
  T. *pedrosianum*
Trichostrongylus
  T. *axei*
  T. *brevis*
  T. *colubriformis*
  T. *instabilis*
  T. *orientalis*
  T. *vitrinus*
Trichothecium
  T. *roseum*
Trichuris
  T. *trichiura*
triglyceride
triiodothyronine
Triodontophorus
  T. *diminutus*
Triphleps insidiosus
triploidy
trisomies
trisomy C, mosaic
trisomy D
trisomy E
trisomy G
trisomy X
trisomy 8
trisomy 13
trisomy 18

tritiated
Trombicula
    T. autumnalis
    T. irritans
    T. tsalsahuatl
    T. vandersandi
Trombiculidae
trophoplasm
trophozoite
TRP — tubular reabsorption of
    phosphate
Truant's stain
Trypanosoma
    T. brucei
    T. cruzi
    T. escomeli
    T. gambiense
    T. rangeli
    T. rhodesiense
trypanosomiasis
trypsin
trypsinogen
tryptase
TSH — thyroid-stimulating
    hormone
tularemia
Tunga
    T. penetrans
turbidimetric
turbidimetry
turbidity
Türk's cell
typhoid
typhus
typing
    ABO t.
    ABO-Rh t.
Tyroglyphus
    T. siro
tyrosine
tyrosinosis
Tzanck test

ubakterealez. See
    Eubacteriales.
ubaktereum. See
    Eubacterium.
Uffelmann's test
Uganda S virus
uglena. See *Euglena.*
uglobulin. See *euglobulin.*
ugonik. See *eugonic.*
ultracentrifugation
unit
    Bessey-Lowry u.
    Bodansky u.
    Gutman u.
    Karmen u's
    King-Armstrong u.
    mouse u.
    rat u.
    Russell u.
    Shinowara-Jones-
      Reinhard u.
    Somogyi u.
    Todd u's
    Wohlgemuth u.
uproktis. See *Euproctis.*
uptake
    RAI u.
    resin u.
urate
urea
ureaplasma
urease
uric
urinalysis
urobilin
urobilinogen
Uronema caudatum
uropepsin
uroporphyrin
uroporphyrinogen I, III
uroreaction
urosheum. See *Eurotium.*

Uruma virus
usimuleum. See *Eusimulium.*
utriatoma. See *Eutriatoma.*
utrombikula. See
 Eutrombicula.
vaccinate
vaccine
vacuolation
vacuole
 autophagic v.
 contractile v.
 plasmocrine v.
 rhagiocrine v.
Vahlkampfia
valine
van den Bergh test
van Gieson's stain
Van Slyke test
Vaquez-Osler disease
Vaquez's disease
VDRL — Venereal Disease
 Research
 Laboratories
VDRL test
VEE virus — Venezuelan
 equine encephalomyelitis
 virus
Veillonella
 V. alcalescens
 V. discoides
 V. orbiculus
 V. parvula
 V. reniformis
 V. vulvovaginitidis
venipuncture
Verticillium
 V. graphii
Vi agglutination
Vi antigen
Vibrio
 V. alginolyticus
 V. bulbulus

Vibrio (continued)
 V. cholerae
 V. cholerae-asiaticae
 V. coli
 V. comma
 V. danubicus
 V. fecalis
 V. fetus
 V. finkleri
 V. ghinda
 V. jejuni
 V. massauah
 V. metchnikovii
 V. niger
 V. parahemolyticus
 V. phosphorescens
 V. proteus
 V. septicus
 V. tyrogenus
vibrio
 Celebes' v.
 cholera v.
 El Tor's v's
 non-agglutinating v's
 paracholera v's
vibrion
 v. septique
Vicia
 V. graminea
Vincent's organism
viral
virology
viruria
virus
 animal v's
 v. animatum
 arbor v's
 attenuated v.
 Australian X disease v.
 bacterial v.
 Brunhilde v.
 Bunyamwera v.

virus (*continued*)

    Bwamba fever v.
    C v.
    CA v.
    Cache valley v.
    California v.
    Chikungunya v.
    Coe v.
    Colorado tick fever v.
    coryza v.
    Coxsackie v.
    croup associated v.
    cytomegalic inclusion
      disease v.
    dengue v.
    eastern equine encephalo-
      myelitis v.
    EBV v.
    ECBO v.
    ECDO v.
    ECHO v.
    ECHO 28 v.
    ECMO v.
    ECSO v.
    EEE v.
    EMC v.
    encephalomyocarditis v.
    enteric orphan v's
    entomopox v.
    epidemic keratoconjunc-
      tivitis v.
    Epstein-Barr v.
    equine encephalomye-
      litis v.
    filterable v.
    fixed v.
    Guaroa v.
    hemadsorption v. types
      1 and 2
    hepatitis v.
    herpangina v.
    herpes v.

virus (*continued*)

    Ilheus v.
    inclusion conjunctivitis v.
    influenza v.
    Japanese B encephalitis v.
    JH v.
    Junin v.
    Kumba v.
    Kyasanur Forest disease v.
    Lansing v.
    Lassa v.
    latent v.
    Leon v.
    lepori pox v.
    louping ill v.
    Lunyo v.
    lymphocytic chorio-
      meningitis v.
    lymphogranuloma
      venereum v.
    masked v.
    Mayaro v.
    Mengo v.
    Murray Valley
      encephalitis v.
    Newcastle disease v.
    O'nyong-nyong v.
    ornithosis v.
    Oropouche v.
    orphan v's
    pappataci fever v.
    parainfluenza v.
    parapox v.
    parrot v.
    pharyngoconjunctival
      fever v.
    pneumonitis v.
    poliomyelitis v.
    polyoma v.
    Powassan v.
    poxvirus v.
    psittacosis v.

virus (*continued*)
    rabies v.
    respiratory syncytial v.
    Rift Valley fever v.
    RS v.
    rubella v.
    Russian spring-summer
      encephalitis v.
    salivary gland v.
    Semliki Forest v.
    Sendai v.
    Simbu v.
    simian v's
    Sindbis v.
    St. Louis encephalitis v.
    street v.
    Teschen v.
    Theiler's v.
    tick-borne v's
    trachoma v.
    2060 v.
    Uganda S v.
    unorganized v.
    Uruma v.
    vaccine v.
    varicella-zoster v.
    variola v.
    VEE v.
    WEE v.
    Wesselsbron v.
    western equine encephal-
      omyelitis v.
    West Nile v.
viscosimeter
    Stormer v.
viscosity
viscous
VMA — vanillylmandelic acid
Voges-Proskauer
    broth
    test
Volhard's test

volumetric
Wade-Fite-Faraco stain
Waldenström's macroglobulin-
    emia
washing
    bronchial w.
Wassermann
    reaction
    test
Watson-Schwartz test
WBC — white blood cell
    white blood count
WBC/hpf — white blood cells
    per high power
    field
WEE virus — Western equine
    encephalomyeli-
    tis virus
Weichselbaum's diplococcus
Weigert's stain
Weil-Felix reaction
Wesselsbron virus
Westergren's sedimentation
    rate
western equine encephalo-
    myelitis virus
West Nile virus
whipworm
Whitmore's bacillus
Widal reaction
Wilkins-Chilgren agar
Wintrobe's sedimentation rate
Wohlgemuth unit
Wright's stain
Wuchereria
    W. bancrofti
    W. malayi
wuchereriasis
xanthochromatic
xanthocyte
xanthomatous
Xanthomonas

X chromosome
X chromatin bodies
Xenopsylla
    X. cheopis
Xenopus
    X. laevis
xeroradiography
D-xylose tolerance test
Y chromosome
Yersinia
    Y. enterocolitica
    Y. pestis
    Y. pseudotuberculosis

Yersinieae
zantho-. See words beginning
    xantho-.
Zenker's fixative
Zeta sedimentation rate
Ziehl-Neelsen's stain
Zoogloea
Zuberella
Zygomyces
Zygomycetes
Zygomycosis
Zymobacterium
zymogen

REFERENCE VALUES IN HEMATOLOGY

	CONVENTIONAL UNITS		FACTOR	S.I. UNITS	NOTES
Acid hemolysis test (Ham)	No hemolysis		—	No hemolysis	
Alkaline phosphatase, leukocyte	Total score 14–100		—	Total score 14–100	
Carboxyhemoglobin	Up to 5% of total		0.01	0.05 of total	a
Cell counts					
Erythrocytes			10^6		
Males	4.6–6.2 million/cu. mm.			$4.6–6.2 \times 10^{12}/l$	
Females	4.2–5.4 million/cu. mm.			$4.2–5.4 \times 10^{12}/l$	
Children (varies with age)	4.5–5.1 million/cu. mm.			$4.5–5.1 \times 10^{12}/l$	
Leukocytes			10^6		
Total	4500–11,000/cu. mm.			$4.5–11.0 \times 10^9/l$	
Differential	*Percentage*	*Absolute*	10^6		b
Myelocytes	0	0/cu. mm.		0/l	
Band neutrophils	3–5	150–400/cu. mm.		$150–400 \times 10^6/l$	
Segmented neutrophils	54–62	3000–5800/cu. mm.		$3000–5800 \times 10^6/l$	
Lymphocytes	25–33	1500–3000/cu. mm.		$1500–3000 \times 10^6/l$	
Monocytes	3–7	300–500/cu. mm.		$300–500 \times 10^6/l$	
Eosinophils	1–3	50–250/cu. mm.		$50–250 \times 10^6/l$	
Basophils	0–0.75	15–50/cu. mm.		$15–50 \times 10^6/l$	
Platelets	150,000–350,000/cu. mm.		10^6	$150–350 \times 10^9/l$	b
Reticulocytes	0.5–1.5% of erythrocytes		10^6	$25–75 \times 10^9/l$	
Coagulation tests					
Bleeding time (Duke)	1–5 min.		—	1–5 min	
Bleeding time (Ivy)	Less than 5 min.		—	Less than 5 min	
Clot retraction, qualitative	Begins in 30–60 min.		—	Begins in 30–60 min	
	Complete in 24 hrs.		—	Complete in 24 h	
Coagulation time (Lee-White)	5–15 min. (glass tubes)		—	5–15 min (glass tubes)	
	19–60 min. (siliconized tubes)		—	19–60 min (siliconized tubes)	
Euglobulin lysis time	2–6 hr. at 37°		—	2–6 h at 37 C	
Factor VIII and other coagulation factors	50–150% of normal		—	0.50–1.5 of normal	a

Fibrin split products (Thrombo-Wellco test)	Negative at 1:4 dilution	—	Negative at 1:4 dilution	c
Fibrinogen	200–400 mg/100 ml.	0.0293	5.9–11.7 μmol/l	
Fibrinolysins	0	—	0	
Partial thromboplastin time, activated (APTT)	35–45 sec.	—	35–45 s	
Prothrombin consumption	Over 80% consumed in 1 hr.	0.01	Over 0.80 consumed in 1 h	a
Prothrombin content	100% (calculated from prothrombin time)	0.01	1.0 (calculated from prothrombin time)	a
Prothrombin time (one stage)	12.0–14.0 sec.	—	12.0–14.0 s	
Thromboplastin generation test	Compared to normal control	—	Compared to normal control	
Tourniquet test	Ten or fewer petechiae in a 2.5 cm. circle after 5 min.	—	Ten or fewer petechiae in a 2.5 cm circle after 5 min	
Cold hemolysin test (Donath-Land-steiner)	No hemolysis	—	No hemolysis	
Coombs test				
Direct	Negative	—	Negative	
Indirect	Negative	—	Negative	
Corpuscular values of erythrocytes (values are for adults; in children, values vary with age)				
M.C.H. (mean corpuscular hemoglobin)	27–31 picogm.	0.0155	0.42–0.48 fmol	d
M.C.V. (mean corpuscular volume)	80–105 cu. micra	1.0	80–105 fl	a
M.C.H.C. (mean corpuscular hemoglobin concentration)	32–36%	0.01	0.32–0.36	
Haptoglobin (as hemoglobin binding capacity)	100–200 mg/100 ml.	0.155	16–31 μmol/l	d
Hematocrit				
Males	40–54 ml/100 ml.	0.01	0.40–0.54	a
Females	37–47 ml/100 ml.		0.37–0.47	
Newborn	49–54 ml/100 ml.		0.49–0.54	
Children (varies with age)	35–49 ml/100 ml.		0.35–0.49	
Hemoglobin				
Males	14.0–18.0 grams/100 ml.	0.155	2.17–2.79 mmol/l	d
Females	12.0–16.0 grams/100 ml.		1.86–2.48 mmol/l	
Newborn	16.5–19.5 grams/100 ml.		2.56–3.02 mmol/l	
Children (varies with age)	11.2–16.5 grams/100 ml.		1.74–2.56 mmol/l	

REFERENCE VALUES IN HEMATOLOGY (Continued)

	CONVENTIONAL UNITS	FACTOR	S.I. UNITS	NOTES
Hemoglobin, fetal	Less than 1% of total	0.01	Less than 0.01 of total	a
Hemoglobin A₁c	3–5% of total	0.01	0.03–0.05 of total	a
Hemoglobin A₂	1.5–3.0% of total	0.01	0.015–0.03 of total	a
Hemoglobin, plasma	0–5.0 mg./100 ml.	0.155	0–0.8 μmol/l	d
Methemoglobin	0–130 mg./100 ml.	0.155	4.7–20 μmol/l	e
Osmotic fragility of erythrocytes	Begins in 0.45–0.39% NaCl	171	Begins in 77–67 mmol/l NaCl	
	Complete in 0.33–0.30% NaCl		Complete in 56–51 mmol/l NaCl	
Sedimentation rate				
Wintrobe: Males	0–5 mm. in 1 hr.	—	0–5 mm/h	
Females	0–15 mm. in 1 hr.	—	0–15 mm/h	
Westergren: Males	0–15 mm. in 1 hr.	—	0–15 mm/h	
Females	0–20 mm. in 1 hr.	—	0–20 mm/h	
(May be slightly higher in children and during pregnancy)				
Bone marrow, differential cell count				

	Range	Average	FACTOR	Range	Average	
Myeloblasts	0.3–5.0%	2.0%	0.01	0.003–0.05	0.02	
Promyelocytes	1.0–8.0%	5.0%		0.01–0.08	0.05	
Myelocytes: Neutrophilic	5.0–19.0%	12.0%		0.05–0.19	0.12	
Eosinophilic	0.5–3.0%	1.5%		0.005–0.03	0.015	
Basophilic	0.0–0.5%	0.3%		0.00–0.005	0.003	
Metamyelocytes	13.0–32.0%	22.0%		0.13–0.32	0.22	
Polymorphonuclear neutrophils	7.0–30.0%	20.0%		0.07–0.30	0.20	
Polymorphonuclear eosinophils	0.5–4.0%	2.0%		0.005–0.04	0.02	
Polymorphonuclear basophils	0.0–0.7%	0.2%		0.00–0.007	0.002	
Lymphocytes	3.0–17.0%	10.0%		0.03–0.17	0.10	
Plasma cells	0.0–2.0%	0.4%		0.00–0.02	0.004	
Monocytes	0.5–5.0%	2.0%		0.005–0.05	0.02	
Reticulum cells	0.1–2.0%	0.2%		0.001–0.02	0.002	
Megakaryocytes	0.3–3.0%	0.4%		0.003–0.03	0.004	
Pronormoblasts	1.0–8.0%	4.0%		0.01–0.08	0.04	
Normoblasts	7.0–32.0%	18.0%		0.07–0.32	0.18	

REFERENCE VALUES FOR BLOOD, PLASMA AND SERUM

(For some procedures the reference values may vary depending upon the method used)

	CONVENTIONAL UNITS	FACTOR	S.I. UNITS	NOTES
Acetoacetate plus acetone, serum				
Qualitative	Negative	—	Negative	
Quantitative	0.3–2.0 mg./100 ml.	10	3–20 mg/l	
Adrenocorticotropin (ACTH), plasma	10–80 picogm./ml.	1.0	10–80 ng/l	
Aldolase, serum	0–11 milliunits/ml. (I.U.) (30°)	1.0	0–11 units/l (30 C)	f
Alpha amino nitrogen, serum	3.0–5.5 mg./100 ml.	0.714	2.1–3.9 mmol/l	
Ammonia, plasma	20–120 mcg./100 ml.	0.554	11–67 μmol/l	
Amylase, serum	Less than 160 Caraway units/100 ml.	—	Less than 160 Caraway units/dl	f
Anion gap	8–16 mEq./l.	1.0	8–16 mmol/l	
Ascorbic acid, blood	0.4–1.5 mg./100 ml.	56.8	23–85 μmol/l	
Base excess, blood	0 ± 2 mEq./liter	1.0	0 ± 2 mmol/l	
Bicarbonate, serum	23–29 mEq./liter	1.0	23–29 mmol/l	
Bile acids, serum	0.3–3.0 mg./dl.	10	3.0–30.0 mg/l	
Bilirubin, serum				
Direct	0.1–0.4 mg./100 ml.	17.1	1.7–6.8 μmol/l	
Indirect	0.2–0.7 mg./100 ml. (Total minus direct)	17.1	3.4–12 μmol/l (Total minus direct)	
Total	0.3–1.1 mg./100 ml.	17.1	5.1–19 μmol/l	
Bromsulphalein (BSP) (Inject 5 mg/kg. body weight, draw sample at 45 min.)	Less than 5%	0.01	Less than 0.05	a
Calcium, serum	4.5–5.5 mEq./liter	0.50	2.25–2.75 mmol/l	
	9.0–11.0 mg./100 ml.	0.25	2.25–2.75 mmol/l	
	(Slightly higher in children)		(Slightly higher in children)	
	(Varies with protein concentration)		(Varies with protein concentration)	
Calcium, ionized, serum	2.1–2.6 mEq./liter	0.50	1.05–1.30 mmol/l	
	4.25–5.25 mg./100 ml.	0.25	1.05–1.30 mmol/l	
Carbon dioxide content, serum				
Adults	24–30 mEq./liter	1.0	24–30 mmol/l	
Infants	20–28 mEq./liter	1.0	20–28 mmol/l	

REFERENCE VALUES FOR BLOOD, PLASMA AND SERUM (Continued)

(For some procedures the reference values may vary depending upon the method used)

	CONVENTIONAL UNITS	FACTOR	S.I. UNITS	NOTES
Carbon dioxide tension (Pco₂), blood	35–45 mm. Hg	—	35–45 mm Hg	
Carotene, serum	50–300 mcg./100 ml.	0.0186	0.93–5.58 μmol/l	g
Ceruloplasmin, serum	23–44 mg./100 ml.	0.0662	1.5–2.9 μmol/l	h
Chloride, serum	96–106 mEq./liter	1.0	96–106 mmol/l	
Cholesterol, serum				
Total	150–250 mg./100 ml.	0.0259	3.9–6.5 mmol/l	
Esters	68–76% of total cholesterol	0.01	0.68–0.76 of total cholesterol	a
Cholinesterase				
Serum	0.5–1.3 pH units	—	0.5–1.3 pH units	f
Erythrocytes	0.5–1.0 pH unit	—	0.5–1.0 pH unit	f
Copper, serum				
Males	70–140 mcg./100 ml.	0.157	11–22 μmol/l	
Females	85–155 mcg./100 ml.	0.157	13–24 μmol/l	
Cortisol, plasma (8 A.M.)	6–29 mcg./100 ml.	27.6	170–635 nmol/l	
Creatine, serum	0.2–0.8 mg./100 ml.	76.3	15–61 μmol/l	
Creatine phosphokinase, serum				
Males	0–50 milliunits/ml. (I.U.) (30°)	1.0	0–50 units/l (30 C)	f
Females	0–30 milliunits/ml. (I.U.) (30°) (Oliver-Rosalki)	1.0	0–30 units/l (30 C) (Oliver-Rosalki)	f
Creatine phosphokinase isoenzymes, serum				
CPK-MM	Present	—	Present	
CPK-MB	Absent	—	Absent	
CPK-BB	Absent	—	Absent	
Creatinine, serum	0.7–1.5 mg./100 ml.	88.4	62–133 μmol/l	
Cryoglobulins, serum	0	—	0	
Fatty acids, total, serum	190–420 mg./100 ml.	0.0352	7–15 mmol/l	
Ferritin, serum	20–200 nanogm./ml.	1.0	20–200 μg/l	i
Fibrinogen, plasma	200–400 mg./100 ml.	0.0293	5.9–11.7 μmol/l	
Folate, serum	5–21 nanogm./ml.	2.27	11–48 nmol/l	c

Test	Conventional value	Factor	SI value	
Follicle stimulating hormone (FSH), plasma				
Males	4–25 milliunits/ml. (I.U.)	1.0	4–25 IU/l	f
Females	4–30 milliunits/ml. (I.U.)		4–30 IU/l	f
Postmenopausal	40–250 milliunits/ml. (I.U.)		40–250 IU/l	
Gamma glutamyltransferase				
Males	6–32 milliunits/ml. (I.U.) (30°)	1.0	6–32 units/l (30 C)	
Females	4–18 milliunits/ml. (I.U.) (30°)	1.0	4–18 units/l (30 C)	
Gastrin, serum	0–200 picogm./ml.	1.0	0–200 ng/l	
Glucose (fasting)				
Blood	60–100 mg./100 ml.	0.0555	3.33–5.55 mmol/l	d
Plasma or serum	70–115 mg./100 ml.	0.0555	3.89–6.38 mmol/l	
Growth hormone, serum	0–10 nanogm./ml.	1.0	0–10 µg/l	f
Haptoglobin, serum	100–200 mg./100 ml.	0.155	16–31 µmol/l	
	(As hemoglobin binding capacity)		(As hemoglobin binding capacity)	
Hydroxybutyric dehydrogenase, serum	0–180 milliunits/ml. (I.U.) (30°) (Rosalki-Wilkinson)	1.0	0–180 units/l (30 C) (Rosalki-Wilkinson)	f, j
17-Hydroxycorticosteroids, plasma	8–18 mcg./100 ml.	0.0276	0.22–0.50 µmol/l	
Immunoglobulins, serum				
IgG	550–1900 mg./100 ml.	0.01	5.5–19.0 g/l	k
IgA	60–333 mg./100 ml.	0.01	0.60–3.3 g/l	
IgM	45–145 mg./100 ml.	0.01	0.45–1.5 g/l	
	(Varies with age in children)		(Varies with age in children)	
Insulin, plasma (fasting)	5–25 microunits/ml.	1.0	5–25 milliunits/l	
Iodine, protein bound, serum	3.5–8.0 mcg./100 ml.	0.0788	0.28–0.63 µmol/l	a
Iron, serum	75–175 mcg./100 ml.	0.179	13–31 µmol/l	l
Iron binding capacity, serum				
Total	250–410 mcg./100 ml.	0.179	45–73 µmol/l	
Saturation	20–55%	0.01	0.20–0.55	
17-Ketosteroids, plasma	25–125 mcg./100 ml.	0.0347	0.87–4.34 µmol/l	
Lactate, blood, venous	0.6–1.8 mEq./liter	1.0	0.6–1.8 mmol/l	
Lactate dehydrogenase, serum	0–300 milliunits/ml. (I.U.) (30°) (Wroblewski modified)	1.0	0–300 units/l (30 C) (Wroblewski modified)	f
	150–450 units/ml. (Wroblewski)	—	150–450 units/ml (Wroblewski)	
	80–120 units/ml. (Wacker)	—	80–120 units/ml (Wacker)	

REFERENCE VALUES FOR BLOOD, PLASMA AND SERUM (Continued)

(For some procedures the reference values may vary depending upon the method used)

	CONVENTIONAL UNITS	FACTOR	S.I. UNITS	NOTES
Lactate dehydrogenase isoenzymes, serum				
LDH₁	22–37% of total	0.01	0.22–0.37 of total	a
LDH₂	30–46% of total		0.30–0.46 of total	
LDH₃	14–29% of total		0.14–0.29 of total	
LDH₄	5–11% of total		0.05–0.11 of total	
LDH₅	2–11% of total		0.02–0.11 of total	
Leucine aminopeptidase, serum	14–40 milliunits/ml. (I.U.) (30°)	1.0	14–40 units/l (30 C)	f
Lipase, total, serum	0–1.5 units (Cherry-Crandall)	—	0–1.5 units (Cherry-Crandall)	f
Lipids, total, serum	450–850 mg/100 ml.	0.01	4.5–8.5 g/l	m
Lutenizing hormone (LH), serum				
Males	6–18 milliunits/ml. (I.U.)	1.0	6–18 IU/l	
Females, premenopausal	5–22 milliunits/ml. (I.U.)	1.0	5–22 IU/l	
midcycle	3 times baseline		3 times baseline	
postmenopausal	Greater than 30 milliunits/ml. (I.U.)		Greater than 30 IU/l	
Magnesium, serum	1.5–2.5 mEq./liter	0.50	0.75–1.25 mmol/l	
5'-Nucleotidase, serum	Less than 1.6 milliunits/ml. (I.U.) (30°)	1.0	Less than 1.6 units/l (30 C)	f
Nitrogen, nonprotein, serum	15–35 mg/100 ml.	0.714	10.7–25.0 mmol/l	
Osmolality, serum	285–295 mOsm./kg. serum water	—	285–295 mmol/kg serum water	n
Oxygen, blood				
Capacity	16–24 vol.% (varies with hemo-globin)	0.446	7.14–10.7 mmol/l (varies with hemoglobin)	o
Content Arterial	15–23 vol.%	0.446	6.69–10.3 mmol/l	o
Venous	10–16 vol.%	0.446	4.46–7.14 mmol/l	o
Saturation Arterial	94–100% of capacity	0.01	0.94–1.00 of capacity	a
Venous	60–85% of capacity	0.01	0.60–0.85 of capacity	a
Tension, pO₂ Arterial	75–100 mm. Hg	—	75–100 mm Hg	g
P₅₀, blood	26–27 mm. Hg	—	26–27 mm Hg	g
pH, arterial, blood	7.35–7.45	—	7.35–7.45	p
Phosphatase, acid, serum	Less than 3 mg/100 ml.	0.0605	Less than 0.18 mmol/l	
	0–7.0 milliunits/ml. (I.U.) (30°)	1.0	0–7.0 units/l (30 C)	f
	1.0–5.0 units (King-Armstrong)	—	1.0–5.0 units (King-Armstrong)	
Phosphatase, alkaline, serum	10–32 milliunits/ml. (I.U.) (30°)	1.0	10–32 units/l (30 C)	f
	5.0–13.0 units (King-Armstrong) (Values are higher in children)	—	5.0–13.0 units (King-Armstrong) (Values are higher in children)	

Test	Conventional Value	Factor	SI Value	
Phosphate, inorganic, serum				
Adults	3.0–4.5 mg/100 ml.	0.323	1.0–1.5 mmol/l	
Children	4.0–7.0 mg/100 ml.		1.3–2.3 mmol/l	
Phospholipids, serum	6–12 mg/100 ml.	0.323	1.9–3.9 mmol/l	
	(As lipid phosphorus)		(As lipid phosphorus)	
Potassium, serum	3.5–5.0 mEq./liter	1.0	3.5–5.0 mmol/l	
Protein, serum				
Total	6.0–8.0 grams/100 ml.	10	60–80 g/l	
Albumin	3.5–5.5 grams/100 ml.	10	35–55 g/l	m
		0.154	0.54–0.85 mmol/l	q
Phosphate, inorganic, serum				
Adults	3.0–4.5 mg/100 ml.	0.323	1.0–1.5 mmol/l	
Children	4.0–7.0 mg/100 ml.		1.3–2.3 mmol/l	
Phospholipids, serum	6–12 mg/100 ml.	0.323	1.9–3.9 mmol/l	
	(As lipid phosphorus)		(As lipid phosphorus)	
Potassium, serum	3.5–5.0 mEq./liter	1.0	3.5–5.0 mmol/l	
Protein, serum				
Total	6.0–8.0 grams/100 ml.	10	60–80 g/l	
Albumin	3.5–5.5 grams/100 ml.	10	35–55 g/l	m
		0.154	0.54–0.85 mmol/l	q
Globulin	2.5–3.5 grams/100 ml.	10	25–35 g/l	q
Electrophoresis				
Albumin	3.5–5.5 grams/100 ml.	10	35–55 g/l	
	52–68% of total	0.01	0.52–0.68 of total	a
Globulin				
Alpha$_1$	0.2–0.4 gram/100 ml.	10	2–4 g/l	m
	2–5% of total	0.01	0.02–0.05 of total	a
Alpha$_2$	0.5–0.9 gram/100 ml.	10	5–9 g/l	m
	7–14% of total	0.01	0.07–0.14 of total	a
Beta	0.6–1.1 grams/100 ml.	10	6–11 g/l	m
	9–15% of total	0.01	0.09–0.15 of total	a
Gamma	0.7–1.7 grams/100 ml.	10	7–17 g/l	m
	11–21% of total	0.01	0.11–0.21 of total	a
Protoporphyrin, erythrocyte	27–61 mcg/100 ml. packed RBC	0.0178	0.48–1.09 µmol/l packed RBC	
Pyruvate, blood	0.01–0.11 mEq./liter	1.0	0.01–0.11 mmol/l	
Sodium, serum	136–145 mEq./liter	1.0	136–145 mmol/l	
Sulfates, inorganic, serum	0.8–1.2 mg/100 ml.	104	83–125 µmol/l	
Testosterone, plasma				
Males	275–875 nanogm./100 ml.	0.0347	9.5–30 nmol/l	
Females	23–75 nanogm./100 ml.	0.0347	0.8–2.6 nmol/l	
Pregnant	38–190 nanogm./100 ml.	0.0347	1.3–6.6 nmol/l	

REFERENCE VALUES FOR BLOOD, PLASMA AND SERUM *(Continued)*

(For some procedures the reference values may vary depending upon the method used)

	CONVENTIONAL UNITS	FACTOR	S.I. UNITS	NOTES
Thyroid stimulating hormone (TSH), serum	0–7 microunits/ml.	1.0	0–7 milliunits/l	
Thyroxine, free, serum	1.0–2.1 nanogm./100 ml.	12.9	13–27 pmol/l	
Thyroxine (T₄), serum	4.4–9.9 mcg./100 ml.	12.9	57–128 nmol/l	
Thyroxine binding globulin (TBG), serum (as thyroxine)	10–26 mcg./100 ml.	12.9	129–335 nmol/l	
Thyroxine iodine, serum	2.9–6.4 mcg./100 ml.	78.8	229–504 nmol/l	k
Tri-iodothyronine (T₃), serum	150–250 nanogm./100 ml.	0.0154	2.3–3.9 nmol/l	a
Tri-iodothyronine (T₃) uptake, resin (T₃RU)	25–38%	0.01	0.25–0.38 uptake	
Transaminase, serum				
SGOT (aspartate aminotransferase)	0–19 millunits/ml. (I.U.) (30°) (Karmen modified)	1.0	0–19 units/l (30 C) (Karmen modified)	f
	15–40 units/ml. (Karmen)		15–40 units/ml (Karmen)	
	18–40 millunits/ml. (Reitman-Frankel)		18–40 units/ml (Reitman-Frankel)	
SGPT (alanine aminotransferase)	0–17 millunits/ml. (I.U.) (30°) (Karmen modified)	1.0	0–17 units/l (30 C) (Karmen modified)	f
	6–35 units/ml. (Karmen)		6–35 units/ml (Karmen)	
	5–35 units/ml. (Reitman-Frankel)		5–35 units/ml (Reitman-Frankel)	
Triglycerides, serum	40–150 mg./100 ml.	0.01	0.4–1.5 g/l	r
Urate (serum)		0.0114	0.45–1.71 mmol/l	
Males	2.5–8.0 mg./100 ml.	0.0595	0.15–0.48 mmol/l	
Females	1.5–7.0 mg./100 ml.	0.0595	0.09–0.42 mmol/l	
Urea				
Blood	21–43 mg./100 ml.	0.167	3.5–7.2 mmol/l	
Plasma or serum	24–49 mg./100 ml.	0.167	4.0–8.2 mmol/l	
Urea nitrogen				
Blood	10–20 mg./100 ml.	0.714	7.1–14.3 mmol/l	
Plasma or serum	11–23 mg./100 ml.	0.714	7.9–16.4 mmol/l	
Vitamin A, serum	20–80 mcg./100 ml.	0.0349	0.70–2.8 μmol/l	
Vitamin B₁₂, serum	180–900 picogrm./ml.	0.738	133–664 pmol/l	k

REFERENCE VALUES FOR URINE

(For some procedures the reference values may vary depending upon the method used)

	CONVENTIONAL UNITS	FACTOR	S.I. UNITS	NOTES
Acetone and acetoacetate, qualitative	Negative	—	Negative	
Addis count				
Erythrocytes	0–130,000/24 hrs.	—	0–130 000/24 h	
Leukocytes	0–650,000/24 hrs.	—	0–650 000/24 h	
Casts (hyaline)	0–2000/24 hrs.	—	0–2000/24 h	
Albumin				
Qualitative	Negative	—	Negative	
Quantitative	10–100 mg./24 hrs.	—	10–100 mg/24 h	q
Aldosterone	3–20 mcg./24 hrs.	0.0154	0.15–1.5 μmol/24 h	
Alpha amino nitrogen	50–200 mg./24 hrs.	2.77	8.3–55 nmol/24 h	
Ammonia nitrogen	20–70 mEq./24 hrs.	0.0714	3.6–14.3 mmol/24 h	
Amylase	35–260 Caraway units/hr.	1.0	35–260 Caraway units/h	
Bilirubin, qualitative	Negative	—	Negative	f
Calcium				
Low Ca diet	Less than 150 mg./24 hrs.	0.025	Less than 3.8 mmol/24 h	
Usual diet	Less than 250 mg./24 hrs.	0.025	Less than 6.3 mmol/24 h	
Catecholamines				
Epinephrine	Less than 10 mcg./24 hrs.	5.46	Less than 55 nmol/24 h	s
Norepinephrine	Less than 100 mcg./24 hrs.	5.91	Less than 590 nmol/24 h	t
Total free catecholamines	4–126 mcg./24 hrs.	5.91	24–745 nmol/24 h	
Total metanephrines	0.1–1.6 mg./24 hrs.	5.07	0.5–8.1 μmol/24 h	
Chloride	110–250 mEq./24 hrs.	1.0	110–250 mmol/24 h	
	(Varies with intake)		(Varies with intake)	
Chorionic gonadotropin	0	—	0	
Copper	0–50 mcg./24 hrs.	0.0157	0–0.80 μmol/24 h	
Creatine				
Males	0–40 mg./24 hrs.	0.00762	0–0.30 mmol/24 h	
Females	0–100 mg./24 hrs.	0.00762	0–0.76 mmol/24 h	
	(Higher in children and during pregnancy)		(Higher in children and during pregnancy)	
Creatinine	15–25 mg./kg. body weight/24 hrs.	0.00884	0.13–0.22 mmol·kg^{-1} body weight/24 h	

REFERENCE VALUES FOR URINE (Continued)

(For some procedures the reference values may vary depending upon the method used)

	CONVENTIONAL UNITS	FACTOR	S.I. UNITS	NOTES
Creatinine clearance				
Males	110–150 ml/min.	—	110–150 ml/min	
Females	105–132 ml/min. (1.73 sq. meter surface area)	—	105–132 ml/min (1.73 m² surface area)	
Cystine or cysteine, qualitative	Negative	—	Negative	
Dehydroepiandrosterone	Less than 15% of total 17-keto-steroids	0.01	Less than 0.15 of total 17-keto-steroids	a
Delta aminolevulinic acid	1.3–7.0 mg./24 hrs.	7.63	10–53 μmol/24 h	
Estrogens				
Males				
Estrone	3–8 μg./24 hrs.	3.70	11–30 nmol/24 h	
Estradiol	0–6 μg./24 hrs.	3.67	0–22 nmol/24 h	
Estriol	1–11 μg./24 hrs.	3.47	3–38 nmol/24 h	
Total	4–25 μg./24 hrs.	3.60	14–90 nmol/24 h	u
Females				
Estrone	4–31 μg./24 hrs.	3.70	15–115 nmol/24 h	
Estradiol	0–14 μg./24 hrs.	3.67	0–51 nmol/24 h	
Estriol	0–72 μg./24 hrs.	3.47	0–250 nmol/24 h	
Total	5–100 μg./24 hrs.	3.60	18–360 nmol/24 h	u
	(Markedly increased during pregnancy)		(Markedly increased during pregnancy)	
Glucose (as reducing substance)	Less than 250 mg/24 hrs.	—	Less than 250 mg/24 h	
Gonadotropins, pituitary	10–50 mouse units/24 hrs.	—	10–50 mouse units/24 h	
Hemoglobin and myoglobin, qualitative	Negative	—	Negative	
Homogentisic acid, qualitative	Negative	—	Negative	
17-Hydroxycorticosteroids				
Males	3–9 mg./24 hrs.	2.76	8.3–25 μmol/24 h	j
Females	2–8 mg./24 hrs.		5.5–22 μmol/24 h	
5-Hydroxyindoleacetic acid				
Qualitative	Negative	—	Negative	
Quantitative	Less than 9 mg/24 hrs.	5.23	Less than 47 μmol/24 h	
17-Ketosteroids				
Males	6–18 mg./24 hrs.	3.47	21–62 μmol/24 h	1
Females	4–13 mg./24 hrs.		14–45 μmol/24 h	
	(Varies with age)		(Varies with age)	

Magnesium	6.0–8.5 mEq./24 hrs.	0.5	3.0–4.3 mmol/24 h
Metanephrines (see Catecholamines)			
Osmolality	38–1400 mOsm./kg. water	—	38–1400 mmol/kg water	n
pH	4.6–8.0, average 6.0	—	4.6–8.0, average 6.0	p
	(Depends on diet)		(Depends on diet)
Phenolsulfonphthalein excretion (PSP)	25% or more in 15 min.	0.01	0.25 or more in 15 min	a
	40% or more in 30 min.		0.40 or more in 30 min
	55% or more in 2 hrs.		0.55 or more in 2 h
	(After injection of 1 ml PSP intra-		(After injection of 1 ml PSP intra-
	venously)		venously)
Phenylpyruvic acid, qualitative	Negative	—	Negative
Phosphorus	0.9–1.3 gm./24 hrs.	32.3	29–42 mmol/24 h
Porphobilinogen			
Qualitative	Negative	—	Negative
Quantitative	0–2 mg./100 ml.	4.42	0–0.9 μmol/l
	Less than 2.0 mg./24 hrs.		Less than 9 μmol/24 h
Porphyrins			
Coproporphyrin	50–250 mcg./24 hrs.	1.53	77–380 nmol/24 h
Uroporphyrin	10–30 mcg./24 hrs.	1.20	12–36 nmol/24 h
Potassium	25–100 mEq./24 hrs.	1.0	25–100 mmol/24 h
	(Varies with intake)		(Varies with intake)
Pregnanediol	0.4–1.4 mg./24 hrs.	3.12	1.2–4.4 μmol/24 h
Males			
Females			
Proliferative phase	0.5–1.5 mg./24 hrs.		1.6–4.7 μmol/24 h
Luteal phase	2.0–7.0 mg./24 hrs.		6.2–22 μmol/24 h
Postmenopausal phase	0.2–1.0 mg./24 hrs.		0.6–3.1 μmol/24 h
Pregnanetriol	Less than 2.5 mg./24 hrs. in adults	2.97	Less than 7.4 μmol/24 h in adults
Protein			
Qualitative	Negative	—	Negative
Quantitative	10–150 mg./24 hrs.	—	10–150 mg/24 h
Sodium	130–260 mEq./24 hrs.	1.0	130–260 mmol/24 h
	(Varies with intake)		(Varies with intake)
Specific gravity	1.003–1.030	—	1.003–1.030
Titratable acidity	20–40 mEq./24 hrs.	1.0	20–40 mmol/24 h
Urate	200–500 mg./24 hrs.	0.00595	1.2–3.0 mmol/24 h
	(With normal diet)		(With normal diet)
Urobilinogen	Up to 1.0 Ehrlich unit/2 hrs.	—	Up to 1.0 Ehrlich unit/2 h
	(1–3 P.M.)		(1–3 P.M.)
Vanillylmandelic acid (VMA)	0–4.0 mg./24 hrs.	—	0–4.0 mg/24 h
(4-hydroxy-3-methoxymandelic acid)	1–8 mg./24 hrs.	5.05	5–40 μmol/24 h	m

REFERENCE VALUES FOR THERAPEUTIC DRUG MONITORING

DRUG	THERAPEUTIC RANGE	TOXIC LEVELS	PROPRIETARY NAMES
Antibiotics			
Amikacin, serum	15–25 mcg./ml.	Peak: > 35 mcg./ml. Trough: > 5 mcg./ml.	Amikin
Chloramphenicol, serum	10–20 mcg./ml.	> 25 mcg./ml.	Chloromycetin
Gentamicin, serum	5–10 mcg./ml.	Peak: > 12 mcg./ml. Trough: > 2 mcg./ml.	Garamycin
Tobramycin, serum	5–10 mcg./ml.	Peak: > 12 mcg./ml. Trough: > 2 mcg./ml.	Nebcin
Anticonvulsants			
Carbamazepine, serum	5–12 mcg./ml.	> 15 mcg./ml.	Tegretol
Ethosuximide, serum	40–80 mcg./ml.	> 150 mcg./ml.	Zarontin
Phenobarbital, serum	10–25 mcg./ml.	Vary widely because of developed tolerance	
Phenytoin, serum (diphenylhydantoin)	10–20 mcg./ml.	> 20 mcg./ml.	Dilantin
Primidone, serum	4–12 mcg./ml.	> 15 mcg./ml.	Mysoline
Valproic acid, serum	50–100 mcg./ml.	> 200 mcg./ml.	Depakene
Anti-inflammatory agents			
Acetaminophen, serum	10–20 mcg./ml.	> 250 mcg./ml.	Tylenol
Salicylate, serum	100–250 mcg./ml.	> 300 mcg./ml.	Datril
Bronchodilator			
Theophylline (aminophylline)	10–20 mcg./ml.	> 20 mcg./ml.	

Cardiovascular drugs		
Digitoxin, serum	15–25 nanogm./ml.	Crystodigin
	(Specimen obtained 12–24 hrs. after last dose) >25 nanogm./ml.	
Digoxin, serum	0.8–2 nanogm./ml.	Lanoxin
	(Specimen obtained 12–24 hrs. after last dose) >2.4 nanogm./ml.	
Disopyramide, serum	2–4 mcg./ml. >7 mcg./ml.	Norpace
Lidocaine, serum	1.5–5 mcg./ml. >7 nanogm./ml.	Anestacon
		Xylocaine
		Pronestyl
Procainamide, serum	4–10 mcg./ml. >16 mcg./ml.	
	*8–16 mcg./ml. *>20 mcg./ml.	
	(*Procainamide + N-Acetyl Procainamide)	
Propranolol, serum	50–100 nanogm./ml. Variable	Inderal
Quinidine, serum	2–5 mcg./ml. >10 mcg./ml.	Cardioquin
		Quinaglute
		Quinidex
		Quinora
Psychopharmacologic drugs		
Amitriptyline, serum	*120–150 nanogm./ml. *>500 nanogm./ml.	Amitril
	(*Amitriptyline + Nortriptyline)	Elavil
		Endep
		Etrafon
		Limbitrol
		Triavil
		Librium
		Norpramin
Chlordiazepoxide, serum	1–3 mcg./ml. >5 mcg./ml.	Pertofrane
Desipramine, serum	*150–250 nanogm./ml. *>500 nanogm./ml.	Valium
	(*Desipramine + Imipramine)	Antipress
Diazepam, serum	0.5–2.5 mcg./ml. >5 mcg./ml.	Imavate
Imipramine, serum	*150–250 nanogm./ml. *>500 nanogm./ml.	Janimine
	(*Imipramine + Desipramine)	Presamine
		Tofranil
Lithium, serum	0.8–1.5 mEq./liter >2.0 mEq./liter	
	(Specimen obtained 12 hrs. after last dose)	
Nortriptyline, serum	50–150 nanogm./ml. >500 nanogm./ml.	Aventyl
		Pamelor

REFERENCE VALUES IN TOXICOLOGY

	CONVENTIONAL UNITS	FACTOR	S.I. UNITS	NOTES
Arsenic, blood	3.5–7.2 mcg/100 ml.	0.133	0.47–0.96 μmol/l	
Arsenic, urine	Less than 100 mcg/24 hrs.	0.0133	Less than 1.3 μmol/24 h	
Bromides, serum	0	1.0	0	a
	Toxic levels:		Toxic levels:	
	Above 17 mEq/liter		Above 17 mmol/l	
Carbon monoxide, blood	Up to 5% saturation	—	Up to 0.05 saturation	
	Symptoms occur with 20% satura-		Symptoms occur with 0.20 satura-	
	tion		tion	
Ethanol, blood	Less than 0.005%	217	Less than 1 mmol/l	
Marked intoxication	0.3–0.4%		65–87 mmol/l	
Alcoholic stupor	0.4–0.5%		87–109 mmol/l	
Coma	Above 0.5%		Above 109 mmol/l	
Lead, blood	0–40 mcg/100 ml.	0.0483	0–2 μmol/l	
Lead, urine	Less than 100 mcg/24 hrs.	0.00483	Less than 0.48 μmol/24 h	
Mercury, urine	Less than 10 mcg/24 hrs.	4.98	Less than 50 nmol/24 h	

REFERENCE VALUES FOR CEREBROSPINAL FLUID

	CONVENTIONAL UNITS	FACTOR	S.I. UNITS	NOTES
Cells	Fewer than 5/cu. mm.; all mono-nuclear	—	Fewer than 5/μl; all mononuclear	
Chloride	120–130 mEq/liter	1.0	120–130 mmol/l	
	(20 mEq./liter higher than serum)		(20 mmol/l higher than serum)	
Electrophoresis	Predominantly albumin	—	Predominantly albumin	
Glucose	50–75 mg/100 ml.	0.0555	2.8–4.2 mmol/l	
	(20 mg./100 ml. less than serum)		(1.1 mmol/l less than serum)	
IgG				
Children under 14	Less than 8% of total protein	—	Less than 0.08 of total protein	a,m
Adults	Less than 14% of total protein		Less than 0.14 of total protein	
Pressure	70–180 mm. water		70–180 mm water	g
Protein, total	15–45 mg./100 ml.	0.01	0.150–0.450 g/l	m
	(Higher, up to 70 mg./100 ml., in elderly adults and children)		(Higher, up to 0.70 g/l, in elderly adults and children)	

REFERENCE VALUES FOR GASTRIC ANALYSIS

	CONVENTIONAL UNITS	FACTOR	S.I. UNITS	NOTES
Basal gastric secretion (1 hour)				
Concentration	(Mean ± 1 S.D.)	1.0	(Mean ± 1 S.D.)	
Males	25.8 ± 1.8 mEq/liter		25.8 ± 1.8 mmol/l	
Females	20.3 ± 3.0 mEq/liter		20.3 ± 3.0 mmol/l	
Output	(Mean ± 1 S.D.)	1.0	(Mean ± 1 S.D.)	
Males	2.57 ± 0.16 mEq/hr.		2.57 ± 0.16 mmol/h	
Females	1.61 ± 0.18 mEq/hr.		1.61 ± 0.18 mmol/h	
After histamine stimulation		1.0		
Normal	Mean output 11.8 mEq/hr.		Mean output 11.8 mmol/h	
Duodenal ulcer	Mean output 15.2 mEq/hr.		Mean output 15.2 mmol/h	
After maximal histamine stimulation		1.0		
Normal	Mean output 22.6 mEq/hr.		Mean output 22.6 mmol/h	
Duodenal ulcer	Mean output 44.6 mEq/hr.		Mean output 44.6 mmol/h	
Diagnex blue (Squibb): Anacidity	0–0.3 mg. in 2 hrs.	—	0–0.3 mg in 2 h	
Doubtful	0.3–0.6 mg. in 2 hrs.	—	0.3–0.6 mg in 2 h	
Normal	Greater than 0.6 mg. in 2 hrs.	—	Greater than 0.6 mg in 2 h	
Volume, fasting stomach content	50–100 ml.	—	0.05–0.11	
Emptying time	3–6 hrs.	—	3–6 h	
Color	Opalescent or colorless	—	Opalescent or colorless	
Specific gravity	1.006–1.009	—	1.006–1.009	
pH (adults)	0.9–1.5	—	0.9–1.5	P

GASTROINTESTINAL ABSORPTION TESTS

	CONVENTIONAL UNITS	FACTOR	S.I. UNITS	NOTES
d-Xylose absorption test	After an 8 hour fast, 10 ml/kg. body weight of a 0.05 solution of d-xylose is given by mouth. Nothing further by mouth is given until the test has been completed. All urine voided during the following 5 hours is pooled, and blood samples are taken at 0, 60, and 120 minutes. Normally 0.26 (range 0.16–0.33) of ingested xylose is excreted within 5 hours, and the serum xylose reaches a level between 25 and 40 mg/100 ml. after 1 hour and is maintained at this level for another 60 minutes.		No change	
Vitamin A absorption	A fasting blood specimen is obtained and 200,000 units of vitamin A in oil is given by mouth. Serum vitamin A level should rise to twice fasting level in 3 to 5 hours.		No change	

REFERENCE VALUES FOR FECES

	CONVENTIONAL UNITS	FACTOR	S.I. UNITS	NOTES
Bulk	100–200 grams/hrs.	—	100–200 g/24 h	
Dry matter	23–32 grams/24 hrs.	—	23–32 g/24 h	
Fat, total	Less than 6.0 grams/24 hrs.	—	Less than 6.0 g/24 h	
Nitrogen, total	Less than 2.0 grams/24 hrs.	—	Less than 2.0 g/24 h	
Urobilinogen	40–280 mg/24 hrs.	—	40–280 mg/24 h	
Water	Approximately 65%	0.01	Approximately 0.65	a

REFERENCE VALUES FOR SEMEN ANALYSIS

	CONVENTIONAL UNITS	FACTOR	S.I. UNITS	NOTES
Volume	2-5 ml.; usually 3-4 ml.	—	2-5 ml; usually 3-4 ml	
Liquefaction	Complete in 15 min.	—	Complete in 15 min	p
pH	7.2-8.0; average 7.8	—	7.2-8.0; average 7.8	
Leukocytes	Occasional or absent	—	Occasional or absent	
Count	60-150 million/ml.	—	60-150 million/ml	
	Below 60 million/ml. is abnormal	—	Below 60 million/ml is abnormal	
Motility	80% or more motile	—	0.80 or more motile	a
Morphology	80-90% normal forms	—	0.80-0.90 normal forms	a

PANCREATIC (ISLET) FUNCTION TESTS

Glucose tolerance tests		
Oral	Patient should be on a diet containing 300 grams of carbohydrate per day for 3 days prior to test. After ingestion of 100 grams of glucose or 1.75 grams glucose/kg. body weight, blood glucose is not more than 160 mg./100 ml. after 60 minutes, 140 mg./100 ml. after 90 minutes, and 120 mg./100 ml. after 120 minutes. Values are for blood; serum measurements are approximately 15% higher.	Cortisone-glucose tolerance test	The patient should be on a diet containing 300 grams of carbohydrate per day for 3 days prior to test. At 8½ and again 2 hours prior to glucose load patient is given cortisone acetate by mouth (50 mg. if patient's ideal weight is less than 160 lb., 62.5 mg. if ideal weight is greater than 160 lb.). An oral dose of glucose, 1.75 grams/kg. body weight, is given and blood samples are taken at 0, 30, 60, 90, and 120 minutes. Test is considered positive if true blood glucose exceeds 160 mg./100 ml. at 60 minutes, 140 mg./100 ml. at 90 minutes, and 120 mg./100 ml. at 120 minutes. Values are for blood; serum measurements are approximately 15% higher.
Intravenous	Blood glucose does not exceed 200 mg./100 ml. after infusion of 0.5 gram of glucose/kg. body weight over 30 minutes. Glucose concentration falls below initial level at 2 hours and returns to preinfusion levels in 3 or 4 hours. Values are for blood; serum measurements are approximately 15% higher.		

REFERENCE VALUES FOR IMMUNOLOGIC PROCEDURES

	CONVENTIONAL UNITS		FACTOR	S.I. UNITS	NOTES
Syphilis serology (RPR and VDRL)	Negative			No change	
Mono screen	Negative			No change	
R.A. test (latex)	1:40	Doubtful		No change	
	1:80–1:160	Positive			
	1:320	Positive			
Rose test	1:10	Negative		No change	
	1:20–1:40	Doubtful			
	1:80	Positive			
Anti-streptolysin O titer	Normal up to 1:128. Single test usually has little significance. Rise in titer or persistently elevated titer is significant.			No change	
Anti-hyaluronidase titer	Less than 1:200. Significant if rising titer can be demonstrated at weekly intervals.			No change	
C-reactive protein	Negative			No change	
Anti-nuclear antibody	One specimen is sufficient, unless the result is inconsistent with the clinical impression. Most patients with active lupus have high ANA titers (160 or greater); some have lower titers (20–40). Patients with inactive lupus may have a negative test. Antinuclear antibodies are occasionally present in patients with no evidence of systemic lupus, usually in lower titers (20–40).			No change	
Febrile agglutinins	Titers of 1:80 or greater may be significant, particularly if subsequent samples show rise in titer.			No change	
Tularemia agglutinins	1:80	Negative		No change	
	1:160	Doubtful			
	1:320	Positive			
Proteus OX-19 agglutinins	Titers of 1:80 or greater may be significant, particularly if subsequent samples show rise in titer.			No change	
Complement fixation tests	Titers of 1:8 or less are usually not significant. Paired sera showing rise in titer of more than two tubes are usually considered significant.			No change	
C3 Test	80–140 mg/100 ml.		0.01	0.80–1.40 g/l	
C4 Test	11–75 mg/100 ml.		0.01	0.11–0.75 g/l	q

NOTES

a. Percentage is expressed as a decimal fraction.

b. Percentage may be expressed as a decimal fraction; however, when the result expressed is itself a variable fraction of another variable, the absolute value is more meaningful. There is no reason, other than custom, for expressing reticulocyte counts and differential leukocyte counts in percentages or decimal fractions rather than in absolute numbers.

c. Molecular weight of fibrinogen = 341,000 daltons.

d. Molecular weight of hemoglobin = 64,500 daltons. Because of disagreement as to whether the monomer or tetramer of hemoglobin should be used in the conversion, it has been recommended that the conventional grams per deciliter be retained. The tetramer is used in the table; values given should be multiplied by 4 to obtain concentration of the monomer.

e. Molecular weight of methemoglobin = 64,500 daltons. See note d above.

f. Enzyme units have not been changed in these tables because the proposed enzyme unit, the katal, has not been universally adopted (1 International Unit = 16.7 nkat).

g. It has been proposed that pressure be expressed in the Pascal (1 mm Hg = 0.133 kPa); however, this convention has not been universally accepted.

h. Molecular weight of ceruloplasmin = 151,000.

i. "Fatty acids" includes a mixture of different aliphatic acids of varying molecular weight. A mean molecular weight of 284 has been assumed in calculating the conversion factor.

j. Based upon molecular weight of cortisol 362.47.

k. The practice of expressing concentration of an organic molecule in terms of one of its constituent elements originated when measurements included a heterogeneous class of compounds (nonprotein nitrogenous compounds, iodine-containing compounds bound to serum proteins). It was carried over to expressing measurements of specific substances (urea, thyroxine), but the practice should be discarded. For iodine and nitrogen 1 mole is taken as the monoatomic form, although they occur as diatomic molecules.

l. Based upon molecular weight of dehydroepiandrosterone 288.41.

m. Weight per volume is retained as the unit because of the heterogeneous nature of the material measured.

n. The proposal that osmolality be reported as freezing point depression using the millikelvin as the unit has not been received with universal enthusiasm. The milliosmole is not an S.I. unit, and the unit used here is the millimole.

o. Volumes per cent might be converted to a decimal fraction; however, this would not permit direct correlation with hemoglobin content, which is possible when oxygen content and capacity are expressed in molar quantities. One millimole of hemoglobin combines with 4 millimoles of oxygen.

p. Hydrogen ion concentration in S.I. units would be expressed in nanomoles per liter; however, this change has not received general approval. Conversion can be calculated as antilog $(-\text{pH})$.

q. Albumin is expressed in grams per liter to be consistent with units used for other proteins.

Concentration of albumin may be expressed in mmol/l also, an expression that permits assessment of binding capacity of albumin for substances such as bilirubin. Molecular weight of albumin is 65,000.

r. Most techniques for quantitating triglycerides measure the glycerol moiety, and the total mass is calculated using an average molecular weight. The factor given assumes a mean molecular weight of 875 for triglycerides.

s. Calculated as norepinephrine, molecular weight 169.18.

t. Calculated as metanephrine, molecular weight 197.23.

u. Conversion factor calculated from molecular weights of estrone, estradiol, and estriol in proportions of 2:1:2.

REFERENCES

1. AMA Drug Evaluations. 4th ed. Chicago, American Medical Association, 1980.
2. Baron, D. N., Broughton, P. M. G., Cohen, M., Lansley, T. S., Lewis, S. M., and Shinton, N. K.: J. Clin. Path. 27:590, 1974.
3. Dybkaer, R.: Am. J. Clin. Path. 52:637, 1969.
4. Goodman, L. S., and Gilman, A.: Pharmacologic Basis of Therapeutics. 5th ed. New York, Macmillan, 1975.
5. Henry, J. B.: Clinical Diagnosis and Management by Laboratory Methods, 16th ed. Philadelphia, W. B. Saunders Company, 1979.
6. Henry, R. J., Cannon, D. C., and Winkleman, J. W.: Clinical Chemistry—Principles and Techniques, 2nd ed. New York, Harper & Row, 1974.
7. International Committee for Standardization in Hematology, International Federation of Clinical Chemistry and World Association of Pathology Societies: Clin. Chem. 19:135, 1973.
8. Lehmann, H. P.: Amer. J. Clin. Path. 65:2, 1976.

9. Miale, J. B.: Laboratory Medicine — Hematology, 5th ed. St. Louis, C. V. Mosby, 1977.

10. Page, C. H., and Vigoureux, P.: The International System of Units (S.I.). U.S. Department of Commerce, National Bureau of Standards, Special Publication 330, 1974.

11. Physicians' Desk Reference. 34th ed. Oradell, N.J., Medical Economics Company, 1980.

12. Scully, R. E., McNeely, B. U., and Galdabini, J. J.: N. Engl. J. Med. *302*:37, 1980.

13. Tietz, N. W.: Fundamentals of Clinical Chemistry, 2nd ed. Philadelphia, W. B. Saunders Company, 1976.

14. Wintrobe, M. D., Lee, G. R., Boggs, D. R., Bithell, T. C., Athens, J. W., and Foerster, J.: Clinical Hematology. 7th ed. Philadelphia, Lea & Febiger, 1974.

15. Young, D. S.: N. Engl. J. Med., *292*:795, 1975.

II

SYSTEMS AND SPECIALTIES

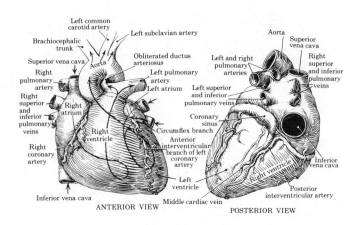

Left common carotid artery

Left subclavian artery

Brachiocephalic trunk

Obliterated ductus arteriosus

Superior vena cava

Aorta

Left pulmonary artery

Right pulmonary artery

Left atrium

Right superior and inferior pulmonary veins

Right atrium

Right ventricle

Circumflex branch

Anterior interventricular branch of left coronary artery

Right coronary artery

Left ventricle

Inferior vena cava

Middle cardiac vein

ANTERIOR VIEW

Aorta

Superior vena cava

Right superior and inferior pulmonary veins

Left and right pulmonary arteries

Left superior and inferior pulmonary veins

Coronary sinus

Right ventricle

Inferior vena cava

Posterior interventricular artery

POSTERIOR VIEW

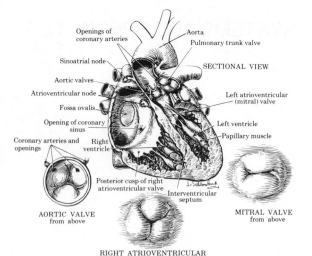

Openings of coronary arteries

Aorta

Pulmonary trunk valve

Sinoatrial node

SECTIONAL VIEW

Aortic valves

Atrioventricular node

Fossa ovalis

Left atrioventricular (mitral) valve

Opening of coronary sinus

Left ventricle

Papillary muscle

Coronary arteries and openings

Right ventricle

Posterior cusp of right atrioventricular valve

Interventricular septum

AORTIC VALVE from above

MITRAL VALVE from above

RIGHT ATRIOVENTRICULAR (TRICUSPID) VALVE from above

DETAILS OF STRUCTURE OF THE HEART

(Courtesy of Dorland's Illustrated Medical Dictionary, 26th ed. Plate XX. Philadelphia, W. B. Saunders Company, 1981.)

CARDIOVASCULAR SYSTEM

A_2 — aortic second sound
AA — ascending aorta
ABE — acute bacterial
      endocarditis
Abée's support
aberrant
Abrams' heart reflex
AC — anodal closure
      anterior chamber
      aortic closure
ACC — anodal closing
      contraction
accelerans
accretio
      a. cordis
      a. pericardii
ACD — absolute cardiac
      dullness
achalasia
acromioclavicular
Adams' disease
Adams-Stokes
    disease
    syncope
    syndrome
Addison's disease
ADG — atrial diastolic gallop
adipositas
      a. cordis

Adson's
    forceps
    hook
    needle
    retractor
adventitious
aerendocardia
AF — aortic flow
    atrial fibrillation
    atrial flutter
AG — atrial gallop
AHD — arteriosclerotic heart
      disease
      atherosclerotic heart
      disease
AI — aortic incompetence
    aortic insufficiency
    apical impulse
Alexander-Farabeuf
    periosteotome
Alfred M. Large's clamp
ALG — antilymphocyte
      globulin
Allen's test
Allison's retractor
allorhythmia
allorhythmic
all or none law
Allport-Babcock searcher

alternans
    a. of the heart
Alvarez' prosthesis
AMI — acute myocardial
    infarction
Amtech-Killeen pacemaker
amyloid
anastomosis
anesthesia. See *General*
    Surgical Terms.
aneurysm
    abdominal a.
    aortic arch a.
    aortic sinusal a.
    arteriovenous a.
    axial a.
    Bérard's a.
    cardiac a.
    cylindroid a.
    cystogenic a.
    dissecting a.
    ectatic a.
    embolic a.
    embolomycotic a.
    endogenous a.
    erosive a.
    exogenous a.
    fusiform a.
    luetic a.
    mycotic a.
    Park's a.
    popliteal a.
    Pott's a.
    Richet's a.
    Rodrigues' a.
    saccular a.
    syphilitic a.
    thoracic a.
    traumatic a.
    ventricular a.
aneurysmal
aneurysmectomy

aneurysmogram
aneurysmoplasty
aneurysmorrhaphy
aneurysmotomy
angialgia
angiasthenia
angiectasis
angiectatic
angiectid
angiectomy
angiectopia
angiemphraxis
angiitis
angileucitis
angina
    a. cordis
    a. decubitus
    a. dyspeptica
    exertional a.
    hysteric a.
    a. inversa
    a. pectoris
    a. pectoris vasomotoria
    Prinzmetal's a.
    a. sine dolore
    variant a. pectoris
anginal
anginiform
anginoid
anginose
anginosis
angioataxia
angioblast
angioblastic
angioblastoma
angiocardiogram
angiocardiography
angiocardiokinetic
angiocardiopathy
angiocarditis
angioclast
angiodiascopy

angiodiathermy
angioedema
angiogenesis
angiogenic
angiogram
angiograph
angiography
angiohypertonia
angiohypotonia
angioinvasive
angiokinesis
angiokinetic
angiolipoma
angiolith
angiolithic
angiologia
angiology
angioma
angiomatosis
angiometer
angiomyocardiac
angioneoplasm
angioneumography
angioneurosis
angioneurotomy
angionoma
angioparalysis
angioparesis
angiopathology
angiopathy
angioplasty
    percutaneous trans-
      luminal a.
angiopressure
angiorrhaphy
angiosclerosis
angiosclerotic
angiospasm
angiostomy
angiotelectasis
angiotensin
angiotribe

angloid
annuloplasty
annulus
anomaly
    Ebstein's a.
anoxemia
anoxia
    myocardial a.
    stagnant a.
anoxic
anteroposterior
anteroseptal
anticoagulant
AO — anodal opening
    aorta
    aortic opening
    opening of the atrio-
      ventricular valves
AOC — anodal opening
      contraction
aorta
    abdominal a.
    a. abdominalis
    a. ascendens
    ascending a.
    a. chlorotica
    a. descendens
    descending a.
    dextropositioned a.
    dynamic a.
    overriding a.
    palpable a.
    primitive a.
    a. sacrococcygea
    straddling a.
    a. thoracalis
    thoracic a.
    a. thoracica
    throbbing a.
    ventral a.
aortae
aortal

aortalgia
aortarctia
aortectasia
aortectasis
aortectomy
aortic
    a. insufficiency
    a. regurgitation
    a. stenosis
aorticopulmonary
aorticorenal
aortism
aortismus
    a. abdominalis
aortitis
    Dohle-Heller a.
    luetic a.
    nummular a.
    rheumatic a.
    syphilitic a.
    a. syphilitica
    a. syphilitica obliterans
aortoclasia
aortogram
    transbrachial arch a.
    translumbar a.
aortography
    retrograde a.
    translumbar a.
aortolith
aortomalacia
aortopathy
aortoptosia
aortorrhaphy
aortosclerosis
aortostenosis
aortotomy
AOS — anodal opening sound
AOT — anodal opening tetanus
AP — angina pectoris
    anteroposterior
    arterial pressure

APB — atrial premature beat
    auricular premature
      beat
APC — atrial premature
      contraction
apex
    a. cordis
apical
apices
apnea
apneic
appendage
    atrial a.
    auricular a.
AR — aortic regurgitation
    artificial respiration
arch
    aortic a.
Arco pacemaker
arcus
    a. aortae
area
    Bamberger's a.
Argyle's catheter
arrest
    cardiac a.
    sinus a.
arrhythmia
    inotropic a.
    nodal a.
    respiratory a.
    sinus a.
    vagus a.
arrhythmic
arterial
arterialization
arteriarctia
arteriasis
arteriectasis
arteriectomy
arterioatony
arteriocapillary

arteriodilating
arteriofibrosia
arteriogram
    femoral a.
    subclavian a.
arteriograph
arteriography
arteriolae
arteriolar
arteriole
arteriolith
arteriolitis
arteriolonecrosis
arteriolosclerosis
arteriolosclerotic
arteriomalacia
arteriometer
arteriomotor
arteriomyomatosis
arterionecrosis
arteriopalmus
arteriopathy
    hypertensive a.
arteriophlebotomy
arterioplania
arterioplasty
arteriorenal
arteriorrhagia
arteriorrhaphy
arteriorrhexis
arteriosclerosis
    cerebral a.
    coronary a.
    decrescent a.
    diffuse a.
    hyaline a.
    hypertensive a.
    infantile a.
    intimal a.
    Mönckeberg's a.
    nodose a.
    nodular a.

arteriosclerosis (*continued*)
    a. obliterans
    peripheral a.
    presenile a.
    senile a.
arteriosclerotic
arteriospasm
arteriostenosis
arteriosteogenesis
arteriostosis
arteriostrepsis
arteriosus
    patent ductus a.
    truncus a.
arteriosympathectomy
arteriotome
arteriotomy
arteriotony
arteriovenous
arterioversion
arteritis
    brachiocephalic a.
    a. deformans
    a. hyperplastica
    necrosing a.
    a. nodosa
    a. obliterans
    temporal a.
    a. umbilicalis
    a. verrucosa
artery
    brachial a.
    brachiocephalic a.
    carotid a.
    celiac a.
    circumflex a.
    coronary a.
    epicardial coronary a.
    esophageal a.
    femoral a.
    iliac a.
    innominate a.

artery (*continued*)
    intercostal a.
    interventricular a.
    marginal a.
    peroneal a.
    preventricular a.
    pulmonary a.
    renal a.
    subclavian a.
    tibial a.
artifact
AS — aortic stenosis
    arteriosclerosis
Aschoff's
    bodies
    node
Aschoff and Tawara node
ascites
ASCVD — arteriosclerotic
          cardiovascular
          disease
        atherosclerotic
          cardiovascular
          disease
ASD — atrial septal defect
asequence
ASH — asymmetrical septal
      hypertrophy
ASHD — arteriosclerotic
      heart disease
ASMI — anteroseptal
      myocardial infarct
ASO — arteriosclerosis
      obliterans
asphygmia
AST — aspartate aminotrans-
      ferase
asthenia
    neurocirculatory a.
asthma
    cardiac a.
    Elsner's a.

asthma (*continued*)
    Heberden's a.
    Rostan's a.
asynchronism
asystole
atelocardia
atheroma
atheromatous
atheronecrosis
atherosclerosis
atresia
    aortic a.
    tricuspid a.
atria
atrial
Atricor pacemaker
atriocommissuropexy
atriomegaly
atrionector
atrioseptopexy
atriotome
atriotomy
atrioventricular
atrium
    common a.
    a. cordis
    a. dextrum
    a. pulmonale
    pulmonary a.
    a. sinistrum
Auenbrugger's sign
auricle
auricula
    a. atrii
    a. atrii dextri
    a. atrii sinistri
    a. cordis
    a. dextra cordis
    a. sinistra cordis
auricular
auriculoventricular
auscultation

auscultatory
Austin Flint murmur
AV or A-V — arteriovenous
                 atrioventricular
AV or A-V
     dissociation
     heart block
avascular
AVR — aortic valve
               replacement
AVRP — atrioventricular
          · refractory period
A wave
awbooshma. See
     embouchment.
AWI — anterior wall infarction
awl
     Rochester's a.
     Wangensteen's a.
AWMI — anterior wall myo-
               cardial infarction
axis
Ayerza's syndrome
azotemia
azygography
azygos
Babinski's syndrome
Bachmann's bundle
bacterial endocarditis
Bahnson's clamp
Bailey-Gibbon rib contractor
Bailey-Glover-O'Neil knife
Bailey-Morse knife
Bailey's
     clamp
     rib contractor
Bainbridge's reflex
ballistocardiogram
ballistocardiograph
ballistocardiography
Bamberger's
     area
     bulbar pulse

Bamberger's (*continued*)
     sign
Bardic's cannula
Barlow's syndrome
Barraya's forceps
Baylor's sump
BE — bacterial endocarditis
Beardsley's dilator
beat
     capture b's
     ectopic b's
     nodal b's
     premature auricular b's
Beau's
     disease
     syndrome
Beck I operation
Beck II operation
Beck's
     clamp
     rasp
     triad
Béhier-Hardy sign
Bengolea's forceps
Bérard's aneurysm
Bernheim's syndrome
Bethune's rib shears
bicuspid
bifurcation
bigeminal
bigeminy
     nodal b.
Biotronik pacemaker
bipolar
bisferious
Bishop's sphygmoscope
biventricular
Björk-Shiley prosthesis
blade
     Cooley-Pontius b.
     DeBakey's b.
Blalock-Hanlen operation
Blalock-Taussig operation

block. See *heart block.*
blood
    deoxygenated b.
blow
    diastolic b.
body
    Aschoff's b's
Boettcher's forceps
Bosher's knife
Botallo's duct
Bouillaud's
    sign
    syndrome
    tinkle
Bouveret's
    disease
    syndrome
BP — blood pressure
brachiocephalic
Bradshaw-O'Neill clamp
bradycardia
    Branham's b.
    cardiomuscular b.
    clinostatic b.
    essential b.
    nodal b.
    postinfective b.
    sinoatrial b.
    sinus b.
    vagal b.
bradycardiac
bradycrotic
bradydiastole
bradydiastolia
bradytachycardia
Branham's
    bradycardia
    sign
Brauer's operation
Braunwald's
    prosthesis
    sign

Bright's murmur
Broadbent's sign
Brockenborough's sign
Brock's
    knife
    operation
    punch
bruit (brwe)
    aneurysmal b.
    b. de canon (brwe duh kahnaw)
    b. de choc (brwe duh shawk)
    b. de craquement (brwe duh krak maw)
    b. de cuir neuf (brwe duh kwer nuf)
    b. de diable (brwe duh de ahbl)
    b. de frolement (brwe duh frolmaw)
    b. de lime (brwe duh lem)
    b. de moulin (brwe duh moola)
    b. de parchemin (brwe duh parshmaw)
    b. de piaulement (brwe duh pyolmaw)
    b. de rape (brwe duh rahp)
    b. de rappel (brwe duh rahpel)
    b. de Roger (brwe duh rozha)
    b. de scie (brwe duh se)
    Roger's b.
    systolic b.
brwe. See *bruit.*
Buerger's disease
bulbus
    b. aortae

bulbus (*continued*)
    b. arteriosus
    b. caroticus
    b. cordis
    b. venae jugularis
bundle
    atrioventricular b.
    a-v. b.
    Bachmann's b.
    b. branch block
    b. of His
    Keith's b.
    Kent-His b.
    Kent's b.
    sino-atrial b.
    b. of Stanley-Kent
    Thorel's b.
Burford's rib spreader
Burger's triangle
bypass
    aortocoronary vein b.
    aortoiliac b.
    cardiopulmonary b.
    coronary artery b.
    femoropopliteal b.
    saphenous vein b.
CA — cardiac arrest
    coronary artery
CAB — coronary artery bypass
CABG — coronary artery
        bypass graft
cachexia
CAD — coronary artery disease
Cameron-Haight elevator
canalization
Cannon's endarterectomy loop
cannula
    Bardic's c.
    Floyd's c.
    Mayo's c.
    Morris' c.
    Rockey's c.

cannula (*continued*)
    Silastic coronary artery c.
    Soresi's c.
    venous c.
cannulate
cannulation
Cape Town prosthesis
capillary
    Meigs' c's
cardiac
cardialgia
cardianastrophe
cardiasthenia
cardiasthma
cardiectasis
cardiectomy
cardioaccelerator
cardioaortic
cardioarterial
cardiocairograph
cardiocele
cardiocentesis
cardiocirrhosis
cardioclasis
cardiodiaphragmatic
cardiodilator
cardiodiosis
cardiogenic
cardiogram
    echo c.
cardiograph
cardiography
Cardio-green
cardiohepatic
cardiohepatomegaly
cardioinhibitory
cardiokinetic
cardiolith
cardiologist
cardiology
cardiolysis
cardiomalacia

cardiomegalia
    c. glycogenica
        circumscripta
cardiomegaly
cardiomelanosis
cardiometer
cardiometry
cardiomotility
cardiomyoliposis
cardiomyopathy
cardiomyopexy
cardiomyotomy
cardionecrosis
cardionector
cardionephric
cardioneural
cardioneurosis
cardio-omentopexy
cardiopalmus
cardiopaludism
cardiopathy
    endocrine c.
cardiopericardiopexy
cardiopericarditis
cardiophone
cardioplegia
cardiopneumograph
cardiopneumonopexy
cardioptosis
cardiopulmonary
cardiorrhaphy
cardiorrhexis
cardioschisis
cardiosclerosis
cardioscope
cardiospasm
cardiosphygmogram
cardiosphygmograph
cardiosplenopexy
cardiosymphysis
cardiotachometer
cardiotomy

cardiotoxic
cardiovalvular
cardiovalvulitis
cardiovalvulotomy
cardiovascular
cardioversion
carditis
    rheumatic c.
    Sterges' c.
Carey-Coombs murmur
Carmalt's forceps
carotid
Carpentier's stent
Carter's retractor
Cartwright's prosthesis
catecholamine
catheter
    Argyle's c.
    Edwards' c.
    Fogarty's c.
    Lehman's c.
    NIH c.
    pigtail c.
    Swan-Ganz c.
    Teflon c.
catheterization
    cardiac c.
    hepatic vein c.
CC – cardiac cycle
CCU – coronary care unit
CD – cardiac disease
    cardiac dullness
    cardiovascular disease
CE – cardiac enlargement
Cegka's sign
cerebrocardiac
CF – cardiac failure
change
    QRS c's
    QRS-T c's
    ST segment c's
    T wave c's

Chardak-Greatbatch pacemaker
CHB — complete heart block
CHD — congenital heart disease
    coronary heart disease
Cheyne-Stokes respiration
CHF — congestive heart failure
choc
    c. en dome
cholesterol
chorda
    c. tendineae cordis
CI — cardiac index
    cardiac insufficiency
    coronary insufficiency
CICU — cardiology intensive
        care unit
       coronary intensive
        care unit
cineangiocardiography
cineangiography
cineradiography
circle
    c. of Willis
circulation
    extracorporeal c.
    systemic c.
circulatory
circulus
    c. arteriosus
    c. arteriosus cerebri
    c. articuli vasculosus
CK — creatine kinase
clamp
    Alfred M. Large's c.
    Bahnson's c.
    Bailey's c.
    Beck's c.
    Bradshaw-O'Neill c.
    bulldog c.
    Cooley's c.
    Crafoord's c.
    Crutchfield's c.

clamp (*continued*)
    Davis' c.
    DeBakey's c.
    Derra's c.
    Diethrich's shunt c.
    Edwards' c.
    Glover's c.
    Gross' c.
    Herbert-Adams c.
    Hopkins' c.
    Hufnagel's c.
    Hume's c.
    Humphries' c.
    Jacobson's c.
    Javid's bypass c.
    Johns Hopkins c.
    Juevenell's c.
    Kantrowicz's c.
    Kapp-Beck c.
    Kelly's c.
    McDonald's c.
    Nichols' c.
    Poppen-Blalock c.
    Poppen's c.
    Potts' c.
    Potts-Niedner c.
    Potts-Smith c.
    Reich-Nechtow c.
    Rienhoff's c.
    Rumel's c.
    Salibi's c.
    Satinsky's c.
    Selverstone's c.
    Shoemaker's c.
    Trendelenburg-
       Crafoord c.
claudication
    intermittent c.
    venous c.
clip
    Scoville-Lewis c.
    Smith's c.

clip (*continued*)
 Sugar's c.
clubbing
CO_2 — carbon dioxide
coarctation
 c. of the aorta
coeur
 c. en sabot
collapse
 hemodynamic c.
collateral
columnae
 c. carneae cordis
commissure
commissurorrhaphy
commissurotomy
communis
 atrioventricularis c.
compensation
complex
 Eisenmenger's c.
 Lutembacher's c.
 QRS c.
 QS c.
 ventricular c.
  (Q,R,S,T waves)
concretio
 c. cordis
conduction
 ventricular c.
congenital
congestion
congestive heart failure
contraction
 anodal closure c.
 anodal opening c.
 atrial premature c.
 automatic ventricular c.
 isometric c.
 nodal premature c.
 supraventricular
  premature c.

conus
 c. arteriosus
conversion
convertin
Cooley-Pontius blade
Cooley's
 clamp
 dilator
 forceps
 prosthesis
 retractor
 scissors
cor
 c. adiposum
 c. arteriosum
 c. biloculare
 c. bovinum
 c. dextrum
 c. hirsutum
 c. juvenum
 c. mobile
 c. pendulum
 c. pseudotriloculare
  biatriatum
 c. pulmonale
 c. sinistrum
 c. taurinum
 c. tomentosum
 c. triatriatum
 c. triloculare biatriatum
 c. triloculare
  biventriculare
 c. venosum
 c. villosum
Coratomic pacemaker
Cordis' pacemaker
Cordis Atricor pacemaker
Cordis-Ectocor pacemaker
Cordis' fixed-rate pacemaker
Cordis Ventricor pacemaker
coronarism
coronaritis

coronary
    c. bypass surgery
Corrigan's
    disease
    pulse
    respiration
    sign
Corvisart's
    disease
    facies
Coryllos'
    raspatory
    retractor
costotome
    Tudor-Edwards c.
counterpulsation
    intra-aortic balloon c.
Cournand's needle
CPB — cardiopulmonary
        bypass
CPI Maxilith pacemaker
CPI Minilith pacemaker
cpm — counts per minute
CPR — cardiopulmonary
        resuscitation
Crafoord's
    clamp
    forceps
Crawford-Cooley tunneler
Crawford's retractor
creatine kinase
crista
    c. supraventricularis
    c. terminalis atrii dextri
crus
    c. fasciculi atrioventri-
        cularis dextrum
    c. fasciculi atrioventri-
        cularis sinistrum
Crutchfield's clamp
Cruveilhier-Baumgarten
    murmur

crux
    c. of heart
cryocardioplegia
CT — cardiothoracic (ratio)
        carotid tracing
CTR — cardiothoracic ratio
Curry's needle
curve
    Traube's c's
Cushing's
    forceps
    needle
cusp
cuspis
    c. anterior valvae
        atrioventricularis
        dextrae
    c. anterior valvae
        atrioventricularis
        sinistrae
    c. anterior valvulae
        bicuspidalis
    c. anterior valvulae
        tricuspidalis
    c. medialis valvulae
        tricuspidalis
    c. posterior valvae
        atrioventricularis
        dextrae
    c. posterior valvae
        atrioventricularis
        sinistrae
    c. posterior valvulae
        bicuspidalis
    c. posterior valvulae
        tricuspidalis
    c. septalis valvae
        atrioventricularis
        dextrae
Cutter-SCDK prosthesis
Cutter-Smeloff prosthesis
CVA — cardiovascular accident

CVA (*continued*)
    cerebrovascular
      accident
CVS — cardiovascular surgery
    cardiovascular system
cyanosis
    shunt c.
    tardive c.
cyanotic
cyst
    pericardial c.
Dacron
    graft
    prosthesis
DAH — disordered action of
      the heart
Davidson's retractor
Davis' clamp
DeBakey-Bahnson forceps
DeBakey-Bainbridge forceps
DeBakey-Balfour retractor
DeBakey-Cooley
    dilator
    forceps
    retractor
DeBakey-Metzenbaum scissors
DeBakey's
    blade
    clamp
    forceps
    graft
    prosthesis
    scissors
    tunneler
decannulation
decompensation
decortication
    arterial d.
defect
    aortic septal d.
    aorticopulmonary d.
    atrial septal d.

defect (*continued*)
    atrioseptal d.
    endocardial cushion d.
    ostium primum d.
    ostium secundum d.
    septal d.
    ventricular septal d.
defibrillated
defibrillation
defibrillator
deflection
    Q-S d's
degeneration
    Mönckeberg's d.
    Quain's d.
Dehio's test
Delorme's operation
de Musset's sign
deoxygenated
depolarization
depressant
    cardiac d.
depression
    ST d.
    systolic d.
Derra's
    clamp
    dilator
    knife
Desault's ligation
devasation
    senile cortical d.
devascularization
deviation
    right axis d.
    ST-T d's
dextrocardia
    mirror-image d.
dextrocardiogram
dextroversion
DG — diastolic gallop
diaphoresis

diastasis
    d. cordis
diastole
diastolic
DIC — diffuse intravascular
      coagulation
      disseminated intra-
      vascular coagulation
Dick's dilator
dicliditis
diclidostosis
diet
    Karell's d.
    Kempner's d.
Diethrich's shunt clamp
Dieuaide's sign
digitalis
digitalism
digitalization
digitalized
dilatation
dilator
    Beardsley's d.
    Cooley's d.
    DeBakey-Cooley d.
    Derra's d.
    Dick's d.
    Gohrbrand's d.
    Jackson-Mosher d.
    Tubbs' d.
    Tucker's d.
diplocardia
disease
    Adams' d.
    Adams-Stokes d.
    Addison's d.
    Beau's d.
    Bouveret's d.
    Buerger's d.
    coronary artery d.
    Corrigan's d.
    Corvisart's d.

disease (*continued*)
    Duroziez's d.
    Eisenmenger's d.
    eosinophilic endomyo-
      cardial d.
    Hamman's d.
    Heller-Döhle d.
    Hodgson's d.
    Lenegre's d.
    Lev's d.
    Libman-Sacks d.
    Lutembacher's d.
    Pick's d.
    pulseless d.
    Raynaud's d.
    rheumatic heart d.
    Roger's d.
    Rummo's d.
    thyrotoxic heart d.
    von Willebrand's d.
    Wenckebach's d.
dissociation
    A-V d.
    auriculoventricular d.
Dittrich's stenosis
diuresis
diuretic
DM — diastolic murmur
DOE — dyspnea on exercise
      dyspnea on exertion
Dohle-Heller aortitis
Doyen's elevator
dressing. See *General Surgical
    Terms.*
Dressler's syndrome
drugs. See *Drugs and
    Chemistry* section.
Drummond's sign
duct
    d. of Botallo
ductus
    d. arteriosus

Duroziez's
    disease
    murmur
    sign
dyskinesia
dyskinetic
dysphagia
dyspnea
    cardiac d.
    exertional d.
    orthostatic d.
    paroxysmal d.
dyspneic
dyspneoneurosis
dyssynergia
dyssystole
Ebstein's anomaly
ECG — electrocardiogram
echo
    metallic e.
echocardiogram
echocardiography
Eck's fistula
Ectocor pacemaker
ectopia
    e. cordis
    e. cordis abdominalis
    e. cordis pectoral
edema
    cardiac e.
    interstitial e.
    pulmonary e.
    subpleural e.
EDP — end-diastolic pressure
Edwards'
    catheter
    clamp
    patch
    prosthesis
efficacy
Effler's ring

effusion
    pericardial e.
Einthoven's
    law
    triangle
Eisenmenger's
    complex
    disease
    syndrome
EKG — electrocardiogram
electrocardiogram
electrocardiograph
electrocardiography
    precordial e.
electrocardiophonogram
electrocardiophonograph
electrocardioscopy
electrocardioversion
electrode
Electrodyne pacemaker
electrofluoroscopy
electrokymography
electrophoresis
electrophysiology
    cardiac e.
electrostethograph
elevation
    ST segment e.
elevator
    Cameron-Haight e.
    Doyen's e.
    Hedblom's e.
    Matson's e.
    Overholt's e.
    Phemister's e.
    Sedillot's e.
elongation
Elsner's asthma
EM — ejection murmur
embolectomy
emboli

embolic
embolism
    air e.
    coronary e.
    paradoxical e.
    plasmodium e.
    pulmonary e.
    venous e.
embolus
embouchment
Emerson's pump
empyema
    e. of pericardium
    pulsating e.
endaortic
endaortitis
    bacterial e.
endarterectomize
endarterectomy
endarterial
endarteritis
    e. deformans
    Heubner's specific e.
    e. obliterans
    e. proliferans
endarterium
endarteropathy
endartery
end-diastolic
endoaneurysmorrhaphy
endocardial
endocarditis
    acute bacterial e.
    e. benigna
    e. chordalis
    e. lenta
    Löffler's e.
    malignant e.
    mural e.
    mycotic e.
    nonbacterial thrombo-e.

endocarditis (*continued*)
    plastic e.
    polypous e.
    pulmonic e.
    pustulous e.
    rheumatic e.
    rickettsial e.
    septic e.
    subacute bacterial e.
    syphilitic e.
    ulcerative e.
    valvular e.
    vegetative e.
    verrucous e.
    viridans e.
endocardium
endophlebitis
    e. hepatica obliterans
    proliferative e.
endostethoscope
endothelium
endovasculitis
engorgement
Engström respirator
enzyme
eparterial
epicardia
epicardiectomy
epicardiolysis
epicardium
Erben's reflex
Erb's point
ergocardiogram
ergocardiography
Erlanger's sphygmomanometer
erythromelalgia
ESM — ejection systolic
        murmur
ethmocarditis
E to F slope
Eustace Smith's murmur

Evans' forceps
Ewart's sign
excitation
    anomalous atrioventri-
        cular e.
extrasystole
    auricular e.
    auriculoventricular e.
    infranodal e.
    interpolated e.
    nodal e.
    retrograde e.
    ventricular e.
facies
    Corvisart's f.
Fallot
    pentalogy of F.
    tetralogy of F.
    trilogy of F.
fascicle
Faught's sphygmomanometer
fenestration
    aortopulmonary f.
feokromositoma. See
    pheochromocytoma.
fever
    rheumatic f.
fiber
    Purkinje's f's
fibrillation
    atrial f.
    auricular f.
    ventricular f.
fibroelastosis
    endocardial f.
fibrosis
    arteriocapillary f.
Fiedler's myocarditis
filter
    Mobin-Uddin umbrella f.
Finochietto's rib spreader
Fisher's murmur

fissure
    Henle's f's
fistula
    arteriovenous f.
    congenital coronary f.
    coronary artery f.
    Eck's f.
Fitzgerald's forceps
Flack's node
fleb-. See words beginning
    phleb-.
Flint's murmur
flowmeter
flow tract
Floyd's cannula
flutter
    atrial f.
    auricular f.
    impure f.
    pure f.
    ventricular f.
flutter-fibrillation
Flynt's needle
Fogarty's catheter
foramen
    Galen's f.
    f. ovale cordis
    f. venae cavae
foramina venarum minimarum
    cordis
forceps
    Adson's f.
    Barraya's f.
    Bengolea's f.
    Boettcher's f.
    Carmalt's f.
    Cooley's f.
    Crafoord's f.
    Cushing's f.
    DeBakey-Bahnson f.
    DeBakey-Bainbridge f.
    DeBakey-Cooley f.

forceps *(continued)*
  DeBakey's f.
  Evans' f.
  Fitzgerald's f.
  Foss' f.
  Glover's f.
  Harken's f.
  Harrington's f.
  Hendren's f.
  Horsley's f.
  Jacobson's f.
  Johns Hopkins f.
  Julian's f.
  Lebsche's f.
  Leland-Jones f.
  Leriche's f.
  Liston-Stille f.
  Love-Gruenwald f.
  McNealy-Glassman-
    Mixter f.
  Mixter's f.
  Mount-Mayfield f.
  O'Shaughnessy's f.
  Potts-Smith f.
  Rienhoff's f.
  Rumel's f.
  Ruskin's f.
  Satinsky's f.
  Sauerbruch's f.
  Selman's f.
  Semb's f.
  Stille-Luer f.
  Stille's f.
  Vanderbilt's f.
Foss' forceps
fossa
  f. ovalis cordis
F & R — force and rhythm
Fraentzel's murmur
fragmentation
  f. of myocardium
Fränkel's treatment

fremitus
  pericardial f.
fren-. See words beginning
    phren-.
Friedreich's sign
frolement
furrow
  atrioventricular f.
F waves
Galen's foramen
ganglia
  cardiac g.
  g. cardiaca
  Wrisberg's g.
gasendarterectomy
General Electric pacemaker
George Lewis technique
Gibbon-Landis test
Gibson's
  murmur
  vestibule
Giertz-Shoemaker rib shears
glomera
  g. aortica
glomus
  g. carotideum
Glover's
  clamp
  forceps
Gluck's rib shears
glycosuria
Gohrbrand's dilator
Goldberg-MPC mediastino-
    scope
Gortex's graft
Gott's prosthesis
Gower's syndrome
gradient
  ventricular g.
graft
  autogenous vein g.
  cross-leg g.

graft (*continued*)
        Dacron g.
        DeBakey's g.
        femoropopliteal bypass g.
        Gortex's g.
        saphenous vein bypass g.
        Weavenit patch g.
Graham Steell murmur
groove
        deltopectoral g.
Gross'
        clamp
        retractor
Gross-Pomeranz-Watkins
        retractor
Hamman's
        disease
        murmur
Harken's
        forceps
        prosthesis
        rib spreader
Harrington-Pemberton
        retractor
Harrington's
        forceps
        operation
        retractor
HB — heart block
HCVD — hypertensive cardio-
        vascular disease
HD — heart disease
HDH — heart disease history
HDL — high density lipo-
        proteins
heart
        armored h.
        athletic h.
        beriberi h.
        bovine h.
        chaotic h.
        encased h.

heart (*continued*)
        extracorporeal h.
        fibroid h.
        flask-shaped h.
        frosted h.
        hyperthyroid h.
        hypoplastic h.
        intracorporeal h.
        irritable h.
        luxus h.
        myxedema h.
        paracorporeal h.
        Quain's fatty h.
        tabby cat h.
        Traube's h.
        triatrial h.
        triocular h.
        vertical h.
        wandering h.
        wooden-shoe h.
heart block
        arborization h.b.
        atrioventricular h.b.
        A-V h.b.
        bundle-branch h.b.
        complete h.b.
        congenital h.b.
        fascicular h.b.
        incomplete h.b.
        interventricular h.b.
        intraventricular h.b.
        Mobitz' h.b.
        partial h.b.
        sino-auricular h.b.
        subjunctional h.b.
        Wenckebach's h.b.
heart failure
        backward h.f.
        congestive h.f.
        forward h.f.
        high output h.f.
        left ventricular h.f.

heart failure (*continued*)
    right ventricular h.f.
heart-lung machine
Heberden's asthma
Hedblom's
    elevator
    retractor
Heller-Döhle disease
hemangioma
hemartoma
hemithorax
hemodynamic
hemopericardium
hemopneumopericardium
hemoptysis
    cardiac h.
hemorrhage
Hendren's forceps
Henle's
    fissures
    membrane
heparinize
Herbert-Adams clamp
hertz
heterograft
Heubner's specific endarteritis
HHD — hypertensive heart
    disease
hiatus
    aortic h.
Hibbs' retractor
His
    bundle of H.
His-Tawara node
Hodgson's disease
holodiastolic
holosystolic
Holter monitor
Holt-Oram syndróme
hook
    Adson's h.
Hope's sign

Hopkins' clamp
Horsley's forceps
Hufnagel's
    clamp
    knife
    operation
    prosthesis
Hume's clamp
Humphries' clamp
HVD — hypertensive vascular
    disease
hydropericarditis
hydropericardium
hydropneumopericardium
hypercalcemia
hypercholesterolemia
hyperemia
hyperkalemia
hyperkinesia
hyperlipidemia
hypertension
    arterial h.
    essential h.
    portal h.
    pulmonary h.
    renovascular h.
    secondary h.
    vascular h.
hypertensive
hypertrophy
    ventricular h.
hyperventilation
hypocalcemia
hypokalemia
hypokinemia
hypokinesia
hyponatremia
hypoproteinemia
hypoprothrombinemia
hypotension
    orthostatic h.
hypothermia

hypovolemia
hypoxia
hysterosystole
hz — hertz
IA — intra-aortic
    intra-arterial
IABP — intra-aortic balloon
       pumping
IAS — interatrial septum
IASD — interatrial septal
      defect
ICC — intensive coronary care
ICCU — intensive coronary
       care unit
ictometer
ictus
    i. cordis
ICU — intensive care unit
idiopathic
idioventricular
IHD — ischemic heart disease
IHSS — idiopathic hyper-
      trophic subaortic
      stenosis
imbalance
    electrolyte i.
IMH — idiopathic myocardial
      hypertrophy
implantation
impressio
    i. cardiaca pulmonis
impulse
    apex i.
    apical i.
    episternal i.
incision. See *General Surgical*
    Terms.
incisura
    i. apicis cordis
incompetence
infarct

infarction
    anterolateral i.
    anteroposterior i.
    anteroseptal i.
    atrial i.
    cardiac i.
    diaphragmatic i.
    myocardial i.
    Roesler-Dressler i.
    septal i.
    subendocardial i.
    transmural i.
inferolateral
infundibular
infundibulum
    i. of heart
inotropic
insufficiency
    aortic i.
    cardiac i.
    coronary i.
    mitral i.
    myocardial i.
    myovascular i.
    pseudoaortic i.
    tricuspid i.
    valvular i.
    venous i.
interatrial
intercostal
interval
    a.-c. i.
    atriocarotid i.
    atrioventricular i.
    auriculocarotid i.
    auriculoventricular i.
    a.-v. i.
    c.-a. i.
    cardioarterial i.
    P-Q i.
    P-R i.

interval (*continued*)
    Q-M i.
    QRST i.
    QT i.
    QU i.
    RS-T i.
    T-P i.
interventricular
intimal
intima-pia
intimectomy
intimitis
intra-aortic balloon
intra-arterial
intra-atrial
intra-auricular
intracardiac
intracoronary
intramural
intramyocardial
intraventricular
inversion
    T-wave i.
Ionescu-Shiley prosthesis
irregularity
    luminal i.
    i. of pulse
ischemia
    i. cordis intermittens
    myocardial i.
ischemic
IVC — inferior vena cava
IVCD — intraventricular
    conduction defect
IVSD — interventricular septal
    defect
IWMI — inferior wall myo-
    cardial infarction
Jackson-Mosher dilator
Jacobson's
    clamp

Jacobson's (*continued*)
    forceps
    scissors
    spatula
Janeway's sphygmomanometer
Javid's
    bypass clamp
    shunt
Johns Hopkins
    clamp
    forceps
Jorgenson's scissors
Judkin's technique
Juevenell's clamp
Julian's forceps
JV — jugular vein
    jugular venous
JVP — jugular venous pulse
kahkekseah. See *cachexia.*
Kantrowicz's clamp
Kapp-Beck clamp
Karell's
    diet
    treatment
Katz-Wachtel phenomenon
Kay-Shiley prosthesis
Kay-Suzuki prosthesis
Keith's bundle
Kelly's clamp
Kempner's diet
Kent-His bundle
Kent's bundle
ker-on-sabo. See *coeur en
    sabot.*
kinking
knife
    Bailey-Glover-O'Neill k.
    Bailey-Morse k.
    Bosher's k.
    Brock's k.
    Derra's k.

knife (*continued*)
    Hufnagel's k.
    Lebsche's k.
    Niedner's k.
    Nunez-Nunez k.
    Rochester's k.
    Sellor's k.
Korotkoff's
    method
    sounds
    test
Krasky's retractor
Kronecker's
    needle
    puncture
Krönig's steps
Kussmaul's
    pulse
    sign
LA — left atrial
    left atrium
lactic dehydrogenase
LAE — left atrial enlargement
LAH — left atrial hypertrophy
LAP — left atrial pressure
law
    all or none l.
    Einthoven's l.
LBBB — left bundle branch
        block
LD — lactic dehydrogenase
LDL — low-density lipoprotein
lead
    precordial l's
    sternal l.
    V l's, 1 through 6
    Wilson's l's
leaflet
Lebsche's
    forceps
    knife
    shears

Lehman's catheter
Leksell's rongeur
Leland-Jones forceps
Lemmon's rib spreader
Lenegre's disease
Leriche's
    forceps
    operation
    syndrome
levoversion
Lev's disease
Libman-Sacks
    disease
    syndrome
ligamentum
    l. arteriosum
ligation
    Desault's l.
    proximal l.
ligature
    Woodbridge's l.
Lilienthal-Sauerbruch rib
    spreader
Lillehei-Kaster prosthesis
limbus
    l. fossae ovalis
line
    midclavicular l.
lipid
lipocardiac
lipoprotein
    low-density l.
Liston-Stille forceps
Litwak's scissors
Livierato's
    reflex
    test
Löffler's endocarditis
loop
    Cannon's endarterec-
        tomy l.
    P l.

Love-Gruenwald forceps
LSM — late systolic murmur
LSV — left subclavian vein
lubb
lubb-dupp
Luken's retractor
lumen
luminal
Lutembacher's
    complex
    disease
    syndrome
luxus
LV — left ventricle
Lyon-Horgan operation
M_2 — mitral second sound
MABP — mean arterial blood
        pressure
machine
    heart-lung m.
Magovern's prosthesis
Makins' murmur
malformation
manometric
manubrium
Marfan's syndrome
Master "2-step" exercise test
Master's two-step test
Matson's elevator
Mayo's cannula
McDonald's clamp
McDowall's reflex
McGinn-White sign
MCI — mean cardiac index
McNealy-Glassman-Mixter
    forceps
MCL — midclavicular line
mediastinal
mediastinitis
mediastinopericarditis
mediastinoscope
    Goldberg-MPC m.

mediastinum
medications. See *Drugs and
    Chemistry* section.
Medtronic pacemaker
Meigs' capillaries
membrane
    Henle's m.
mesaortitis
mesarteritis
mesoaortitis
    m. syphilitica
mesocardia
mesocardium
method
    Korotkoff's m.
    Orsi-Grocco m.
Meyerding's retractor
MI — mitral incompetence
    mitral insufficiency
    myocardial infarction
microvascular
mitral
    m. insufficiency
    m. stenosis
mitrale
    P m.
mitralization
mitroarterial
Mixter's forceps
Mobin-Uddin umbrella filter
Mobitz' heart block
Mönckeberg's
    arteriosclerosis
    degeneration
monitor
    Holter m.
Monneret's pulse
Moore's operation
Morgagni's sinus
Morris' cannula
Morse's scissors
Mount-Mayfield forceps

Moure-Coryllos rib shears
MR — mitral reflux
    mitral regurgitation
MRF — mitral regurgitant flow
MS — mitral stenosis
MSL — midsternal line
multifocal
mural
murmur
    amphoric m.
    aneurysmal m.
    aortic m.
    apex m.
    apical diastolic m.
    arterial m.
    attrition m.
    Austin Flint m.
    basal diastolic m.
    bellows m.
    blowing m.
    Bright's m.
    cardiac m.
    cardiopulmonary m.
    cardiorespiratory m.
    Carey-Coombs m.
    continuous m.
    cooing m.
    crescendo m.
    Cruveilhier-Baumgarten
      m.
    decrescendo m.
    deglutition m.
    diamond-shaped m.
    diastolic m.
    Duroziez's m.
    dynamic m.
    ejection m.
    endocardial m.
    Eustace Smith's m.
    exocardial m.
    expiratory m.
    Fisher's m.

murmur (*continued*)
    Flint's m.
    Fraentzel's m.
    friction m.
    functional m.
    Gibson's m.
    grade 1, 2, 3, 4, 5, or 6 m.
    Graham Steell m.
    Hamman's m.
    harsh m.
    hemic m.
    holosystolic m.
    hour-glass m.
    humming-top m.
    inorganic m.
    inspiratory m.
    lapping m.
    machinery m.
    Makins' m.
    mitral m.
    musical m.
    nun's m.
    obstructive m.
    organic m.
    pansystolic m.
    Parrot's m.
    pericardial m.
    pleuropericardial m.
    prediastolic m.
    presystolic m.
    pulmonic m.
    reduplication m.
    regurgitant m.
    respiratory m.
    Roger's m.
    sea-gull m.
    seesaw m.
    Steell's m.
    stenosal m.
    Still's m.
    subclavicular m.
    systolic m.

murmur (*continued*)
    to-and-fro m.
    Traube's m.
    tricuspid m.
    vascular m.
    venous m.
    vesicular m.
    water-wheel m.
muscle
    papillary m.
    pectinate m.
Mustard's operation
MV – mitral valve
MVP – mitral valve prolapse
Myer's stripper
myocardial infarction
myocardiogram
myocardiograph
myocardiopathy
    idiopathic m.
myocardiorrhaphy
myocarditis
    acute bacterial m.
    Fiedler's m.
    fragmentation m.
    giant cell m.
    indurative m.
    interstitial m.
    parenchymatous m.
    m. scarlatinosa
    toxic m.
myocardium
myocardosis
    Riesman's m.
myofibrosis
    m. cordis
myomalacia
    m. cordis
myopathia
    m. cordis
myxedema
myxoma

Nathan's pacemaker
needle
    Adson's n.
    Cournand's n.
    Curry's n.
    Cushing's n.
    Flynt's n.
    Kronecker's n.
    Parhad-Poppen n.
    Retter's n.
    Rochester's n.
    Sanders-Brown-Shaw n.
    Seldinger's n.
    Sheldon-Spatz n.
    Smiley-Williams n.
    Tuohy's n.
    Wood's n.
neoplasm
nephrectomy
nephritis
nerve
    parasympathetic n.
    sympathetic n.
    vagus n.
network
    Purkinje's n.
Nichols' clamp
Niedner's knife
NIH catheter
nitroglycerin
nodal
node
    Aschoff's n.
    n. of Aschoff and Tawara
    atrioventricular n.
    Flack's n.
    His-Tawara n.
    Osler's n's
    sinoatrial n.
Noonan's syndrome
notch
    Sibson's n.

NPB — nodal premature beat
NSR — normal sinus rhythm
Nunez-Nunez knife
obstruction
    vena cava o.
occlusion
    coronary o.
    thrombotic o.
occlusive
Oertel's treatment
Öhnell
    X wave of O.
omentopexy
OMI — old myocardial
    infarction
Omni-Atricor pacemaker
Omni-Ectocor pacemaker
Omni-Stanicor pacemaker
operation
    Beck I o.
    Beck II o.
    Blalock-Hanlen o.
    Blalock-Taussig o.
    Brauer's o.
    Brock's o.
    Delorme's o.
    Harrington's o.
    Hufnagel's o.
    Leriche's o.
    Lyon-Horgan o.
    Moore's o.
    Mustard's o.
    Potts' o.
    Potts-Smith-Gibson o.
    Rastelli's o.
    Vineberg's o.
Orsi-Grocco method
orthopnea
orthopneic
orthostatic
oscillation
oscillograph

oscillometer
oscillometric
oscillometry
oscilloscope
O'Shaughnessy's forceps
Osler's
    nodes
    sign
ostia
    o. atrioventricularia
        dextrum
    o. atrioventricularis
        sinistrum
    o. venarum pulmonalium
ostium
    o. aortae
    o. arteriosum cordis
    o. cardiacum
    o. primum
    o. secundum
    sinusoidal o.
    o. trunci pulmonalis
    o. venosum cordis
Overholt's elevator
oximetry
oxygen
oxygenate
oxygenator
P_2 — pulmonic second sound
PAC — premature auricular
    contraction
pacemaker
    Amtech-Killeen p.
    Arco p.
    artificial p.
    asynchronous p.
    Atricor p.
    bifocal demand p.
    Biotronik p.
    bipolar p.
    Chardak-Greatbatch p.
    Coratomic p.

pacemaker (*continued*)
  Cordis' p.
  Cordis Atricor p.
  Cordis-Ectocor p.
  Cordis' fixed rate p.
  Cordis Ventricor p.
  CPI Maxilith p.
  CPI Minilith p.
  demand p.
  Ectocor p.
  Electrodyne p.
  endocardial bipolar p.
  epicardial p.
  General Electric p.
  implantable p.
  lithium p.
  Medtronic p.
  Nathan's p.
  nuclear p.
  Omni-Atricor p.
  Omni-Ectocor p.
  Omni-Stanicor p.
  radio frequency p.
  Stanicor p.
  Starr-Edwards p.
  Telectronic p.
  transvenous p.
  unipolar p.
  Ventricor p.
  wandering p.
  Zoll's p.
  Zyrel's p.
  Zytron p.
PAH — pulmonary artery
  hypertension
palpitation
panangiitis
  diffuse necrotizing p.
panarteritis
pansphygmograph
paracentesis
  p. cordis

paracentesis (*continued*)
  p. pericardii
paradoxical
parasternal
parasystole
Parhad-Poppen needle
paries
  p. caroticus cavi tympani
Park's aneurysm
paroxysmal
Parrot's murmur
PAT — paroxysmal atrial
  tachycardia
patch
  Edwards' p.
  Teflon p.
patent
patent ductus arteriosus
paulocardia
PDA — patent ductus
  arteriosus
pectoral
pectoralis
pentalogy
  p. of Fallot
perfusion
periaortitis
periarteritis
  p. nodosa
periatrial
periauricular
pericardial
  p. peel
pericardicentesis
pericardiectomy
pericardiocentesis
pericardiolysis
pericardiomediastinitis
pericardiophrenic
pericardiopleural
pericardiorrhaphy
pericardiostomy

pericardiosymphysis
pericardiotomy
pericarditis
    acute fibrinous p.
    adhesive p.
    amebic p.
    bacterial p.
    p. calculosa
    p. callosa
    carcinomatous p.
    constrictive p.
    p. with effusion
    p. epistenocardiaca
    p. externa et interna
    fibrous p.
    hemorrhagic p.
    idiopathic p.
    localized p.
    mediastinal p.
    neoplastic p.
    p. obliterans
    obliterating p.
    purulent p.
    rheumatic p.
    serofibrinous p.
    p. sicca
    suppurative p.
    tuberculous p.
    uremic p.
    p. villosa
pericardium
    adherent p.
    bread-and-butter p.
    calcified p.
    p. fibrosum
    fibrous p.
    parietal p.
    p. serosum
    serous p.
    shaggy p.
    visceral p.
pericardosis

pericardotomy
period
    Wenckebach's p.
periosteotome
    Alexander-Farabeuf p.
peripericarditis
peripheral
periphlebitis
petechia
Phemister's elevator
phenomenon
    Katz-Wachtel p.
    Raynaud's p.
pheochromocytoma
phlebangioma
phlebarteriectasia
phlebarteriodialysis
phlebasthenia
phlebectasia
phlebectomy
phlebectopia
phlebemphraxis
phlebexairesis
phlebismus
phlebitis
phlebocarcinoma
phlebocholosis
phlebogram
phlebography
phlebolith
phlebolithiasis
phlebomanometer
phlebomyomatosis
phlebophlebostomy
phlebopiezometry
phleboplasty
phleborrhagia
phleborrhaphy
phleborrhexis
phlebosclerosis
phlebosis
phlebostasis

phlebostenosis
phlebostrepsis
phlebothrombosis
phlebotome
phlebotomy
phonocardiogram
phonocardiograph
phonocardiographic
phonocardiography
    intracardiac p.
phonoelectrocardioscope
phonogram
phrenocardia
phrenopericarditis
Pick's
    disease
    syndrome
plethora
plethysmograph
plethysmography
plethysmometer
plethysmometry
pleuropericardial
pleuropericarditis
plexus
    cardiac p.
    p. cardiacus profundus
    p. cardiacus superficialis
    p. caroticus communis
    p. caroticus externus
    p. caroticus internus
    p. coronarius cordis
    vascular p.
    p. venosus caroticus
      internus
    venous p.
P loop
PMI – point of maximal
      impulse
P mitrale
PND – paroxysmal nocturnal
      dyspnea

pneumatocardia
pneumocardial
pneumohemia
pneumohemopericardium
pneumohydropericardium
pneumopericardium
pneumoprecordium
pneumopyopericardium
point
    Erb's p.
polyarteritis
polycythemia
    p. hypertonica
    p. vera
polyunsaturated fat
poodrazh. See *poudrage.*
Poppen-Blalock clamp
Poppen's clamp
porcine
    p. heterograft
    p. xenograft
position. See *General Surgical*
    Terms.
postmyocardial infarction
potassium
Pott's aneurysm
Potts'
    clamp
    operation
    rib shears
    scissors
Potts-Niedner clamp
Potts-Smith
    clamp
    forceps
    scissors
Potts-Smith-Gibson operation
poudrage
P-pulmonale
P-Q interval
P-Q segment
precardiac

precordial
precordium
preponderance
    ventricular p.
presbycardia
presystolic
preventriculosis
preventriculus
P-R interval
Prinzmetal's angina
prolapse
    mitral valve p.
propranolol
prosthesis (valves & grafts)
    Alvarez' p.
    Björk-Shiley p.
    Braunwald's p.
    caged-ball p.
    Cape Town p.
    Cartwright's p.
    Cooley's p.
    Cutter-SCDK p.
    Cutter-Smeloff p.
    Dacron p.
    DeBakey's p.
    discoid aortic p.
    Edwards' p.
    Gott's p.
    Harken's p.
    Hufnagel's p.
    Ionescu-Shiley p.
    Kay-Shiley p.
    Kay-Suzuki p.
    Lillehei-Kaster p.
    Magovern's p.
    Smeloff-Cutter p.
    Starr-Edwards p.
    tilting disk p.
    tri-leaflet aortic p.
    Wada's p.
    Weavenit's p.
    Wesolowski's p.

protodiastolic
P-R segment
pseudoanemia
    p. angiospastica
pseudoangina
pseudoangioma
pseudocoarctation
pseudotruncus arteriosus
pulmonale
    P. p.
pulmonary
pulmonic stenosis
pulsate
pulsatile
pulsation
    expansile p.
    suprasternal p.
pulse
    allorhythmic p.
    anacrotic p.
    anadicrotic p.
    anatricrotic p.
    arachnoid p.
    auriculovenous p.
    Bamberger's bulbar p.
    bigeminal p.
    bisferious p.
    cannon ball p.
    catacrotic p.
    catadicrotic p.
    catatricrotic p.
    centripetal venous p.
    collapsing p.
    cordy p.
    Corrigan's p.
    coupled p.
    decurtate p.
    dicrotic p.
    digitalate p.
    elastic p.
    entopic p.
    filiform p.

pulse (*continued*)
    formicant p.
    gaseous p.
    guttural p.
    high-tension p.
    hyperdicrotic p.
    jugular p.
    Kussmaul's p.
    Monneret's p.
    monocrotic p.
    mouse tail p.
    paradoxical p.
    pedal p.
    pistol-shot p.
    plateau p.
    polycrotic p.
    pulmonary p.
    quadrigeminal p.
    Quincke's p.
    Riegel's p.
    thready p.
    tremulous p.
    tricrotic p.
    trigeminal p.
    undulating p.
    vagus p.
    ventricular venous p.
    vermicular p.
    vibrating p.
    water-hammer p.
pulsus
    p. alternans
    p. bigeminus
    p. bisferiens
    p. celer
    p. contractus
    p. cordis
    p. debilis
    p. deficiens
    p. deletus
    p. differens
    p. duplex

pulsus (*continued*)
    p. durus
    p. filiformis
    p. formicans
    p. frequens
    p. heterochronicus
    p. intercurrens
    p. irregularis perpetuus
    p. magnus et celer
    p. mollis
    p. monocrotus
    p. oppressus
    p. paradoxus
    p. parvus et tardus
    p. plenus
    p. pseudo-intermittens
    p. rarus
    p. tardus
    p. trigeminus
    p. undulosus
    p. vacuus
    p. venosus
    p. vibrans
pump
    Emerson's p.
punch
    Brock's p.
puncture
    Kronecker's p.
Purkinje's
    fibers
    network
PVC — premature ventricular
    contraction
PVS — premature ventricular
    systole
PVT — paroxysmal ventricular
    tachycardia
P wave
pyelophlebitis
pyemia
    arterial p.

pyemia (*continued*)
    portal p.
pyopneumopericardium
Q-M interval
QRS changes
QRS complex
QRS-T changes
QRST interval
QRS wave
QS complex
Q-S deflections
QT interval
Quain's
    degeneration
    fatty heart
Quénu-Muret sign
Quincke's pulse
QU interval
Q wave
RA — right atrial
    right atrium
radicle
ramus
rankenangioma
raphe
rasp
    Beck's r.
raspatory
    Coryllos' r.
Rastelli's operation
ratio
    R/S r.
Raynaud's
    disease
    phenomenon
RBBB — right bundle branch
    block
RCD — relative cardiac dullness
reanastomosis
reflex
    Abrams' heart r.
    Bainbridge's r.

reflex (*continued*)
    bregmocardiac r.
    carotid-sinus r.
    Erben's r.
    Livierato's r.
    McDowall's r.
    oculocardiac r.
    psychocardiac r.
    pulmonocoronary r.
    viscerocardiac r.
regurgitant
regurgitation
    aortic r.
    mitral r.
    pulmonic r.
Reich-Nechtow clamp
respiration
    Cheyne-Stokes' r.
    Corrigan's r.
respirator
    Engström r.
resuscitation
    cardiopulmonary r.
rete
    r. arteriosum
    r. mirabile
    r. vasculosum
    r. venosum
retractor
    Adson's r.
    Allison's r.
    Carter's r.
    Cooley's r.
    Coryllos' r.
    Crawford's r.
    Davidson's r.
    DeBakey-Balfour r.
    DeBakey-Cooley r.
    Gross' r.
    Gross-Pomeranz-
      Watkins r.
    Harrington-Pemberton r.

retractor (*continued*)
 Harrington's r.
 Hedblom's r.
 Hibbs' r.
 Krasky's r.
 Lukens' r.
 Meyerding's r.
 Richardson's r.
 Ross' r.
 Sauerbruch's r.
 Semb's r.
 Walter-Deaver r.
Retter's needle
revascularization
 myocardial r.
RF — rheumatic fever
RHD — rheumatic heart
 disease
rheumapyra
rheumatic heart disease
rhythm
 atrial r.
 auriculoventricular r.
 cantering r.
 coupled r.
 gallop r.
 idioventricular r.
 nodal r.
 pendulum r.
 reversed r.
 sinus r.
 triple r.
 ventricular r.
rhythmophone
rib contractor
 Bailey-Gibbon r.c.
 Bailey's r.c.
 Sellor's r.c.
rib shears
 Bethune's r.s.
 Giertz-Shoemaker r.s.
 Gluck's r.s.

rib shears (*continued*)
 Moure-Coryllos r.s.
 Potts' r.s.
 Sauerbruch's r.s.
 Shoemaker's r.s.
rib spreader
 Burford's r.s.
 Finochietto's r.s.
 Harken's r.s.
 Lemmon's r.s.
 Lilienthal-Sauerbruch r.s.
 Rienhoff-Finochietto r.s.
 Tuffier's r.s.
 Wilson's r.s.
Richardson's retractor
Richet's aneurysm
Riegel's pulse
Rienhoff-Finochietto rib
 spreader
Rienhoff's
 clamp
 forceps
Riesman's myocardosis
ring
 atrial r.
 Effler's r.
 vascular r.
Riva-Rocci sphygmoma-
 nometer
Rochester's
 awl
 knife
 needle
Rockey's cannula
Rodrigues' aneurysm
roentgenocardiogram
roentgenography
Roesler-Dressler infarction
Roger's
 bruit
 disease
 murmur

Roger's (*continued*)
    sphygmomanometer
rongeur
    Leksell's r.
rooma-. See words beginning
    rheuma-.
Rose's tamponade
Ross' retractor
Rostan's asthma
Rotch's sign
Roth's spots
RSR — regular sinus rhythm
R/S ratio
RS-T interval
rumble
    diastolic r.
Rumel's
    clamp
    forceps
    tourniquet
Rummo's disease
Ruskin's forceps
RV — right ventricle
RVE — right ventricular
        enlargement
RVH — right ventricular
        hypertrophy
R wave
Salibi's clamp
Sanders-Brown-Shaw needle
sanguis
Sansom's sign
saphenofemoral
saphenous
sarcoid
sarcoidosis
    s. cordis
Satinsky's
    clamp
    forceps
    scissors
saturated fat

Sauerbruch's
    forceps
    retractor
    rib shears
SBE — subacute bacterial
        endocarditis
scan
    cardiac s.
scanner
scissors
    Cooley's s.
    DeBakey-Metzenbaum s.
    DeBakey's s.
    Jacobson's s.
    Jorgenson's s.
    Litwak's s.
    Morse's s.
    Potts' s.
    Potts-Smith s.
    Satinsky's s.
    Thorek-Feldman s.
    Thorek's s.
    Toennis' s.
scleroderma
sclerosis
    arterial s.
sclerotic
Scoville-Lewis clip
Scribner's shunt
searcher
    Allport-Babcock s.
Sedillot's elevator
segment
    P-Q s.
    P-R s.
    S-T s.
    T-P s.
Seldinger's needle
Sellor's
    knife
    rib contractor
Selman's forceps

Selverstone's clamp
Semb's
     forceps
     retractor
semilunar
septa
septal defects
septum
     s. atriorum cordis
     s. atrioventriculare cordis
     interatrial s.
     s. interatriale cordis
     interauricular s.
     interventricular s.
     s. interventriculare cordis
     s. membranaceum ven-
        triculorum cordis
     s. musculare ventric-
        ulorum cordis
     s. primum
     s. secundum
     s. ventriculorum cordis
serrefine
sfigmo-. See words beginning
     sphygmo-.
SGOT — serum glutamic-oxalic
         transaminase
         serum glutamic-oxalo-
           acetic transaminase
Shaw's stripper
shears
     Lebsche's s.
Sheldon-Spatz needle
Shoemaker's
     clamp
     rib shears
shunt
     arteriovenous s.
     cardiovascular s.
     cavamesenteric s.
     Javid's s.
     left-to-right s.

shunt (*continued*)
     portacaval s.
     portarenal s.
     postcaval s.
     right-to-left s.
     Scribner's s.
     ventriculoatrial s.
     ventriculoperitoneal s.
     Warren's s.
Sibson's
     notch
     vestibule
sign
     Auenbrugger's s.
     Bamberger's s.
     Béhier-Hardy s.
     Bouillaud's s.
     Branham's s.
     Braunwald's s.
     Broadbent's s.
     Brockenborough's s.
     Cegka's s.
     Corrigan's s.
     de Musset's s.
     Dieuaide's s.
     Drummond's s.
     Duroziez's s.
     Ewart's s.
     Friedreich's s.
     Hope's s.
     Kussmaul's s.
     McGinn-White s.
     Osler's s.
     Quénu-Muret s.
     Rotch's s.
     Sansom's s.
     Sterles' s.
     Traube's s.
     vital s's
     Wenckebach's s.
Silastic coronary artery
     cannula

silhouette
>cardiovascular s.
sinistrocardia
sinoatrial
sinoauricular
sinospiral
sinoventricular
sinus
>carotid s.
>s. caroticus
>coronary s.
>s. of Morgagni
>s. transversus pericardii
>s. of Valsalva
sinusoid
>myocardial s's
slope
>E to F s.
Smeloff-Cutter prosthesis
Smiley-Williams needle
Smith's clip
Soresi's cannula
souffle
>cardiac s.
sound
>bellows s.
>flapping s.
>heart s's; first s.,
>>second s.
>Korotkoff's s's
>pistol-shot s.
>tick-tack s's
Southey-Leech tubes
spasm
>coronary-artery s.
spatula
>Jacobson's s.
sphygmobologram
sphygmobolometer
sphygmocardiogram
sphygmocardiograph
sphygmocardioscope

sphygmodynamometer
sphygmogram
sphygmography
sphygmomanometer
>Erlanger's s.
>Faught's s.
>Janeway's s.
>Riva-Rocci s.
>Rogers' s.
>Staunton's s.
>Tycos' s.
sphygmomanometroscope
sphygmometer
sphygmometrograph
sphygmometroscope
sphygmo-oscillometer
sphygmopalpation
sphygmophone
sphygmoplethysmograph
sphygmoscope
>Bishop's s.
sphygmosignal
sphygmosystole
sphygmotonogram
sphygmotonograph
sphygmotonometer
sphygmoviscosimetry
splenosis
>pericardial s.
spot
>Roth's s's
standstill
>atrial s.
>auricular s.
>cardiac s.
>respiratory s.
>ventricular s.
Stanicor pacemaker
Stanley-Kent bundle
Starr-Edwards
>pacemaker
>prosthesis

stasis
    venous s.
Staunton's
    sphygmomanometer
ST depression
steal
    subclavian s.
Steell's murmur
stellectomy
stenocardia
stenosis
    aortic s.
    Dittrich's s.
    mitral s.
    preventricular s.
    pulmonary s.
    pulmonic s.
    subaortic s.
    tricuspid s.
stenotic
stent
    Carpentier's s.
step
    Krönig's s's
Sterges' carditis
Sterles' sign
sternopericardial
sternotomy
sternum
stethoscope
Stille-Luer forceps
Stille's forceps
Still's murmur
stimulation
    vagus s.
stress test
striation
    tabby cat s.
    tigroid s.
stripper
    Myer's s.
    Shaw's s.

stripper (*continued*)
    Wylie's s.
S-T segment
ST segment
    changes
    elevation
ST-T deviations
study
    opacification s.
stylet
subclavian
subclavicular
sublingual
suffusion
Sugar's clip
sulcus
    s. aorticus
    atrioventricular s.
    s. coronarius cordis
    interventricular s. of
        heart
    longitudinal s. of heart
    s. of subclavian artery
    transverse s. of heart
sump
    Baylor's s.
support
    Abée's s.
supraclavicular
surgical procedures. See
    operation.
suture. See *General Surgical
    Terms.*
SVC – superior vena cava
Swan-Ganz catheter
S wave
sympathectomy
sympathetic
    s. ganglia
    s. nerves
symphysis
    cardiac s.

synanastomosis
synchronous
syncopal
syncope
    Adams-Stokes s.
    s. anginosa
    carotid s.
    vasovagal s.
syndrome
    Adams-Stokes s.
    Ayerza's s.
    Babinski's s.
    Barlow's s.
    Beau's s.
    Bernheim's s.
    Bouillaud's s.
    Bouveret's s.
    bradycardia-tachycardia
        s.
    cardiofacial s.
    click-murmur s.
    Dressler's s.
    Eisenmenger's s.
    floppy valve s.
    Gower's s.
    Holt-Oram s.
    Leriche's s.
    Libman-Sacks s.
    Lutembacher's s.
    Marfan's s.
    Noonan's s.
    Pick's s.
    sick-sinus s.
    "stiff-heart" s.
    straight back s.
    Takayasu's s.
    Taussig-Bing s.
    Wolff-Parkinson-White s.
system
    cardiovascular s.
    conduction s.
    vascular s.

systole
    aborted s.
    arterial s.
    atrial s.
    auricular s.
    catalectic s.
    extra s.
    frustrate s.
    hemic s.
    ventricular s.
systolic
systolometer
tachycardia
    atrial t.
    alternating bidirectional t.
    auricular t.
    nodal t.
    orthostatic t.
    paroxysmal ventricular t.
    sinus t.
    supraventricular t.
    ventricular t.
tachycardiac
tachypnea
tachysystole
    atrial t.
    auricular t.
taeni
    t. terminalis
Takayasu's syndrome
takipnea. See *tachypnea.*
tamponade
    cardiac t.
    pericardial t.
    Rose's t.
Taussig-Bing syndrome
technique
    George Lewis t.
    Judkin's t.
Teflon
    catheter
    patch

telangiectasis
telangiosis
telecardiogram
telecardiography
Telectronic pacemaker
telelectrocardiogram
telelectrocardiograph
test
     Allen's t.
     Dehio's t.
     Gibbon-Landis t.
     Korotkoff's t.
     lipid t.
     Livierato's t.
     Master "2-step"
       exercise t.
     Master's two-step t.
     radioactive fibrinogen
       uptake t.
     regitine t.
     serum enzyme t.
     stress t.
     Trendelenburg's t.
tetrad
tetralogy
     t. of Fallot
thebesian
theca
     t. cordis
thoracentesis
Thorek-Feldman scissors
Thorek's scissors
Thorel's bundle
thrill
     aneurysmal t.
     aortic t.
     diastolic t.
     presystolic t.
     systolic t.
thrombectomy
thromboangiitis
     t. obliterans

thromboarteritis
     t. purulenta
thromboclasis
thromboembolism
thromboendarterectomy
thromboendarteritis
thromboendocarditis
thrombokinesis
thrombolymphangitis
thrombolysis
thrombophlebitis
     iliofemoral t.
     t. migrans
     t. purulenta
     t. saltans
thrombopoiesis
thrombosis
     coronary t.
thrombus
TI — tricuspid incompetence
     tricuspid insufficiency
tinkle
     Bouillaud's t.
Toennis' scissors
tortuosity
tourniquet
     Rumel's t.
T-P interval
T-P segment
trabeculae
     t. carneae cordis
     flesh t. of heart
trabecular
transient
transplant
transposition
     t. of great vessels
transseptal
transventricular
Traube-Hering waves
Traube's
     curves

Traube's (*continued*)
    heart
    murmur
    sign
treatment
    Fränkel's t.
    Karell's t.
    Oertel's t.
Trendelenburg-Crafoord
  clamp
Trendelenburg's test
triad
    Beck's t.
triangle
    Burger's t.
    cardiohepatic t.
    Einthoven's t.
tricuspid
trifascicular
trigeminy
triglyceride
trigona
    t. fibrosa cordis
trilogy
    t. of Fallot
truncus
    t. arteriosus
    t. brachiocephalicus
    t. fasciculi atrioventric-
      ularis
trunk
    brachiocephalic t.
Tubbs' dilator
tube
    nasogastric t.
    Southey-Leech t's
Tucker's dilator
Tudor-Edwards costotome
Tuffier's rib spreader
tunica
    t. adventitia vasorum
    t. externa vasorum
    t. intima vasorum

tunica (*continued*)
    t. media vasorum
    t. vasculosa
tunneler
    Crawford-Cooley t.
    DeBakey's t.
Tuohy's needle
turgescent
turgid
turgor
    t. vitalis
T wave
    changes
    inversion
Tycos' sphygmomanometer
ultrasound
unipolar
U wave
Valsalva's sinus
valve
    aortic v.
    atrioventricular v.
    auriculoventricular v.
    ball-type v.
    bicuspid v.
    cardiac v's
    caval v.
    v. of coronary sinus
    eustachian v.
    mitral v.
    pulmonary v.
    semilunar v's
    thebesian v.
    tricuspid v.
valvotome
valvotomy
    mitral v.
valvula
    v. bicuspidalis
    v. semilunaris dextra
      aortae
    v. semilunaris posterior
      aortae

valvula *(continued)*
    v. semilunaris sinistra
      aortae
    v. sinus coronarii
    v. tricuspidalis
    v. venae cavae inferioris
    v. venosa
    v. vestibuli
valvulae semilunares aortae
valvular
valvulitis
    rheumatic v.
valvuloplasty
valvulotome
valvulotomy
Vanderbilt's forceps
variceal
varices
varicose
    v. vein
varicosity
varix
    aneurysmal v.
    arterial v.
vascular
vascularity
vascularization
vasculature
vasculitis
vasoconstriction
vasoconstrictor
vasodepression
vasodilation
vasodilator
vasoinhibitor
vasomotor
vasopressin
vasospasm
    refractory ergonovine-
      induced v.
VDG — ventricular diastolic
      gallop

vector
vectorcardiogram
vectorcardiography
    spatial v.
vegetation
    bacterial v's
    verrucous v's
vein
    cephalic v.
    portal v.
    pulmonary v.
    saphenous v.
    varicose v.
vena cava
    inferior v.c.
    superior v.c.
vena cavagram
venae cavae
venipuncture
venoauricular
venofibrosis
venogram
venography
veno-occlusive
venosinal
venostasis
venotomy
venous
ventricle
Ventricor pacemaker
ventricular
    v. septal defect
ventriculography
ventriculomyotomy
ventriculonector
ventriculotomy
ventriculus
    v. cordis
    v. dexter cordis
    v. sinister cordis
venule
vessel

vestibule
> Gibson's v.
> Sibson's v.

Vineberg's operation

vitium
> v. cordis

VLDL — very low-density
> lipoprotein

V leads, 1 through 6

von Willebrand's disease

VPC — ventricular premature
> contraction

VSD — ventricular septal
> defect

Wada's prosthesis

Walter-Deaver retractor

Wangensteen's awl

Warren's shunt

wave
> A w.
> arterial w.
> delta w.
> dicrotic w.
> F w's
> fibrillary w's
> oscillation w.
> overflow w.
> P w.
> percussion w.
> peridicrotic w.
> predicrotic w.
> pre-excitation w.
> Q w.
> QRS w.
> R w.
> recoil w.
> respiratory w.
> S w.

wave (*continued*)
> T w.
> tidal w.
> transverse w.
> Traube-Hering w's
> tricrotic w.
> U w.
> vasomotor w.
> ventricular w.
> X w. of Öhnell

Weavenit's
> patch graft
> prosthesis

Wenckebach's
> disease
> heart block
> period
> sign

Wesolowski's prosthesis

Willis' circle

Wilson's
> leads
> rib-spreader

Wolff-Parkinson-White
> syndrome

Woodbridge's ligature

Wood's needle

WPW — Wolff-Parkinson-
> White (syndrome)

Wrisberg's ganglia

Wylie's stripper

xenograft

xiphoid process

X wave of Öhnell

zenograft. See *xenograft.*

Zoll's pacemaker

Zyrel's pacemaker

Zytron pacemaker

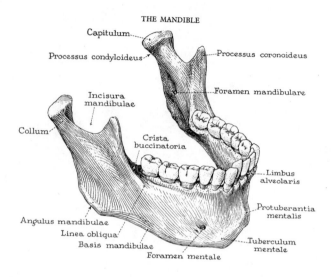

THE MANDIBLE

Capitulum

Processus condyloideus

Processus coronoideus

Incisura mandibulae

Foramen mandibulare

Collum

Crista buccinatoria

Limbus alveolaris

Protuberantia mentalis

Angulus mandibulae

Linea obliqua

Basis mandibulae

Foramen mentale

Tuberculum mentale

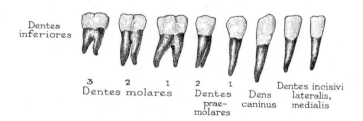

Dentes inferiores

3   2   1
Dentes molares

2   1
Dentes praemolares

Dens caninus

Dentes incisivi lateralis, medialis

(Courtesy of Anson, B. J.: Atlas of Human Anatomy. Philadelphia, W. B. Saunders Company, 1950.)

DENTISTRY

AB — axiobuccal
ABC — axiobuccocervical
ABG — axiobuccogingival
ABL — axiobuccolingual
abocclusion
abrasio
    a. dentium
abscess
    apical a.
    dentoalveolar a.
    periodontal a.
abstraction
abutment
AC — axiocervical
acrylic
AD — axiodistal
adamantine
adamantinocarcinoma
adamas
    a. dentis
Adams' clasp
ADC — axiodistocervical
ADG — axiodistogingival
adhesive
    denture a.
ADI — axiodistoincisal
ADO — axiodisto-occlusal
AG — axiogingival
AI — axioincisal
Ainsworth's punch

AL — axiolingual
ALA — axiolabial
ALAG — axiolabiogingival
ALAL — axiolabiolingual
ALC — axiolinguocervical
ALG — axiolinguogingival
alignment
Allen's root pliers
alloy
ALO — axiolinguo-occlusal
alveolalgia
alveolar
alveolectomy
alveolitis
    a. sicca dolorosa
alveoloclasia
alveolocondylean
alveolodental
alveololabial
alveololabialis
alveololingual
alveolomerotomy
alveolonasal
alveolopalatal
alveoloplasty
alveolotomy
alveolus
alveolysis
AM — axiomesial
amalgam

AMC — axiomesiocervical
AMD — axiomesiodistal
amelodentinal
amelogenesis
    a. imperfecta
AMG — axiomesiogingival
AMI — axiomesioincisal
AMO — axiomesio-occlusal
anchorage
anesthesia. See *General Surgical Terms.*
angina
    Ludwig's a.
ankylosis
anodontia
anteroclusion
antrum
    a. of Highmore
AO — axio-occlusal
AP — axiopulpal
apex
    a. radicis dentis
apical
apices
apicitis
apicoectomy
apicolocator
apicostome
apicostomy
apoxemena
apoxesis
appliance
    Crozat's a.
    Hawley's a.
apposition
arch
    maxillary a.
    zygomatic a.
arch bar
    Erich's a.b.
    Jelanko's a.b.
    Winter's a.b.

arcus
    a. dentalis
    a. zygomaticus
articulator
atresia
attachment
    Gottlieb's epithelial a.
attrition
Austin's
    knife
    retractor
avulsion
axiodistal
axiodistogingival
axiodisto-occlusal
axiogingival
axioincisal
axiolabial
axiolabiogingival
axiolingual
axiolinguogingival
axiomesial
axiomesiogingival
axiomesio-occlusal
axio-occlusal
axiopulpal
BA — buccoaxial
BAC — buccoaxiocervical
BAG — buccoaxiogingival
BC -- buccocervical
BD — buccodistal
bell-crowned
bevel
BG — buccogingival
bicuspid
bicuspidal
bicuspidate
bicuspoid
bimaxillary
bitegage
bitelock
biteplate

bite-rim
bite-wing
BL — buccolingual
block
    infraorbital b.
BM — buccomesial
BO — bucco-occlusal
BP — buccopulpal
bridge
    cantilever b.
    dentin b.
    removable b.
    stationary b.
bridgework
broach
    root-canal b.
Brophy's operation
bruxism
buccal
buccoaxial
buccoaxiocervical
buccoaxiogingival
buccocervical
buccoclination
buccoclusion
buccodistal
buccogingival
buccolingual
buccomesial
bucco-occlusal
buccoplacement
buccopulpal
buccoversion
bunodont
bunolophodont
bunoselenodont
bur
    round b.
CA — cervicoaxial
cacodontia
calcification
calculus

Caldwell-Luc operation
canal
    root c.
canine
carcinoma
caries
carious
Carmichael's crown
cartilage
    gingival c.
carver
catheter
    nasotracheal c.
cavitas
    c. dentis
Cavitron
cellulitis
cementation
cementoperiostitis
cementosis
cementum
ceramics
    dental c.
ceramodontics
cervicoaxial
check-bite
cheilosis
cheilotomy
cingulum
clasp
    Adams' c.
    ball c.
cleoid
coagulate
coagulation
collum
    c. dentis
Commando operation
comminution
condylar
condyle
    c. of mandible

contrusion
corona
    c. dentis
coronal
coronoid
crepitation
crepitus
crevice
    gingival c.
crevicular
crista
    c. buccinatoria
Crombie's ulcer
crossbite
crown
    Carmichael's c.
    Davis' c.
    dowel c.
Crozat's appliance
crusta
    c. petrosa dentis
Cryer's elevator
crypt
curet
    Goldman's c.
    Gracey's c.
    Moult c.
curettage
    subgingival c.
cuspid
cyst
    radicular c.
cytology
dam
    rubber d.
Davis' crown
DB — distobuccal
DBO — distobucco-occlusal
DBP — distobuccopulpal
DC — distocervical
debridement
debris

deciduous
dedentition
def
deglutition
dens
    d. axis
    d. epistrophei
    d. in dente
    d. invaginatus
    d. sapientiae
    d. serotinus
dentagra
dental
dentata
dentate
dentes
    d. acustici
    d. canini
    d. decidui
    d. incisivi
    d. molares
    d. permanentes
    d. premolares
dentia
    d. praecox
    d. tarda
dentibuccal
denticle
    interstitial d.
denticulated
dentification
dentifrice
dentigerous
dentilabial
dentilingual
dentimeter
dentin
    adventitious d.
    circumpulpar d.
    cover d.
    hereditary opalescent d.
    interglobular d.

dentin (*continued*)
    intermediate d.
    irregular d.
    mantle d.
    opalescent d.
    primary d.
    reparative d.
    sclerotic d.
    secondary d.
    sensitive d.
    tertiary d.
    transparent d.
dentinalgia
dentinogenesis
    d. imperfecta
dentinoma
dentinosteoid
dentist
dentition
    deciduous d.
    precocious d.
    predeciduous d.
    transitional d.
dentoalveolar
dentoalveolitis
dentofacial
dentosurgical
dentulous
denture
detrition
DG — distogingival
diastema
diazone
dilaceration
diphyodont
discoid
disease
    Fauchard's d.
    periodontal d.
    Spira's d.
disocclude
displacement

dissection
    blunt d.
    sharp d.
distal
distobuccal
distobucco-occlusal
distobuccopulpal
distocervical
distoclination
distoclusion
distogingival
distolabial
distolabioincisal
distolingual
distolinguoincisal
distolinguo-occlusal
distolinguopulpal
distomolar
disto-occlusal
distoplacement
distopulpal
distopulpolabial
distopulpolingual
distoversion
distraction
DLA — distolabial
DLAI — distolabioincisal
DLI — distolinguoincisal
DLO — distolinguo-occlusal
DLP — distolinguopulpal
DO — disto-occlusal
DP — distopulpal
DPL — distopulpolingual
drill
    Hall's surgical d.
    Lentulo spiral d.
    Spirec d.
    Stryker d.
drip
    succinylcholine d.
drugs. See *Drugs and Chemistry* section.

duct
    parotid d.
    submandibular d.
    submaxillary d.
    Wharton's d.
dysodontiasis
eburnation
eburnitis
edentulous
ekselsimosis. See *exelcymosis.*
eksognatheon. See
    exognathion.
eksolever. See *exolever.*
electrocautery
elevator
    Cryer's e.
embrasure
enamel
enameloma
enamelum
endodontics
endodontist
endodontium
enucleation
enula
epiglottis
epulis
epulofibroma
equilibration
    occlusal e.
Erich's arch bar
erosion
eruption
erythrodontia
ethmoid
evulsed
excavation
excavator
excementosis
excursion
    protrusive e.
    retrusive e.

exelcymosis
exodontics
exodontology
exognathion
exolever
extirpation
extraction
extrude
extrudoclusion
extrusion
exudation
exuviation
farinks. See *pharynx.*
fatno-. See words beginning
    phatno-.
Fauchard's disease
fetor
    f. exore
    f. oris
fibromatosis
    f. gingivae
fibrosarcoma
    odontogenic f.
fistula
fistulous
flange
    buccal f.
    labial f.
    lingual f.
Fleischmann's hygroma
fluoridation
fluoride
fluoridization
fluorosis
follicular
foramen
    mandibular f.
    mental f.
    Scarpa's f.
Fournier teeth
frena
frenectomy

frenum
　　labial f.
　　lingual f.
furca
furcae
Fusobacterium
　　F. plauti-vincenti
fusospirillary
fusospirillosis
G – gingival
GA – gingivoaxial
GBA – gingivobuccoaxial
Gilmer's splint
gingiva
　　alveolar g.
　　areolar g.
　　buccal g.
　　cemented g.
　　interdental g.
　　labial g.
　　lingual g.
　　marginal g.
　　septal g.
gingival
gingivectomy
　　Ochsenbein's g.
gingivitis
　　eruptive g.
　　fusospirochetal g.
　　herpetic g.
　　marginal g.
　　necrotizing ulcerative g.
gingivoaxial
gingivobuccoaxial
gingivoglossitis
gingivolabial
gingivolinguoaxial
gingivoplasty
gingivosis
gingivostomatitis
　　herpetic g.
GLA – gingivolinguoaxial

gland
　　lingual g.
　　palatine g.
　　parotid g.
　　salivary g.
　　sublingual g.
　　submandibular salivary g.
　　submaxillary g.
glaze
glossoncus
glossopexy
glossorrhaphy
glossotomy
Goldman's curet
gomphiasis
gomphosis
Goslee tooth
Gottlieb's epithelial
　　attachment
Gracey's curet
granuloma
gubernaculum
　　g. dentis
gutta-percha
Hall's surgical drill
Hawley's appliance
headgear
　　Kloehn's h.
hemisection
hemorrhage
herpes
　　h. labialis
herpetic
Highmore's antrum
Horner's teeth
Huschke's auditory teeth
Hutchinson's teeth
hydrotherapy
hygienist
　　dental h.
hygroma
　　Fleischmann's h.

hypercementosis
hyperdontia
hyperkeratosis
hyperplasia
hypoconid
hypoconule
hypoconulid
hypoplasia
I & D — incision and drainage
imbrication
immobilization
impacted
impaction
incisal
incisive
incisolabial
incisolingual
incisoproximal
incisor
infection
    Vincent's i.
infrabulge
injection
    nasopalatine i.
inlay
interdigitation
intermaxillary
interocclusal
interosseous
interspace
intraoral
intrapulpal
Ivy wire
jackscrew
Jelanko's arch bar
Kirkland's knife
Kirschner's wire
Kloehn's headgear
knife
    Austin's k.
    Kirkland's k.
LA — linguoaxial

labial
labiogingival
labioglossopharyngeal
labioincisal
LAG — labiogingival
LAI — labioincisal
larynx
LD — linguodistal
ledging
Lentulo spiral drill
leptodontous
leukoplakia
LI — linguoincisal
line
    Salter's incremental l's
lingual
linguoaxial
linguocervical
linguoclination
linguoclusion
linguodental
linguodistal
linguogingival
linguoincisal
linguomesial
linguo-occlusal
linguopapillitis
linguoplacement
linguoplate
    palatal l.
linguopulpal
linguotrite
linguoversion
LM — linguomesial
LO — linguo-occlusal
LP — linguopulpal
Ludwig's angina
macrodontia
malalignment
malar
maleruption
malformation

malocclusion
malposition
malturned
malunion
mamelon
mandible
mandibular
marsupialization
mass
    Stent's m.
masseteric
mastication
matrix
maxilla
maxillary
maxillodental
maxillomandibular
MB – mesiobuccal
MBO – mesiobucco-occlusal
MBP – mesiobuccopulpal
medication. See *Drugs and Chemistry* section.
membrane
    Nasmyth's m.
    peridental m.
mesial
mesiobuccal
mesiobucco-occlusal
mesiobuccopulpal
mesiocervical
mesioclination
mesioclusion
mesiodens
mesiodistal
mesiogingival
mesioincisodistal
mesiolabial
mesiolabioincisal
mesiolingual
mesiolinguoincisal
mesiolinguo-occlusal
mesiolinguopulpal

mesio-occlusal
mesio-occlusodistal
mesiopalatal
mesiopulpal
mesiopulpolabial
mesiopulpolingual
mesioversion
metacone
metaconid
metaconule
metaplasia
    m. of pulp
metodontiasis
MG – mesiogingival
microdontia
micrognathia
MID – mesioincisodistal
ML – mesiolingual
MLA – mesiolabial
MLAI – mesiolabioincisal
MLI – mesiolinguoincisal
MLO – mesiolinguo-occlusal
MLP – mesiolinguopulpal
MO – mesio-occlusal
MOD – mesio-occlusodistal
molar
Moon's teeth
Moorehead's retractor
Moult curet
mouth prop
MP – mesiopulpal
MPL – mesiopulpolingual
MPLA – mesiopulpolabial
mucobuccal
mucocele
mucoid
mucoperiosteal
mucoperiosteum
mucosa
    buccal m.
    retromolar m.
    retrotuberosity m.

Mummery
    pink tooth of M.
muscle
    buccinator m.
    glossopalatine m.
    masseter m.
    masticatory m.
    mylohyoid m.
    platysma m.
    pterygoid m.
    sternocleidomastoid m.
mylohyoid
Nasmyth's membrane
neck
    surgical n. of tooth
necrosis
neoplasm
nerve
    alveolar n.
    lingual n.
    palatine n.
nonocclusion
nonunion
NUG — necrotizing ulcerative
    gingivitis
numatizashun. See
  pneumatization.
OC — occlusocervical
occlude
occlusal
occlusion
    afunctional o.
    buccal o.
    centric o.
    class I, II, III o.
    eccentric o.
    edge-to-edge o.
    functional o.
    lingual o.
    mesial o.
    skeletal o.
    traumatogenic o.

occlusocervical
Ochsenbein's gingivectomy
odontagra
odontalgia
    phantom o.
odontatrophia
odontectomy
odontexesis
odontiasis
odontoblast
odontoblastoma
odontobothrion
odontobothritis
odontocele
odontoceramic
odontocia
odontoclasis
odontoclast
odontogen
odontogenesis
    o. imperfecta
odontogenous
odontoglyph
odontogram
odontography
odontohyperesthesia
odontoiatria
odontoid
odontolith
odontolithiasis
odontologist
odontology
odontoloxia
odontolysis
odontoma
odontonecrosis
odontoneuralgia
odontoparallaxis
odontoplasty
odontoplerosis
odontoptosis
odontoradiograph

odontorrhagia
odontoschism
odontoscope
odontoscopy
odontoseisis
odontosis
odontosteophyte
odontotheca
odontotomy
odontotripsis
odontotrypy
oligodontia
oolo-. See words beginning
    ulo-.
operation
    Brophy's o.
    Caldwell-Luc o.
    Commando o.
operculum
    dental o.
oral
orale
orolingual
oromandibular
oromaxillary
oronasal
oropharyngeal
oropharynx
orthodontic
orthodontics
orthodontist
ostectomy
osteoma
    o. dentale
osteoperiostitis
    alveolodental o.
osteotome
osteotomy
overbite
PA — pulpoaxial
pack
    oropharyngeal p.

packing
    vaginal p.
palatal
palate
    cleft p.
palatine
palatoplasty
papillae
papillomatosis
paracone
paraconid
paradental
parallelometer
pararhizoclasia
parodontal
parodontid
parotid
PBA — pulpobuccoaxial
PD — pulpodistal
pedodontics
pemphigus
perforation
    root p.
periapical
pericementitis
    apical p.
pericementoclasia
pericementum
pericoronitis
peridens
periodontal
periodontics
periodontist
periodontitis
periodontium
periodontoclasia
periodontosis
periosteal
periosteum
    p. alveolare
pharyngeal
pharynx

phatnoma
phatnorrhagia
pick
    Rhein's p's
pioreah. See *pyorrhea.*
PL — pulpolingual
PLA — pulpolabial
    pulpolinguoaxial
plaque
pliers
    Allen's root p.
    crown-crimping p.
PM — pulpomesial
pneumatization
poikilodentosis
polyodontia
pontic
porcelain
pouch
    Rathke's p.
premolar
process
    mastoid p.
profile
    prognathic p.
    retrognathic p.
prognathism
prognathous
prophylactodontics
prophylaxis
prosthesis
prosthetic
prosthion
prosthodontics
protrusion
proximobuccal
proximolabial
proximolingual
pulp
    coronal p.
    mummified p.
    necrotic p.

pulp (*continued*)
    radicular p.
pulpa
    p. dentis
pulpalgia
pulpectomy
pulpitis
pulpoaxial
pulpobuccoaxial
pulpodistal
pulpolabial
pulpolingual
pulpolinguoaxial
pulpomesial
pulpotomy
punch
    Ainsworth's p.
purchase point
putrescence
pyorrhea
    p. alveolaris
    paradental p.
    Schmutz p.
pyorrheal
quadricuspid
radectomy
radicular
radiectomy
radiolucency
radiopacity
radix
    r. dentis
ramus
ranula
raphe
    palatine r.
    pterygomandibular r.
Rathke's pouch
reattachment
reciprocation
replantation
    intentional r.

reposition
restoration
    crown r.
retractor
    Austin's r.
    Moorehead's r.
retromolar
retrusion
Retzius' parallel striae
Rhein's picks
rhizodontrophy
rhizoid
Risdon's wire
rongeur
root canal
rubber dam
rugae
saliva
salivary
salivation
Salter's incremental lines
saprodontia
scaler
scaling
Scarpa's foramen
Schmutz pyorrhea
Schreger's striae
separator
septa
    s. interalveolaria
      maxillae
septum
    gingival s.
    s. interradiculare
sequestrectomy
sequestrum
shelf
    buccal s.
    dental s.
sialadenitis
sialolithiasis
singulum. See *cingulum.*

socket
    dry s.
spicule
Spira's disease
Spirec drill
splint
    acrylic s.
    canine-to-canine lingual s.
    Gilmer's s.
stenocompressor
Stent's mass
Stim-U-Dents
stomatitis
    aphthous s.
    herpetic s.
    necrotizing ulcerative s.
    s. venenata
    Vincent's s.
    vulcanite s.
stomatorrhagia
    s. gingivarum
stratum
    s. adamantinum
    s. eboris
striae
    Retzius' parallel s.
    Schreger's s.
Stryker drill
stylomyloid
sublingual
submandibular
submaxillary
substantia
    s. adamantina dentis
    s. dentalis propria
    s. eburnea dentis
    s. intertubularis dentis
    s. propria dentis
    s. vitrea dentis
sulcus
    alveolabial s.
    alveolingual s.

sulcus (*continued*)

    buccal s.

    gingival s.

    labiodental s.

    lingual s.

supernumerary

suppuration

    alveodental s.

supraclusion

surgical procedures. See
    operation.

symphysis

teeth. See *tooth.*

template

temporomandibular

temporomaxillary

thecodont

tic

    t. douloureux (doo-loo-
      roo)

tongue

tooth (teeth)

    accessional t.

    acrylic resin t.

    anatomic t.

    ankylosed t.

    auditory t. of Huschke

    t. of axis

    barred t.

    bicuspid t.

    brown opalescent t.,
      hereditary

    buccal t.

    canine t.

    cheek t.

    cheoplastic t.

    chiaie t.

    connate t.

    cross-bite t.

    cross-pin t.

    cuspid t.

    cuspless t.

tooth (teeth) (*continued*)

    deciduous t.

    diatoric t.

    embedded t.

    t. of epistropheus

    Fournier t.

    fused t.

    geminate t.

    Goslee t.

    hag t.

    hair t.

    Horner's t.

    Hutchinson's t.

    impacted t.

    incisor t.

    labial t.

    malacotic t.

    malposed t.

    mandibular t.

    maxillary t.

    metal insert t.

    milk t.

    molar t.

    Moon's t.

    morsal t.

    mottled t.

    mulberry t.

    neonatal t.

    nonanatomic t.

    peg t.

    permanent t.

    pink t. of Mummery

    pinless t.

    plastic t.

    posterior t.

    predeciduous t.

    premilk t.

    premolar t.

    primary t.

    pulpless t.

    rake t.

    rootless t.

tooth (teeth) (*continued*)
 sclerotic t.
 screwdriver t.
 shell t.
 snaggle t.
 stomach t.
 straight-pin t.
 submerged t.
 succedaneous t.
 successional t.
 superior t.
 supernumerary t.
 temporary t.
 tube t.
 Turner's t.
 vital t.
 wandering t.
 wisdom t.
 wolf t.
 zero degree t.
tooth-borne
tophus
 dental t.
tork-. See words beginning
 torq-.
torque
torquing
torsion
torsiversion
torus
 t. mandibularis
 t. palatinus
trachea
tracheostomy
transversion
trigonid
triple-angle
trismus
tube
 endotracheal t.
 nasogastric t.
tuberosity

Turner's tooth
ulcer
 Crombie's u.
ulectomy
ulemorrhagia
ulitis
ulocace
ulocarcinoma
uloglossitis
ulokahse. See *ulocace.*
uloncus
ulorrhagia
ulorrhea
ulotomy
ultrasonic
uvula
uvulectomy
vermilion
vestibular
vestibuloplasty
Vincent's
 infection
 stomatitis
Vitallium
vomer
vulcanite
Wharton's duct
Winter's arch bar
wire
 continuous loop w.
 interdental w.
 intraoral w.
 Ivy w.
 Kirschner's w.
 Risdon's w.
xanthodontus
zanthodontus. See
 xanthodontus.
zygoma
zygomatic

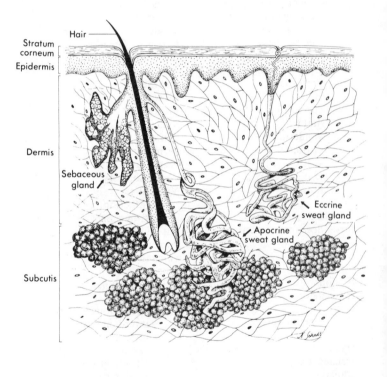

Hair

Stratum corneum

Epidermis

Dermis

Sebaceous gland

Eccrine sweat gland

Apocrine sweat gland

Subcutis

DERMATOLOGY AND ALLERGY

Abernethy's sarcoma
abscess
    Monro's a.
    Paget's a.
Absidia
Abt-Letterer-Siwe syndrome
acanthokeratodermia
acantholysis
    a. bullosa
acanthoma
    a. adenoides cysticum
    a. inguinale
    a. tropicum
    a. verrucosa seborrhoeica
acanthosis
    a. nigricans
    a. papulosa nigra
    a. seborrhoeica
    a. verrucosa
acanthotic
acariasis
    chorioptic a.
    demodectic a.
    psoroptic a.
    sarcoptic a.
acarodermatitis
    a. urticarioides
Acarus
    A. folliculorum
    A. gallinae

Acarus (continued)
    A. hordei
    *A. rhyzoglypticus
      hyacinthi*
    A. scabiei
    A. tritici
acetonasthma
achor
achromatosis
achromia
    congenital a.
    a. parasitica
achromoderma
achromotrichia
acladiosis
acne
    adenoid a.
    a. aggregata seu
      conglobata
    a. agminata
    a. albida
    a. artificialis
    a. atrophica
    bromine a.
    a. cachecticorum
    a. cheloidique
    a. ciliaris
    common a.
    a. conglobata
    cystic a.

acne (*continued*)
    a. decalvans
    a. disseminata
    a. dorsalis
    epileptic a.
    a. erythematosa
    a. excoriee des jeunes
      filles
    a. frontalis
    a. generalis
    halogen a.
    halowax a.
    a. hordeolaris
    a. hypertrophica
    a. indurata
    iodine a.
    a. keloid
    lupoid a.
    a. mentagra
    a. necrotica miliaris
    a. necroticans et
      exulcerans serpiginosa
      nasi
    a. neonatorum
    pancreatic a.
    a. papulosa
    petroleum a.
    a. picealis
    a. punctata
    a. pustulosa
    a. rodens
    a. rosacea
    a. scorbutica
    a. scrofulosorum
    a. seborrheica
    a. simplex
    a. syphilitica
    tar a.
    a. tarsi
    a. varioliformis
    a. vulgaris
acnegenic

acneiform
acrochordon
acrocyanosis
acrodermatitis
    a. chronica atrophicans
    a. continua
    a. enteropathica
    Hallopeau's a.
    a. hiemalis
    a. perstans
    a. vesiculosa tropica
acrodermatoses
acrodermatosis
acrodynia
acrokeratosis
    a. verruciformis
acroscleroderma
acrosclerosis
actinic
actinocutitis
actinodermatitis
actinomycosis
adamantinoma
Addison-Gull disease
Addison's
    disease
    keloid
adenoma
    a. sebaceum
adermia
adermogenesis
adiponecrosis
adipose
adjuvant
    Freund's a.
    mycobacterial a.
aftha. See *aphtha.*
agammaglobulinemia
agglutination
agglutinin
agglutinogen
agranulocytosis

agria
agrius
albinism
albinismus
    a. conscriptus
    a. totalis
    a. universalis
albino
Albright's syndrome
Alibert-Bazin syndrome
Alibert's
    disease
    mentagra
allergen
allergenic
allergic
allergy
alopecia
    androgenetic a.
    a. areata
    a. capitis totalis
    cicatricial a.
    a. cicatrisata
    a. circumscripta
    congenital a.
    a. congenitalis
    a. disseminata
    drug a.
    female pattern a.
    follicular a.
    a. follicularis
    a. hereditaria
    hereditary a.
    a. liminaris
    male pattern a.
    marginal a.
    a. marginalis
    a. medicamentosa
    a. mucinosa
    a. orbicularis
    a. perinevica
    physiologic a.

alopecia (*continued*)
    postpartum a.
    a. prematura
    a. presenilis
    pressure a.
    roentgen a.
    a. seborrheica
    senile a.
    a. senilis
    symptomatic a.
    a. symptomatica
    syphilitic a.
    a. syphilitica
    a. totalis
    toxic a.
    a. toxica
    traction a.
    traumatic a.
    a. traumatica
    a. triangularis
        congenitalis
    a. universalis
    x-ray a.
alopecic
alphodermia
alphos
altauna
amboceptor
amelanotic
ameloblastoma
Amico's
    drill
    extractor
    nail nipper
    skin lifter
amyloid
amyloidosis
    cutaneous a.
    a. cutis
anagen
anagen to telogen ratio
anaphylactic

anaphylactoid
anaphylaxis
Andrews' disease
anergy
anesthesia. See *General
Surgical Terms.*
anetoderma
angiocavernous
angiodermatitis
angiofibroma
angiokeratoma
angiolupoid
angioma
    a. pigmentosum
    plexiform a.
    a. serpiginosum
anhidrosis
anonychia
anthema
anthracia
anthracoid
anthrax
antibody
    antinuclear a's
antifungal
antifungoid
antigen
antiserum
    Reenstierna a.
antitoxigen
antitoxin
antitoxinogen
aphtha
aphthoid
aphthous
apiotherapy
apisination
appendage
areatus
areola
    Chaussier's a.
    vaccinal a.

areolitis
arevareva
argyria
ariboflavinosis
Arndt-Gottron disease
Arthus phenomenon
Asboe-Hansen's disease
aspergillosis
asteatosis
    a. cutis
asthma
    Millar's a.
asthmatic
Asturian leprosy
atheroma
    a. cutis
atheromasia
atheromatosis
    a. cutis
atheromatous
atopen
atopic
atopy
atrichia
atrichosis
atrophie
    a. blanche
atrophodermatosis
aurantiasis
aurid
Auspitz's dermatosis
autoantibody
autoantigen
autodermic
autodesensitization
autoeczematization
autoimmunization
autoinoculation
Aveeno bath
bacillus
    Ducrey's b.
    Hansen's b.

bacterid
    pustular b.
Baerensprung's erythrasma
bandage. See *General Surgical Terms.*
Barber's dermatosis
Bard-Parker dermatome
Barker Vacu-tome dermatome
basal layer
bath
    Aveeno b.
Bazin's disease
Beau's lines
Becker's nevus
bejel
Besnier-Boeck disease
Besnier's prurigo
Biett's collar
biopsy
    punch b.
biotripsis
blastomycosis
    cutaneous b.
    systemic b.
bleb
blef-. See words beginning *bleph-.*
blennorrhagia
blennorrhea
blepharitis
blepharochalasis
blister
Bloch's reaction
blotch
    palpebral b.
Bockhart's impetigo
body
    Leishman-Donovan b's
    Lipschütz's b's
Boeck's
    disease
    itch

Boeck's (*continued*)
    sarcoid
    scabies
boil
boot
    Unna's b.
Bowen's
    disease
    precancerous dermatosis
bromhidrosis
Brooke's disease
Brown's dermatome
Bruck's test
bubo
    Frei's b.
bubon
    b. d'emblée
Buerger's disease
bulla
bullous
Buschke-Ollendorff syndrome
Buschke's scleredema
café-au-lait
calcinosis
    c. circumscripta
    c. cutis
callosity
callous
callus
calor
    c. mordax
    c. mordicans
calva
calvities
calvitium
canceroderm
cancroid
cancrum
Candida
    C. albicans
candidiasis
canities

canker
Cantlie's foot tetter
capillary
carbuncle
carbuncular
carbunculosis
carcinelcosis
carcinomelcosis
carotenemia
carotenodermia
Carrión's disease
caruncle
caruncula
Casal's necklace
caseation
Castellani's paint
cativi
causalgia
Cazenave's
　　　disease
　　　lupus
　　　vitiligo
cell
　　　basal c.
　　　horny c.
　　　keratinized c.
　　　Langhans' c's
　　　Lipschütz's c.
　　　malpighian c's
　　　mast c.
　　　Paget's c.
　　　prickle c.
　　　squamous c.
　　　Touton giant c's
　　　Tzank c.
cellulitis
　　　streptococcus c.
cellulocutaneous
Celsus'
　　　kerion
　　　papules
　　　vitiligo

centrocyte
chalazia
chalazion
chancre
　　　fungating c.
　　　indurated c.
　　　Ricord's c.
　　　Rollet's c.
　　　sporotrichotic c.
　　　sulcus c.
chancriform
chancroid
chapped
Chaussier's aerola
cheilitis
　　　actinic c.
　　　c. actinica
　　　apostematous c.
　　　commissural c.
　　　exfoliativa c.
　　　glandularis apostematosa
　　　　　c.
　　　impetiginous c.
　　　migrating c.
　　　c. venenata
cheiropompholyx
chigger
chigoe
chilblain
　　　necrotized c.
chloasma
　　　c. hepaticum
　　　c. periorale virginium
　　　c. phthisicorum
　　　c. traumaticum
chloracne
chlorosis
cholesterosis
　　　c. cutis
chondrodermatitis
　　　c. nodularis chronica
　　　　　helicis

chromatophore
chromatosis
chromhidrosis
chromoblastomycosis
chromomycosis
chromophytosis
chrotoplast
Ciarrocchi's disease
cicatrix
cimicosis
circinate
Civatte's poikiloderma
clavus
    c. syphiliticus
Coccidioides
    C. immitis
coccidioidomycosis
Cole's herpetiform lesion
collagen
collagenosis
collar
    Biett's c.
    c. of pearls
    c. of Venus
collarette
Collins' dynamometer
comedo
comedones
complex
    EAHF c.
condyloma
    c. acuminatum
    c. latum
    c. subcutaneum
confluent
congelation
conjunctivitis
corium
Corlett's pyosis
corneum
cornification
cornified

cornu
    c. cutaneum
corona
    c. seborrheica
    c. veneris
Coxsackie virus
croup
crustosus
cryocautery
cryotherapy
cryptococcosis
cuniculus
curet
    Fox's c.
    Piffard's c.
    Walsh's c.
cutaneous
cuticle
cuticularization
cutireaction
cutis
    c. anserina
    c. elastica
    c. hyperelastica
    c. laxa
    c. marmorata
    c. pendula
    c. pensilis
    c. rhomboidalis nuchae
    c. testacea
    c. unctuosa
    c. vera
    c. verticis gyrata
cutisector
cutitis
cutization
cyasma
cylindroma
cyst
    dermoid c.
dactylitis
    d. strumosa

dactylitis (*continued*)
    d. syphilitica
    d. tuberculosa
dander
dandruff
Danielssen's disease
Danlos' syndrome
Darier-Roussy sarcoid
Darier's disease
Darier's sign
dartre
dartrous
deallergization
debride
debridement
    enzymatic d.
    surgical d.
decalvant
decongestant
decongestive
decubital
decubitus
deficiency
    riboflavin d.
deflorescence
defluxio
    d. capillorum
    d. ciliorum
defurfuration
Degos-Delort-Tricot syndrome
Demodex
    D. folliculorum
depigmentation
depilate
depilation
depilatory
derma
dermabrader
    Iverson's d.
    sandpaper d.
dermabrasion
dermad

dermadrome
dermagen
dermal
dermalaxia
dermametropathism
dermamyiasis
    d. linearis migrans
      oestrosa
dermanaplasty
dermapostasis
dermatalgia
dermataneuria
dermatauxe
dermatergosis
dermathemia
dermatic
dermatitides
dermatitis
    actinic d.
    d. aestivalis
    allergic d.
    d. ambustionis
    ancylostome d.
    arsphenamine d.
    d. artefacta
    atopic d.
    d. atrophicans
    berloque d.
    bhiwanol d.
    blastomycetic d.
    brucella d.
    d. bullosa
    d. calorica
    d. combustionis
    d. congelationis
    contact d.
    d. contusiformis
    cosmetic d.
    dhobie mark d.
    d. dysmenorrhoeica
    eczematous d.
    d. epidemica

dermatitis (*continued*)
- d. erythematosa
- d. escharotica
- d. excoriativa infantum
- d. exfoliativa
- d. exfoliativa epidemica
- d. exfoliativa infantum
- exudative discoid and lichenoid d.
- d. factitia
- d. gangrenosa
- d. gangrenosa infantum
- d. hemostatica
- d. herpetiformis
- d. hiemalis
- d. hypostatica
- d. infectiosa eczematoides
- Jacquet's d.
- Leiner's d.
- livedoid d.
- d. medicamentosa
- d. multiformis
- mycotic d.
- d. nodosa
- d. nodularis necrotica
- d. papillaris capillitii
- d. pediculoides ventricosus
- pigmented purpuric lichenoid d.
- poison ivy d.
- poison oak d.
- poison sumac d.
- precancerous d.
- d. psoriasiformis nodularis
- purpuric pigmented lichenoid d.
- d. repens
- roentgen-ray d.
- schistosome d.

dermatitis (*continued*)
- seborrheic d.
- d. seborrheica
- d. simplex
- d. skiagraphica
- d. solaris
- stasis d.
- d. traumatica
- uncinarial d.
- d. vegetans
- d. venenata
- d. verrucosa
- weeping d.

dermatoarthritis
dermatoautoplasty
dermatobiasis
dermatocandidiasis
dermatocele
dermatocellulitis
dermatochalasis
dermatoconiosis
dermatoconjunctivitis
dermatocyst
dermatodysplasia
- d. verruciformis

dermatofibroma
- d. protuberans

dermatofibrosarcoma
- d. protuberans

dermatofibrosis
- d. lenticularis disseminata

dermatogen
dermatogenous
dermatograph
dermatographia
dermatoheteroplasty
dermatoid
dermatokelidosis
dermatologic
dermatologist
dermatology

dermatolysis
    d. palpebrarum
dermatoma
dermatome
    Bard-Parker d.
    Barker Vacu-tome d.
    Brown's d.
    Hall's d.
    Hood's d.
    Meek-Wall d.
    Padgett's d.
    Reese's d.
    Stryker's d.
dermatomegaly
dermatomucosomyositis
dermatomycosis
    blastomycetic d.
    d. furfuracea
    d. microsporina
    d. trichophytina
dermatomyiasis
dermatomyoma
dermatomyositis
dermatoneurology
dermato-ophthalmitis
dermatopathic
dermatopathy
dermatophiliasis
Dermatophilus
    D. penetrans
dermatophylaxis
dermatophyte
dermatophytid
dermatophytosis
    d. furfuracea
dermatoplastic
dermatoplasty
dermatopolyneuritis
dermatorrhagia
dermatorrhea
dermatorrhexis
dermatoscopy

dermatosis
    acarine d.
    angioneurotic d.
    Auspitz's d.
    Barber's d.
    Bowen's precancerous d.
    lichenoid d.
    d. papulosa nigra
    precancerous d.
    progressive pigmentary d.
    Schamberg's d.
    stasis d.
    subcorneal pustular d.
    Unna's d.
dermatostomatitis
dermatotherapy
dermatotome
dermatotropic
dermatozoonosus
dermepenthesis
dermis
dermitis
dermoanergy
dermoblast
dermograph
dermographia
dermohemia
dermoid
dermoidectomy
dermolipoma
dermolysis
dermomycosis
dermopathy
dermophlebitis
dermostenosis
dermostosis
dermosynovitis
dermosyphilography
dermosyphilopathy
dermotactile
dermotropic
dermovaccine

dermovascular
desensitize
desiccation
    electric d.
desquamation
    furfuraceous d.
    membranous d.
    siliquose d.
Devergie's disease
diamonds
diaphoresis
diascope
diascopy
Dick test
discoid
disease
    Addison-Gull d.
    Addison's d.
    Alibert's d.
    Andrews' d.
    Arndt-Gottron d.
    Asboe-Hansen's d.
    Bazin's d.
    Besnier-Boeck d.
    Boeck's d.
    Bowen's d.
    Brooke's d.
    Buerger's d.
    Carrión's d.
    Cazenave's d.
    Ciarrocchi's d.
    Danielssen's d.
    Darier's d.
    Devergie's d.
    Duhring's d.
    Fordyce's d.
    Fox-Fordyce d.
    Frei's d.
    Gaucher's d.
    Gibert's d.
    Gilchrist's d.
    Hailey and Hailey d.

disease (*continued*)
    Hallopeau's d.
    Hand-Schüller-Christian
      d.
    Hansen's d.
    Hartnup's d.
    Hebra's d.
    Hodgkin's d.
    Hutchinson's d.
    Hyde's d.
    Jadassohn's d.
    Kaposi's d.
    Köbner's d.
    Landouzy's d.
    Leiner's d.
    Leloir's d.
    Letterer-Siwe d.
    Lipschütz's d.
    Lortat-Jacobs d.
    Lutz-Miescher d.
    Majocchi's d.
    Mibelli's d.
    Neumann's d.
    Nicolas-Favre d.
    Niemann-Pick d.
    Osler's d.
    Osler-Vaquez d.
    Pollitzer's d.
    Puente's d.
    Quincke's d.
    Quinquaud's d.
    Rayer's d.
    Raynaud's d.
    Recklinghausen's d.
    Reiter's d.
    Robinson's d.
    Schamberg's d.
    Senear-Usher d.
    Sticker's d.
    Sutton's d.
    Taenzer's d.
    Urbach-Oppenheim d.

disease (*continued*)
    Weber-Christian d.
    Weber's d.
    White's d.
disseminated
distichia
DLE — discoid lupus
    erythematosus
dopaoxidase
dracunculiasis
dressing. See *General Surgical Terms.*
drill
    Amico's d.
    Ralks' d.
drugs. See *Drugs and Chemistry* section.
D & S — dermatology and
    syphilology
Ducrey's bacillus
Duhring's
    disease
    pruritus
dynamometer
    Collins' d.
dyschromia
dyshidrosis
    trichophytic d.
dyskeratosis
    d. congenita
    d. follicularis
dyspigmentation
dystrophy
    median canaliform d. of
    the nail
EAHF — eczema, asthma,
    hay fever
ecchymosis
ECHO (enteric cytopathogenic
    human orphan) virus
ecthyma
    e. contagiosum

ecthyma (*continued*)
    e. gangrenosum
    e. syphiliticum
ectoderm
ectodermosis
    e. erosiva pluriorificialis
ectothrix
Ectotrichophyton
ectropion
ectylotic
eczema
    allergic e.
    e. articulorum
    atopic e.
    e. barbae
    e. capitis
    e. craquelé
    e. crustosum
    e. diabeticorum
    e. epilans
    e. epizootica
    e. erythematosum
    flexural e.
    e. herpeticum
    e. hypertrophicum
    infantile e.
    e. intertrigo
    lichenoid e.
    linear e.
    e. madidans
    e. marginatum
    e. neuriticum
    e. nummulare
    e. papulosum
    e. parasiticum
    e. pustulosum
    e. rubrum
    e. scrofuloderma
    e. seborrhoeicum
    e. siccum
    solar e.
    e. solare

eczema (*continued*)
    e. squamosum
    stasis e.
    e. tyloticum
    e. vaccinatum
    e. verrucosum
    e. vesiculosum
    weeping e.
eczematid
eczematization
eczematoid
eczematosis
eczematous
edema
    angioneurotic e.
efelis. See *ephelis.*
effluvium
    anagen e.
    telogen e.
efidrosis. See *ephidrosis.*
Ehlers-Danlos syndrome
eksan-. See words beginning
    exan-.
ekzema. See *eczema.*
elastosis
    e. senilis
electrodermogram
electrodermography
electrodesiccation
elephantiasis
    e. arabicum
    e. asturiensis
    e. filariensis
    e. graecorum
    e. leishmaniana
    lymphangiectatic e.
    e. telangiectodes
elevator
    Ralks' e.
emaculation
emollient
emphlysis

emphractic
emulsion
    Pusey's e.
encrusted
endothelioma
    e. capitis
    e. cutis
endothrix
endotoxin
enzyme
eosinophilia
ephelis
ephidrosis
    e. cruenta
epidermal
epidermatitis
epidermatoplasty
epidermicula
epidermidosis
epidermis
epidermitis
epidermization
epidermodysplasia
    e. verruciformis
epidermoid
epidermolysis
    e. acquisita
    e. bullosa
    e. bullosa dystrophica
    polydysplastic e. bullosa
    toxic bullous e.
epidermoma
epidermomycosis
epidermophytid
Epidermophyton
    E. floccosum
epidermophytosis
    e. cruris
    e. interdigitale
epidermosis
epilation
epilatory

epiparonychia
epithelial
epithelialization
epithelioid
epithelioma
    e. adenoides cysticum
    e. capitis
    e. molluscum
epitheliomatosis
epitheliomatous
epithelium
epithelization
eponychia
eponychium
ergodermatosis
erisipelas. See *erysipelas.*
erosion
erubescence
eruption
    bullous e.
    creeping e.
    crustaceous e.
    erythematous e.
    Kaposi's varicelliform e.
    macular e.
    papular e.
    petechial e.
    pustular e.
    squamous e.
    serum e.
    tubercular e.
eruptive
erysipelas
    ambulant e.
    gangrenous e.
    e. grave internum
    idiopathic e.
    migrant e.
    e. perstans
    phlegmonous e.
    e. pustulosum
    e. verrucosum

erysipelas (*continued*)
    e. vesiculosum
    zoonotic e.
erysipelatous
erysipeloid
erythema
    e. abigne
    acrodynic e.
    e. annulare
    e. annulare centrifugum
    e. annulare rheumaticum
    e. bullosum
    e. caloricum
    e. circinatum
    e. elevatum diutinum
    e. exudativum
    e. figuratum
    e. fugax
    e. gyratum
    e. induratum
    e. infectiosum
    e. intertrigo
    e. iris
    Jacquet's e.
    e. marginatum
    Milian's e.
    e. multiforme
    e. neonatorum
    e. neonatorum toxicum
    e. nodosum
    e. nodosum syphiliticum
    palmar e.
    e. paratrimma
    e. pernio
    e. perstans
    e. pudicitiae
    e. punctatum
    e. scarlatiniforme
    e. simplex
    e. solare
    e. streptogenes
    e. toxicum

erythema (*continued*)
    e. traumaticum
    e. venenatum
erythematosus
    discoid lupus e.
    systemic lupus e.
erythematous
erythra
erythralgia
erythrasma
    Baerensprung's e.
erythredema polyneuropathy
erythrocyanosis
    e. crurum puellaris
    e. frigida crurum
      puellarum
    e. supramalleolaris
erythroderma
    atopic e.
    congenital ichthyosiform
      e.
    e. desquamativum
    exfoliative e.
    e. ichthyosiforme
      congenitum
    lymphomatous e.
    e. psoriaticum
    Sézary e.
    e. squamosum
erythrodermatitis
erythromelia
erythroplasia
    e. of Queyrat
eschar
eskar. See *eschar.*
esthiomene
evanescent
exanthem
    vesicular e.
exanthema
    e. subitum
exanthematous

excoriation
    neurotic e.
excrescence
excrescent
exfoliation
exfoliative
exocrine
extractor
    Amico's e.
    comedo e.
    Saalfield's e.
    Schamberg's e.
    Unna's e.
    Walton's e.
exudate
exudation
exulceratio
    e. simplex
exuviae
fajedenah. See *phagedena.*
FANA — fluorescent anti-
      nuclear antibody
favid
favus
    f. circinatus
    f. herpeticus
    f. herpetiformis
    f. pilaris
felon
fester
fever
    scarlet f.
fiber
    Herxheimer's f's
fibroblast
fibroma
    f. cutis
    f. lipomatodes
    f. pendulum
    telangiectatic f.
    f. xanthoma
fibrosis

fissure
fitofotodermatitis. See
    phytophotodermatitis.
flare
flumen
flumina pilorum
fluorescence
follicle
    sebaceous f.
follicular
folliculitis
    f. abscedens et
      suffodiens
    agminate f.
    f. barbae
    f. cheloidalis
    f. decalvans
    f. decalvans et lichen
      spinulosus
    f. gonorrhoeica
    f. keloidalis
    f. nares perforans
    f. ulerythematosa
      reticulata
    f. varioliformis
foot tetter
    Cantlie's f.t.
Fordyce's
    disease
    spots
formication
formiciasis
Foshay's test
Fox-Fordyce disease
Fox's
    curet
    impetigo
fragilitas
    f. crinium
    f. unguium
frambesia
frambesioma

freckle
    melanotic f. of Hutchison
Frei's
    bubo
    disease
    test
frenulum
frenum
Freund's adjuvant
fulguration
fulgurize
fungal
fungate
fungous
fungus
furfur
furfuraceous
furuncle
furuncular
furunculoid
furunculosis
furunculus
    f. vulgaris
ganglion
gangrene
    cutaneous g.
    disseminated cutaneous
      g.
    gaseous g.
    Raynaud's g.
gangrenous
Gaucher's disease
Gennerich's treatment
genodermatology
genodermatosis
Gibert's
    disease
    pityriasis
Gilchrist's disease
gingivitis
gingivoglossitis
glabrous

gland
    sebaceous g.
    sweat g.
globulin
    antidiphtheritic g.
    antitoxic g.
    gamma g's
    immune serum g.
glomus
    cutaneous g.
    digital g.
    neuromyoarterial g.
glossitis
    g. areata exfoliativa
    g. dissecans
    Hunter's g.
    Moeller's g.
    g. parasitica
    parenchymatous g.
    rhomboid g.
    g. rhomboidea mediana
goatpox
Goeckerman treatment
gonitis
    fungous g.
gonococcus
gonorrhea
gonorrheal
Gougerot's syndrome
granular
granulation
granuloma
    g. annulare
    g. endemicum
    eosinophilic g.
    g. fungoides
    g. gangraenescens
    Hodgkin's g.
    g. inguinale
    lipoid g.
    lycopodium g.
    Majocchi's g.

granuloma (*continued*)
    g. malignum
    g. pyogenicum
    g. sarcomatodes
    g. telangiectaticum
    g. trichophyticum
    g. venereum
granulomatosis
    Miescher-Leder g.
gumma
gutta
    g. rosacea
guttate
Hailey and Hailey disease
Hallopeau's
    acrodermatitis
    disease
Hall's dermatome
hamartoma
hamartomatosis
hamartomatous
Hand-Schüller-Christian disease
Hansen's
    bacillus
    disease
haplodermatitis
Hartnup's disease
Hebra's
    disease
    ointment
    pityriasis
hemangioma
    capillary h.
    cavernous h.
    h. congenitale
    h. hypertrophicum cutis
    h. simplex
hemangiomatosis
hematid
hematidrosis
hemochromatosis
hemorrhage

heparin
herpangina
herpes
    h. catarrhalis
    h. digitalis
    h. facialis
    h. farinosus
    h. febrilis
    h. generalisatus
    h. genitalis
    h. gestationis
    h. iris
    h. labialis
    h. menstrualis
    h. mentalis
    nasal h.
    h. oticus
    h. phlyctaenodes
    h. praeputialis
    h. progenitalis
    h. recurrens
    h. simplex
    h. simplex recurrens
    h. tonsurans
    h. tonsurans maculosus
    h. vegetans
    h. zoster
    h. zoster ophthalmicus
    h. zoster oticus
    h. zoster varicellosus
herpetic
herpetiform
Herxheimer's
    fibers
    reaction
    spirals
heterochromia
heterodermic
heterophil
heterophilic
heterotrichosis
    h. supercilliorum

hidradenitis
    h. suppurativa
hidrocystoma
hidrorrhea
hidrosadenitis
    h. axillaris
    h. destruens suppurativa
hidroschesis
hidrosis
hirsuties
hirsutism
histaminase
histamine
histaminia
histiocyte
histiocytoma
    lipoid h.
histiocytomatosis
histiocytosis
histoplasmosis
Hodgkin's
    disease
    granuloma
hodi-potsy
holocrine
homme
    h. rouge
homograft
homologous
Hood's dermatome
hornification
horny
horripilation
Hunter's glossitis
Hutchinson's
    disease
    freckle
    mask
    triad
hyalin
hyaline
hyatid

Hyde's disease
hydration
hydroa
    h. aestivale
    h. febrile
    h. gestationis
    h. gravidarum
    h. puerorum
    h. vacciniforme
    h. vesiculosum
hydrocystoma
hydrotherapy
hygroma
    h. colli
    cystic h.
    h. cysticum
hyperergia
hyperergy
hypergammaglobulinemia
hyperhidrosis
hyperkeratosis
    h. congenitalis palmaris
      et plantaris
    epidermolytic h.
    h. excentrica
    h. figurata centrifuga
      atrophica
    h. follicularis in cutem
      penetrans
    h. follicularis vegetans
    h. linguae
    h. penetrans
    h. subungualis
    h. universalis congenita
hyperpigmentation
hypersarcosis
hypersensibility
hypersensitiveness
hypersensitivity
hypersensitization
hypertrichiasis
hypertrichophrydia

hypertrichosis
hypha
hyphomycetic
hyphomycosis
hypochromotrichia
hypodermis
hypodermolithiasis
hypoergia
hypogammaglobulin
hypogammaglobulinemia
hyponychium
hyponychon
hyposensitive
hyposensitization
ichthyismus
    i. exanthematicus
ichthyosis
    i. congenita
    i. cornea
    follicular i.
    i. follicularis
    i. hystrix
    i. intrauterina
    linear i.
    i. linguae
    nacreous i.
    i. palmaris
    i. palmaris et plantaris
    i. plantaris
    i. sauroderma
    i. scutulata
    i. sebacea cornea
    i. serpentina
    i. simplex
    i. spinosa
    i. thysanotrichica
    i. uteri
    i. vulgaris
icterus
I & D — incision and drainage
idiosyncrasy
iksodiahsis. See *ixodiasis.*

ikthe-. See words beginning
   ichthy-.
immunity
immunization
immunochemical
immunodiagnosis
immunoelectrophoresis
immunofluorescent
immunoglobulin
immunohistochemical
immunology
immunoreaction
immunotherapy
impetiginization
impetiginous
impetigo
   Bockhart's i.
   i. bullosa
   bullous i.
   i. contagiosa
   i. eczematodes
   follicular i.
   Fox's i.
   furfuraceous i.
   i. herpetiformis
   i. neonatorum
   i. simplex
   i. staphylogenes
   i. syphilitica
   i. variolosa
incontinentia
   i. pigmenti
induration
infestation
infiltrate
infiltration
   adipose i.
   cellular i.
   inflammatory i.
   lymphocytic i.
inflammation
integument

integumentary
integumentum
   i. commune
intertriginous
intertrigo
   i. labialis
   i. saccharomycetica
intimitis
   proliferative i.
intracutaneous
intradermal
intradermoreaction
intraepidermal
intraepithelial
itch
   Boeck's i.
   dhobie i.
   grain i.
   Moeller's i.
   seven-year i.
   swimmers' i.
itching
Ito-Reenstierna test
Iverson's dermabrader
ixodiasis
Jacquet's
   dermatitis
   erythema
Jadassohn-Bloch test
Jadassohn-Lewandosky law
Jadassohn's
   disease
   nevus
Jarisch-Herxheimer reaction
Jarisch's ointment
jaundice
jigger
Jones-Mote reaction
kalazea. See *chalazia*.
kalazeon. See *chalazion*.
Kaposi's
   disease

Kaposi's (*continued*)
    sarcoma
    varicelliform eruption
    xeroderma
Keller's ultraviolet test
keloid
    Addison's k.
keloidosis
keratiasis
keratin
keratinocyte
keratinous
keratoacanthoma
keratoderma
    k. blennorrhagica
    k. palmaris et plantaris
keratodermatitis
keratohyalin
keratohyaline
keratolysis
    k. exfoliativa
    k. neonatorum
keratoma
    k. diffusum
    k. hereditaria mutilans
    k. malignum congenitale
    k. palmare et plantare
    k. plantare sulcatum
    k. senile
keratomycosis
    k. linguae
keratonosis
keratoprotein
keratosis
    actinic k.
    k. blennorrhagica
    k. diffusa fetalis
    k. follicularis
    k. follicularis contagiosa
    gonorrheal k.
    k. labialis
    k. linguae

keratosis (*continued*)
    nevoid k.
    k. nigricans
    k. obturans
    k. palmaris et plantaris
    k. pilaris
    k. punctata
    seborrheic k.
    k. seborrheica
    senile k.
    k. senilis
    k. suprafollicularis
    k. vegetans
keratotic
kerion
    k. celsi
    Celsus' k.
Keyes' dermal punch
kilitis. See *cheilitis.*
kiropomfoliks. See
    cheiropompholyx.
kloazma. See *chloasma.*
klor-. See words beginning
    chlor-.
Köbner's disease
Koebner's phenomenon
KOH — potassium hydroxide
koilonychia
Kolmer's test
kondro-. See words beginning
    chondro-.
kraurosis
    k. penis
    k. vulvae
Kveim test
lacuna
Landouzy's
    disease
    purpura
Langhans'
    cells
    layer

lanugo
larva
    l. migrans
Lassar's paste
law
    Jadassohn-Lewandosky l.
layer
    Langhans' l.
    malpighian l.
LE — lupus erythematosus
Leiner's
    dermatitis
    disease
leiodermia
leiomyoma
    l. cutis
Leishman-Donovan bodies
leishmaniasis
Leloir's disease
lenticula
lentigines
lentigo
    l. maligna malignant
lentigomelanosis
lepidosis
lepothrix
lepra
    l. alba
    l. alphoides
    l. alphos
    l. anaesthetica
    l. arabum
    l. conjunctivae
    l. graecorum
    l. maculosa
    l. mutilans
    l. nervorum
    l. nervosa
    l. tuberculoides
    Willan's l.
leprid
leproma

lepromatous
leprosy
    Asturian l.
    cutaneous l.
    lazarine l.
    lepromatous l.
    Lombardy l.
    macular l.
    maculoanesthetic l.
    neural l.
    nodular l.
    trophoneurotic l.
    tuberculoid l.
leprotic
leprous
leptochroa
lesion
    Cole's herpetiform l.
    disseminated l.
    initial syphilitic l.
Letterer-Siwe disease
leukoderma
    l. acquisitum
        centrifugum
leukodermatous
leukonychia
leukoplakia
Lewandowsky's nevus elasticus
Libman-Sacks syndrome
lichen
    l. albus
    l. amyloidosus
    l. annularis
    l. chronicus simplex
    l. corneus hypertrophicus
    l. fibromucinoidosus
    l. frambesianus
    l. leprosus
    l. myxedematosus
    l. nitidus
    l. obtusus corneus
    l. pilaris

lichen (*continued*)
    l. planopilaris
    l. planus
    l. planus, acute bullous
    l. planus et acuminatus
      atrophicans
    l. planus, hypertrophic
    l. planus hypertrophicus
    l. ruber acuminatus
    l. ruber moniliformis
    l. ruber planus
    l. sclerosus et atrophicus
    l. scrofulosorum
    l. simplex chronicus
    l. spinulosus
    l. striatus
    l. urticatus
licheniasis
lichenification
lichenization
lichenoid
light
    Wood's l.
line
    Beau's l's
lipoatrophy
lipoblast
lipocyte
lipoidosis
lipoidproteinosis
lipoma
lipomatosis
liposarcoma
Lipschütz's
    bodies
    cell
    disease
    ulcer
lipsotrichia
livedo
    l. annularis
    l. racemosa

livedo (*continued*)
    l. reticularis
    l. reticularis iodiopathica
    l. reticularis
      symptomatica
    l. telangiectatica
livedoid
livid
Lombardy leprosy
Lortat-Jacob's disease
louse
lues
    l. nervosa
    l. tarda
    l. venerea
lunula
    l. of nail
    l. unguis
lupoid
lupus
    Cazenave's l.
    l. erythematodes
    l. erythematosus
    l. erythematosus
      discoides
    l. erythematosus
      disseminatus
    l. livido
    l. pernio
    l. tuberculosus
    l. tumidus
    l. verrucosus
    l. vorax
    l. vulgaris
Lutz-Miescher disease
Lutz-Splendore-de Almeida
    syndrome
Lyell's syndrome
lymphadenitis
lymphangioma
    l. cavernosum
    l. circumscriptum

lymphangioma (*continued*)
    l. cysticum
    l. tuberosum multiplex
    l. xanthelasmoideum
lymphangitis
    l. carcinomatosa
lymphedema
lymphocytoma
lymphodermia
lymphogranuloma
    l. benignum
    l. inguinale
    l. venereum
lymphogranulomatosis
    l. cutis
    l. inguinalis
    l. maligna
lymphoma
lymphosarcoma
lymphosarcomatosis
maceration
macroglobulinemia
macula
    m. solaris
maculae
    m. atrophicae
    m. caeruleae
macular
maculate
maculation
macule
maculopapular
maculopapule
maduromycosis
Majocchi's
    disease
    granuloma
    purpura
Malpighi rete
malpighian
    cells
    layer

mange
    demodectic m.
    follicular m.
Mantoux test
mask
    Hutchinson's m.
matrix
    nail m.
    m. unguis
matrixitis
Mauriac's syndrome
measles
medications. See *Drugs and Chemistry* section.
Meek-Wall dermatome
melanin
melanism
melanocyte
melanoderma
    m. cachecticorum
    senile m.
melanodermatitis
melanoleukoderma
    m. colli
melanoma
    malignant m.
    subungual m.
melanomatosis
melanomatous
melanonychia
melanopathy
melanosis
    m. lenticularis progressiva
    Riehl's m.
melanotrichia
melasma
    m. universale
Melkersson-Rosenthal syndrome
membrane
    basement m.

mentagra
    Alibert's m.
Mibelli's disease
microsporosis
    m. capitis
Microsporum
    M. audouini
    M. canis
    M. furfur
    M. lanosum
Miescher-Leder granulomatosis
Milian's
    erythema
    sign
    syndrome
miliaria
    m. pustulosa
    m. rubra
milium
    colloid m.
Millar's asthma
Milton's urticaria
Moeller's
    glossitis
    itch
mole
molluscum
    cholesterinic m.
    m. contagiosum
    m. epitheliale
    m. fibrosum
    m. lipomatodes
    m. pendulum
    m. sebaceum
    m. simplex
    m. varioliformis
    m. verrucosum
monilethrix
Monilia
moniliasis
Monro's abscess
morbilliform

morphea
    acroteric m.
    m. alba
    m. atrophica
    m. flammea
    m. guttata
    herpetiform m.
    m. linearis
    m. nigra
mucinosis
    follicular m.
    papular m.
mucocutaneous
mucodermal
mycetoma
mycid
Mycobacterium
    M. leprae
mycoderma
mycodermatitis
mycology
mycosis
    cutaneous m.
    m. cutis chronica
    m. favosa
    m. framboesioides
    m. fungoides
    m. interdigitalis
myiasis
myoepithelium
myringodermatitis
myxodermia
myxoma
nail
    double-edge n's
    eggshell n.
    hang n.
    ingrown n.
    parrot beak n.
    reedy n.
    spoon n.
    turtle-back n.

nail nipper
> Amico's n.n.

necklace
> Casal's n.

necrobiosis
> n. lipoidica
>> diabeticorum

necrosis

necrotic

neoplasm

Neumann's disease

neurodermatitis
> n. disseminata

neurodermatosis

neurodermite

neurofibromatosis

nevi
> epithelial n.

nevocarcinoma

nevose

nevoxanthoendothelioma

nevus
> amelanotic n.
> n. anemicus
> n. angiectodes
> n. angiomatodes
> n. arachnoideus
> n. araneosus
> n. araneus
> n. avasculosus
> bathing trunk n.
> Becker's n.
> blue n.
> n. cavernosus
> cellular blue n.
> n. cerebelliformis
> n. comedonicus
> compound n.
> connective-tissue n.
> n. depigmentosus
> dermoepidermal n.

nevus (*continued*)
> n. elasticus of
>> Lewandowsky
> epidermal n.
> epithelial n.
> n. fibrosus
> n. flammeus
> n. follicularis
> n. fusco-caeruleus
>> ophthalmo-maxillaris
> giant pigmented n.
> hairy n.
> halo n.
> Jadassohn's n.
> junctional n.
> linear n.
> n. lipomatosus
> n. lymphaticus
> n. maternus
> melanocytic n.
> n. mollusciformis
> n. morus
> multiplex n.
> n. nervosus
> nevocytic n.
> nonpigmented n.
> Ota's n.
> n. papillaris
> n. papillomatosus
> n. pigmentosus
> n. pilosus
> polyploid n.
> n. sanguineus
> sebaceous n. of
>> Jadassohn
> n. spilus
> spindle cell n.
> Spitz' n.
> n. spongiosus albus
>> mucosae
> strawberry n.

nevus (*continued*)
    n. syringocystadenosus
      papilliferus
    n. unius lateralis
    Unna's n.
    n. vasculosus
    n. venosus
    n. verrucosus
    n. vinosus
Nicolas-Favre disease
Niemann-Pick disease
Nikolsky's sign
Nocardia
    N. madurae
nocardiosis
nodose
nodosity
nodular
nodulus
noli-me-tangere
nonallergic
Norwegian scabies
nummular
oidiomycosis
ointment
    Hebra's o.
    Jarisch's o.
    Whitfield's o.
onchocerciasis
onikalja. See *onychalgia.*
onikatrofea. See
    onychatrophia.
onikawksis. See *onychauxis.*
onikea. See *onychia.*
onikeksalaksis. See *onychexal-*
    laxis.
onikektome. See *onychectomy.*
onikitis. See *onychitis.*
oniko-. See words beginning
    onycho-.
onychalgia

onychatrophia
onychauxis
onychectomy
onychexallaxis
onychia
    o. lateralis
    o. maligna
    o. parasitica
    o. periungualis
    o. sicca
onychitis
onychoclasis
onychocryptosis
onychodynia
onychodystrophy
onychogenic
onychograph
onychogryphosis
onychogryposis
onychohelcosis
onycholysis
onychoma
onychomadesis
onychomalacia
onychomycosis
onychonosus
onychopathic
onychopathology
onychopathy
onychophagia
onychophagist
onychophyma
onychophysis
onychoptosis
onychorrhexis
onychoschizia
onychosis
onychotillomania
onychotomy
ophryitis
Osler's disease

Osler-Vaquez disease
Ota's nevus
Otomyces
    O. hageni
    O. purpureus
otomycosis
otopathy
oxyuriasis
pachyderma
    p. lymphangiectatica
pachydermatocele
pachydermatosis
pachydermatous
pachydermic
pachydermoperiostosis
    p. plicata
pachyhymenic
pachylosis
pachymenia
pachymenic
pachyonychia
Padgett's dermatome
Paget's
    abscess
    cell
paint
    Castellani's p.
panniculitis
    nodular nonsuppurative
       p.
panniculus
    p. adiposus
papilla
papillary
papillocarcinoma
papilloma
    p. diffusum
    intracanalicular p.
    p. lineare
papular
papule
    Celsus' p's

papule (*continued*)
    pearly penile p.
    prurigo p.
papuliferous
papuloerythematous
papuloid
papulopustular
papulopustule
papulosis
    lymphomatoid p.
papulosquamous
papulovesicular
paracanthosis
paracoccidioidomycosis
paraeponychia
parakeratosis
    p. ostracea
    p. psoriasiformis
    p. scutularis
    p. variegata
parapsoriasis
    p. atrophicans
    p. varioliformis
parasite
paronychia
    p. tendinosa
paronychial
paronychosis
paste
    Lassar's p.
    Veiel's p.
peau
    p. d'orange
pediculation
Pediculoides
    P. ventricosus
pediculosis
    p. capillitii
    p. capitis
    p. corporis
    p. inguinalis
    p. palpebrarum

pediculosis (*continued*)
    p. pubis
    p. vestimenti
    p. vestimentorum
Pediculus
    P. humanus capitis
    P. humanus corporis
    P. inguinalis
    P. pubis
pellagra
pemphigoid
    bullous p.
pemphigus
    p. acutus
    p. erythematosus
    p. foliaceus
    p. gangrenosus
    p. hemorrhagicus
    p. malignus
    p. neonatorum
    p. syphiliticus
    p. vegetans
    p. vulgaris
periadenitis
    p. mucosa necrotica
      recurrens
periarteritis
    p. gummosa
    p. nodosa
periderm
perifollicular
perifolliculitis
    p. capitis abscedens et
      suffodiens
    superficial pustular p.
perionychia
perionychium
perionyx
perionyxis
periphery
perlèche
perlesh. See *perlèche*.

perna
pernio
petechia
petechial
petechiasis
peteke-. See words beginning
    petechi-.
phacoanaphylaxis
phagedena
    sloughing p.
    tropical p.
phenomenon
    p. of Arthus
    Koebner's p.
    Raynaud's p.
Phialophora
    P. verrucosa
photodermatitis
photosensitive
photosensitization
phthiriasis
    p. inguinalis
    pubic p.
Phthirus
    P. pubis
phthisic
phytophotodermatitis
piedra
Piffard's curet
pigment
pigmentation
pili
    p. multigemini
pilonidal
pilosebaceous
pilus
    p. annulatus
    p. cuniculatus
    p. incarnatus recurvus
    p. tortus
pimple
pinta

pintado
pintid
pityriasic
pityriasis
    p. alba
    p. amiantacea
    p. capitis
    p. circinata
    p. circinata et marginata
    p. furfuracea
    Gibert's p.
    Hebra's p.
    p. lichenoides
    p. lichenoides et
      varioliformis acuta
    p. linguae
    p. maculata
    p. pilaris
    p. rosea
    p. rotunda
    p. rubra
    p. rubra pilaris
    p. sicca
    p. simplex
    p. steatoides
    p. versicolor
pityroid
Pityrosporon
    P. orbiculare
    P. ovale
plaque
po dorahnj. See *peau d'orange.*
poikiloderma
    p. atrophicans vasculare
    Civatte's p.
    p. congenitale
poikilodermatomyositis
poliosis
    p. eccentrica
pollen
pollinosis
Pollitzer's disease

polyonychia
polyp
pomphoid
pompholyx
pomphus
porokeratosis
porphyria
    p. cutanea tarda
      hereditaria
PPD — purified protein
      derivative
PPD test
pressure ring
    Walsh's p. r.
prophylaxis
prurigo
    p. agria
    Besnier's p.
    p. chronica multiformis
    p. estivalis
    p. ferox
    p. mitis
    p. nodularis
    p. simplex
    p. universalis
pruritic
pruritus
    p. ani
    Duhring's p.
    p. hiemalis
    p. scroti
    p. senilis
    p. vulvae
pseudoxanthoma
    p. elasticum
psora
psoralen
psorelcosis
psoriasiform
psoriasis
    p. annularis
    p. arthropathica

psoriasis (*continued*)
- p. buccalis
- p. circinata
- p. diffusa
- p. discoides
- p. figurata
- p. follicularis
- p. guttata
- p. gyrata
- p. inveterata
- p. linguae
- p. nummularis
- p. ostracea
- p. palmaris et plantaris
- p. punctata
- pustular p.
- p. rupioides
- p. universalis
- volar p.

psoriatic
psoric
psorospermosis
- p. follicularis

psorous
psydracium
pterygium
- p. unguis

Puente's disease
Pulex
- *P. irritans*

pulicosis
punch
- Keyes' dermal p.

punctiform
punctum
purpura
- allergic p.
- anaphylactoid p.
- p. angioneurotica
- p. annularis telangiectodes
- p. bullosa

purpura (*continued*)
- p. cachectica
- p. fulminans
- p. hemorrhagica
- p. hyperglobulinemica
- p. iodica
- Landouzy's p.
- p. maculosa
- Majocchi's p.
- orthostatic p.
- p. pulicosa
- p. rheumatica
- Schönlein-Henoch p.
- Schönlein's p.
- p. senilis
- p. simplex
- p. symptomatica
- thrombocytopenic p.
- p. urticans
- p. variolosa

purpuric
purulent
purupuru
pus
Pusey's emulsion
pustula
- p. maligna

pustular
pustulation
pustule
pustulocrustaceous
pustulosis
- p. palmaris
- p. vacciniformis acuta

pyemia
pyoderma
- p. chancriforme faciei
- p. faciale
- p. gangrenosum
- p. ulcerosum tropicalum
- p. vegetans
- p. verrucosum

pyodermatitis
    p. vegetans
pyodermatosis
pyodermitis
    p. vegetans
pyogenic
pyonychia
pyosis
    Corlett's p.
Queyrat's erythroplasia
Quincke's disease
Quinquaud's disease
racemose
radioepidermitis
ragadez. See *rhagades.*
rakoma. See *rhacoma.*
Ralks'
    drill
    elevator
rash
Rayer's disease
Raynaud's
    disease
    gangrene
    phenomenon
reaction
    Bloch's r.
    dopa r.
    Herxheimer's r.
    Jarisch-Herxheimer r.
    Jones-Mote r.
    Sanarelli-Shwartzman r.
    Schultz-Charlton r.
    Schultz-Dale r.
Recklinghausen's disease
Reenstierna antiserum
Reese's dermatome
Reiter's disease
rete
    dermal r.
    r. Malpighi

reticulosis
    Sézary r.
rhacoma
rhagades
rhinophyma
rhinoscleroma
Rhus
    R. diversiloba
    R. toxicodendron
    R. venenata
Ricord's chancre
Riehl's melanosis
ringworm
rino-. See words beginning
    rhino-.
Robinson's disease
Rollet's chancre
rosacea
roseola
rosette
rubefacient
rubella
rubeola
ruber
rubescent
rupia
    r. escharotica
Saalfield's extractor
Saccharomycetes
saccharomycosis
Sanarelli-Shwartzman reaction
sarcoid
    Boeck's s.
    Darier-Roussy s.
    Spiegler-Fendt s.
sarcoidosis
sarcoma
    Abernethy's s.
    adipose s.
    Kaposi's s.
sarcomagenic

sarcomatosis
    s. cutis
satellite
sauriasis
sauriderma
sauriosis
scabetic
scabicide
scabies
    Boeck's s.
    Norwegian s.
scabrities
    s. unguium
scale
scaly
scarification
scarlatiniform
Schamberg's
    dermatosis
    disease
    extractor
Schick test
schistosomiasis
Schönlein-Henoch purpura
Schönlein's purpura
Schultz-Charlton reaction
Schultz-Dale reaction
scleredema
    Buschke's s.
    s. neonatorum
sclerema
    s. neonatorum
sclerodactylia
    s. annularis ainhumoides
sclerodactyly
scleroderma
sclerodermatitis
scleromyxedema
scleronychia
scrofuloderma
    s. gummosa

scrofuloderma (*continued*)
    papular s.
    pustular s.
    tuberculous s.
    ulcerative s.
    verrucous s.
scrofulophyma
scurf
scutulum
sebaceous
seborrhea
    s. adiposa
    s. capitis
    s. congestiva
    s. corporis
    eczematoid s.
    s. faciei
    s. furfuracea
    s. generalis
    s. nigricans
    s. oleosa
    s. sicca
    s. squamo neonatorum
seborrheic
sebum
Senear-Usher disease
sensibilisinogen
sensitinogen
sensitization
serpiginous
Sézary
    erythroderma
    reticulosis
    syndrome
shanker. See *chancre.*
shankreform. See *chancriform.*
shankroid. See *chancroid.*
shingles
shock
    anaphylactic s.
siazma. See *cyasma.*

sidraseum. See *psydracium.*
sign

>Darier's s.
>Milian's s.
>Nikolsky's s.
>Silex's s.

Silex's sign
Sjögren's syndrome
skin lifter

>Amico's s. l.

SLE – systemic lupus
>erythematosus
slough
sluf. See *slough.*
solenonychia
solum

>s. unguis

sora. See *psora.*
soreatik. See *psoriatic.*
sorelkosis. See *psorelcosis.*
soriasis. See *psoriasis.*
sorik. See *psoric.*
sorospermosis. See
>*psorospermosis.*
sorus. See *psorous.*
Spiegler-Fendt sarcoid
spiloplania
spiloplaxia
spiradenoma
spiral

>Herxheimer's s's

Spitz' nevus
sporotrichosis
Sporotrichum

>*S. schenckii*

spot

>Fordyce's s's

squamous
Staphylococcus

>*S. epidermidis*

staphyloderma
staphylodermatitis

steatoma
steatomatosis
Stevens-Johnson syndrome
Sticker's disease
stigmatosis
stomatitis
strata
stratified
stratum

>s. basale epidermidis
>s. corneum epidermidis
>s. corneum unguis
>s. filamentosum
>s. germinativum
>epidermidis
>s. germinativum unguis
>s. granulosum
>epidermidis
>s. malpighii

Streptothrix
streptotrichosis
stria
striae

>Wickham's s.

Stryker-Halbeisen syndrome
Stryker's dermatome
subcutaneous
subungual
sudamen
sudoriferous
sudorrhea
sudozanthoma. See
>*pseudoxanthoma.*
sumac

>swamp s.

Sutton's disease
Sweet's syndrome
sycoma
sycosis

>bacillogenic s.
>s. barbae
>coccogenic s.

sycosis (*continued*)
    s. contagiosa
    s. framboesia
    s. framboesiaeformis
    hyphomycotic c.
    lupoid s.
    nonparasitic s.
    s. nuchae necrotisans
    parasitic s.
    s. staphylogenes
    s. vulgaris
synanthema
syndrome
    Abt-Letterer-Siwe s.
    Albright's s.
    Alibert-Bazin s.
    antibody deficiency s.
    Buschke-Ollendorff s.
    Danlos' s.
    Degos-Delort-Tricot s.
    Ehlers-Danlos s.
    Gougerot's s.
    Libman-Sacks s.
    Lutz-Splendore-de
      Almeida s.
    Lyell's s.
    Mauriac's s.
    Melkersson-Rosenthal s.
    Milian's s.
    Sézary s.
    Sjögren's s.
    Stevens-Johnson s.
    Stryker-Halbeisen s.
    Sweet's s.
    Waterhouse-Friderichsen
      s.
    Weber-Christian s.
syphilid
syphilis
syphilitic
syphiloderm
syphilophyma

syringadenoma
syringocystadenoma
syringocystoma
syringoma
system
    integumentary s.
tache
    t's bleuâtres
tachetic
Taenzer's disease
tegument
telangiectasia
telangiectasis
telangiectatic
telogen
teratoma
terijeum. See *pterygium.*
test
    agglutination t.
    basophil degranulation t.
    Bruck's t.
    coccidioidin skin t.
    complement-fixation t.
    Dick t.
    fluorescent antinuclear
      antibody t.
    Foshay's t.
    Frei's t.
    in vitro t.
    Ito-Reenstierna t.
    Jadassohn-Bloch t.
    Keller's ultraviolet t.
    Kolmer's t.
    Kveim t.
    lepromin t.
    Mantoux t.
    mast cell degranulation t.
    patch t.
    PPD t. – purified protein
      derivative
    Schick t.
    scratch t.

test (*continued*)

    tine t.
    tuberculin t.
    Tzank t.
    Vollmer's t.
    Wassermann-fast t.
    Wassermann reaction t.

tetter

    brawny t.
    honeycomb t.

thenar eminence

thiriasis. See *phthiriasis.*

thrush

tinea

    t. amiantacea
    t. axillaris
    t. barbae
    t. capitis
    t. ciliorum
    t. circinata
    t. corporis
    t. cruris
    t. decalvans
    t. favosa
    t. furfuracea
    t. glabrosa
    t. imbricata
    t. inguinalis
    t. kerion
    t. nigra
    t. nodosa
    t. pedis
    t. profunda
    t. sycosis
    t. tarsi
    t. tonsurans
    t. unguium
    t. versicolor

tizik. See *phthisic.*

tophus

    t. syphiliticus

Torula

toruli

    t. tactiles

toruloma

torulosis

torulus

Touton giant cells

toxicoderma

toxicodermatitis

treatment

    Gennerich's t.
    Goeckerman t.

Treponema

triad

    Hutchinson's t.

trichiasis

trichitis

trichoepithelioma

    t. papillosum multiplex

trichofibroacanthoma

trichofibroepithelioma

trichoglossia

trichoid

trichologia

trichomadesis

trichomatosis

Trichomonas

trichomycosis

    t. axillaris
    t. chromatica
    t. favosa
    t. nigra
    t. nodosa
    t. palmellina
    t. pustulosa
    t. rubra

trichonocardiasis

trichonodosis

trichonosis

    t. furfuracea

trichopathic

trichophytid

Trichophyton

trichophytosis
    t. barbae
    t. capitis
    t. corporis
    t. cruris
    t. unguium
trichorrhea
trichorrhexis
    t. nodosa
trichoschisis
trichostasis spinulosa
Trichothecium
    T. roseum
trichotillomania
Triphleps insidiosus
Trombicula
tubercle
tubercular
tuberculid
    papulonecrotic t.
    rosacea-like t.
tuberculoderm
tuberculosis
    t. papulonecrotica
tularemia
Tunga
    T. penetrans
tungiasis
turgor
tylosis
    t. ciliaris
    t. palmaris et plantaris
Tzank
    cell
    test
ulcer
    decubitus u.
    Lipschütz's u.
ulceration
ulcus
    u. ambulans
    u. ambustiforme

ulcus (*continued*)
    u. durum
    u. interdigitale
    u. molle cutis
    u. scorbuticum
    u. syphiliticum
    u. vulvae acutum
ulerythema
    u. acneiforma
    u. centrifugum
    u. ophryogenes
    u. sycosiforme
ulodermatitis
uloid
ungual
unguinal
unguis
    u. incarnatus
Unna's
    boot
    dermatosis
    extractor
    nevus
Urbach-Oppenheim disease
urethritis
    gonorrheal u.
urhidrosis
urtica
urticaria
    u. bullosa
    cholinergic u.
    endemic u.
    u. endemica
    u. epidemica
    u. factitia
    u. gigantea
    u. hemorrhagica
    heredofamilial u.
    u. medicamentosa
    Milton's u.
    papular u.
    u. papulosa

urticaria (*continued*)
    u. perstans
    u. photogenica
    u. pigmentosa
    solar u.
    u. solaris
    u. subcutanea
    subcutaneous u.
urticarial
urticate
vaccination
vaccinia
varicella
    v. gangrenosa
    pustular v.
    v. pustulosa
varicelliform
    Kaposi's v. eruption
variola
    v. crystallina
    v. inserta
    v. miliaris
    v. mitigata
    v. pemphigosa
    v. siliquosa
    v. vera
    v. verrucosa
vasculitis
    nodular v.
Veiel's paste
vellus
Venus
    collar of V.
verruca
    v. acuminata
    v. digitata
    v. filiformis
    v. glabra
    v. necrogenica
    v. peruana
    v. peruviana
    v. plana

verruca (*continued*)
    v. plana juvenilis
    v. plantaris
    v. seborrheica
    v. senilis
    v. simplex
    v. tuberculosa
    v. vulgaris
verrucae
verruciform
verrucose
verrucosis
verruga
    v. peruana
vesication
vesicle
vesicular
vesiculation
vesiculobullous
vesiculopapular
vesiculopustular
virus
    Coxsackie v.
    ECHO v. — enteric
      cytopathogenic
      human orphan v.
vitiligo
    v. capitis
    Cazenave's v.
    Celsus' v.
    circumscribed v.
    perinevic v.
Vollmer's test
vulgaris
Walsh's
    curet
    pressure ring
Walton's extractor
wart
    anatomical w.
    filiform w.
    mosaic w.

wart (*continued*)
    mucocutaneous w.
    necrogenic w.
    periungual w.
    pitch w.
    plantar w.
    seborrheic w.
    telangiectatic w.
    tuberculous w.
    venereal w.
Wassermann-fast test
Wassermann reaction test
Waterhouse-Friderichsen
    syndrome
Weber-Christian
    disease
    syndrome
Weber's disease
wen
wheal
White's disease
Whitfield's ointment
Wickham's striae
Willan's lepra
Wood's light
xanthelasma
xanthoderma
xanthoma
    x. diabeticorum
    x. disseminatum
    x. eruptivum
    x. multiplex

xanthoma (*continued*)
    x. planum
    x. striatum palmare
    x. tuberosum
    x. tuberosum multiplex
xanthomatosis
xanthomatous
xanthosis
    x. cutis
XDP — xeroderma
       pigmentosum
xeroderma
    follicular x.
    Kaposi's x.
    x. pigmentosum
xerodermatic
xerodermosteosis
xerosis
    x. cutis
XP — xeroderma pigmentosum
yaws
zan-. See words beginning
    Xan-.
zero-. See words beginning
    xero-.
zoacanthosis
zona
    z. dermatica
    z. epithelioserosa
    z. facialis
zosteriform
zosteroid

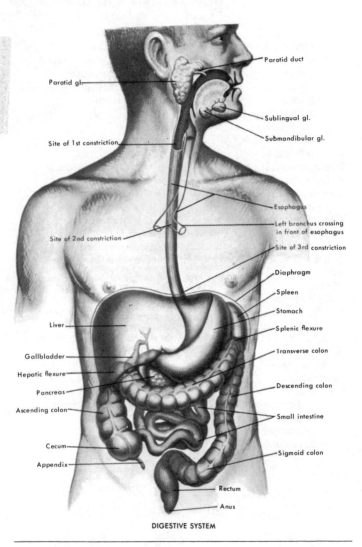

Parotid duct

Parotid gl.

Sublingual gl.

Submandibular gl.

Site of 1st constriction

Esophagus

Left bronchus crossing in front of esophagus

Site of 2nd constriction

Site of 3rd constriction

Diaphragm

Spleen

Stomach

Liver

Splenic flexure

Gallbladder

Transverse colon

Hepatic flexure

Pancreas

Descending colon

Ascending colon

Small intestine

Cecum

Appendix

Sigmoid colon

Rectum

Anus

DIGESTIVE SYSTEM

GASTROENTEROLOGY

a-beta-lipoproteinemia
abscess
    subphrenic a.
absorption
a.c. — before meals (ante
      cibum)
achalasia
achlorhydria
    a. apepsia
acholia
acholic
achylia
    a. gastrica haemorrhagica
    a. pancreatica
achylous
acid
    amino a.
    hydrochloric a.
acidity
acidosis
ACMI gastroscope
adenasthenia
    a. gastrica
adenia
    angibromic a.
adenitis
    mesenteric a.
adenocarcinoma
adenohypersthenia
    a. gastrica

adenoma
    papillary a.
    villous a.
adenomyoma
adhesion
adipolysis
aerenterectasia
aerocoly
aerogastria
aerogastrocolia
aeroperitoneum
aerophagia
aerophagy
agastroneuria
aglutition
akahlazea. See *achalasia.*
akilea. See *achylia.*
akilus. See *achylous.*
aklorhidreah. See *achlorhydria.*
akoleah. See *acholia.*
akolic. See *acholic.*
alimentary tract
alimentation
alkaline
alkalosis
ALP — alkaline phosphatase
amino acid
Althausen's test
amebiasis
    intestinal a.

333

ampulla
    a. hepatopancreatica
    a. of Vater
amylase
amyloidosis
anacidity
analysis
    gastric a.
anapepsia
anastomosis
    Braun's a.
    Billroth I a.
    Billroth II a.
    enteric a.
    peristaltic a.
    Roux-en-Y a.
Andresen's diet
anesthesia. See *General Surgical Terms.*
angina
    abdominal a.
    a. abdominalis
    a. dyspeptica
    intestinal a.
angiocholecystitis
angiocholitis
    a. proliferans
angulation
angulus
annular
anoplasty
anorectal
anorexia
antacid
anticholagogic
anticholinergic
antidiarrheal
antimesenteric
antiperistalsis
antispasmodic
    biliary a.
antral

antrectomy
antrum
anus
    imperforate a.
apepsia
    achlorhydria a.
apepsinia
aperistalsis
appendectomy
appendicitis
appendix
    vermiform a.
arachnogastria
arch
    Treitz's a.
argentaffinoma
Argyle's tube
ascariasis
ascites
aspiration
atony
atresia
atrophy
    gastric mucosal a.
awbarra. See *embarras.*
Ba — barium
bacteriocholia
BaE — barium enema
Baker's tube
Banti's syndrome
barium
Barrett's syndrome
belching
Benedict's gastroscope
bezoar
bile
biliary
bilidigestive
bilihumin
bilious
biliousness
biliprasin

bilirubin
bilirubinemia
Billroth
     I anastomosis
     II anastomosis
Billroth's hypertrophy
Blakemore's tube
blood
     occult b.
Blumer's shelf
Boas' test meal
bolus
borborygmi
borborygmus
bougie
bowel
     greedy b.
Boyden's test meal
bradypepsia
bradystalsis
brash
Braun's anastomosis
Brinton's disease
bronchoscope
Browne-McHardy dilator
bruit
brwe. See *bruit.*
bulb
     duodenal b.
calculi
canaliculus
Cannon's ring
Cantor's tube
cap
     phrygian c.
capotement
capsule
     Glisson's c.
caput
     c. medusae
carcinoid
carcinoma

carcinomatosis
     c. peritonei
cardia
     c. of stomach
cardialgia
cardiospasm
carminative
Carnot's test
carreau
CAT – computed axial
     tomography
catabolism
cecitis
cecocolon
cecocolostomy
cecoileostomy
cecopexy
cecosigmoidostomy
cecostomy
cecotomy
cecum
celiac
celiocentesis
celiomyalgia
celiomyomotomy
celioparacentesis
celiopathy
celiopyosis
celioscope
celitis
Chevalier Jackson gastroscope
cholagogic
cholagogue
cholaligenic
cholaneresis
cholangeitis
cholangiectasis
cholangioadenoma
cholangiocarcinoma
cholangiocholecystocholedo-
     chectomy
cholangioenterostomy

cholangiogastrostomy
cholangiogram
cholangiography
    operative c.
cholangiohepatitis
cholangiohepatoma
cholangiojejunostomy
    intrahepatic c.
cholangiole
cholangiolitis
cholangioma
cholangiostomy
cholangiotomy
cholangitis
    catarrhal c.
    c. lenta
cholecyst
cholecystalgia
cholecystatony
cholecystectasia
cholecystectomy
cholecystenteric
cholecystenteroanastomosis
cholecystenterorrhaphy
cholecystenterostomy
cholecystic
cholecystis
cholecystitis
    acute c.
    chronic c.
    c. emphysematosa
    emphysematous c.
    follicular c.
    gaseous c.
    c. glandularis proliferans
cholecystocholangiogram
cholecystocolonic
cholecystocolostomy
cholecystocolotomy
cholecystoduodenostomy
cholecystogastric
cholecystogastrostomy

cholecystogram
cholecystography
cholecystoileostomy
cholecystojejunostomy
cholecystokinetic
cholecystokinin
cholecystolithiasis
cholecystolithotripsy
cholecystopathy
cholecystoptosis
cholecystorrhaphy
cholecystosis
    hyperplastic c.
cholecystostomy
cholecystotomy
choledochal
choledochectomy
choledochitis
choledochocele
choledochocholedochostomy
choledochoduodenostomy
choledochoenterostomy
choledochogastrostomy
choledochogram
choledochography
choledochohepatostomy
choledochoileostomy
choledochojejunostomy
choledocholith
choledocholithiasis
choledocholithotomy
choledocholithotripsy
choledochoplasty
choledochorrhaphy
choledochoscope
choledochostomy
choledochotomy
choledochus
cholelithiasis
cholelithotomy
cholelithotripsy
cholemesis

cholemimetry
cholepathia
    c. spastica
choleperitoneum
cholepoiesis
cholepoietic
cholera
    bilious c.
    c. morbus
    c. nostras
cholerrhagia
cholestasis
cholesterol
choloscopy
chromoscopy
    gastric c.
chyle
chymase
chyme
chymification
chymorrhea
cicatricial
cirrhosis
    biliary c.
    calculus c.
    cardiac c.
    Maixner's c.
claudication
    intermittent c.
clysma
clyster
colectomy
colic
    biliary c.
    bilious c.
    crapulent c.
    gallstone c.
    hepatic c.
    mucous c.
    pancreatic c.
    pseudomembranous c.
    saburral c.

colic (*continued*)
    stercoral c.
    vermicular c.
    verminous c.
colicky
colicolitis
colitis
    adaptive c.
    amebic c.
    balantidial c.
    c. cystica profunda
    c. cystica superficialis
    fulminating c.
    granulomatous c.
    c. gravis
    mucous c.
    myxomembranous c.
    c. polyposa
    pseudomembranous c.
    segmental c.
    transmural c.
    ulcerative c.
colloid
coloclyster
colocutaneous
colodyspepsia
coloenteritis
colon
    ascending c.
    descending c.
    distal c.
    irritable c.
    lead-pipe c.
    proximal c.
    sigmoid c.
    spastic c.
    transverse c.
    unstable c.
colonorrhea
colonoscope
    fiberoptic c.
colonoscopy

colonotomy
coloproctitis
colorectal
colorectitis
colorectostomy
colorrhea
colostomy
      end-to-side ileotransverse
         c.
Congo red test
coniasis
constipation
      gastrojejunal c.
copremia
coprolith
coprostasis
Corner's tampon
Courvoisier-Terrier syndrome
craigiasis
crater
crepitus
Crohn's disease
crura
Cruveilhier's disease
curvature
      greater c.
      lesser c.
defecation
deglutition
Degos' disease
dehydration
dehydrocholaneresis
dehydrogenase
      lactic d.
demucosatio
      d. intestini
Diagnex blue test
diaphragm
diarrhea
diastalsis
diastase
      pancreatic d.
diathesis

diet
      Andresen's d.
      Giordano-Giovannetti d.
      gluten free d.
      Jarotsky's d.
      Meulengracht's d.
      Sippy d.
Dieulafoy's erosion
digestion
digestive
dilatation
dilator
      Browne-McHardy d.
      Einhorn's d.
      esophageal d.
dis-. See also words beginning
    dys-.
disease
      Brinton's d.
      celiac d.
      Crohn's d.
      Cruveilhier's d.
      Degos' d.
      Hanot's d.
      hepatobiliary tract d.
      Hirschsprung's d.
      Menetrier's d.
      Myà's d.
      Patella's d.
      Payr's d.
      Reichmann's d.
      Whipple's d.
distention
distomiasis
      intestinal d.
diverticula
      jejunal d.
diverticulitis
diverticulosis
      jejunal d.
diverticulum
      epiphrenic d.
      hepatic d.

diverticulum (*continued*)
  hypopharyngeal d.
  Meckel's d.
  midesophageal d.
  Zenker's d.
Dock's test meal
drip
  intragastric d.
drugs. See *Drugs and Chemistry* section.
Dubin-Johnson syndrome
duct
  biliary d.
  common bile d.
  extrahepatic bile d.
  hepatic d.
ductus
  d. choledochus
duodenal
duodenectomy
duodenitis
duodenocholangitis
duodenocholecystostomy
duodenocholedochotomy
duodenocolic
duodenocystostomy
duodenoduodenostomy
duodenoenterostomy
duodenogram
duodenohepatic
duodenoileostomy
duodenojejunostomy
duodenolysis
duodenorrhaphy
duodenoscope
duodenoscopy
duodenostomy
duodenotomy
duodenum
D-xylose absorption test
dyschezia

dysentery
  amebic d.
dyskinesia
  biliary d.
dyspepsia
dysperistalsis
dysphagia
  sideropenic d.
dyspragia
  d. intermittens angiosclerotica intestinalis
D-*zylose*. See D-*xylose*.
ecterograph
ectocolon
ectoperitonitis
edema
  alimentary e.
edematous
Ehrmann's alcohol test meal
Einhorn's dilator
electrogastrogram
electrogastrography
embarras
  e. gastrique
empyema
emulsification
endocolitis
endoenteritis
endogastric
endogastritis
endometriosis
  e. of colon
endoscopy
enema
  barium e.
enteraden
enteradenitis
enteral
enteralgia
enterauxe

enterectasis
enterectomy
enterelcosis
enteric
enteritides
enteritis
    choleriform e.
    cicatrizing e.
    e. cystica chronica
    granulomatous e.
    e. gravis
    myxomembranous e.
    e. necroticans
    e. nodularis
    pellicular e.
    phlegmonous e.
    e. polyposa
    protozoan e.
    pseudomembranous e.
    regional e.
    segmental e.
    streptococcus e.
enteroanastomosis
enteroapokleisis
enterobiasis
enterobiliary
enterocele
enterocentesis
enterochirurgia
enterocholecystostomy
enterocholecystotomy
enterocinesia
enterocinetic
enterocleisis
enteroclysis
enterocoele
enterocolectomy
enterocolitis
    hemorrhagic e.
    necrotizing e.
    pseudomembranous e.
    regional e.

enterocolostomy
enterocutaneous
enterocyst
enterocystocele
enterocystoma
enterodynia
enteroenterostomy
enteroepiplocele
enterogastric
enterogastritis
enterogenous
enterogram
enterograph
enterography
enterohepatitis
enterohepatopexy
enteroidea
enterointestinal
enterokinase
enterokinesia
enterokinetic
enterokinin
enterolith
enterolithiasis
enterology
enterolysis
enteromegaly
enteromere
enteromycosis
    e. bacteriaceae
enteromyiasis
enteron
enteroneuritis
enteronitis
    polytropous e.
enteroparesis
enteropathogen
enteropathogenesis
enteropathogenic
enteropathy
    gluten e.
    protein-losing e.

enteropeptidase
enteropexy
enteroplasty
enteroplegia
enteroptosis
enteroptychia
enterorrhagia
enterorrhaphy
enterorrhea
enterorrhexis
enteroscope
enterosepsis
enterosorption
enterospasm
enterostasis
enterostaxis
enterostenosis
enterostomal
enterostomy
    gun-barrel e.
enterotome
enterotomy
enterotoxin
enterovirus
enzyme
epigastralgia
epigastric
epigastrium
epigastrocele
epiploon
epithalaxia
erepsin
erosion
    Dieulafoy's e.
eructation
    nervous e.
esofa-. See words beginning
    esopha-.
esogastritis
esophagalgia
esophageal

esophagectasia
esophagism
esophagitis
    e. dissecans superficialis
    peptic e.
    reflux e.
esophagocologastrostomy
esophagoduodenostomy
esophagodynia
esophagoenterostomy
esophagofundopexy
esophagogastrectomy
esophagogastric
esophagogastroanastomosis
esophagogastromyotomy
esophagogastroplasty
esophagogastroscopy
esophagogastrostomy
esophagogram
esophagography
esophagojejunogastrostomosis
esophagojejunogastrostomy
esophagojejunoplasty
esophagojejunostomy
esophagoscope
    Jesberg's e.
esophagoscopy
esophagospasm
esophagostenosis
esophagus
etiology
euchlorhydria
eucholia
euchylia
eupepsia
evacuation
Ewald's test meal
excrement
excrementitious
excreta
excretion

fecalith
feces
feculent
fiberscope
    Hirschowitz's f.
    Olympus f.
fibroblast
Finney's pyloroplasty
Fischer's test meal
fistula
    enterocolic f.
    enteroenteric f.
    gastrojejunocolic f.
    jejunocolic f.
fitobezor. See *phytobezoar.*
flatulence
flatulent
flatus
flexure
    splenic f.
flora
    intestinal f.
fluke
    intestinal f's
flux
    bilious f.
    celiac f.
foramen
    Winslow's f.
fossa
    Treitz's f.
freezing
    gastric f.
fundus
GA – gastric analysis
Galeati's glands
gall
gallbladder
gallstone
gastradenitis
gastralgia
    appendicular g.

gastralgokenosis
gastraneuria
gastrasthenia
gastratrophia
gastrectasia
gastrectomy
    Roux-en-Y g.
gastric
gastricism
gastricsin
gastrin
gastritic
gastritis
    antral g.
    atrophic g.
    catarrhal g.
    cirrhotic g.
    erosive g.
    exfoliative g.
    follicular g.
    giant hypertrophic g.
    g. granulomatosa
        fibroplastica
    hyperpeptic g.
    hypertrophic g.
    interstitial g.
    mycotic g.
    phlegmonous g.
    polypous g.
    pseudomembranous g.
    purulent g.
    suppurating g.
gastroalbuminorrhea
gastroatonia
gastroblennorrhea
gastrobrosis
gastrocamera
gastrocardiac
gastrocele
gastrochronorrhea
gastrocolic
gastrocolitis

gastrocoloptosis
gastrocolostomy
gastrocolotomy
gastrocutaneous
gastrodialysis
gastrodiaphane
gastrodiaphany
gastroduodenal
gastroduodenitis
gastroduodenoscopy
gastroduodenostomy
gastrodynia
gastroenteralgia
gastroenteric
gastroenteritis
gastroenteroanastomosis
gastroenterocolic
gastroenterocolitis
gastroenterocolostomy
gastroenterologist
gastroenterology
gastroenteropathy
gastroenteroplasty
gastroenteroptosis
gastroenterostomy
gastroenterotomy
gastroepiploic
gastroesophageal
gastroesophagitis
gastroesophagostomy
gastrogalvanization
gastrogastrostomy
gastrogavage
gastrogenic
Gastrografin
gastrograph
gastrohelcoma
gastrohelcosis
gastrohepatic
gastrohepatitis
gastrohydrorrhea
gastrohyperneuria

gastrohypertonic
gastrohyponeuria
gastroileitis
gastroileostomy
gastrointestinal
gastrojejunocolic
gastrojejunostomy
gastrokinesograph
gastrolienal
gastrolith
gastrolithiasis
gastrologist
gastrology
gastrolysis
gastromalacia
gastromegaly
gastromycosis
gastromyotomy
gastromyxorrhea
gastrone
gastronesteostomy
gastropancreatitis
gastroparalysis
gastroperiodynia
gastroperitonitis
gastropexy
gastrophotography
gastrophrenic
gastrophthisis
gastroplasty
gastroplication
gastroptosis
gastroptyxis
gastropylorectomy
gastropyloric
gastroradiculitis
gastrorrhagia
gastrorrhaphy
gastrorrhea
    g. continua chronica
gastrorrhexis
gastroschisis

gastroscope
    ACMI g.
    Benedict's g.
    Chevalier Jackson g.
    fiberoptic g.
    flexible g.
    Hirschowitz's g.
    Housset Debray g.
    Wolf-Schindler g.
gastroscopic
gastroscopy
gastrosia
    g. fungosa
gastrospasm
gastrosplenic
gastrostaxis
gastrostenosis
gastrostogavage
gastrostolavage
gastrostoma
gastrostomy
    Ssabanejew-Frank g.
    Stamm's g.
gastrosuccorrhea
    digestive g.
    g. mucosa
gastrotome
gastrotomy
gastrotonometer
gastrotoxin
gastroxynsis
    g. fungosa
gavage
geotrichosis
GET — gastric emptying time
GET½ — gastric emptying
    half-time
GI — gastrointestinal
Giardia
    G. lamblia
giardiasis
Giordano-Giovannetti diet

gland
    Galeati's g's
    Theile's g's
Glénard's syndrome
Glisson's capsule
globus
    g. hystericus
glucose
glycogen
glycogenesis
glycogenolysis
glycolysis
glyconeogenesis
GM — gastric mucosa
Gmelin's test
Goldstein's hematemesis
granulation
granulomatosis
    lipophagic intestinal g.
GU — gastric ulcer
guaiac
gutter
    paracolic g.
Hanot-Rössle syndrome
Hanot's disease
Hartmann's pouch
haustra of colon
haustral
haustrum
heartburn
Heineke-Mikulicz pyloroplasty
helminthemesis
hematemesis
    Goldstein's h.
    h. puellaris
hematobilia
hematochezia
hemidiaphragm
hemocholecystitis
hemolysis
hemoperitoneum
hemoptysis

hemorrhage
    petechial h.
Henoch's purpura
hepar
hepatitis
    anicteric h.
    serum h.
    viral h.
hepatobiliary
hepatocholangeitis
hepatocholangioduodenostomy
hepatocolic
hepatocystic
hepatoenteric
hepatogastric
hepatolithiasis
hepatomegaly
hepatorrhea
hepatosplenomegaly
hernia
    diaphragmatic h.
    hiatal h.
    spigelian h.
    Treitz's h.
herniorrhaphy
herniotomy
heterochylia
hiatus
    esophageal h.
hiccup
Hirschowitz's
    fiberscope
    gastroscope
Hirschsprung's disease
Hoguet's maneuver
hologastroschisis
Housset-Debray gastroscope
Hueter's maneuver
hydraeroperitoneum
hydragogue
hydrepigastrium

hydrochloric
hydrocholecystis
hydrocholeresis
hydrolysis
hydroperitoneum
hydrops
    h. abdominis
hyperbilirubinemia
hyperchlorhydria
hypercholia
hyperemesis
    h. hiemis
hyperemic
hyperglycemia
hyperpepsia
hyperpepsinia
hyperperistalsis
hypersecretion
    gastric h.
hypertrophy
    Billroth's h.
hypochloremia
hypochlorhydria
hypochondrium
hypochylia
hypogammaglobulinemia
hypogastric
hypogastrium
hypogastroschisis
hypoglycemia
hypokalemia
hypomagnesemia
hyponatremia
hypoxia
hypopepsia
hypopepsinia
hypoperistalsis
hypophrenium
hyposteatolysis
hypothermia
IC — irritable colon

ichthyismus
    i. exanthematicus
icterus
ileal
ileectomy
ileitis
    regional i.
    terminal i.
ileocecal
ileocecum
ileocolitis
    i. ulcerosa chronica
ileocolostomy
ileojejunitis
    granulomatous i.
    nongranulomatous i.
ileoproctostomy
ileorectal
ileosigmoid
ileostomy
ileum
    terminal i.
ileus
    adynamic i.
    meconium i.
    paralytic i.
    spastic i.
iliohypogastric
ilioinguinal
iliopectineal
impaction
    fecal i.
incision. See *General Surgical Terms.*
incontinence
    fecal i.
indigestion
inertia
    colonic i.
infarction
ingestion

inructation
insufficiency
    pancreatic i.
insulin
intestinal
intestine
intestinum
intubated
intubation
intussusception
ischemia
    mesenteric i.
    midgut i.
ischochymia
ischocholia
isko-. See words beginning *ischo-*.
IVC — intravenous cholangiogram
Jarotsky's diet
jaundice
    obstructive j.
jejunal
jejunitis
jejunoileitis
jejunoileostomy
jejunojejunostomy
jejunostomy
jejunum
Jesberg's esophagoscope
junction
    esophagogastric j.
juxtapyloric
kapotmaw. See *capotement.*
karro. See *carreau.*
Kehr's sign
kil. See *chyle.*
kim. See *chyme.*
kimas. See *chymase.*
kimifikashun. See *chymification.*

kimorea. See *chymorrhea.*
kolange-. See words beginning *cholangi-.*
kole-. See words beginning *chole-.*
kolera. See *cholera.*
lamp
    Wood's l.
laparotomy
lavage
    gastric l.
leiomyoma
leiomyosarcoma
Leube's test meal
leukocytosis
Levin tube
ligament
    falciform l.
    gastrohepatic l.
    Treitz's l.
linitis
    l. plastica
liomioma. See *leiomyoma.*
liomiosarkoma. See *leiomyosarcoma.*
lipase
lipodystrophia
    l. intestinalis
lipodystrophy
    intestinal l.
lipoid
lipolysis
lipophagia
    l. granulomatosis
liver
    biliary cirrhotic l.
loop
    afferent l.
    efferent l.
    jejunal l.
    terminal ileal l.
lumen

lymphangiectasia
lymphenteritis
lymphoma
lysozyme
macrogastria
Maixner's cirrhosis
malabsorption
Mallory-Weiss syndrome
maneuver
    Hoguet's m.
    Hueter's m.
mastication
McArthur's method
meal
    barium m.
Meckel's diverticulum
medications. See *Drugs and Chemistry* section.
megacolon
megadolichocolon
megaduodenum
megaesophagus
megalobulbus
melena
melenemesis
Menetrier's disease
mesenteric adenitis
mesenteriolum
mesenteritis
mesenterium
mesentery
mesoappendicitis
mesoappendix
mesocecum
mesocolon
metaduodenum
metadysentery
meteorism
method
    McArthur's m.
    Nimeh's m.
Meulengracht's diet

micelle
mikso-. See words beginning
    myxo-.
Miller-Abbott tube
motility
Moynihan's test
mucopolysaccharide
mucoprotein
mucosa
    antral m.
    duodenal m.
    gastric m.
    gastroduodenal m.
    jejunal m.
mucus
Murphy's
    sign
    treatment
muscle
    Treitz's m.
Myà's disease
myasthenia
    m. gastrica
mycogastritis
mycosis
    m. intestinalis
myenteron
myocelialgia
myocelitis
myoneurosis
    colic m.
    intestinal m.
myxoneurosis
    intestinal m.
myxorrhea
    m. intestinalis
nerve
    splanchnic n.
    vagus n.
neurectomy
    gastric n.
neurogastric

neurogenic
NG — nasogastric
Nimeh's method
node
    Troisier's n.
    Virchow's n.
NPO — nothing by mouth
    (nulla per os)
numo-. See words beginning
    pneumo-.
obstipation
obstruction
    biliary tract o.
    intestinal o.
occlusion
occult blood
OCG — oral cholecystogram
Ochsner's
    ring
    treatment
Oddi's sphincter
odditis
oil breakfast
oligocholia
oligochylia
oligochymia
oligopepsia
Olympus fiberscope
omentum
operation. See *General
    Surgical Terms.*
Osler's syndrome
pancreas
pancreatectomy
pancreatic
pancreaticoduodenal
pancreaticoduodenostomy
pancreaticoenterostomy
pancreaticogastrostomy
pancreaticojejunostomy
pancreatitis
pancreatoduodenectomy

pancreatoduodenostomy
pancreatogenic
pancreatography
pancreatolith
pancreatolithectomy
pancreatolithiasis
pancreatolithotomy
pancreatotomy
pancreolithotomy
pancreopathy
pancreotherapy
papilla
    duodenal p.
paracholia
paracolitis
parenteral
parepigastric
parietography
    gastric p.
pars
    p. superior duodeni
Patella's disease
Paterson-Brown-Kelly
  syndrome
Payr's disease
p.c. — after meals (post cibum)
pellagra
pepsin
pepsinogen
peptic
perforation
    pyloroduodenal p.
pericecal
pericecitis
pericholangitis
pericholecystitis
    gaseous p.
pericolic
pericolitis
perigastric
perigastritis

peristalsis
peristaltic
peristole
peristolic
peritoneal
peritoneoscope
peritoneoscopy
peritoneum
    visceral p.
peritonitis
    chylous p.
perityphlitis
    p. actinomycotica
periumbilical
petechial
Peutz-Jeghers syndrome
phytobezoar
pleurocholecystitis
plexus
    enteric p.
    myenteric p.
Plummer-Vinson syndrome
pneumatosis
    p. cystoides intestinalis
    p. cystoides intestinorum
    p. intestinales
pneumocholecystitis
pneumocolon
pneumoenteritis
pneumogastric
pneumogastrography
pneumogastroscopy
pneumoperitoneum
pneumoperitonitis
PO — by mouth (per os)
polycholia
polygastria
polyp
    adenomatous p.
    sessile p.
polyphagia

polypoid
polyposis
     p. coli
     p. gastrica
     p. intestinalis
     p. ventriculi
porta
     p. hepatis
portal
postprandial
pouch
     Hartmann's p.
p.p. — after meals (post-
    prandial)
proctoclysis
proctologist
protoduodenitis
protoduodenum
pseudodiverticula
pseudoleukemia
     p. gastrointestinalis
pseudomegacolon
pseudomyxoma
     p. peritonei
pseudopolyp
psorenteria
psychogenic
PU — peptic ulcer
purpura
     p. abdominalis
     Henoch's p.
     Schönlein-Henoch p.
pylephlebitis
pyloralgia
pyloric
pyloristenosis
pyloritis
pyloroduodenitis
pyloromyotomy
pyloroplasty
     Finney's p.
     Heineke-Mikulicz p.

pyloroptosis
pylorospasm
pylorotomy
pylorus
pyochezia
pyrosis
rectostenosis
rectum
reflex
     epigastric r.
     gastroileac r.
     ileogastric r.
     myenteric r.
reflux
regurgitation
Reichmann's disease
renninogen
rentgenograhfe. See
    roentgenography.
resection
     antral r.
     gastric r.
retrocecal
Riegel's test meal
rigidity
ring
     Cannon's r.
     Ochsner's r.
     Schatzki's r.
roentgenography
Roux-en-Y
     anastomosis
     gastrectomy
Rubin's tube
ruga
     r. gastrica
rugae
rugitus
Sahli's test
Salomon's test
Salzer's test meals
sarcoma

scan
    CAT s.
Schatzki's ring
Schilling test
Schönlein-Henoch purpura
scirrhous
scleroderma
sclerosis
    gastric s.
scoretemia
Sengstaken's tube
sepsis
    s. intestinalis
serosal
serosanguineous
serotonin
shelf
    Blumer's s.
sialoaerophagy
sialorrhea
    s. pancreatica
sigmoid
sigmoidoscope
sigmoidoscopic
sigmoidoscopy
sign
    Kehr's s.
    Murphy's s.
    Trousseau's s.
    Zugsmith's s.
sikwa. See *siqua.*
singultus
    s. gastricus nervosus
Sippy diet
siqua
sirrosis. See *cirrhosis.*
skirus. See *scirrhous.*
sorenterea. See *psorenteria.*
sphincter
    esophagogastric s.
    Oddi's s.
    pyloric s.

splanchnolith
splanchnologia
splanchnomegaly
splanchnomicria
splanchnopathy
splanchnopleure
splanchnoptosis
splanchnosclerosis
splanchnostaxis
splank-. See words beginning
    splanch-.
splenomegaly
splenopancreatic
splenopathy
splenorrhagia
sprue
    tropical s.
Ssabanejew-Frank gastrostomy
Stamm's gastrostomy
stasis
    ileal s.
    venous s.
status
    s. gastricus
steatorrhea
stenosis
    pyloric s.
stoma
stomach
    cup-and-spill s.
    leather bottle s.
stool
    s. culture
    s. guaiac
    lienteric s.
strangulation
stratum
    s. longitudinale tunicae
        muscularis coli
    s. longitudinale tunicae
        muscularis intestini
        tenuis

stricture
submucosa
succus
    s. entericus
    s. gastricus
    s. pancreaticus
succussion
    s. splash
sudo-. See words beginning
    pseudo-.
sulcus
    s. intermedius
suppository
    glycerin s.
swallow
    barium s.
syndrome
    Banti's s.
    Barrett's s.
    blind loop s.
    Courvoisier-Terrier s.
    Dubin-Johnson s.
    dumping s.
    gastrocardiac s.
    Glénard's s.
    Hanot-Rössle s.
    malabsorption s.
    Mallory-Weiss s.
    Osler's s.
    Paterson-Brown-Kelly s.
    Peutz-Jeghers s.
    Plummer-Vinson s.
    Wermer's s.
    Zollinger-Ellison s.
system
    portal s.
Szabo's test
tabes
    t. mesenterica
tampon
    Corner's t.
tamponade
    esophageal t.

telangiectasia
    hemorrhagic t.
telephium
tenesmus
tenia
    t. mesocolica
    t. omentalis
test
    alkaline phosphatase t.
    Althausen's t.
    Carnot's t.
    Congo red t.
    Diagnex blue t.
    D-xylose absorption t.
    fecal fat t.
    glucose absorption t.
    Gmelin's t.
    histamine t.
    liver function t.
    Moynihan's t.
    Sahli's t.
    Salomon's t.
    Schilling t.
    secretin t.
    secretin-pancreozymin t.
    serum bilirubin t.
    stool guaiac t.
    string t.
    Szabo's t.
    Topfer's t.
    Udránszky's t.
    vitamin A absorption t.
test meal
    Boas' t. m.
    Boyden's t. m.
    Dock's t. m.
    Ehrmann's alcohol t. m.
    Ewald's t. m.
    Fischer's t. m.
    Leube's t. m.
    motor t. m.
    Riegel's t. m.
    Salzer's t. m's

Theile's glands
tif-. See words beginning
    typh-.
tomography
    computed t.
Topfer's test
torsion
tract
    alimentary t.
    biliary t.
    gastrointestinal t.
treatment
    Murphy's t.
    Ochsner's t.
Treitz's
    arch
    fossa
    hernia
    ligament
    muscle
trichobezoar
Trichuris
    T. trichiura
Troisier's node
Trousseau's sign
trunci
    t. intestinales
truncus
    t. celiacus
tube
    Argyle's t.
    Baker's t.
    Blakemore's t.
    Cantor's t.
    duodenal t.
    Levin t.
    Miller-Abbott t.
    nasogastric t.
    Rubin's t.
    Sengstaken's t.
    Wangensteen's t.

tuberculosis
    intestinal t.
tumor
    islet cell t.
tunica
    t. fibrosa hepatis
    t. fibrosa lienis
    t. mucosa ventriculi
    t. mucosa vesicae felleae
    t. muscularis coli
    t. muscularis intestini
        tenuis
    t. muscularis recti
    t. muscularis ventriculi
    t. serosa
    t. serosa coli
    t. serosa hepatis
    t. serosa intestini tenuis
    t. serosa lienis
    t. serosa peritonei
    t. serosa ventriculi
    t. serosa vesicae felleae
typhlenteritis
typhlitis
typhlocholecystitis
typhlocolitis
Udránszky's test
UGI — upper gastrointestinal
ukilea. See *euchylia*.
uklorhidrea. See *euchlorhydria*.
ukolea. See *eucholia*.
ulcer
    duodenal u.
    esophageal u.
    gastric u.
    jejunal u.
    peptic u.
    postbulbar u.
    stomal u.
ulceration
ultrasonography

umbilicus
unrest
    peristaltic u.
upepsea. See *eupepsia.*
urease
vagal
vagotomy
vagus
varices
    esophageal v.
vasospasm
Vater's ampulla
vermiform
villi
    jejunal v.
villus
Virchow's node
viscus
vitamin A absorption test
volvulus

vomit
vomitus
    v. cruentus
    v. matutinus
Wangensteen's tube
Wermer's syndrome
Whipple's disease
Winslow's foramen
Wolf-Schindler gastroscope
Wood's lamp
xiphoid
Zenker's diverticulum
zifoid. See *xiphoid.*
Zollinger-Ellison syndrome
Zugsmith's sign
zymogen
    lab z.
zymosis
    z. gastrica

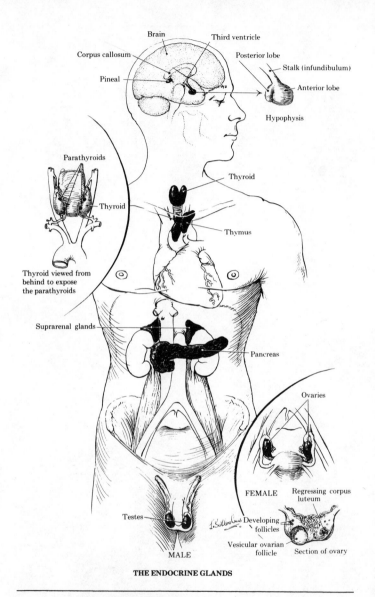

THE ENDOCRINE GLANDS

(Courtesy of Dorland's Illustrated Medical Dictionary, 26th ed. Plate XIX. Philadelphia, W. B. Saunders Company, 1981.)

INTERNAL MEDICINE

Abderhalden-Fanconi
   syndrome
abdomen
abdominal
abdominalgia
Abercrombie's syndrome
abetalipoproteinemia
Abrami's disease
Abrikossoff's tumor
abscess
      caseocavernous a.
      epidural a.
      Pautrier's a.
acalcerosis
acanthocheilonema perstans
acanthocheilonemiasis
acanthocytosis
acantholysis
acanthosis
     a. nigricans
acapnia
acariasis
acatalasia
acaulinosis
achalasia
Achard-Thiers syndrome
achondroplasia
achroacytosis
achylanemia
acidosis
     diabetic a.

acidosis (*continued*)
     hypercapnic a.
     hyperchloremic a.
     metabolic a.
     nonrespiratory a.
     renal tubular a.
     respiratory a.
     starvation a.
     uremic a.
aciduria
acinus
acne
     a. pustulosa
     a. vulgaris
Acosta's disease
acremoniosis
acrocyanosis
acrodynia
acromegaly
acropachyderma
ACTH — adrenocorticotropic
        hormone
actinomycosis
adamantinoma
     pituitary a.
     a. polycysticum
Adams-Stokes
     disease
     syndrome
addisonian
Addison's disease

adenalgia
adenia
    leukemic a.
adenine
adenitis
    acute epidemic infectious
        a.
    acute salivary a.
    cervical a.
    phlegmonous a.
adenoacanthoma
adenoangiosarcoma
adenocarcinoma
adenocystoma
    papillary a. lympho-
        matosum
adenofibroma
adenohypophysis
adenoma
    acidophilic a.
    adamantinum a.
    chromophobe a.
    chromophobic a.
    langerhansian a.
    pituitary a.
adenomata
    colloid a.
    follicular a.
adenomatosis
adenomeloblastoma
adenomyoepithelioma
adenomyofibroma
adenomyomatosis
adenopathy
adenosarcoma
adenosarcorhabdomyoma
adenosclerosis
adenosis
adenotyphus
adenovirus
ADH — antidiuretic hormone

adiposis
    a. dolorosa
    a. hepatica
    a. tuberosa simplex
    a. universalis
adjuvant
adrenal
    a. cortex
    a. gland
    Marchand's a's
    a. medulla
    a. virilism
adrenalectomize
adrenaline
adrenalism
adrenalitis
adrenalopathy
adrenalotropic
adrenarche
adrenergic
adrenic
adrenin
adreninemia
adrenitis
adrenocortical
adrenocorticomimetic
adrenocorticotrophic
adrenocorticotropic
adrenogenous
adrenogram
adrenokinetic
adrenolytic
adrenomedullotropic
adrenomegaly
adrenopathy
adrenopause
adrenoprival
adynamia
    a. episodica hereditaria
aerophagia
afazea. See *aphasia.*

afibrinogenemia
aftha. See *aphtha.*
agalactia
agalactous
agalorrhea
agammaglobulinemia
aglutition
agranulemia
agranulocytopenia
agranulocytosis
agranulosis
ague
      brass-founders' a.
      catenating a.
      dumb a.
      quartan a.
      quintan a.
      quotidian a.
      shaking a.
      tertian a.
Ahumada–Del Castillo
      syndrome
akalazea. See *achalasia.*
akawlinosis. See *acaulinosis.*
akilahnemea. See *achylanemia.*
akinesia
akondroplazea. See
      achondroplasia.
akroahsitosis. See
      achroacytosis.
akromikrie
alastrim
Albers-Schönberg's syndrome
albinism
Albright's syndrome
albuminemia
albuminuria
albumosuria
alcaptonuria
alcoholic
alcoholism
aldosterone

aldosteronism
Aldrich's syndrome
aleukemia
aleukia
      a. hemorrhagica
alkaloid
      plant a.
alkalosis
alkylating agent
allantiasis
allergy
alopecia
alpha-fetoprotein
alveolar
alymphocytosis
alymphoplasia
amanitotoxin
amaurosis
      albuminuric a.
amebiasis
      hepatic a.
ameboma
ameloblastoma
amenorrhea
amine
      aromatic a.
amino acid
aminoaciduria
AML – acute monocytic
      leukemia
      acute myeloblastic
      leukemia
      acute myelocytic
      leukemia
AMML – acute myelomono-
      cytic leukemia
amnesia
amyloidosis
amylosuria
amyotrophy
      diabetic a.
anabolism

anafil-. See words beginning
   anaphyl-.
analbuminemia
anaphylactia
anaphylactic
anaphylactoid
anaphylaxis
anaplasia
anaplasmosis
anaplastic
ancylostomiasis
Anders' disease
Andersen's disease
androgen
anemia
   achrestic a.
   aplastic a.
   Bagdad Spring a.
   Biermer-Ehrlich a.
   Chvostek's a.
   congenital nonsphero-
     cytic hemolytic a.
   Cooley's a.
   Dresbach's a.
   Edelmann's a.
   glucose-6-phosphate
     dehydrogenase de-
     ficiency a.
   hemolytic a.
   Herrick's a.
   hypochromic a.
   hypoplastic a.
   icterohemolytic a.
   Lederer's a.
   Mediterranean a.
   megaloblastic a.
   myelophthisic a.
   normochromic a.
   normocytic a.
   pernicious a.
   sickle cell a.
   sideroblastic a.

anemia (*continued*)
   sideropenic a.
   spherocytic a.
   thrombopenic a.
anergy
aneurysm
angiitis
   visceral a.
angina
   a. cordis
   monocytic a.
   a. nervosa
   a. pectoris
   Plaut's a.
   Schultz's a.
   vasomotor a.
angiohemophilia
angiokeratoma
   a. corporis diffusum
angiolupoid
angioma
angiomatosis
   hemorrhagic familial a.
angiomatous
angiomyosarcoma
angioneuralgia
angioneurosis
angiopancreatitis
anhidrosis
anhydremia
anisocytosis
anisuria
ANLL — acute nonlympho-
        cytic leukemia
anomaly
   Ebstein's a.
   Hegglin's a.
   May-Hegglin a.
   Pelger-Huët a.
   Undritz' a.
anorexia
   a. nervosa

anorexic
anoxemia
anoxia
ansilostomiasis. See
   ancylostomiasis.
antagonist
   metabolic a.
anthracosis
   a. linguae
anthrax
anthrocosilicosis
antibiotic
antidiuretic hormone (ADH)
antifolate
antigen
   carcinoembryonic a.
antimetabolite
antipurine
antipyrimidine
anuria
aortitis
apancrea
apancreatic
aparathyrosis
aphasia
aphtha
APL – acute promyelocytic
    leukemia
aplasia
aplastic
apnea
apoplexy
appendicitis
ARA-C – cytosine arabinoside
arachnodactyly
arachnoiditis
Arakawa-Higashi syndrome
areolitis
arginosuccinicaciduria
Arias' syndrome
ariboflavinosis

Armanni-Ehrlich's
   degeneration
Armstrong's disease
arrhythmia
arsenical
arteriosclerosis
arteritis
arthralgia
   a. saturnina
arthritis
   degenerative a.
   gouty a.
   a. hiemalis
   hypertrophic a.
   juvenile a.
   a. nodosa
   rheumatoid a.
   tuberculous a.
arthrogryposis
arthropathia
   a. ovaripriva
   a. psoriatica
arthrosis
asbestos
asbestosis
ascariasis
Ascher's syndrome
ascites
ascorbemia
Aseli's pancreas
asfiksea. See *asphyxia.*
Asiatic cholera
asiderosis
asinus. See *acinus.*
aspergillosis
asphyxia
aspiration
assay
   estrogen receptor n.
astereognosis
asterixis

asthenia
    a. gravis hypo-
        physeogenea
asthma
    Heberden's a.
astrocyte
astrocytoma
ataxia
atelectasis
atherosclerosis
athetosis
athyreosis
atrophy
    Sudeck's a.
Aufrecht's disease
Australian X disease
autolysis
avitaminosis
Ayerza's
    disease
    syndrome
azmah. See *asthma.*
azotemia
Baber's syndrome
babesiosis
Babinski's sign
bacillemia
bacilluria
bacteremia
bacteriocidal
bacteriuria
Bagdad Spring anemia
balantidiasis
Balo's disease
Balser's fatty necrosis
Banti's
    disease
    syndrome
Bard-Pic syndrome
Bar's syndrome
bartonellosis
Bartter's syndrome

basaloma
Basedow's disease
basiloma
Bassen-Kornzweig syndrome
bath
    paraffin b.
BCNU — bischloroethylnitro-
        sourea
Bearn-Kunkel syndrome
Beauvais' disease
Begbie's disease
Behçet's disease
Behr's disease
Bell's palsy
benign
Bennett's disease
benzpyrene
beriberi
Bernard's syndrome
Bernard-Sergent syndrome
berylliosis
Besnier-Boeck disease
Biermer-Ehrlich anemia
Biett's disease
bilharziasis
bilirubinemia
biofeedback
biopsy
    bone marrow b.
    excisional b.
    incisional b.
    needle b.
bischloroethylnitrosourea
bisinosis. See *byssinosis.*
blastomycosis
Bloom's syndrome
Blumenthal's disease
Blum's syndrome
BMR — basal metabolic rate
Boeck's
    disease
    sarcoid

botulism
Bouchard's nodes
Bouillaud's syndrome
Bowen's disease
Bradley's disease
bradycardia
Brill-Symmer's disease
Brill-Zinsser disease
Brinton's disease
bromohyperhidrosis
bronchiectasis
bronchiolitis
bronchitis
bronchopneumonia
brucellosis
Bruhl's disease
bruit
     Verstraeten's b.
Brunsting's syndrome
brwe. See *bruit.*
bubonalgia
bubonulus
Budd-Chiari syndrome
Budd's cirrhosis
Buerger's disease
Burkitt's
    lymphoma
    tumor
bursitis
Busse-Buschke disease
Butter's cancer
BX — biopsy
byssinosis
CA — cancer
cachexia
café au lait spots
caisson disease
calcemia
calcinosis
    c. interstitialis
    c. universalis
calcitonin

calcium
California encephalitis
calor
    c. febrilis
    c. fervens
    c. innatus
    c. internus
cancer
    acinous c.
    adenoid c.
    c. atrophicans
    Butter's c.
    cellular c.
    cerebriform c.
    dendritic c.
    dermoid c.
    endothelial c.
    epidermal c.
    epithelial c.
    fungous c.
    glandular c.
    hematoid c.
    c. in situ
    Lobstein's c.
    medullary c.
    melanotic c.
    retrograde c.
    scirrhous c.
    solanoid c.
    spider c.
    tubular c.
    villous duct c.
    withering c.
canceration
canceremia
cancericidal
cancerous
cancroid
candidiasis
candidosis
Caplan's syndrome
carcinogen

carcinogenesis
carcinogenic
carcinoid
carcinolytic
carcinoma
 acinous c.
 adenocystic c.
 adenoid cystic c.
 c. adenomatosum
 alveolar c.
 anaplastic c.
 basal cell c.
 c. basocellulare
 basosquamous cell c.
 bronchioalveolar c.
 bronchiolar c.
 bronchogenic c.
 cerebriform c.
 chorionic c.
 colloid c.
 comedo c.
 corpus c.
 cribriform c.
 c. cutaneum
 cylindrical c.
 cylindrical cell c.
 ductal c.
 c. durum
 embryonal c.
 encephaloid c.
 c. en cuirasse
 epibulbar c.
 epidermoid c.
 epithelial c.
 c. epitheliale adenoides
 erectile c.
 exophytic c.
 c. exulcere
 c. fibrosum
 gelatiniform c.
 gelatinous c.
 giant cell c.

carcinoma (*continued*)
 c. gigantocellulare
 glandular c.
 granulosa cell c.
 hair-matrix c.
 hematoid c.
 Hürthle cell c.
 hyaline c.
 hypernephroid c.
 infiltrating ductal cell c.
 c. in situ
 intraepidermal c.
 intraepithelial c.
 Kulchitzky-cell c.
 lenticular c.
 c. lenticulare
 lipomatous c.
 lobular c.
 c. mastitoides
 c. medullare
 c. melanodes
 melanotic c.
 c. molle
 mucinous c.
 c. muciparum
 c. mucocellulare
 mucoepidermoid c.
 c. mucosum
 c. myxomatodes
 c. nigrum
 oat cell c.
 c. ossificans
 osteoid c.
 papillary c.
 periportal c.
 preinvasive c.
 prickle cell c.
 pultaceous c.
 renal cell c.
 c. sarcomatodes
 schneiderian c.
 scirrhous c.

carcinoma (*continued*)
    c. scroti
    signet-ring cell c.
    c. simplex
    solanoid c.
    spheroidal cell c.
    spindle cell c.
    c. spongiosum
    squamous c.
    squamous cell c.
    string c.
    c. telangiectaticum
    c. telangiectodes
    transitional cell c.
    c. tuberosum
    tuberous c.
    verrucous c.
    c. villosum
carcinomata
carcinomatoid
carcinomatosis
carcinomatous
carcinosarcoma
carcinosis
cardiac
cardiospasm
cardiothyrotoxicosis
carotenemia
Carrión's disease
Castellani's disease
catabolism
cataplexy
catecholamine
causalgia
CEA — carcinoembryonic
    antigen
celialgia
celiopathy
cell
    bone marrow c's
    daughter c.
    germinal c's

cell (*continued*)
    parent c.
    somatic c's
cellulitis
cephalalgia
cestodiasis
Chagas' disease
chancre
chancroid
Charcot's cirrhosis
Chédiak-Higashi syndrome
cheilosis
CHEM — chemotherapy
chemotaxis
chemotherapeutic
chemotherapy
    combination c.
Cheyne-Stokes respiration
Chiari-Frommel syndrome
chickenpox
Chinese restaurant syndrome
chloremia
chlorosis
chloruremia
cholangiogram
cholangiography
cholangiohepatoma
cholangiole
cholangiolitis
cholangioma
cholangitis
    catarrhal c.
    c. lenta
cholecystitis
cholecystolithiasis
choledocholithiasis
cholelithiasis
cholemia
    familial c.
    Gilbert's c.
cholepathia
    c. spastica

choleperitoneum
cholera
    Asiatic c.
    bilious c.
    c. morbus
    c. nostras
cholestasis
cholestatic
cholesteremia
cholesterol
cholesteroleresis
cholesterolosis
cholesteroluria
cholesterosis
chondriosome
chondritis
chondromalacia
chondrosarcoma
chordoma
chorea
choriocarcinoma
chorioepithelioma
    c. malignum
choriomeningitis
    lymphocytic c.
    pseudolymphocytic c.
Christmas disease
chromoblastomycosis
chromosome
Chvostek's anemia
Chvostek-Weiss sign
cirrhosis
    alcoholic s.
    atrophic c.
    Budd's c.
    Charcot's c.
    Cruveilhier-Baumgarten c.
    Glisson's c.
    Hanot's c.
    Laennec's c.
    Maixner's c.
    portal c.
    Todd's c.

claudication
    intermittent c.
climacteric
climacterium
    c. praecox
clonorchiasis
clostridia
CMF − Cytoxan, methotrex-
    ate, 5-fluorouracil
CML − chronic myelocytic
    leukemia
    chronic myelogenous
    leukemia
coccidioidomas
coccidioidomycosis
coccidiosis
code
    genetic c.
    molecular c.
colibacillosis
colic
    renal c.
    stercoral c.
    ureteral c.
    uterine c.
colisepsis
colitis
Colorado tick fever virus
comedocarcinoma
communicable
Concato's disease
Conn's syndrome
constipation
contracture
    Dupuytren's c.
convulsion
Cooley's anemia
Cooper's disease
COP − Cytoxan, Oncovin,
    prednisone
COPD − chronic obstructive
    pulmonary disease
coproporphyria

cor
- c. pulmonale
- c. triatriatum

cortex
- adrenal c.

corticoid
corticosteroid
cortisol
cortisone
coryza
Coxsackie virus
cretinism
Crohn's disease
croup
CRS — Chinese restaurant syndrome
Cruveilhier-Baumgarten
- cirrhosis
- syndrome

cryoglobulinemia
cryosurgery
cryptococcosis
culture
Curschmann's disease
cushingoid
Cushing's syndrome
CVA — cerebrovascular accident
CVP — Cytoxan, vincristine, prednisone
cyanosis
cycle
- growth c.

cylindroma
cyst
cystadenocarcinoma
cystadenoma
cystadenosarcoma
cystathioninuria
cystic
cysticercosis
cystinemia

cystinosis
cystinuria
cystitis
cystoadenoma
cystocarcinoma
cystomyoma
cystomyxoadenoma
cystomyxoma
cystosarcoma
- c. phylloides

cytology
- exfoliative c.

cytomycosis
cytoplasm
cytosine arabinoside
dactylolysis
- d. spontanea

Darier-Roussy sarcoid
Darling's disease
Debove's disease
decalcification
dedifferentiated
dedifferentiation
degeneration
- amyloid d.
- Armanni-Ehrlich's d.
- hepatolenticular d.
- hyaline d.

Degos'
- disease
- syndrome

dehydration
Déjerine-Sottas disease
delirium
- d. tremens

De Morgan's spots
dengue
deoxyribonucleic acid
deoxyribose
deradenitis
deradenoncus
dermalaxia

dermametropathism
dermamyiasis
dermataneuria
dermatitis
dermatomucosomyositis
dermatomycosis
dermatophytid
dermatophytosis
dermatosis
DES — diethylstilbestrol
desequestration
deshydremia
dethyroidism
detoxification
DHL — diffuse histocytic
       lymphoma
DI — diabetes insipidus
diabetes
    d. alternans
    d. insipidus
    Lancereaux's d.
    latent d.
    d. mellitus
diabetic
    brittle d.
dialysis
diaphoresis
diaphoretic
diaphragm
diaphragma
diarrhea
diaspironecrobiosis
diaspironecrosis
diathermy
diathesis
diet
    Ebstein's d.
diethylstilbestrol
differentiated
differentiation
    cellular d.
diffuse

difilobothriasis. See
    diphyllobothriasis.
difth-. See words beginning
    diphth-.
digitalization
DiGuglielmo's syndrome
diphtheria
diphtheroid
diphyllobothriasis
diplegia
diplococcemia
diplopia
dis-. See words beginning
    dys-.
disease
    Abrami's d.
    Acosta's d.
    acute demyelinating d.
    Adams-Stokes d.
    Addison's d.
    Anders' d.
    Andersen's d.
    angiospasmodic d.
    Armstrong's d.
    Aufrecht's d.
    Australian X d.
    autoimmune d.
    Ayerza's d.
    Baló's d.
    Banti's d.
    Basedow's d.
    Beauvais' d.
    Begbie's d.
    Behçet's d.
    Behr's d.
    Bennett's d.
    Besnier-Boeck d.
    Biett's d.
    Blumenthal's d.
    Boeck's d.
    Bowen's d.
    Bradley's d.

disease (*continued*)

Brill-Symmer's d.
Brill-Zinsser d.
Brinton's d.
Bruhl's d.
Buerger's d.
Busse-Buschke d.
caisson d.
Carrión's d.
Castellani's d.
cat-scratch d.
celiac d.
Chagas' d.
Christmas d.
collagen d.
combined immuno-
deficiency d.
Concato's d.
Cooper's d.
Crohn's d.
Curschmann's d.
Darling's d.
Debove's d.
Degos' d.
Déjerine-Sottas d.
demyelinating d.
Dressler's d.
Durand's d.
Ebstein's d.
Economo's d.
Fabry's d.
Fenwick's d.
Filatov's d.
Flajani's d.
Friedländer's d.
Gamna's d.
Gandy-Nanta d.
Gaucher's d.
Gilbert's d.
Gilchrist's d.
glycogen storage d.
Graves' d.

disease (*continued*)

Hand-Schüller-Christian
d.
Hanot's d.
Hansen's d.
Hartnup's d.
Hashimoto's d.
Heberden's d.
Heerfordt's d.
hemolytic d.
heredoconstitutional d.
Hers' d.
Hirschsprung's d.
Hodgkin's d.
Horton's d.
Huchard's d.
Huntington's d.
Hutinel's d.
Kahler's d.
Kirkland's d.
Krabbe's d.
Landouzy's d.
Letterer-Siwe d.
Lignac's d.
Luft's d.
Marie's d.
mast cell d.
Mathieu's d.
Meleda d.
Meniere's d.
Mikulicz's d.
Möbius' d.
Monge's d.
Morquio's d.
Nicolas-Favre d.
Niemann-Pick d.
Niemann's d.
Ollier's d.
Opitz's d.
Osler's d.
Osler-Vaquez d.
Paget's d.

disease (*continued*)
    parenchymatous d.
    Parkinson's d.
    Parrot's d.
    Parry's d.
    Parsons' d.
    Pavy's d.
    Pfeiffer's d.
    Pick's d.
    Plummer's d.
    Pompe's d.
    Poncet's d.
    Pott's d.
    pulseless d.
    Raynaud's d.
    Refsum's d.
    Reiter's d.
    rheumatic heart d.
    Riedel's d.
    Rokitansky's d.
    Runeberg's d.
    San Joaquin Valley d.
    Schaumann's d.
    Sheehan's d.
    Simmonds' d.
    Smith-Strang d.
    Sternberg's d.
    Stuart-Bras d.
    Symmers' d.
    Tangier d.
    tsutsugamushi d.
    von Gierke's d.
    von Willebrand's d.
    Weil's d.
    Werner's d.
    Wernicke's d.
    Widal-Abrami d.
    Willis' d.
    Wilson's d.
    zymotic d.
dissection
    block d.

distomiasis
    hemic d.
    hepatic d.
diuresis
diverticulitis
diverticulosis
diverticulum
    Meckel's d.
DM — diabetes mellitus
DNA — deoxyribonucleic acid
DNA virus
dormant
dracunculiasis
Dresbach's
    anemia
    syndrome
Dressler's disease
dropsy
drugs. See *Drugs and*
    Chemistry section.
Dupuytren's contracture
Durand's disease
dwarfism
    pituitary d.
dwarfs
    achondroplastic d.
    hypopituitary d.
dysarthria
dyscrasia
    blood d.
    lymphatic d.
dyscrinism
dysdiemorrhysis
dysdipsia
dysendocrisiasis
dysentery
    amebic d.
dysesthesia
dysgammaglobulinemia
dysglobulinemia
dyshepatia
dyshidrosis

dyskeratosis
dyskinesia
dyspancreatism
dysparathyroidism
dyspareunia
dyspepsia
dysphagia
dyspinealism
dyspituitarism
dysplasia
dyspnea
dysponderal
dyspragia
dysproteinemia
dyssebacea
dysthyroidism
dystonia
dysuria
eastern equine encephalo-
    myelitis
Ebstein's
        anomaly
        diet
        disease
EBV — Epstein-Barr virus
ecchymosis
eccyclomastoma
echinococcosis
echinostomiasis
echovirus
eclampsia
Economo's disease
ecphyma
        e. globulus
ectasia
ecthyma
ectodermosis
        e. erosiva pluriorificialis
ectopia
eczema
Edelmann's anemia

edema
    Milroy's e.
    nonpitting e.
    pedal e.
    Pirogoff's e.
    prehepatic e.
edematous
edentulous
Ehlers-Danlos syndrome
ekfima. See *ecphyma.*
ekimosis. See *ecchymosis.*
ekino-. See words beginning
    echino-.
eksanthema. See *exanthema.*
eksiklomastoma. See
    eccyclomastoma.
ekthima. See *ecthyma.*
ekzema. See *eczema.*
elastofibroma
    e. dorsi
elastoma
elastosis
electrocauterization
electrocautery
electrolysis
electrolyte
electromyography
electrophoresis
electropyrexia
elephantiasis
ellipsoid
    e. of spleen
elliptocytosis
emaciation
embolemia
embolism
embolomycotic
embolus
EMC — encephalomyocarditis
emetatrophia
emphysema

empyema
encapsulated
encephalitis
    acute disseminated e.
    acute necrotizing e.
    California e.
    hemorrhagic e.
    Japanese B e.
    Murray Valley e.
    Russian spring-summer e.
    e. siderans
    St. Louis e.
    Strümpell-Leichtenstern
      e.
    West Nile e.
encephalomyelitis
    eastern equine e.
    Venezuelan equine e.
    western equine e.
encephalopathy
    hepatic e.
    Wernicke's e.
enchondromatosis
endarteritis
endocarditis
    bacterial e.
endocrine
endocrinosis
endometriosis
endothelioangiitis
endothelioblastoma
endotheliocytosis
endotheliomatosis
endotheliomyoma
endotheliomyxoma
endotoxicosis
enkondromatosis. See
    enchondromatosis.
ensefal-. See words beginning
    encephal-.

entamebiasis
enteritis
    e. necroticans
enterobiasis
enterovirus
enzyme
eosinophilia
    Löffler's e.
epidemic
epidermodysplasia
epidermoid
epidermophytosis
epididymis
epididymitis
epilepsy
epiloia
epinephrine
epistaxis
    Gull's renal e.
epithelial
epithelioblastoma
epithelioma
epituberculosis
Epstein-Barr virus
ER — estrogen receptors
Erb's sign
erethism
ergotism
erisipela de la costa
erysipelas
erythema
    e. multiforme
    e. nodosum
    e. toxicum
erythematous
erythralgia
erythrasma
erythremia
erythroblastoma
erythroblastomatosis

erythroblastopenia
erythroblastosis
erythrocyanosis
erythrocythemia
erythrocytosis
    leukemic e.
    e. megalosplenica
erythroderma
erythrogenesis
    e. imperfecta
erythroleukemia
erythroleukosis
erythromelalgia
erythromelia
erythroneocytosis
erythropenia
erythropoiesis
eschar
esophagitis
estriasis. See *oestriasis.*
estrogen
eunuchism
    pituitary e.
euthanasia
euthyroid
euthyroidism
exanthema
    e. subitum
Exc. — excision
exfoliative
exhaustion
exogenous
exophthalmos
exophthalmometry
exostosis
expectoration
exsanguination
Faber's syndrome
Fabry's disease
facies
    Parkinson's f.

fagositosis. See *phagocytosis.*
Fallot's tetralogy
Falta's triad
Fanconi's syndrome
farinjitis. See *pharyngitis.*
Farre's tubercles
fasciolopsiasis
fatigue
favism
FBS — fasting blood sugar
Felty's syndrome
fenetidinurea. See
    phenetidinuria.
fenilketonurea. See
    phenylketonuria.
feno-. See words beginning
    pheno-.
Fenwick's disease
feo-. See words beginning
    pheo-.
fetor
    f. hepaticus
fever
    etiocholanolone f.
    Haverhill f.
    hay f.
    hemorrhagic f.
    Malta f.
    Oroya f.
    phlebotomus f.
    Q f.
    quartan f.
    quinine f.
    quintana f.
    quotidian f.
    rat-bite f.
    rheumatic f.
    Rift Valley f.
    Rocky Mountain spotted
      f.
    San Joaquin f.

fever (*continued*)
 scarlet f.
 South American
  hemorrhagic f.
 Southeast Asian
  mosquito-borne
  hemorrhagic f.
 streptobacillary f.
 typhoid f.
 undulant f.
 West Nile f.
 yellow f.
fibrillation
fibrinogenemia
fibrinogenopenia
fibrinolysis
fibrinopenia
fibroadamantoblastoma
fibroadenia
fibroadenoma
fibroadenosis
fibroblastoma
fibrocyst
fibrocystic
fibrocystoma
fibroelastosis
fibrolymphoangioblastoma
fibroma
fibromatoid
fibromatosis
fibromyoma
fibromyositis
fibromyxosarcoma
fibrosarcoma
fibrosis
 cystic f.
fibrositis
fikomycosis. See
 phycomycosis.
filariasis
Filatov's disease
Fitz-Hugh-Curtis syndrome

Fitz's
 law
 syndrome
flagellosis
Flajani's disease
flebitis. See *phlebitis.*
flebo-. See words beginning
 phlebo-.
fleckmilz
5-fluorouracil
folic acid
follicle-stimulating hormone
follicular
folliculitis
food poisoning
 Bacillus cereus f. p.
 enterococcal f. p.
Forbes-Albright syndrome
fractionation
fragilitas
 f. sanguinis
fragilocytosis
Friedländer's disease
Friedmann's vasomotor
 syndrome
frostbite
fructosuria
FSH — follicle-stimulating
 hormone
FU — fluorouracil
fungating
furunculosis
G-1 period
G-2 period
Ga — gallium
Gaisböck's syndrome
galactorrhea
galactosemia
gallstones
Gamna's disease
Gandy-Gamna
 nodules

Gandy-Gamna (*continued*)
    spleen
Gandy-Nanta disease
ganglion
    Troisier's g.
ganglioneuroma
gangrene
    Raynaud's g.
Gardner's syndrome
gargoylism
gastrectasia
gastroma
Gaucher's
    disease
    splenomegaly
generation time
genes
genetic code
geotrichosis
German measles
germinal
giardiasis
gigantism
Gilbert's
    cholemia
    disease
Gilchrist's
    disease
    mycosis
gland
    adrenal g.
    endocrine g.
    exocrine g.
    parathyroid g.
    pineal g.
    pituitary g.
    suprarenal g.
    thymus g.
    thyroid g.
glanders
Glanzmann's syndrome
Glisson's cirrhosis

globulinemia
globus
    g. hystericus
glomangioma
glomerulitis
glomerulonephritis
glomerulosclerosis
    intercapillary g.
glossitis
glucagon
glucocorticoid
gluconeogenesis
glucose
glucosuria
glycemia
glycogen
glycopenia
glycopolyuria
glycosuria
goiter
    adenomatous g.
    colloid g.
    endemic g.
    exophthalmic g.
    fibrous g.
    follicular g.
    intrathoracic g.
    nodular g.
    papillomatous g.
    parenchymatous g.
    substernal g.
    toxic g.
gonadotropic hormone
gonadotropin
gongylonemiasis
gonorrhea
Goodpasture's syndrome
Gopalan's syndrome
gout
    abarticular g.
    articular g.
    calcium g.

gout (*continued*)
    chalky g.
    latent g.
    lead g.
    misplaced g.
    oxalic g.
    polyarticular g.
    retrocedent g.
    rheumatic g.
    saturnine g.
    tophaceous g.
gouty
grading
Graefe's sign
granuloblastosis
granulocytopenia
granulocytosis
granuloma
    amebic g.
    Hodgkin's g.
granulomatosis
    g. siderotica
    Wegener's g.
Graves' disease
grippe
growth
    g. cycle
    g. fraction
    g. hormone
GTT — glucose tolerance test
guanine
Gubler's icterus
Guillian-Barré syndrome
Gull's renal epistaxis
gumma
Günther's syndrome
gynecomastia
hamartoma
hamartomatosis
Hamman-Rich syndrome
Hand-Schüller-Christian
  disease

Hanger-Rose skin test
Hanot's
    cirrhosis
    disease
Hansen's disease
Harris' syndrome
Hartnup's disease
Hashimoto's
    disease
    struma
Haverhill fever
Hayem's icterus
Hayem-Widal syndrome
HD — Hodgkin's disease
headache
    cluster h.
    Horton's h.
    migraine h.
heartburn
Heberden's
    asthma
    disease
    nodes
    rheumatism
Heerfordt's
    disease
    syndrome
Hegglin's anomaly
Heidenhaim's syndrome
helical
helminthiasis
    cutaneous h.
    h. elastica
    h. wuchereri
hemangioblastoma
hemangioma
hemangiosarcoma
hemarthrosis
hematemesis
hematogenesis
hematoma
    epidural h.

hematomycosis
hematomyelia
hematopenia
hematoporphyria
hematuria
hemiparesis
hemiplegia
hemisporosis
hemobilinuria
hemoblastosis
hemochromatosis
hemocytoblastoma
hemodialysis
hemoglobinemia
hemoglobinuria
hemophilia
hemopneumothorax
hemoptysis
hemosiderosis
hemuresis
hepar
    h. adiposum
    h. lobatum
hepatalgia
hepatargia
hepatatrophia
hepatic
hepatism
hepatitis
    anicteric h.
    infectious h.
    serum h.
    viral h.
hepatocele
hepatocirrhosis
hepatodynia
hepatodystrophy
hepatoglobinemia
hepatohemia
hepatolienal
hepatoma
hepatomalacia

hepatomegaly
hepatomphalos
hepatonephritis
hepatonephromegaly
hepatoperitonitis
hepatophyma
hepatoportal
hepatoptosis
hepatorrhagia
hepatorrhexis
hepatosis
hepatosplenitis
hepatosplenomegaly
hepatotoxicity
heredity
heredopathia
    h. atactica
        polyneuritiformis
hermaphroditism
herpangina
herpes
    h. catarrhalis
    h. generalisatus
    h. labialis
    h. meningoencephalitis
    h. simplex
    h. zoster
herpesvirus
Herrick's anenia
Hers' disease
heteradenia
heteropancreatism
heterophyiasis
HGF — hyperglycemic-glyco-
        genolytic factor
HGH — human growth
        hormone
hibernoma
hiccup
Hickey-Hare test
hidradenitis
    h. suppurativa

hidrorrhea
hidrosadenitis
   h. axillaris
   h. destruens suppurativa
hidrosis
Hines-Bannick syndrome
Hirschsprung's disease
hirsutism
histiocytomatosis
histiocytosis
   h. X
histoplasmosis
Hodgkin's
   disease
   granuloma
Homans' sign
homeostasis
homocystinuria
hookworm
hormone
Horton's
   disease
   headache
   syndrome
host cell
Huchard's disease
Hunter's syndrome
Huntington's disease
Hurler's syndrome
Hürthle cell carcinoma
Hutchinson's triad
Hutinel's disease
hyaloserositis
hydatid
hydatidoma
hydatidosis
hydremia
hydrocarbon
   aromatic h.
hydrocephalus
hydrocortisone
hydrophobia

hydrops
hydroxyprolinemia
hyloma
hymenolepiasis
hyperaminoaciduria
hyperbilirubinemia
hypercalcemia
hypercalciuria
hypercapnia
hyperchloremia
hypercholesterolemia
hypercholesterolia
hyperchromatic
hyperchromatism
   macrocytic h.
hyperchromia
hyperemesis
   h. hiemis
hyperemia
hyperesthesia
hyperfibrinogenemia
hypergammaglobulinemia
hypergenesis
hyperglobulinemia
hyperglycemia
hyperglycemic-glycogenolytic
   factor
hyperglyceridemia
hyperglycinemia
hyperglycinuria
hypergonadism
hyperhidrosis
   h. lateralis
hyperhistidinemia
hyperinsulinemia
hyperinsulinism
hyperkalemia
hyperkeratomycosis
hyperkeratosis
hyperketonemia
hyperketonuria
hyperkinemia

hyperlipemia
hyperlipidemia
hyperlipoproteinemia
hyperliposis
hypernatremia
hypernephroma
hypernitremia
hypernormocytosis
hyperoxaluria
hyperoxemia
hyperparathyroidism
hyperpathia
hyperpepsinemia
hyperphosphatemia
hyperphosphaturia
hyperphosphoremia
hyperpituitarism
    basophilic h.
    eosinophilic h.
hyperplasia
hyperpnea
hyperpotassemia
hyperprolinemia
hyperproteinemia
hyperpyrexia
hypersecretion
hypersplenism
hypertension
hypertensive
hyperthermia
hyperthrombinemia
hyperthrombocytemia
hyperthyroidism
hypertrichiasis
hypertriglyceridemia
hypertrophy
    Marie's h.
hyperuricemia
hypervalinemia
hyperventilation
hypervitaminosis
hypervolemia

hypoadrenalemia
hypoadrenalism
hypoalbuminemia
hypoalbuminosis
hypoaldosteronemia
hypoaminoacidemia
hypocalcemia
hypocapnia
hypochloremia
hypochromasia
hypochromemia
    idiopathic h.
hypochromia
hypochrosis
hypocrinism
hypocythemia
hypodermoclysis
hypodermolithiasis
hypoendocrinism
hypoestrogenemia
hypofibrinogenemia
hypogammaglobulinemia
hypoglycemia
hypogonadism
hypogonadotrophism
hypogranulocytosis
hypohepatia
hypoinsulinemia
hypoinsulinism
hypokalemia
hypolepidoma
hypoleukocytosis
hypolipidemia
hyponatremia
hyponeocytosis
hyponitremia
hypoparathyroidism
hypophosphatasia
hypophosphatemia
hypophyseal
hypophysis
hypopiesia

hypopiesis
hypopituitarism
hypoplasia
hypoproteinemia
hypoprothrombinemia
hyposecretion
hyposialadenitis
hyposthenuria
hypotension
    orthostatic h.
hypothalamus
hypothermia
    endogenous h.
hypothrombinemia
hypothyroidism
hypotonic
hypoventilation
hypovitaminosis
hypovolemia
hypoxemia
hypoxia
IADH — inappropriate anti-
    diuretic hormone
ichthyosarcotoxism
ichthyosis
icteric
icteroanemia
icterohepatitis
icterus
    acholuric hemolytic i.
      with splenomegaly
    bilirubin i.
    i. castrensis gravis
    i castrensis levis
    i catarrhalis
    cythemolytic i.
    i. gravis
    Gubler's i.
    Hayem's i.
    i. hemolyticus
    i. infectiosus
    i. praecox

icterus (*continued*)
    i. simplex
    spirochetal i.
    i. typhoides
    urobilin i.
    i. viridans
ictus
iksodiasis. See *ixodiasis.*
ikterik. See *icteric.*
iktero-. See words beginning
    ictero-.
ikterus. See *icterus.*
iktheosarkotoksizm. See
    ichthyosarcotoxism.
iktheosis. See *ichthyosis.*
iktus. See *ictus.*
immune response
immunity
immunization
impetigo
impotence
inappropriate antidiuretic
    hormone
incarnatio
    i. unguis
incontinentia
    i. pigmenti
incubation
Indian tick typhus
indoluria
inebriation
inert
infarction
    myocardial i.
infection
infectious
infertility
infestation
infiltrative
inflammation
inflammatory
influenza

infundibuloma
inguinodynia
inhibition
    contact i.
inoculation
inocystoma
in situ
insomnia
insulin
insulinemia
insulinogenesis
insulinoma
insuloma
intersexuality
interstitialoma
intertrigo
intestine
intussusception
invasive
in vitro
in vivo
iodine
ionic
ionizing
iritis
    diabetic i.
    gouty i.
irradiation
ischemia
islet
    i's of Langerhans
isonormocytosis
isopathy
isosthenuria
isotope
isthmus
ixodiasis
Janeway's spots
Japanese B encephalitis
jaundice
    hemolytic j.
    obstructive j.

Job's syndrome
K — potassium
kahkeksea. See *cachexia.*
Kahler's disease
kala-azar
kalemia
kaliopenia
Kallmann's syndrome
Kartagener's syndrome
karyotype
katzenjammer
Kayser-Fleischer ring
kemotherape. See
    chemotherapy.
keratitis
keratoderma
    k. blennorrhagica
keratoma
keratomalacia
keratosis
kernicterus
ketoacidosis
ketonuria
ketosis
kifosis. See *kyphosis.*
kilosis. See *cheilosis.*
Kimmelstiel-Wilson syndrome
kinetics
    cell population k.
kinetosis
Kirkland's disease
Kleine-Levin syndrome
Klinefelter's syndrome
klor-. See words beginning
    chlor-.
Kocher's syndrome
koksake. See *Coxsackie.*
kolange-. See words beginning
    cholangi-.
kole-. See words beginning
    chole-.
kolera. See *cholera.*

koles-. See words beginning
  choles-.
kondritis. See *chondritis.*
kondro-. See words beginning
  chondro-.
König's syndrome
kopf-tetanus
kordoma. See *chordoma.*
korea. See *chorea.*
koreo-. See words beginning
  chorio-.
Krabbe's disease
kromoblastomikosis. See
  chromoblastomycosis.
Kulchitzky-cell carcinoma
Kundrat's lymphosarcoma
kwashiorkor
kyphosis
lactogenic hormone
Laennec's cirrhosis
la grippe
Lancereaux's diabetes
Landouzy's
    disease
    purpura
Langerhans
    islets of L.
laparotomy
    staging l.
laryngitis
latent
Laurence-Moon-Biedl
    syndrome
law
    Fitz's l.
Läwen-Roth syndrome
LE – lupus erythematosus
LED – lupus erythematosus
        disseminatus
Lederer's anemia
leiomyoma
leiomyosarcoma

leishmaniasis
leprosy
leptoprosopia
leptospirosis
    l. icterohemorrhagica
Leriche's syndrome
Lesch-Nyhan syndrome
lethal
Letterer-Siwe disease
leukemia
    acute nonlymphocytic l.
    acute promyelocytic l.
    aleukocythemic l.
    basophilic l.
    blast cell l.
    l. cutis
    embryonal l.
    eosinophilic l.
    granulocytic l.
    hemocytoblastic l.
    histiocytic l.
    leukopenic l.
    lymphatic l.
    lymphoblastic l.
    lymphocytic l.
    lymphogenous l.
    lymphoid l.
    lymphoidocytic l.
    lymphosarcoma cell l.
    mast cell l.
    megakaryocytic l.
    micromyeloblastic l.
    monocytic l.
    myeloblastic l.
    myelocytic l.
    myelogenous l.
    myeloid granulocytic l.
    plasma cell l.
    plasmacytic l.
    promyelocytic l.
    Rieder cell l.
    Schilling's l.

leukemia (*continued*)
> splenomedullary l.
> splenomyelogenous l.
> stem cell l.
> subleukemic l.
> undifferentiated cell l.

leukocyte
leukocytosis
leukodystrophy
leukolymphosarcoma
leukopenia
leukoplakia
LH — luteinizing hormone
Lignac-Fanconi syndrome
Lignac's disease
line
> Sergent's white l.

linitis
> l. plastica

liomioma. See *leiomyoma*.
liomiosarcoma. See
> *leiomyosarcoma*.

lipemia
lipiduria
lipoblastosis
lipochondrodystrophy
lipodystrophia
> l. progressiva

lipodystrophy
lipoma
lipomatosis
lipoproteinemia
> A-beta l.

liposarcoma
liver
> amyloid l.
> brimstone l.
> cirrhotic l.
> lardaceous l.

Loa
> *L. loa*

loaiasis
Lobstein's cancer
Löffler's
> eosinophilia
> syndrome

lordosis
LTH — luteotropic hormone
lues
> l. hepatis

Luft's
> disease
> syndrome

lumbago
> ischemic l.

lupus
> l. erythematosus
> l. nephritis
> l. pernio

luteinizing hormone
lymphadenectasis
lymphadenhypertrophy
lymphadenia
> l. ossea

lymphadenitis
> caseous l.
> paratuberculous l.

lymphadenocyst
lymphadenogram
lymphadenography
lymphadenoid
lymphadenoleukopoiesis
lymphadenoma
lymphadenopathy
> giant follicular l.

lymphadenosis
lymphadenovarix
lymphangiectasis
lymphangioendothelioblastoma
lymphangioendothelioma
lymphangiofibroma
lymphangiogram

lymphangiosarcoma
lymphangitis
lymphatic
lymphatism
lymphedema
    l. praecox
lymphemia
lymphoblastoma
    giant follicular l.
lymphoblastomatosis
lymphocystosis
lymphocyte
lymphocythemia
lymphocytoma
lymphocytopenia
lymphocytosis
lymphodermia
lymphogranuloma
lymphogranulomatosis
lymphoidotoxemia
lymphoma
    Burkitt's l.
    clasmocytic l.
    giant follicular l.
    granulomatous l.
    lymphoblastic l.
    lymphocytic l.
    stem-cell l.
lymphomatosis
lymphopathia
    l. venereum
lymphopenia
lymphosarcoleukemia
lymphosarcoma
    Kundrat's l.
    lymphocytic l.
lymphosarcomatosis
lymphotoxemia
lysemia
M period
MacLeod's capsular
  rheumatism

macrodystrophia
    m. lipomatosa progressiva
macrogenitosomia
    m. praecox
macroglobulinemia
    Waldenström's m.
macrosomatia
    m. adiposa congenita
maculation
    pernicious m.
maduromycosis
Maixner's cirrhosis
mal
    m. de mer
malabsorption
maladie
malaise
malaria
malignancy
malignant
mali-mali
malnutrition
Malta fever
mamillary
mamillitis
mamma
mammogram
mammoplasia
marasmus
Marchand's adrenals
Marchiafava-Micheli syndrome
Marfan's syndrome
Marie's
    disease
    hypertrophy
    sign
    syndrome
Maroteaux-Lamy syndrome
mastadenoma
mastalgia
mastatrophy
mastauxe

masthelcosis
mastitis
mastocarcinoma
mastochondroma
mastocytosis
mastoiditis
mastoncus
mastopathia
    m. cystica
mastopathy
mastoplastia
mastoptosis
Mathieu's disease
May-Hegglin anomaly
measles
    German m.
Meckel's diverticulum
mediastinitis
mediastinum
medications. See *Drugs and Chemistry* section.
Mediterranean anemia
medulla
    adrenal m.
medullary
medulloblastoma
megacolon
megakaryoblastoma
megakaryocytosis
megalerythema
megalgia
melanocyte
melanoma
melanosis
melanuria
melasma
    m. addisonii
    m. suprarenale
melatonin
Meleda disease
melena

melenemesis
melioidosis
membrane
    nuclear m.
menarche
Meniere's
    disease
    syndrome
meningitis
meningoblastoma
meningococcemia
meningoencephalitis
meningopneumonitis
meningotyphoid
meniscocytosis
menopause
menstruation
meralgia
    m. paresthetica
6-mercaptopurine
Merseburg triad
metabolic
metabolism
metagonimiasis
metamorphosis
    fatty m.
metaplasia
    myeloid m.
metastases
metastasis
metastasize
metastatic
methemoglobinemia
methionine
mets — metastases
microcephaly
microcythemia
microlithiasis
micturition
mielo-. See words beginning
    myelo-.

migraine
miks-. See words beginning
   myx-.
mikso-. See words beginning
   myxo-.
Mikulicz's
   disease
   syndrome
miliaria
Milroy's edema
mineralocorticoids
Minkowski-Chauffard
   syndrome
mirinjitis. See *myringitis.*
mitochondria
mitochondrion
mitosis
mittelschmerz
Möbius'
   disease
   sign
modality
molecule
Monge's disease
moniliasis
mononucleosis
   infectious m.
MOPP — nitrogen mustard,
        Oncovin, pred-
        nisone, procarba-
        zine
morbidity
morbilliform
Morquio's
   disease
   syndrome
MP — mercaptopurine
mRNA — messenger RNA
MS — multiple sclerosis
MTX — methotrexate
mucinous
mucopolysaccharidosis

mucopolysacchariduria
mucopurulent
mucormycosis
mucosanguineous
mucositis
   m. necroticans
      agranulocytica
mucoviscidosis
mumps
Münchausen's syndrome
murmur
   heart m.
Murray Valley encephalitis
mutagen
mutagenesis
mutagenic
mutation
   spontaneous genetic m.
myalgia
myasthenia
   m. gravis
myasthenic
myatonia
   m. congenita
myatrophy
mycethemia
mycetismus
mycobacteriosis
Mycobacterium
   M. tuberculosis
mycosis
   Gilchrist's m.
   splenic m.
mycotoxicosis
myelemia
myelitis
myeloblastemia
myeloblastoma
myeloblastomatosis
myeloblastosis
myelocythemia
myelocytoma

myelocytomatosis
myelofibrosis
myeloma
     giant cell m.
     multiple m.
myelomatosis
myelosarcoma
myelosarcomatosis
myelosclerosis
myelosis
myelosuppression
myelotoxicosis
myiasis
myoblastoma
myocardia
myocardiac
myocardial
myocarditis
     acute bacterial m.
myocardosis
myoglobinuria
myoglobulinuria
myolysis
     m. cardiotoxica
myoma
myositis
myotonia
myringitis
myxadenitis
myxadenoma
myxangitis
myxasthenia
myxedema
myxoblastoma
myxochondrofibrosarcoma
myxochondroma
myxochondrosarcoma
myxodermia
myxofibrosarcoma
myxoidedema
myxoma
myxomatosis

myxosarcoma
myxovirus
Na — sodium
nanism
     Paltauf's n.
narcolepsy
natremia
natriuresis
nausea
necrobiosis
     n. lipoidica
     n. lipoidica diabeticorum
necrosis
     Balser's fatty n.
     decubital n.
     icteric n.
necrotic
NED — no evidence of disease
nefritis. See nephritis.
*nefro-. See words beginning
     nephro-.*
nemathelminthiasis
nematodiasis
neoplasia
neoplasm
nephritis
nephrocalcinosis
nephrocirrhosis
nephrocystitis
nephrocystosis
nephrolithiasis
nephropyelitis
nephrosclerosis
nephrosis
NER — no evidence of recur-
         rence
NERD — no evidence of recur-
         rent disease
neuralgia
neurasthenia
neuritis
neuroamebiasis

neuroblastoma
neurofibroma
neurohypophysis
neuroma
    acoustic n.
neuromyositis
neurosyphilis
neutropenia
neutrophilia
Nicolas-Favre disease
Niemann-Pick disease
Niemann's
    disease
    splenomegaly
Nikolsky's sign
nocardiosis
noctalbuminuria
nocturia
node
    Bouchard's n's
    Heberden's n's
    lymph n's
    Osler's n's
    Parrot's n.
nodular
nodule
    cold n.
    Gandy-Gamna n's
Noonan's syndrome
noradrenaline
norepinephrine
NPDL — nodular, poorly
        differentiated
        lymphocytes
nucleic acid
nucleolus
nucleoprotein
nucleotide
nucleus
numo-. See words beginning
    pneumo-.
nystagmus

obesity
    endogenous o.
    exogenous o.
ochrodermatosis
ochrodermia
ochronosis
odon-eki
odoriferous
oestriasis
ofthal-. See words beginning
    ophthal-.
17-OHS — 17-hydroxycortico-
        steroid
okro-. See words beginning
    ochro-.
oksalosis. See *oxalosis.*
okseuriasis. See *oxyuriasis.*
oligemia
oligochromemia
oligocythemia
oligophrenia
    phenylpyruvic o.
oligoplasmia
oligoptyalism
oligotrophia
oliguria
Ollier's disease
onchocerciasis
oncogenesis
oncogenic
oncology
onyalai
onychomycosis
oophoritis
    o. parotidea
ophthalmia
ophthalmoplegia
opisthorchiasis
opisthotonos
Opitz's disease
orchitis
    o. parotidea

orchitis (*continued*)
    o. variolosa
orf
ornithosis
Oroya fever
orthopnea
Osler's
    disease
    nodes
    sign
    syndrome
Osler-Vaquez disease
osteitis
    o. fibrosa cystica
osteoarthritis
osteolysis
osteoma
osteomalacia
osteomyelitis
osteopetrosis
osteoporosis
osteosarcoma
osteosarcomatous
osteosclerosis
ovaries
ovary
overhydration
oxalosos
oxytocin
oxyuriasis
pachydermoperiostosis
pachymeningitis
Paget's disease
pake-. See words beginning
    pachy-.
palpitation
palsy
    Bell's p.
Paltauf's nanism
pancreas
    Aseli's p.
    p. divisum

pancreas (*continued*)
    Willis' p.
    Winslow's p.
pancreatalgia
pancreatemphraxis
pancreathelcosis
pancreatitis
pancytopenia
panencephalitis
panhypopituitarism
panneuritis
    p. epidemica
panniculus
pansitopenea. See
    pancytopenia.
pantatrophia
pantatrophy
papilla
papillary
papilledema
papillitis
papilloadenocystoma
papillocarcinoma
papilloma
papillomatosis
papillomatous
papillosarcoma
Pap smear
Papanicolaou smear
papular
papule
papuloerythematous
papulosquamous
paracentesis
paracoccidioidomycosis
paragonimiasis
paragranuloma
parahemophilia
parakeratosis
paralysis
parascarlatina
parasite

parasitemia
parasitic
parathormone
parathyroid
parathyroidoma
parathyroprival
parathyroprivia
parathyrotoxicosis
paresis
paresthesia
Parkinson's
    disease
    facies
    syndrome
parkinsonian
parkinsonism
    postencephalitis p.
paroksizm. See *paroxysm.*
paroksizmal. See
    paroxysmal.
parotid
parotidoscirrhus
parotidosclerosis
parotitis
    p. phlegmonosa
paroxysm
paroxysmal
Parrot's
    disease
    node
    ulcer
Parry's disease
Parsons' disease
pasteurellosis
pathoglycemia
Paterson-Brown-Kelly
    syndrome
Paul's treatment
Pautrier's abscess
Pavy's disease
PBI — protein-bound iodine
peadra. See *piedra.*

pectenosis
pectoralgia
pediculosis
pedunculated
Pel-Ebstein pyrexia
Pelger-Huët anomaly
pellagra
pelohemia
pemfigoid. See *pemphigoid.*
pemfigus. See *pemphigus.*
pemphigoid
pemphigus
    p. erythematosus
    p. foliaceus
    p. neonatorum
    p. vegetans
    p. vulgaris
penicilliosis
pentastomiasis
pentatrichomoniasis
pentosemia
pentosuria
periarteritis
    p. nodosa
pericarditis
peritoneoscopy
peritonitis
perityphlitis
perlingual
pertussis
pestilence
pestis
    p. ambulans
    p. bubonica
    p. siderans
petechia
petechiasis
Pfeiffer's disease
Pfuhl's sign
phagocytosis
pharmacology
pharmacokinetics

pharyngitis
phenetidinuria
phenolemia
phenoluria
phenomenon
    Raynaud's p.
    Rumpel-Leede p.
phenylketonuria
pheochromoblastoma
pheochromocytoma
phlebitis
phleboclysis
phlebothrombosis
phosphate
photophobia
photoscan
phototherapy
phycomycosis
pian
    p. bois
piarhemia
pica
Pick's disease
pickwickian syndrome
piedra
pineal
pinocytosis
Pirogoff's edema
pituitarism
pituitary
pituitrism
pityriasis
placebo
plague
plasmapheresis
Plaut's angina
pleocytosis
pleomastia
pleomorphic
pleura
pleuralgia
pleurisy

pleurocholecystitis
pleurodynia
plombage
Plummer's disease
Plummer-Vinson syndrome
PND — paroxysmal nocturnal
    dyspnea
pneumococcemia
pneumococcosis
pneumococcus
pneumoconiosis
pneumonia
    pneumococcal p.
pneumonitis
pneumothorax
podagra
podalgia
poikilocytosis
poikiloderma
poikilodermatomyositis
poisoning
    mushroom p.
polioencephalitis
poliomyelencephalitis
poliomyelitis
    bulbar p.
poliothrix
poliovirus
pollinosis
polyadenitis
polyadenosis
polyarteritis
polyarthritis
polychondritis
polycythemia
    myelopathic p.
    splenomegalic p.
    p. vera
polycytosis
polydipsia
polydysplasia
polyemia

polymyositis
polyneuritis
polyneuropathy
    erythredema p.
polyp
polyphagia
polypoid
polyposis
    p. coli syndrome
polypus
polyradiculitis
polyradiculoneuritis
polyrrhea
polysarcia
polyserositis
polyuria
POMP — prednisone, Oncovin,
        methotrexate,
        6-mercaptopurine
Pompe's disease
Poncet's
    disease
    rheumatism
porphyria
Pott's disease
Prader-Willi syndrome
preeclampsia
PRL — prolactin
proctalgia
    p. fugax
proctencleisis
proctitis
    epidemic gangrenous p.
proctodynia
proctorrhagia
proctorrhea
proctoscopy
proctosigmoidoscopy
progeria
progesterone
progestin
prolactin

protein
proteinemia
proteinosis
proteinuria
    orthostatic p.
proteolysis
prothrombin
prothrombinopenia
protocol
protocoproporphyria
protoporphyria
prurigo
pruritus
psammocarcinoma
psammoma
psammosarcoma
pseudoacanthosis
    p. nigricans
pseudoaldosteronism
pseudohemophilia
    p. hepatica
pseudohermaphrodism
pseudohyperkalemia
pseudohyponatremia
pseudohypoparathyroidism
pseudoleukemia
    p. lymphatica
pseudoproteinuria
pseudo-pseudohypopara-
    thyroidism
pseudoxanthoma
    p. elasticum
psilosis
psittacosis
psoriasis
PTH — parathormone
        parathyroid hormone
ptosis
pulpa
    p. lienis
PUO — pyrexia of unknown
        origin

purine
purpura
    p. cachectica
    p. hemorrhagica
    idiopathic p.
    Landouzy's p.
    orthostatic p.
    p. rheumatica
    Schönlein-Henoch p.
    thrombocytopenic p.
    p. variolosa
pyarthrosis
pyelitis
pylonephritis
pyelonephrosis
pyemia
    cryptogenic p.
pyrexia
    Pel-Ebstein p.
pyrimidine
pyrogenic
pyroglobulinemia
pyruvemia
pyuria
Q fever
quarantine
rabdomioma. See
    rhabdomyoma.
rabdomyosarcoma. See
    rhabdomyosarcoma.
rabies
rachitis
radiation
    ionizing r.
    non-ionizing r.
radioactivity
radiocurable
radioimmunoassay
radioiodine
radioisotope
radioneuritis
radioresistant

radiosensitive
radiotherapy
RAI — radioactive iodine
RAIU — radioactive iodine
    uptake
rakitis. See *rachitis.*
ranula
    pancreatic r.
RAtx — radiation therapy
Raynaud's
    disease
    gangrene
    phenomenon
receptor
    estrogen r.
recrudescence
Refsum's disease
regimen
regurgitation
    aortic r.
Reifenstein's syndrome
Reiter's
    disease
    syndrome
remission
Rénon-Delille syndrome
replication
resection
    block r.
respiration
    Cheyne-Stokes r.
resuscitation
reticulocytosis
reticuloendothelioma
reticuloendotheliosis
    leukemic r.
reticulosarcoma
reticulum
    endoplasmic r.
retinitis
retinoblastoma
Reye's syndrome

rhabdomyoma
rhabdomyosarcoma
rheumapyra
rheumarthritis
rheumatalgia
rheumatic
rheumatism
      Heberden's r.
      MacLeod's capsular r.
      Poncet's r.
rheumatoid
      r. arthritis
rhinitis
rhinophyma
rhinorrhea
rhinosporidiosis
rhonchi
RIA − radioimmunoassay
ribonucleic acid
ribose
ribosome
rickets
rickettsial
rickettsialpox
rickettsiosis
Riedel's
      disease
      struma
Rieder cell leukemia
Rift Valley fever
ring
      Kayser-Fleischer r.
rinitis. See rhinitis.
rino-. See words beginning rhino-.
RNA − ribonucleic acid
RNA-dependent DNA polymerase
RNA reverse transcriptase
RNA virus
Rocky Mountain spotted fever
Rokitansky's disease

Romaña's sign
Romberg-Paessler syndrome
Romberg's sign
rongki. See rhonchi.
rooma-. See words beginning rheuma-.
Rosenbach's syndrome
roseola
roseolus
Rotor's syndrome
roundworm
rubella
      r. scarlatinosa
rubeola
      r. scarlatinosa
rubor
rubra
Rumpel-Leede phenomenon
Runeberg's
      disease
      type
rupia
Russian spring-summer encephalitis
S period
St. Louis encephalitis
salmonellosis
samokarsinoma. See psammocarcinoma.
samoma. See psammoma.
samosarkoma. See psammosarcoma.
Sanfilippo's syndrome
San Joaquin fever
San Joaquin Valley disease
sarcocarcinoma
sarcoid
      s. of Boeck
      Darier-Roussy s.
      Schaumann's s.
      Spiegler-Fendt s.
sarcoidosis

sarcoma
    meningeal s.
    osteogenic s.
    reticulum cell s.
sarcomphalocele
sarcosepsis
sarcosis
SBE — subacute bacterial
    endocarditis
scabies
scalenus anticus syndrome
scan
    brain s.
    CT (computed tomog-
      raphy) s.
    thyroid s.
scarlatina
Schaumann's
    disease
    sarcoid
    syndrome
Scheie's syndrome
Schilling's leukemia
schistosomiasis
    cutaneous s.
    hepatic s.
Schmidt's syndrome
Schönlein-Henoch purpura
Schultz's angina
schwannoma
scirrhoma
scirrhous
scleredema
sclerodactylia
    s. annularis ainhumoides
scleroderma
scleromalacia
sclerosis
    amyotrophic lateral s.
    multiple s.
scoleciasis
scopulariopsosis

scotodinia
scotoma
scrofula
scrofuloderma
scurvy
sefalaljeah. See *cephalalgia.*
seizure
self-replication
sella turcica
seminoma
Senear-Usher syndrome
senile
    s. dementia
sepsis
    s. lenta
    puerperal s.
septicemia
septicophlebitis
septicopyemia
Sergent's white line
serous
sessile
Sézary's syndrome
sferositosis. See *spherocytosis.*
shangker. See *chancre.*
shangkroid. See *chancroid.*
Sheehan's disease
shigellosis
shingles
shock
    insulin s.
sialadenitis
sialoadenitis
sialoangiitis
sialorrhea
    s. pancreatica
sickle cell anemia
sign
    Babinski's s.
    Chvostek-Weiss s.
    Erb's s.
    Graefe's s.

sign (*continued*)
    Homans' s.
    Marie's s.
    Möbius' s.
    Nikolsky's s.
    Osler's s.
    Pfuhl's s.
    Romaña's s.
    Romberg's s.
    Stellwag's s.
    Troisier's s.
    Trousseau's s.
    Unschuld's s.
silicatosis
silicosis
silicotuberculosis
silosis. See *psilosis.*
Simmonds' disease
singultus
sinusitis
sirrosis. See *cirrhosis.*
sitakosis. See *psittacosis.*
Sjögren's syndrome
skistosomiasis. See
    schistosomiasis.
SLE — systemic lupus
    erythematosus
smallpox
smear
    Papanicolaou (Pap) s.
Smith-Strang disease
somatotropin
sootsoogamooshe. See
    tsutsugamushi.
soriasis. See *psoriasis.*
South African tick typhus
South American hemorrhagic
    fever
Southeast Asian mosquito-
    borne hemorrhagic fever
spherocytosis

Spiegler-Fendt sarcoid
spina bifida
spirochetosis
spleen
    accessory s.
    Gandy-Gamna s.
    lardaceous s.
splenadenoma
splenalgia
splenatrophy
splenauxe
splenculus
splenectasis
splenectomy
splenectopia
splenelcosis
splenemia
splenemphraxis
spleneolus
splenepatitis
splenetic
splenic
splenicterus
splenitis
    spodogenous s.
splenocele
splenocleisis
splenocolic
splenocyte
splenodynia
splenogenous
splenogram
splenogranulomatosis
    s. siderotica
splenography
splenohepatomegaly
splenokeratosis
splenolymphatic
splenolysin
splenolysis
splenoma

splenomalacia
splenomedullary
splenomegaly
 Gaucher's s.
 hemolytic s.
 hypercholesterolemic s.
 myelophthisic s.
 Niemann's s.
 siderotic s.
 spodogenous s.
splenometry
splenomyelogenous
splenomyelomalacia
splenoncus
splenonephric
splenonephroptosis
splenopancreatic
splenoparectasis
splenopathy
splenopexy
splenophrenic
splenoptosis
splenorrhagia
splenosis
splenotoxin
splenotyphoid
splenulus
spondylitis
 von Bechterew-
  Strümpell s.
spondylosis
sporotrichosis
spot
 café au lait s's
 De Morgan's s's
 Janeway's s's
squamous
st — stage (of disease)
stage
 Tanner s.
staging
staphylococcus

status
 s. asthmaticus
 s. choleraicus
 s. degenerativus
 s. epilepticus
 s. lymphaticus
 s. parathyreoprivus
 s. praesens
 s. thymicolymphaticus
steatorrhea
Stein-Leventhal syndrome
Stellwag's sign
stenosis
 aortic s.
 mitral s.
sterility
Sternberg's disease
sternutatio
 s. convulsiva
steroid
Stevens-Johnson syndrome
stomatitis
stomatocytosis
Strachan-Scott syndrome
streptococcus
stridor
strongyloidiasis
struma
 s. basedowificata
 Hashimoto's s.
 s. lymphomatosa
 Riedel's s.
Strümpell-Leichtenstern
 encephalitis
Stuart-Bras disease
stuporous
sucrosemia
Sudeck's atrophy
sudo-. See words beginning
 pseudo-.
sulfhemoglobinemia
sunstroke

Sutton-Rendu-Osler-Weber
    syndrome
Symmers' disease
sympathomimetic
syncope
    carotid sinus s.
syndrome
    Abderhalden-Fanconi s.
    Abercrombie's s.
    Achard-Thiers s.
    Adams-Stokes s.
    addisonian s.
    adrenogenital s.
    Ahumada-Del Castillo s.
    Albers-Schönberg's s.
    Albright's s.
    Aldrich's s.
    aortic arch s.
    Arakawa-Higashi s.
    argentaffinoma s.
    Arias' s.
    Ascher's s.
    Ayerza's s.
    Baber's s.
    Banti's s.
    Bard-Pic s.
    Bar's s.
    Bartter's s.
    basal cell nevus s.
    Bassen-Kornzweig s.
    Bearn-Kunkel s.
    Bernard's s.
    Bernard-Sergent s.
    Bloom's s.
    Blum's s.
    Bouillaud's s.
    Brunsting's s.
    Budd-Chiari s.
    Caplan's s.
    carcinoid s.
    carpal tunnel s.
    cervical rib s.

syndrome (*continued*)
    Chédiak-Higashi s.
    Chiari-Frommel s.
    Chinese restaurant s.
    Conn's s.
    Cruveilhier-Baumgarten s.
    Cushing's s.
    defibrination s.
    Degos' s.
    DiGuglielmo's s.
    Dresbach's s.
    dysglandular s.
    ectopic ACTH s.
    Ehlers-Danlos s.
    Faber's s.
    Fanconi's s.
    Felty's s.
    Fitz-Hugh-Curtis s.
    Fitz's s.
    Forbes-Albright s.
    Friedmann's vasomotor s.
    Gaisböck's s.
    Gardner's s.
    Glanzmann's s.
    Goodpasture's s.
    Gopalan's s.
    Guillain-Barré s.
    Günther's s.
    Hamman-Rich s.
    Harris' s.
    Hayem-Widal s.
    Heerfordt's s.
    Heidenhaim's s.
    hemopleuropneumonic s.
    hepatorenal s.
    Hines-Bannick s.
    Horton's s.
    Hunter's s.
    Hurler's s.
    hydralizine lupus s.
    hyperventilation s.
    hyperviscosity s.

syndrome (*continued*)
  Job's s.
  Kallmann's s.
  Kartagener's s.
  Kimmelstiel-Wilson s.
  Kleine-Levin s.
  Klinefelter's s.
  Kocher's s.
  König's s.
  Laurence-Moon-Biedl s.
  Läwen-Roth s.
  Leriche's s.
  Lesch-Nyhan s.
  Lignac-Fanconi s.
  Löffler's s.
  Luft's s.
  lymphoproliferative s.
  malabsorption s.
  Marchiafava-Micheli s.
  Marfan's s.
  Marie's s.
  Maroteaux-Lamy s.
  Meniere's s.
  Mikulicz's s.
  Minkowski-Chauffard s.
  Morquio's s.
  Münchausen's s.
  neurocutaneous s.
  nevoid basalioma s.
  Noonan's s.
  Osler's s.
  pancreaticohepatic s.
  parkinsonian s.
  Parkinson's s.
  Paterson-Brown-Kelly s.
  pickwickian s.
  Plummer-Vinson s.
  polyglandular s.
  polyposis coli s.
  Prader-Willi s.
  Reifenstein's s.
  Reiter's s.

syndrome (*continued*)
  Rénon-Delille s.
  Reye's s.
  Romberg-Paessler s.
  Rosenbach's s.
  Rotor's s.
  rubella s.
  Sanfilippo's s.
  scalenus anticus s.
  Schaumann's s.
  Scheie's s.
  Schmidt's s.
  Senear-Usher s.
  Sézary's s.
  Sjögren's s.
  Stein-Leventhal s.
  Stevens-Johnson s.
  Strachan-Scott s.
  Sutton-Rendu-Osler-
    Weber s.
  Takayasu's s.
  Tietze's s.
  toxic shock s.
  Troisier-Hanot-
    Chauffard s.
  Troisier's s.
  Turner's s.
  Wallenberg's s.
  Waterhouse-Friderichsen
    s.
  Weil's s.
  Werner's s.
  Willebrand's s.
  Wiskott-Aldrich s.
synovioma
synthesis
  DNA s.
  protein s.
syphilis
system
  TNM staging s.
T_3 – triiodothyronine

T_4 — thyroxine
tabes
    diabetic t.
    t. dorsalis
tachycardia
Takayasu's syndrome
Tangier disease
Tanner stage
Tc — technetium
telalgia
telangiectasia
telangiectasis
template
tenesmus
tenosynovitis
teratoma
test
    alpha-fetoprotein t.
    beta-HCG t.
    CEA (carcinoembryonic
      antigen) t.
    estrogen receptor assay t.
    Hanger-Rose skin t.
    Hickey-Hare t.
testes
testosterone
tetanus
tetany
    hyperventilation t.
    parathyroid t.
    parathyroprival t.
    rheumatic t.
    thyroprival t.
tetralogy
    t. of Fallot
thalassemia
thrombasthenia
thromboangiitis
    t. obliterans
thromboarteriosclerosis
    t. obliterans
thrombocytasthenia

thrombocythemia
thrombocytopenia
thrombocytopenic purpura
thrombocytosis
thrombopenia
thrombophlebitis
thrombosis
thrush
thymine
thymoma
thymus
thyrocalcitonin
thyroid
thyroid-stimulating hormone
thyroidism
thyroiditis
    ligneous t.
thyromegaly
thyrophyma
thyroprival
thyrotoxicosis
thyroxine
tic
    t. douloureux (doo-loo-
      roo)
Tietze's syndrome
time
    generation t.
tinnitus
TNM — tumor, nodes,
      metastases
TNM staging system
Todd's cirrhosis
tomography
tonsillitis
tophus
    t. syphiliticus
torticollis
torulosis
tosis. See *ptosis.*
toxemia
toxic

toxicity
toxicology
toxicosis
toxocariasis
toxoplasmosis
tracheitis
trachelagra
trachoma
transplantation
    allogeneic marrow t.
treatment
    Paul's t.
    Yeo's t.
trematodiasis
treponematosis
treponemiasis
triad
    Falta's t.
    Hutchinson's t.
    Merseburg t.
trichinosis
trichocephaliasis
trichoglossia
trichomoniasis
trichophytosis
trichostrongylosis
trichuriasis
triiodothyronine
trikinosis. See trichinosis.
triko-. See words beginning
    tricho-.
trikuriasis. See trichuriasis.
trismus
trisomy 13, 18, 21, 22
tRNA — transfer RNA
trofedema. See trophedema.
Troisier-Hanot-Chauffard
    syndrome
Troisier's
    ganglion
    sign
    syndrome

trophedema
Trousseau's sign
TSH — thyroid-stimulating
    hormone
trypanosomiasis
tsutsugamushi disease
tubercle
    Farre's t's
tuberculin
tuberculosis
tularemia
tumor
    Abrikossoff's t.
    Burkitt's t.
    fungating t.
    islet cell t.
    mixed-tissue t's
    mucinous t.
    nonresponsive t.
    radiocurable t.
    radioresistant t.
    radiosensitive t.
    responsive t.
    serous t.
    solid t.
    Wilms' t.
Turner's syndrome
type
    Runeberg's t.
typhoid
typhoidette
typhus
    Indian tick t.
    South African tick t.
ulcer
    Parrot's u.
ulcerating
ulceration
ultrasonography
uncinariasis
undifferentiated
Undritz' anomaly

undulant fever
Unschuld's sign
unsinariasis. See *uncinariasis.*
unukizm. See *eunuchism.*
uptake
    radioactive iodine u.
uracil
uremia
uremic
urethritis
URI – upper respiratory
      infection
uricosuria
urobilinemia
urobilinuria
urolithiasis
urticaria
uthanazea. See *euthanasia.*
uthiroid. See *euthyroid.*
uthiroidism. See *euthyroidism.*
vaccination
    smallpox v.
vaccine
valine
varicella
variola
varix
vasopressin
Venezuelan equine
   encephalomyelitis
vermiculous
verrucous
Verstraeten's bruit
vertigo
vinyl chloride
viremia
viricidal
virilism
    adrenal v.
    prosopopilary v.
virion

virology
virus
    Colorado tick fever v.
    Coxsackie v.
    DNA v.
    Epstein-Barr v.
    herpes v.
    oncogenic v.
    RNA v.
vitiligo
vitium
    v. conformationis
    v. primae formationis
von Bechterew-Strümpell
   spondylitis
von Gierke's disease
von Willebrand's disease
vookereriasis. See
   wuchereriasis.
Waldenström's
   macroglobulinemia
Wallenberg's syndrome
Waterhouse-Friderichsen
   syndrome
Wegener's granulomatosis
Weil's
    disease
    syndrome
Werner's
    disease
    syndrome
Wernicke's
    disease
    encephalopathy
West Nile
    encephalitis
    fever
western equine
   encephalomyelitis
whooping cough
Widal-Abrami disease

Willebrand's syndrome
Willis'
    disease
    pancreas
Wilms' tumor
Wilson's disease
Winslow's pancreas
Wiskott-Aldrich syndrome
wuchereriasis
xanthelasma
xanthogranuloma
xanthoma
    x. diabeticorum
xanthomatosis
xanthosis
    x. diabetica

xeroderma pigmentosum
xerophthalmia
xerosis
yaws
yellow fever
Yeo's treatment
zan.- See words beginning *xan-.*
zantho-. See words beginning *xantho-.*
zerofthalmea. See *xerophthalmia.*
zerosis. See *xerosis.*
zymolysis

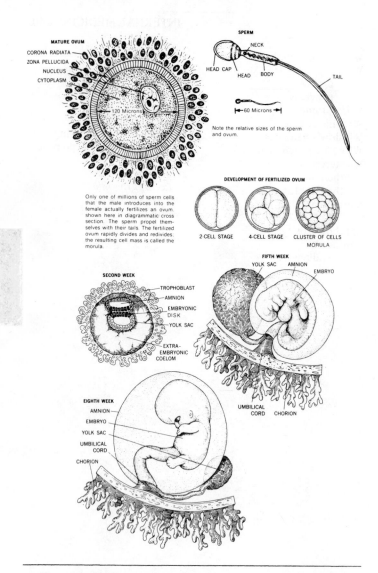

MATURE OVUM

CORONA RADIATA
ZONA PELLUCIDA
NUCLEUS
CYTOPLASM

120 Microns

SPERM

NECK
HEAD CAP
HEAD
BODY
TAIL

60 Microns

Note the relative sizes of the sperm and ovum.

Only one of millions of sperm cells that the male introduces into the female actually fertilizes an ovum. shown here in diagrammatic cross section. The sperm propel themselves with their tails. The fertilized ovum rapidly divides and redivides. the resulting cell mass is called the morula.

DEVELOPMENT OF FERTILIZED OVUM

2-CELL STAGE

4-CELL STAGE

CLUSTER OF CELLS
MORULA

SECOND WEEK

TROPHOBLAST
AMNION
EMBRYONIC DISK
YOLK SAC
EXTRA-EMBRYONIC COELOM

FIFTH WEEK

YOLK SAC
AMNION
EMBRYO

UMBILICAL CORD
CHORION

EIGHTH WEEK

AMNION
EMBRYO
YOLK SAC
UMBILICAL CORD
CHORION

(Courtesy of Miller, B. F., and Keane, C. B.: Encyclopedia and Dictionary of Medicine, Nursing and Allied Health, 2nd ed. Philadelphia, W. B. Saunders Company, 1978.)

OBSTETRICS AND GYNECOLOGY

AB — abortion
abactio
abactus venter
abdominal
abdominohysterectomy
abdominohysterotomy
Abell's operation
ablatio
    a. placentae
ABO incompatibility
abort
aborticide
abortifacient
abortion
    afebrile a.
    ampullar a.
    cervical a.
    complete a.
    contagious a.
    criminal a.
    epizootic a.
    habitual a.
    imminent a.
    incomplete a.
    inevitable a.
    infectious a.
    justifiable a.
    missed a.
    septic a.

abortion *(continued)*
    spontaneous a.
    therapeutic a.
    threatened a.
    tubal a.
    vibrio a.
abortionist
abortive
abortus
abruptio
    a. placentae
    a. placentae marginalis
abscess
Aburel's operation
acanthosis
accouchement
    a. force
accoucheur
acephalocystis racemosa
Achard-Thiers syndrome
acrocyanosis
acrohysterosalpingectomy
Adair's tenaculum
adenitis
adenoacanthoma
adenocarcinoma
adenofibroma
adenoma
    a. endometrioides ovarii

adenoma *(continued)*
    a. ovarii testiculare
    a. tubulare testiculare
      ovarii
adenomyofibroma
adenomyoma
adenomyomatosis
adenomyometritis
adenomyosis
adenomyositis
adenopathy
adhesion
   filamentous a.
adnexa
    a. uteri
adnexal
adnexectomy
adnexitis
adnexogenesis
adnexopexy
adnexorganogenic
aerocolpos
afibrinogenemia
after-birth
after-coming head
after-pains
agenitalism
Ahlfeld's sign
Ahumada-Del Castillo
   syndrome
AID — artificial insemination
      donor
aidoiitis
albuginea
    a. ovarii
albumin
Aldrich's operation
Alexander-Adams operation
Alexander's operation
algomenorrhea
Allen-Masters syndrome

All-Flex diaphragm
Allis'
    clamp
    forceps
alopecia
   postpartum a.
amenia
amenorrhea
   absolute a.
   dysponderal a.
   hypothalamic a.
   lactation a.
   ovarian a.
   physiologic a.
   pituitary a.
   premenopausal a.
   primary a.
   relative a.
   secondary a.
amenorrheal
ametria
amniocentesis
amniochorial
amniogenesis
amniogram
amniography
amnioma
amnion
amnionic
amnionitis
amniorrhea
amniorrhexis
amniotic
   a. fluid
amniotin
amniotome
   Baylor's a.
   Beacham's a.
amniotomy
ampule
ampulla

anastomosis
      ureterotubal a.
android
anesthesia. See *General
      Surgical Terms.*
angle
      costovertebral a.
anisocytosis
ankylocolpos
anovaginal
anovaria
anovarism
anovular
anovulation
anovulatory
anovulia
anovulomenorrhea
anoxia
      a. neonatorum
anteflexed
anteflexio
      a. uteri
anteflexion
antenatal
antepartal
antepartum
anteversion
anteverted
anthropoid
antihypertensive
A & P repair — anterior and
                  posterior
                  repair
Apgar
      rating
      score
aplasia
apoplexia
      a. uteri
apoplexy
      uterine a.
      uteroplacental a.

applicator
      Ernst's a.
      Fletcher's loading a.
arcuate
areno-. See words beginning
      arrheno-.
areola
areolar
Arey's rule
Arias-Stella's phenomenon
Arnoux's sign
arrhenoblastoma
arrhenogenic
arrhenoma
arrhenomimetic
artery
      hypogastric a.
      iliac a.
      ilioinguinal a.
      ovarian a.
      pudendal a.
      umbilical a.
      uterine a.
ascensus
      a. uteri
Aschheim-Zondek test
ascites
Asherman's syndrome
aspiration
      vacuum a.
aspirator
      blue tip a.
      red tip a.
      vacuum a.
      yellow tip a.
assimilation
asynclitism
Atlee's dilator
atony
      uterine a.
atopomenorrhea
atresia

atrium
    a. vaginae
atrophy
atypical
Auerbach's plexus
augmentation
ausculatory
Auvard-Remine speculum
Auvard's
    cranioclast
    weighted speculum
avascular
axillary
Ayerst's knife
AZ test – Aschheim-Zondek
        test
Babcock's clamp
Backhaus towel clamp
Baer's vesicle
bag
    Champetier de Ribes b.
    Voorhees' b.
Bailey-Williamson forceps
balanic
Baldwin's operation
Baldy's operation
Baldy-Webster operation
Balfour's retractor
Ballantine's clamp
ballotable
ballottement
Ball's operation
Bandl's ring
Bard-Parker blade
Barkow
    colliculus of B.
barren
Barrett-Allen forceps
Barrett's
    forceps
    tenaculum
bartholinitis

Bartholin's
    cyst
    gland
Barton's
    forceps
    traction handle
Basedow's disease
basiotripsy (fetal)
Basset's operation
Baudelocque's operation
Baylor's amniotome
Beacham's amniotome
Beatson's operation
Beccaria's sign
Beck. See *Boeck.*
Beclard's sign
Bellow's pack
Bel-O-Pak
Benaron's forceps
benign
Berlind-Auvard speculum
Berry's forceps
Beuttner's method
bicornuate
bifid
bilirubin
Billroth's forceps
Bill's traction handle
bimanual
Biocept-G test
biopsies
biopsy
    bite b.
    cervical b.
    cold knife conization b.
    cone b.
    endometrial b.
    excisional b.
    four point b.
    multiple b.
    needle b.
    punch b.

biopsy *(continued)*
 sponge b.
 wedge b.
Birnberg's bow
Bischoff's operation
Bissell's operation
bivalve
Black-Wylie dilator
bladder
 b. blade
 dome of b.
 b. flap
blade
 Bard-Parker b.
 bistoury b.
 bladder b.
blennorrhea
block
 paracervical b.
 pudendal b.
blood
 cord b.
Blot's perforator
Boeck's sarcoidosis
boggy
Bolt's sign
Bond's forceps
Bonnaire's method
Bonney's hysterectomy
bosselated
Bouilly's operation
Bovie unit
bow
 Birnberg's b.
Bowen's disease
box
 Stockholm b.
Bozeman's
 forceps
 operation
Braasch's forceps
Bracht's maneuver

Brandt-Andrews maneuver
Brandt's
 brassiere
 technique
 treatment
Brantley-Turner retractor
brassiere
 Brandt's b.
Braune's canal
Braun-Fernwald sign
Braun-Jardine-DeLee hook
Braun's
 cranioclast
 hook
 scissors
 tenaculum
Braxton-Hicks
 contraction
 sign
 version
breech. See also presentation.
 b. delivery
 b. extraction
 b. presentation
Breisky's
 disease
 pelvimeter
Brenner's tumor
Brentano's syndrome
Breu's mole
Brewer's speculum
Bricker's operation
Broder's classification
Brouha's test
bruit
Brunschwig's operation
brwe. See *bruit.*
Buie clamp
bulbus
 b. vestibuli vaginae
Bumm's curet
Burch's operation

BUS glands — Bartholin's,
 urethral, and Skene's
 glands
Buxton clamp
cachectic
cachexia
 c. ovariopriva
calculation
 Johnson's c.
canal
 Braune's c.
 cervical c.
 endocervical c.
 c. of Nuck
canalis
 c. cervicis uteri
cannula
 Holman-Mathieu c.
 Hudgins' c.
 Jarcho's c.
 Kahn's c.
 Neal's c.
 Rubin's c.
caput
 c. medusae
 c. succedaneum
carcinoma
 comedo c.
 cylindromatous c.
 ductal c.
 embryonal c.
 epidermoid c.
 granulosa cell c.
 gyriform c.
 infiltrating c.
 c. in situ
 intraepithelial c.
 invasive c.
 macrofolliculoid c.
 microfolliculoid c.
 parenchymatous c.
 squamous cell c.

carcinomatosis
carcinophilic
carcinosarcoma
carina
 c. fornicis
 c. urethralis vaginae
caruncle
 hymenal c's
 urethral c.
carunculae hymenales
catamenia
catamenial
catamenogenic
catheter
 Foley c.
 French c.
 Fritsch's c.
 indwelling c.
 Wurd's c.
cauterization
cauterized
cautery
 Percy's c.
cavity
 endometrial c.
cavum
 c. uteri
CDC — calculated date of
 confinement
celiocolpotomy
celiohysterectomy
celiohysterotomy
celiosalpingectomy
celiosalpingotomy
celiotomy
 vaginal c.
cell
 atypical c.
 bank c.
 basket c.
 ciliated c.
 clue c.

cell *(continued)*
    cornified c.
    decidual c.
    endocervical c.
    endometrial c.
    epithelial c.
    epithelioid c.
    hilar c.
    intercalary c.
    keratinized c.
    Langhan's c.
    luteum c.
    mesothelial c.
    navicular c.
    Paget's c.
    parabasal c.
    precornified c.
    superficial c.
    syncytial c.
    "tadpole" c.
    target c.
    tart c.
    theca lutein c.
    Walthard's c.
cephalad
cephalic
cephalometry
cephalopelvic disproportion
cerclage
cervical
    c. biopsy
    c. canal
    c. conization
    c. fascia
    c. os
cervicectomy
cervicitis
    granulomatous c.
    traumatic c.
cervicocolpitis
    c. emphysematosa
cervicovaginal

cervicovaginitis
cervicovesical
cervimeter
cervitome
    Milex c.
cervix
    conglutination of c.
    incompetent c.
    c. uteri
cesarean. See under *section.*
CGT − chorionic gonadotropin
Chadwick's sign
Chamberlen's forceps
Champetier de Ribes bag
chancroid
Chiari-Frommel syndrome
chloasma
    c. gravidarum
    c. uterinum
chlorosis
    c. vulvae
chondromalacia
    c. fetalis
chorioadenoma
    c. destruens
chorioamnionitis
choriocarcinoma
chorioepithelioma
chorion
    c. frondosum
chorionic
    c. gonadotropin
    c. villi
chorioplacental
chromohydrotubation
cicatrix
circumcision
circumoral
clamp
    Allis' c.
    Babcock's c.
    Backhaus towel c.

clamp *(continued)*
    Ballantine's c.
    Buie c.
    Buxton c.
    Heaney's c.
    Kane's c.
    Kelly's c.
    Kocher's c.
    Lahey's c.
    Ochsner's c.
    Pennington's c.
    Reich's c.
    Willett's c.
    Yellan c.
classification
    Broder's c.
Claudius' fossa
cleidotomy (fetal)
cleidotripsy
climacteric
climacterium
    c. praecox
clip
    Hulka's c.
clitoral
clitoridauxe
clitoridean
clitoridectomy
clitoriditis
clitoridotomy
clitoris
    bifid c.
    crura of c.
    prepuce of c.
clitorism
clitoritis
clitoromania
clitorotomy
cloaca
Cloquet's node
closure
    Latzko's c.

Coffey's operation
coil
    Margulles' c.
coitophobia
coitus
    c. á la vache
    c. incompletus
    c. interruptus
    c. reservatus
coleocele
coleocystitis
coleoptosis
coleospastia
coleotomy
colliculus
    c. of Barkow
    cervical c. of female
      urethra
Collin's
    forceps
    pelvimeter
    speculum
Collyer's pelvimeter
colostrum
    c. gravidarum
    c. puerperarum
colovaginal
colpalgia
colpatresia
colpectasia
colpectasis
colpectomy
colpeurysis
colpismus
colpitic
colpitis
    c. emphysematosa
    emphysematous c.
    c. granulosa
    c. mycotica
colpocele
colpoceliocentesis

colpoceliotomy
colpocleisis
colpocystitis
colpocystocele
colpocystoplasty
colpocystotomy
colpocystoureterocystotomy
colpocytogram
colpocytology
colpodynia
colpoepisiorrhaphy
colpohyperplasia
colpohysterectomy
colpohysteropexy
colpohysterorrhaphy
colpohysterotomy
colpolaparotomy
colpomicroscope
colpomicroscopic
colpomicroscopy
colpomycosis
colpomyomectomy
colpoperineoplasty
colpoperineorrhaphy
colpopexy
colpoplasty
colpopoiesis
colpopolypus
colpoptosis
colporectopexy
colporrhagia
colporrhaphy
colporrhexis
colposcope
colposcopy
colpospasm
colpostat
colpostenosis
colpostenotomy
colpotherm
colpotomy
colpoureterocystotomy

colpoureterotomy
colpoxerosis
comedocarcinoma
commissura
    c. labiorum anterior
    c. labiorum posterior
    c. labiorum pudendi
commissure
    anterior c. of labia
    posterior c. of labia
compatible
conception
conceptus
conduplicato
    c. corpore
condyloma
    c. acuminatum
    c. latum
    c. subcutaneum
condylomatoid
condylomatosis
condylomatous
condylotomy
configuration
    arcuate c.
confinement
conglutinatio
    c. orificii externi
conglutination
conization
    cold knife c.
conjugata
    c. vera obstetrica
conjugate
    diagonal c.
    obstetric c.
contraception
contraceptive
contraction
    Braxton-Hicks c.
    premonitory c's
Coombs' test

copious
copulation
cord
>medullary c's
>ovigerous c's
>umbilical c.

cord blood
Corey's forceps
Corner-Allen test
cornu
cornua
cornual
corpora atretica
corpus
>c. albicans
>c. cavernosum clitoridis
>c. clitoridis
>c. glandulosum
>c. hemorrhagicum
>c. luteum
>c. spongiosum urethrae
>muliebris
>c. uteri
>uterine c.

cortex
costovertebral
cotyledon
Couvelaire uterus
CPD — cephalopelvic dispro-
>portion
cranioclasis (fetal)
cranioclast
>Auvard's c.
>Braun's c.
>Zweifel-DeLee c.

craniotome
craniotomy (fetal)
Credé's method
cretin
cribriform
crista
>c. urethralis femininae

crista (continued)
>c. urethralis muliebris

crura
crus
>c. clitoridis
>c. of clitoris
>c. glandis clitoridis

cryostat
cryosurgery
cryotherapy
cryptomenorrhea
crystalline
CS — cesarean section
C-section — cesarean section
cul-de-sac
>Douglas' c.d.s.

culdocentesis
culdoscope
>Decker's c.

culdoscopy
Cullen's sign
cumulus
>c. oophorus
>ovarian c.
>c. ovaricus

cuneihysterectomy
curet
>banjo c.
>Bumm's c.
>Greene's c.
>Gusberg's c.
>Hannon's c.
>Heaney's c.
>Holden's c.
>Holtz's c.
>Hunter's c.
>Kelly-Gray c.
>Kelly's c.
>Kevorkian's c.
>Kushner-Tandatnick c.
>Lounsbury's c.
>Novak's c.

curet *(continued)*
  Randall's c.
  Récamier's c.
  Reich-Nechtow c.
  serrated c.
  Sims' c.
  Skene's c.
  Thomas' c.
curettage
  fractional c.
  suction c.
curette. See *curet*.
curettement
Curtius' syndrome
Cusco's speculum
CVA — costovertebral angle
CWP — childbirth without pain
cyanotic
cycle
  aberrant c.
  anovulatory c.
  endometrial c.
  genesial c.
  gonadotropic c.
  menstrual c.
  myometrial c.
  oogenetic c.
  ovarian c.
  reproductive c.
  sexual c.
cyclic
cyema
cyesedema
cyesiognosis
cyesiology
cyesis
cyestein
cyogenic
cyonin
cyophoria
cyophoric
cyotrophy

cyst
  atheromatous c.
  Bartholin's c.
  blue dome c.
  chocolate c.
  chorionic c.
  corpus luteum c.
  dermoid c.
  embryonal c.
  endometrial c.
  epoophoron c.
  follicular c.
  gartnerian c.
  granulosa lutein c.
  hemorrhagic c.
  hymenal c.
  inclusion c.
  inflammatory c.
  lutein c.
  c. of Morgagni
  morgagnian c.
  nabothian c.
  Naboth's c's
  oophoritic c.
  ovarian c.
  paroophoritic c.
  parovarian c.
  pedicled c.
  polycystic c.
  retention c.
  Sampson's c.
  sebaceous c.
  theca-lutein c.
  tubo-ovarian c.
  vaginal inclusion c.
  wolffian c.
cystadenocarcinoma
cystadenoma
  mucinous c.
  pseudomucinous c.
  serous c.
cystic mastitis

cystocele
cystoelytroplasty
cystolutein
cystoma
    myxoid c.
    c. serosum simplex
cystomatitis
cystomatous
cystometrogram
cystosarcoma
    c. phylloides
cystourethrocele
cytogenic
Dacron shield
Dalkon shield
Danforth's
    method
    sign
David's disease
Davis' operation
D & C – dilatation and
          curettage
    diagnostic D & C
    suction D & C
De Alvarez's forceps
Deaver's retractor
decidua
    basal d.
    d. basalis
    capsular d.
    d. capsularis
    menstrual d.
    d. menstrualis
    parietal d.
    d. parietalis
    reflex d.
    d. reflexa
    d. serotina
    d. vera
decidual
decidualitis
deciduate

deciduation
deciduitis
deciduoma
deciduomatosis
decipara
Decker's
    culdoscope
    operation
defervesced
deflection
    vesicouterine d.
defundation
defundectomy
DeLee's
    forceps
    maneuver
    pelvimeter
    retractor
    tenaculum
delivery
    breech d.
    low forceps d.
    mid forceps d.
    spontaneous d.
denidation
depression
    reactive d.
dermoplast spray
DES – diethylstilbestrol
descensus
    d. uteri
    uterine d.
desensin
Desjardin's forceps
desultory
detachment
    annular d.
Deventer's
    diameter
    pelvis
Devilbiss' speculum
Devilbiss-Stacey speculum

Dewees' sign
Dewey's forceps
dextroposition
dextrorotation
dextrostix
dextroverted
diagnostic D & C
diameter
    Deventer's d.
    Löhlein's d.
diaphragm
    All-Flex d.
    Ramses' d.
diastasis
    d. recti abdominis
Diday's law
didelphia
didelphic
Dienst's test
dihysteria
dilatation
dilatation and curettage
dilated
dilation
dilation and curettage
dilator
    Atlee's d.
    Black-Wylie d.
    Goodell's d.
    Hank-Bradley d.
    Hank's d.
    Hegar's d.
    Hurtig's d.
    Jolly's d.
    Kelly's d.
    Palmer's d.
    Pratt's d.
    Reich-Nechtow d.
    Starlinger's d.
    Wylie's d.
diovulatory
diphasia

dis-. See also words beginning
    dys-.
discission
discrete
disease
    Basedow's d.
    Bowen's d.
    Breisky's d.
    David's d.
    fibrocystic d.
    Fox-Fordyce d.
    Halban's d.
    Lignac-Fanconi d.
    Maher's d.
    Niemann-Pick d.
    Paget's d.
    pelvic inflammatory d.
    Schroeder's d.
    Valsuani's d.
disproportion
    cephalopelvic d.
dissection
Doderlein's operation
Doleris' operation
Donald-Fothergill operation
Donald's operation
doptone
douche
Douglas'
    cul-de-sac
    fold
    line
    method
    pouch
douglascele
douglasitis
Dow-Corning implant
Down's syndrome
Doyen's
    operation
    retractor
    scissors

Doyen's *(continued)*
    vaginal hysterectomy
drain
        Penrose d.
drip
        pitocin d.
drugs. See *Drugs and
    Chemistry* section.
DUB — dysfunctional uterine
        bleeding
Dubovitz's syndrome
duct
        Gartner's d.
        mesonephric d.
        mullerian d.
        omphalomesenteric d.
        ovarian d.
        Reichel's cloacal d.
        Skene's d.
        vitelline d.
        wolffian d.
ductuli transversi epoophori
ductus
        d. epoophori
            longitudinalis
Dudley's
        hook
        operation
Dührssen's
        operation
        tampon
duipara
Duncan's mechanism
Duplay's
        hook
        tenaculum
D 5 & W — 5% dextrose and
            water
dye
        Indigo carmine d.
dysfunction

dysfunctional
dysgerminoma
dyskaryosis
dyskinesia
        uterine d.
dysmenorrhea
        d. intermenstrualis
        plethoric d.
        psychogenic d.
dyspareunia
dysplasia
dysponderal
dystocia
Eastman's retractor
easy-pulls
EBL — estimated blood loss
eclampsia
ectocervix
ectopic
EDC — estimated date of
            confinement
        expected date of
            confinement
Eder's forceps
effaced
effacement
electrometrogram
elephantiasis
        e. of vulva
elevator
        Soonawalla uterine e.
Elliott's
        forceps
        treatment
emansio mensium
embryo
embryoctony
embryogenesis
embryogenetic
embryogenic
embryonal

embryonate
embryonic
embryoniform
embryonism
embryonization
embryonoid
embryopathia
    e. rubeolaris
embryopathology
embryopathy
embryotocia
embryotome
embryotomy
emesis
    e. gravidarum
emmenagogic
emmenagogue
emmenia
emmenic
emmeniopathy
emmenology
Emmert-Gellhorn pessary
Emmet's
    hook
    operation
    retractor
    scissors
Emmet-Studdiford perineor-
    rhaphy
en bloc
encephalopathy
    bilirubin e.
endocervical
    e. canal
    e. mucosa
    e. polyp
endocervicitis
endocervix
endocolpitis
endometrectomy
endometria

endometrioid
endometrioma
endometriosis
    e. externa
    e. interna
    ovarian e.
    e. ovarii
    e. uterina
    e. vesicae
endometriotic
endometritis
    bacteriotoxic e.
    decidual e.
    e. dissecans
    exfoliative e.
    glandular e.
    membranous e.
    puerperal e.
    syncytial e.
endometrium
    hyperplastic e.
    secretory e.
    Swiss-cheese e.
endosalpingitis
endosalpingoma
endosalpingosis
endosalpinx
endotoxic
endouterine
engorge
engorgement
entad
ental
enterocele
enucleated
epichorion
epimenorrhagia
epimenorrhea
episioclisia
episioelytrorrhaphy
episioperineoplasty

episioperineorrhaphy
episioplasty
episiorrhaphy
episiostenosis
episiotomy
    Matsner e.
epithelial
epithelialized
epithelioid
epithelioma
    e. of Malherbe
epoophorectomy
epoophoron
    e. cyst
Ernst's applicator
eroded
erosion
erythroblastosis
    e. fetalis
    e. neonatorum
escutcheon
Estes' operation
esthiomene
estradiol
estrogen
etrohysterectomy
EUA — examination under
    anesthesia
eutocia
eversion
evert
examination
    bimanual e.
    gynecologic e.
    hanging drop e.
    postpartal e.
    speculum e.
    vaginorectal e.
exenteration
exercise
    Kegel's e.

exfetation
exometritis
exophytic
external os
extraction
    breech e.
extraperitoneal
extrauterine
extravaginal
falciform
Falk-Shukuris operation
Falk's operation
fallectomy
fallopian tube
fallostomy
fallotomy
Falope's ring
Farre's line
Farris' test
fascia
    cervical f.
    pubovesicocervical f.
    subvesical f.
fecalith
fenestrated
fenestration
Ferguson's scissors
Fergusson's speculum
ferning
Ferris' forceps
fertile
fertility
fertilization
fetal
    f. asphyxia
    f. distress
    f. heart sound
    f. heart tone
    f. hydrops
    f. monitor
    f. oophoritis

fetal position
 LFA — left fronto-anterior
 LFP — left fronto-posterior
 LFT — left fronto-transverse
 LMA — left mento-anterior
 LMP — left mento-posterior
 LMT — left mento-transverse
 LOA — left occipito-anterior
 LOP — left occipito-posterior
 LOT — left occipito-transverse
 LSA — left sacroanterior
 L. Sc. A. — left scapulo-anterior
 L. Sc. P. — left scapulo-posterior
 LSP — left sacroposterior
 LST — left sacro-transverse
 RFA — right fronto-anterior
 RFP — right fronto-posterior
 RFT — right fronto-transverse
 RMA — right mento-anterior
 RMP — right mento-posterior
 RMT — right mento-transverse
 ROA — right occipito-anterior

fetal position *(continued)*
 ROP — right occipito-posterior
 ROT — right occipito-transverse
 RSA — right sacro-anterior
 R. Sc. A. — right scapulo-anterior
 R. Sc. P. — right scapulo-posterior
 RSP — right sacro-posterior
 RST — right sacro-transverse
fetation
feticide
feticulture
fetogram
fetography
fetometry
fetoplacental
fetus
 f. acardiacus
 f. amorphus
 calcified f.
 f. compressus
 harlequin f.
 f. in fetu
 macerated f.
 mummified f.
 paper-doll f.
 papyraceous f.
 f. papyraceus
 parasitic f.
 f. sanguinolentis
 sireniform f.
Feulgen stain
FHS — fetal heart sound
FHT — fetal heart tone
fibroadenoma

fibrocystic
fibroid
fibroidectomy
fibroma
fibromyoma
fibromyomata
fibromyomectomy
filamentous
fimbria
    ovarian f.
    f. ovarica
fimbriae of uterine tube
fimbriae tubae uterinae
fimbriated
fimbriocele
fistula
    rectolabial f.
    rectovaginal f.
    ureterovaginal f.
    vaginoperineal f.
    vesicocervical f.
    vesicovaginal f.
    vulvorectal f.
Fitz-Hugh's syndrome
flebitis. See *phlebitis.*
Fleming's
    knife
    operation
Fletcher's
    loading applicator
    suit
Fletcher-Van Doren forceps
fluffs
fluid
    amniotic f.
    crystalline f.
fluor
    f. albus
Foerster's forceps
fold
    Douglas' f.
    Pawlik's f.

Foley catheter
follicle
    graafian f's
    nabothian f's
    Naboth's f's
    ovarian f.
    primordial f.
follicle-stimulating hormone
follicular
folliculoma
fontanelle
forceps
    Allis' f.
    Bailey-Williamson f.
    Barrett-Allen f.
    Barrett's f.
    Barton's f.
    Benaron's f.
    Berry's f.
    Billroth's f.
    Bond's f.
    Bozeman's f.
    Braasch's f.
    Chamberlen's f.
    Collin's f.
    Corey's f.
    De Alvarez's f.
    DeLee's f.
    Desjardin's f.
    Dewey's f.
    Eder's f.
    Elliott's f.
    Ferris' f.
    Fletcher-Van Doren f.
    Foerster's f.
    Garrigue's f.
    Gaylor's f.
    Gellhorn's f.
    Gelpi-Lowrie f.
    Glenner's f.
    Gordon's f.
    Gutglass' f.

forceps *(continued)*
Hale's f.
Hartman's f.
Hawkins' f.
Hawks-Dennen f.
Heaney-Ballantine f.
Heaney-Kanter f.
Heaney-Rezek f.
Heaney's f.
Heise's f.
Henrotin's f.
Hirst-Emmett f.
Hodge's f.
Iowa f.
Jacobs' f.
Jarcho's f.
Kelly's f.
Kennedy's f.
Kielland-Luikart f.
Kielland's f. (Kjelland's f.)
Kittner's f.
Krause's f.
Laufe-Barton-Kielland f.
Laufe-Piper f.
Laufe's f.
Levret's f.
Long Island f.
Long's f.
Luikart's f.
Luikart-Simpson f.
Maier's f.
Mann's f.
Maryan's f.
McLane's f.
McLane-Tucker f.
McLane-Tucker-Luikart f.
Mitchell-Diamond f.
mouse-tooth f.
Mundie's f.
Newman's f.

forceps *(continued)*
O'Hanlon's f.
Overstreet's f.
ovum f.
Palmer's f.
Pean's f.
Phaneuf's f.
Piper's f.
placental f.
polyp f.
Randall's stone f.
ring f.
Rochester-Carmalt f.
Rochester-Ochsner f.
Rochester-Pean f.
Russell's f.
Schroeder's f.
Schubert's f.
Schwartz's f.
Schweizer's f.
Segond's f.
Senn f.
Simpson-Luikart f.
Simpson's f.
Skene's f.
Smith's f.
Somers' f.
sponge f.
Staude-Moore f.
Staude's f.
stone f.
Tarnier's f.
Teale's f.
Thoms' f.
Thoms-Allis f.
Thoms-Gaylor f.
Tischler's f.
tissue f.
Tucker-McLean f.
Van Doren f.
vulsellum f.
Walton's f.

forceps *(continued)*
    Walton-Schubert f.
    Weisman's f.
    Wertheim-Cullen f.
    Wertheim's f.
    Willett's f.
    Wittner's f.
    Yeoman's f.
forewaters
fornices
fornix
fossa
    Claudius' f.
    navicular f.
    f. navicularis
    obturator f.
    f. of vestibule of vagina
    ovarian f.
    f. ovarica
    f. vestibuli vaginae
Fothergill's operation
fourchette
Fox-Fordyce disease
fractional
Frangenheim-Goebell-Stoeckel
    operation
frenal
French catheter
frenulum
    f. labiorum pudendi
    f. of clitoris
frenum
    f. of labia
Freund's
    law
    operation
Friedman-Lapham test
Friedman's
    retractor
    test
frigid
frigidity

Fritsch-Asherman syndrome
Fritsch's
    catheter
    operation
Frommel's operation
FSH – follicle stimulating
        hormone
FTLB – full term living birth
FTND – full term normal
         delivery
fulcrum
fulguration
fundectomy
fundus
    f. of uterus
    f. of vagina
    f. uteri
    f. vaginae
fungating
funis
Gabastou's hydraulic method
galactorrhea
Galli-Mainini test
gamete
Gariel's pessary
Garrigue's
    forceps
    speculum
Gartner's duct
gastrocolpotomy
Gauss's sign
Gaylor's forceps
GC – gonococcus
       gonorrhea
Gehrung pessary
Gellhorn's
    forceps
    pessary
Gelpi-Lowrie forceps
Gelpi's retractor
genesial
genitalia

genitourinary
Genupak tampon
gestation
gestational
gestosis
Gigli's operation
Gilliam-Doleris' operation
Gilliam's operation
Giordano's operation
gland
    Bartholin's g.
    BUS g's
    Littre's g's
    Naboth's g's
    Skene's g.
    urethral g.
    vestibular g.
glans
    g. clitoridis
    g. of clitoris
Glenner's
    forceps
    retractor
Goebel-Stoeckel operation
Goffe's operation
Golden's sign
gonad
gonadotrophic
gonadotropin
gonococcus
gonorrhea
Goodall-Power operation
Goodell's
    dilator
    law
    sign
Gordan-Overstreet syndrome
Gordon's forceps
Gottschalk's operation
graafian
    g. follicle
    g. ovule

Grant-Ward operation
granulosa
    g. lutein
Graves' speculum
gravid
gravida I, II, III, etc.
gravidic
gravidism
graviditas
    g. examnialis
    g. exochorialis
gravidity
gravidocardiac
gravidopuerperal
Grawitz's tumor
Green-Armytage operation
Greene's curet
grip
    Pawlik's g.
Gusberg's curet
Gutglass' forceps
Guttmann's
    retractor
    speculum
GYN — gynecology
gynandrism
gynandroblastoma
gynatresia
gynecogen
gynecography
gynecoid
    g. pelvis
gynecoil
gynecologic
gynecological
gynecologist
gynecology
gynecopathy
gynecotokology
gyneduct
gynogamon
gynomerogon

gynomerogony
gynopathic
gynopathy
gynoplastics
gynoplasty
Haase's rule
Halban's
    disease
    sign
Hale's forceps
Halsted's radical mastectomy
Hamilton's method
Hank-Bradley dilator
Hank's dilator
Hannon's curet
Hardy-Duddy speculum
Harrison's method
Hartman's forceps
Haultaim's operation
Hawkins' forceps
Hawks-Dennen forceps
HCG — human chorionic
    gonadotropin
Heaney-Ballantine forceps
Heaney-Kanter forceps
Heaney-Rezek forceps
Heaney's
    clamp
    curet
    forceps
    needle holder
    retractor
    vaginal hysterectomy
Heaney-Simon retractor
Hegar's
    dilator
    operation
    sign
Heise's forceps
hematocele
    parametric h.

hematocele *(continued)*
    pudendal h.
    retrouterine h.
    vaginal h.
hematochlorine
hematocolpometra
hematocolpos
hematoma
hematome
hematometra
hematosalpinx
hemelytrometra lateralis
hemorrhage
hemostasis
Henrotin's
    forceps
    speculum
herpes
    h. genitalis
    h. gestationis
    h. menstrualis
    h. progenitalis
Hicks'
    sign
    version
hilar
hilus
    h. of ovary
    h. ovarii
Hirst-Emmett forceps
Hirst's operation
hirsutism
His' rule
Hodge's
    forceps
    maneuver
    pessary
Hoehne's sign
Hogben's test
Holden's curet
Holman-Mathieu cannula

Holtz's curet
hood
    Rock-Mulligan h.
hook
    Braun-Jardine-DeLee h.
    Braun's h.
    Dudley's h.
    Duplay's h.
    Emmet's h.
    Kelly's h.
    Mayo's h.
    Newman's h.
    Schwartz's h.
hormonal
hormone
hormonotherapy
horn
    h. of clitoris
    h. of uterus
Horrocks' maieutic
HSG – hysterosalpingogram
Hudgins' cannula
Huffman-Graves speculum
Huhner's test
Hulka's clip
human chorionic gonadotropin
Hunter's
    curet
    ligament
Huntington's operation
Hurtig's dilator
hyaline
Hyam's operation
hydatid
    h. of Morgagni
hydatidiform
hydramnios
hydrocele
    h. feminae
    h. muliebris
    Nuck's h.
hydrocephalus

hydrocolpos
hydroparasalpinx
hydrops
    h. fetalis
    h. folliculi
hydrorrhea
    h. gravidarum
hydrosalpinx
    h. follicularis
    intermittent h.
    h. simplex
hydrotubation
hydroureter
hydrovarium
hymen
    annular h.
    h. bifenestratus
    h. biforis
    circular h.
    cribriform h.
    denticular h.
    falciform h.
    fenestrated h.
    imperforate h.
    infundibuliform h.
    lunar h.
    septate h.
    h. septus
    h. subseptus
hymenal
    h. band
    h. ring
hymenectomy
hymenitis
hymenorrhaphy
hymenotome
hymenotomy
hyperbilirubinemia
hyperemesis
    h. gravidarum
hyperestrogenism
hyperflexion

hypermenorrhea
hypernephroma
hyperovaria
hyperovarianism
hyperovarism
hyperplasia
    adenomatous h.
    endometrial h.
    postmenopausal h.
    proliferative h.
    stromal h.
hyperthecosis
hypertonic
hypertrophy
hypofibrinogenemia
hypofunction
hypogalactia
hypomastia
hypomenorrhea
hypo-ovaria
hypoplasia
hypospadias
    female h.
hypothalamic
hypotonic
hypovaria
hypovarianism
hysteralgia
hysteratresia
hysterectomy
    abdominal h.
    Bonney's h.
    cesarean h.
    chemical h.
    complete h.
    Doyen's vaginal h.
    Heaney's vaginal h.
    Latzko's radical h.
    Mayo-Ward vaginal h.
    paravaginal h.
    partial h.
    Porro's h.

hysterectomy *(continued)*
    radical h.
    Ries-Wertheim h.
    Schauta-Amreich vaginal
      h.
    Schauta's radical vaginal
      h.
    Spalding-Richardson h.
    subtotal h.
    supracervical h.
    supravaginal h.
    total abdominal h.
    total h.
    vaginal h.
    Ward-Mayo vaginal h.
    Wertheim's radical h.
hystereurynter
hystereurysis
hysterobubonocele
hysterocarcinoma
hysterocele
hysterocervicotomy
hysterocleisis
hysterocolpectomy
hysterocolposcope
hysterocystic
hysterocystopexy
hysterocytocleisis
hysterodynia
hysterogastrorrhaphy
hysterogram
hysterograph
hysterography
hysterolaparotomy
hysterolith
hysterology
hysterolysis
hysterometer
hysterometry
hysteromyoma
hysteromyomectomy
hysteromyotomy

hystero-oophorectomy
hystero-ovariotomy
hysteropathy
hysteropexia
hysteropexy
hysteroptosia
hysteroptosis
hysterorrhaphy
hysterorrhexis
hysterosalpingectomy
hysterosalpingogram
hysterosalpingography
hysterosalpingo-
    oophorectomy
hysterosalpingostomy
hysteroscope
hysteroscopy
hysterospasm
hysterostat
hysterostomatocleisis
hysterostomatome
hysterostomatomy
hysterothermometry
hysterotome
hysterotomotokia
hysterotomy
hysterotrachelectasia
hysterotrachelectomy
hysterotracheloplasty
hysterotrachelorrhaphy
hysterotrachelotomy
hysterotubography
hysterovaginoenterocele
idiometritis
ileus
I.M. cocktail — intramuscular
                cocktail
implant
    Dow-Corning i.
implantation
incision. See *General Surgical
    Terms.*

incompatibility
incontinence
    stress i.
index
    Mengert's i.
indices
Indigo carmine dye
induced
induction
inertia
    uterine i.
infarction
infertilitas
    i. feminis
infertility
infundibula
infundibular
infundibuliform
infundibulum
    i. of fallopian tube
    i. of uterine tube
    i. tubae uterinae
inguinolabial
insemination
    artificial i. donor
    heterologous i.
    homologous i.
in situ
insufflation
    methylene blue i.
    tubal i.
insufflator
    Kidde's tubal i.
intercalary
intercourse
intermenstrual
intermural
internal os
interstitial
intracervical
intrafetation
intraligamentous

intramural
intranatal
intraovarian
intrapartum
intraplacental
intratubal
intrauterine device (IUD)
    bow IUD
    coil IUD
    copper-7 IUD
    Mazlin spring IUD
intravaginal
introitus
    marital i.
    parous i.
    i. vaginae
in utero
inversion
    i. of uterus
involution
Iowa forceps
IPD — inflammatory pelvic
       disease
Irving's operation
Isaac's differential distortion
    divergent method
ischiopubic
ischiopubiotomy
ischiorectal
ischiovaginal
isoimmunization
isthmica nodosa
isthmus
    i. of fallopian tube
    i. of uterus
    i. tubae uterinae
    i. uteri
IU — international unit
IUD — intrauterine device
IV cocktail — intravenous
       cocktail
Jackson's retractor

Jacobs'
    forceps
    tenaculum
Jacquemier's sign
Jarcho's
    cannula
    forceps
Johnson's calculation
Jolly's dilator
Jonas-Graves speculum
Jones' operation
Jungbluth
    vasa propria of J.
Kahn-Graves speculum
Kahn's
    cannula
    tenaculum
kakektic. See *cachectic.*
kakexia. See *cachexia.*
Kane's clamp
Kanter's sign
Kapeller-Adler test
Kegel's exercise
Keith's needle
Kelly-Gray curet
Kelly's
    clamp
    curet
    dilator
    forceps
    hook
    operation
    scissors
Kennedy's
    forceps
    operation
keratinized
Kergaradec's sign
kernicterus
Kerr's cesarean section
Kevorkian's curet
Kidde's tubal insufflator

Kielland-Luikart forceps
Kielland's forceps (Kjelland's
    forceps)
Kittner's forceps
Klinefelter's syndrome
Kline's flocculation test
kloasma. See *cloasma.*
Klotz's syndrome
Kluge's method
knife
    Ayerst's k.
    Fleming's k.
    Pace's k.
kocherization
kocherized
Kocher's clamp
Kocks's operation
koleo-. See words beginning
    coleo-.
kolostrum. See *colostrum.*
kolp-, kolpo-. See words
    beginning *colp-, colpo-.*
kondilo-. See words beginning
    condylo-.
kondro-. See words beginning
    chondro-.
korio-. See words beginning
    chorio-.
kotiledon. See *cotyledon.*
kraurosis
    k. vulva
Krause's forceps
Kristeller's method
Kroener's operation
Kronig's cesarean section
Krukenberg's tumor
krura. See *crura.*
kryo-. See words beginning
    cryo-.
kuldo-. See words beginning
    culdo-.
Kupperman's test

Kushner-Tandatnick curet
Küstner's
    law
    operation
    sign
kyphosis
    dorsal k.
kyphotic
labia
    l. majora
    l. majus
    l. minora
labial
labium
labor
    atonic l.
    desultory l.
    dyskinetic l.
    habitual l.
    induced l.
    instrumental l.
    mimetic l.
    obstructed l.
    postponed l.
    precipitate l.
    prodromal l.
    protracted l.
    spontaneous l.
laceration
    fishmouth l.
lactation
lacteal
lactic
lactogen
    human placental l.
lactogenic
lacuna
    intervillous l.
Ladin's sign
Lahey's clamp
Laminaria tent
lamination

Landou's sign
Langhan's
    cell
    stria
laparocolpohysterotomy
laparocystotomy
laparohysterectomy
laparohystero-oophorectomy
laparohysterosalpingo-
    oophorectomy
laparohysterotomy
laparokelyphotomy
laparomonodidymus
laparomyomectomy
laparosalpingectomy
laparosalpingo-oophorectomy
laparosalpingotomy
laparoscope
laparoscopic
laparoscopy
laparotomy
    exploratory l.
laparotrachelotomy
laparouterotomy
Lash's operation
Latzko's
    cesarean section
    closure
    operation
    radical hysterectomy
Laufe-Barton-Kielland forceps
Laufe-Piper forceps
Laufe's forceps
law
    Diday's l.
    Freund's l.
    Goodell's l.
    Küstner's l.
    Leopold's l.
    Levret's l.
    Pajot's l.
LeFort's operation

leiomyoma
    l. uteri
leiomyomata
    l. uteri
leiomyosarcoma
Leopold's
    law
    maneuver
    operation
Lerous's method
leukocytosis
leukokraurosis
leukophlegmasia
leukoplakia
    l. vulvae
leukorrhea
levator ani
level
    pregnanediol l.
Levret's
    forceps
    law
LFA — left frontoanterior
LFP — left frontoposterior
LFT — left frontotransverse
LH — luteinizing hormone
libido
ligament
    anterior l.
    broad l.
    cardinal l.
    Hunter's l.
    infundibulopelvic l.
    keystone l.
    lacunar l.
    lateral l.
    Mackenrodt's l.
    ovarian l.
    posterior l.
    rectouterine l.
    round l.
    sacrogenital l.

ligament *(continued)*
    sacrouterine l.
    suspensory l.
    uterosacral l.
    vesicouterine l.
ligamenta
    l. ovarii proprium
    l. teres uteri
ligation
    tubal l.
Lignac-Fanconi disease
line
    Douglas' l.
    Farre's l.
linea
    l. nigra
lio-. See words beginning *leio-.*
lipoid
Lippes' loop
liquor
    l. amnii
    l. chorii
    l. folliculi
lithopedion
Littre's glands
littritis
Litzmann's obliquity
LMA – left mentoanterior
LMP – last menstrual period
    left mentoposterior
LMT – left mentotransverse
LNMP – last normal menstrual
    period
LOA – left occipitoanterior
lochia
    l. alba
    l. cruenta
    l. purulenta
    l. rubra
    l. sanguinolenta
lochial
lochiocolpos

lochiocyte
lochiometra
lochiometritis
lochiopyra
lochiorrhagia
lochiorrhea
lochioschesis
lochiostasis
lochometritis
lochoperitonitis
Löhlein's diameter
Long Island forceps
Long's forceps
loop
    Lippes' l.
LOP – left occipitoposterior
LOT – left occipitotransverse
Lounsbury's curet
Løvset's maneuver
LSA – left sacroanterior
L. Sc. A. – left scapuloanterior
L. Sc. P. – left scapulo-
    posterior
LSP – left sacroposterior
LS ratio – lecithin-sphingo-
    myelin ratio
LST – left sacrotransverse
Lugol's stain
Luikart-Bill traction handle
Luikart's forceps
Luikart-Simpson forceps
lumen
    vaginal l.
lumpectomy
luteal
luteectomy
lutein
luteinic
luteinization
luteoid
luteoma
luteum

lying-in
lymphogranuloma
    l. benignum
    Schaumann's benign l.
    venereal l.
    l. venereum
lyo-. See words beginning *leio-*.
lyra
    l. uteri
    l. uterina
    l. vaginae
lyre
    l. of uterus
    l. of vagina
maceration
Mackenrodt's
    ligament
    operation
macula
    m. gonorrhoeica
    Saenger's m.
Madlener operation
Maher's disease
Maier's forceps
maieusiomania
maieusiophobia
maieutic
    Horrocks' m.
Malherbe
    epithelioma of M.
malposition
malpresentation
mammary
mammectomy
mammogram
mammoplasty
Manchester
    operation
    ovoid
maneuver. See also *method*.
    Bracht's m.
    Brandt-Andrews m.

maneuver *(continued)*
    DeLee's m.
    Hodge's m.
    Leopold's m.
    Løvset's m.
    Massini's m.
    Mauriceau's m.
    Mauriceau-Smellie m.
    Mauriceau-Smellie-Veit
      m.
    McDonald's m.
    Müller-Hillis m.
    Munro-Kerr m.
    Phaneuf's m.
    Pinard's m.
    Prague m.
    Ritgen m.
    Saxtorph's m.
    Scanzoni's m.
    Schatz's m.
    Van Hoorn's m.
    Wigand's m.
manner
    Pomeroy's m.
Mann's forceps
Marchetti test
Marckwald's operation
Margulles' coil
Marshall-Marchetti-Krantz
    operation
Marshall-Marchetti operation
marsupialization
Martin's
    operation
    pelvimeter
Martius' operation
Maryan's forceps
masculinovoblastoma
Mason-Auvard speculum
Massini's maneuver
mastectomy
    Halsted's radical m.

mastectomy *(continued)*
    Willy Meyer radical m.
mastitis
    cystic m.
mastodynia
mastogram
mastography
Matsner episiotomy
maturation
Mauriceau's maneuver
Mauriceau-Smellie maneuver
Mauriceau-Smellie-Veit
    maneuver
Mayer-Rokitansky-Küster
    syndrome
Mayer's speculum
Mayo-Fueth operation
Mayo-Harrington scissors
Mayor's sign
Mayo's
    hook
    needle
    scissors
Mayo-Sims scissors
Mayo-Ward vaginal
    hysterectomy
maza
mazic
Mazlin spring IUD
McCall-Schuman operation
McCall's operation
McDonald's
    maneuver
    operation
McDowell's operation
McIndoe operation
McLane's forceps
McLane-Tucker forceps
McLane-Tucker-Luikart
    forceps
meatus
    urinary m.

mechanism
    Duncan's m.
    Schultze's m.
meconium
medications. See *Drugs and
    Chemistry* section.
megaloclitoris
Meigs-Cass syndrome
Meigs' syndrome
melanoma
melasma
    m. gravidarum
membrane
    hyaline m.
    mucous m.
menalgia
menarche
menarchial
Mengert's index
Menge's
    operation
    pessary
menhidrosis
menolipsis
menometrorrhagia
menopausal
menopause
menophania
menoplania
menorrhagia
menorrhalgia
menorrhea
menorrheal
menoschesis
menosepsis
menostasis
menostaxis
menotoxic
menotoxin
menoxenia
menses
menstrual

menstruant
menstruate
menstruation
 anovular m.
 anovulatory m.
 nonovulational m.
 ovulatory m.
 regurgitant m.
 retrograde m.
 scanty m.
 supplementary m.
 suppressed m.
 vicarious m.
menstruous
menstruum
mesenchymal
mesometritis
mesometrium
mesonephric
mesonephroma
mesosalpinx
mesothelial
mesothelioma
mesovarium
metacyesis
metaplasia
 squamous m.
method. See also *maneuver.*
 Beuttner's m.
 Bonnaire's m.
 Credé's m.
 Danforth's m.
 Douglas' m.
 Gabastou's hydraulic m.
 Hamilton's m.
 Harrison's m.
 Isaac's differential
  distortion divergent m.
 Kluge's m.
 Kristeller's m.
 Lerous's m.

method *(continued)*
 Pajot's m.
 Puzo's m.
 rhythm m.
 Schultze's m.
 Schuman's m.
 Smellie's m.
 Watson's m.
methylene blue insufflation
metra
metralgia
metranoikter
metratonia
metratrophia
metrechoscopy
metrectasia
metrectomy
metrectopia
metreurynter
metreurysis
metria
metritis
 m. dissecans
 dissecting m.
 puerperal m.
metrocampsis
metrocarcinoma
metrocele
metrocolpocele
metrocystosis
metrocyte
metrodynia
metroendometritis
metrofibroma
metrogenous
metrogonorrhea
metrography
metroleukorrhea
metromalacia
metromalacoma
metromenorrhagia

metroparalysis
metropathia
    m. haemorrhagica
metropathic
metropathy
metroperitoneal
metroperitonitis
metrophlebitis
metroplasty
metroptosis
metrorrhagia
    m. myopathica
metrorrhea
metrorrhexis
metrosalpingitis
metrosalpingogram
metrosalpingography
metroscope
metrostaxis
metrostenosis
metrotome
metrotomy
metrotoxin
metrotubography
Metzenbaum scissors
MH — marital history
micturition
Milex cervitome
Miller's
    operation
    speculum
Millin-Read operation
Mitchell-Diamond forceps
mitotic
mittelschmerz
mole
    Breu's m.
    hydatidiform m.
molimen
molimina
mongoloid
monilial

monocyesis
mons
    m. pubis
    m. ureteris
    m. veneris
Montgomery strap
morcellated
morcellation
morcellement
Morgagni
    cyst of M.
    hydatid of M.
mosaicism
Moschcowitz's operation
motile
mucinous
mucosa
    endocervical m.
Mueller's needle
Müller-Hillis maneuver
müllerian
müllerianoma
müllerianosis
mülleriosis
Müller's operation
multigravida
multiloculated
multipara
multiparity
multiparous
Mundie's forceps
Munnell's operation
Munro-Kerr maneuver
muscle
    levator ani m.
    pubovaginal m.
    pyramidalis m.
    recti m.
    rectouterine m.
    sphincter ani m.
myoma
myomagenesis

myomata
    m. uteri
myomatectomy
myomatosis
myomatous
myomectomy
myometrial
myometritis
myometrium
myomohysterectomy
myomotomy
myosalpingitis
myosalpinx
myosarcoma
mytotic. See *mitotic.*
nabothian
Naboth's
    cysts
    follicles
    glands
    ovules
    vesicles
Nägele's
    obliquity
    pelvis
    rule
navicular
NB — newborn
Neal's cannula
necrosis
necrotic
needle
    Keith's n.
    Mayo's n.
    Mueller's n.
    Pereyra n.
    Shirodkar n.
    Touhey's n.
    Verres' n.
    Vim-Silverman n.
    Voorhees' n.

needle holder
    Heaney's n.h.
Nelson's scissors
neonatal
neonate
neonatologist
neonatology
nerve
    ilioinguinal n.
    pudendal n.
    uterine n.
neumo-. See words beginning
    pneumo-.
neurectomy
    presacral n.
Newman's
    forceps
    hook
Nickerson's medium smear
Niemann-Pick disease
node
    Cloquet's n.
nodule
    discrete n.
noma
    n. pudendi
    n. vulvae
norethindrone test
norethynodrel test
Nott's speculum
Novak's curet
Nuck
    canal of N.
    hydrocele of N.
nulligravida
nullipara
nulliparity
nulliparous
numo-. See words beginning
    pneumo-.
nympha

nymphae
nymphectomy
nymphitis
nymphocaruncular
nymphohymeneal
nymphomania
nymphomaniac
nymphoncus
nymphotomy
OB — obstetrics
OB-GYN — obstetrics and
        gynecology
obliquity
    Litzmann's o.
    Nägele's o.
    Roederer's o.
obliteration
obstetrical
obstetrician
obstetrics
occipital
occipitoanterior
occipitoposterior
Ochsner's clamp
octigravida
octipara
O'Hanlon's forceps
oligohydramnios
oligohypermenorrhea
oligohypomenorrhea
oligomenorrhea
oligo-ovulation
Olshausen's
    operation
    sign
oocyesis
oocyte
oocytin
oogenesis
oogenetic
oophoralgia
oophorectomize

oophorectomy
oophoritis
oophorocystectomy
oophorocystosis
oophorogenous
oophorohysterectomy
oophoroma
oophoron
oophoropathy
oophoropeliopexy
oophoropexy
oophoroplasty
oophororrhaphy
oophorosalpingectomy
oophorosalpingitis
oophorostomy
oophorotomy
oophorrhagia
operation
    Abell's o.
    Aburel's o.
    Aldrich's o.
    Alexander-Adams o.
    Alexander's o.
    Baldwin's o.
    Baldy's o.
    Baldy-Webster o.
    Ball's o.
    Basset's o.
    Baudelocque's o.
    Beatson's o.
    Bischoff's o.
    Bissell's o.
    Bouilly's o.
    Bozeman's o.
    Bricker's o.
    Brunschwig's o.
    Burch's o.
    Coffey's o.
    Davis' o.
    Decker's o.
    Doderlein's o.

operation *(continued)*
  Doleris' o.
  Donald-Fothergill o.
  Donald's o.
  Doyen's o.
  Dudley's o.
  Dührssen's o.
  Emmet's o.
  Estes' o.
  Falk's o.
  Falk-Shukuris o.
  Fleming's o.
  Fothergill's o.
  Frangenheim-Goebell-
    Stoeckel o.
  Freund's o.
  Fritsch's o.
  Frommel's o.
  Gigli's o.
  Gilliam-Doleris' o.
  Gilliam's o.
  Giordano's o.
  Goebel-Stoeckel o.
  Goffe's o.
  Goodall-Power o.
  Gottschalk's o.
  Grant-Ward o.
  Green-Armytage o.
  Haultaim's o.
  Hegar's o.
  Hirst's o.
  Huntington's o.
  Hyam's o.
  interposition o.
  Irving's o.
  Jones' o.
  Kelly's o.
  Kennedy's o.
  Kocks's o.
  Kroener's o.
  Küstner's o.
  Lash's o.

operation *(continued)*
  Latzko's o.
  LeFort's o.
  Leopold's o.
  Mackenrodt's o.
  Madlener o.
  Manchester o.
  Marckwald's o.
  Marshall-Marchetti o.
  Marshall-Marchetti-
    Krantz o.
  Martin's o.
  Martius' o.
  Mayo-Fueth o.
  McCall's o.
  McCall-Schuman o.
  McDonald's o.
  McDowell's o.
  McIndoe o.
  Menge's o.
  Miller's o.
  Millin-Read o.
  Moschcowitz's o.
  Müller's o.
  Munnell's o.
  Olshausen's o.
  O'Sullivan's o.
  Oxford's o.
  Pean's o.
  Peterson's o.
  Pomeroy's o.
  Porro's o.
  Porro-Veit o.
  Pozzi's o.
  Récamier's o.
  Ries-Wertheim o.
  Rizzoli's o.
  Rubin's o.
  Saenger's o.
  Scanzoni's o.
  Schauffler's o.
  Schauta's o.

operation *(continued)*
    Schauta-Wertheim o.
    Schröder's o.
    Schuchardt's o.
    Shirodkar o.
    Simon's o.
    Spalding-Richardson o.
    Spinelli's o.
    Strassman-Jones o.
    Sturmdorf's o.
    Taussig-Morton o.
    Taussig's o.
    Te Linde o.
    Thomas' o.
    Torpin's o.
    Tuffier's o.
    Twombly's o.
    Twombly-Ulfelder's o.
    Uchida's o.
    Vernon-David o.
    Warren's o.
    Water's o.
    Watkins' o.
    Watkins-Wertheim o.
    Webster's o.
    Wertheim's o.
    Wertheim-Schauta o.
    Wharton's o.
    Whitacre's o.
    William's o.
    Williams-Richardson o.
    Wylie's o.
orifice
    abdominal o. of uterine
      tube
    external urethral o.
    hymenal o.
    o. of uterus
    vaginal o.
orificium
    o. externum uteri
    o. hymenis

orificium *(continued)*
    o. internum uteri
    o. vaginae
os
Osiander's sign
ostium
    o. abdominale tubae
      uterinae
    o. uteri
    o. uterinum tubae
      uterinae
    o. vaginae
O'Sullivan-O'Connor
    retractor
    speculum
O'Sullivan's operation
outlet
    marital o.
ova
ovarian
ovariectomy
ovaries
ovarin
ovariocele
ovariocentesis
ovariocyesis
ovariodysneuria
ovariogenic
ovariohysterectomy
ovarioncus
ovariopathy
ovariopexy
ovariorrhexis
ovariosalpingectomy
ovariosteresis
ovariostomy
ovariotestis
ovariotherapy
ovariotomist
ovariotomy
ovariotubal
ovariprival

ovaritis
ovarium
ovarotherapy
ovary
Overstreet's forceps
oviduct
ovoid
     Manchester o.
ovotestis
ovotherapy
ovula
ovulate
ovulation
ovulatory
ovule
     graafian o's
     Naboth's o's
     primitive o.
     primordial o.
ovulogenous
ovulum
ovum
     blighted o.
Oxford's operation
oxytocic
oxytocin
oxyuriasis
Pace's knife
pack
     Bellow's p.
packing
     iodoform gauze p.
Pagano-Levin medium smear
Paget's
     cell
     disease
Pajot's
     law
     method
Palmer's
     dilator
     forceps

palpation
pampiniform
panhysterectomy
panhystero-oophorectomy
panhysterosalpingectomy
panhysterosalpingo-
     oophorectomy
Papanicolaou's
     smear
     stain
papilla
Pap test
papyraceous
para — primipara
para 0, I, II, III, etc.
paracentesis
paracolpitis
paracolpium
paracyesis
paragomphosis
parametrial
parametric
parametritic
parametritis
parametrium
parasalpingeal
parasalpingitis
paratubal
parauterine
paravaginal
paravaginitis
parenchymatous
paries
       p. anterior vaginae
parietal
paroophoric
paroophoritis
paroophoron
parous
parovarian
parovariotomy
parovaritis

parovarium

pars

    p. fetalis placentae

    p. uterina placentae

    p. uterina tubae uterinae

partes genitales externae
muliebres

partes genitales femininae
externae

parturient

parturifacient

parturiometer

parturition

partus

    p. agrippinus

    p. caesareus

    p. immaturus

    p. maturus

    p. precipitatus

    p. prematurus

    p. serotinus

    p. siccus

patent

path — pathology

patulous

pavilion

    p. of the oviduct

Pawlik's

    fold

    grip

    triangle

Pean's

    forceps

    operation

Pederson's speculum

pedicle

pediculosis

pedunculated

pelvic

pelvicellulitis

pelvicephalography

pelvicephalometry

pelvicliseometer

pelvifixation

pelvigraph

pelvilithotomy

pelvimeter

    Breisky's p.

    Collin's p.

    Collyer's p.

    DeLee's p.

    Martin's p.

    Thoms' p.

    William's p.

pelvimetry

pelvis

    p. aequabiliter justo
major

    p. aequabiliter justo
minor

    android p.

    p. angusta

    anthropoid p.

    beaked p.

    brachypellic p.

    contracted p.

    Deventer's p.

    dolichopellic p.

    funnel-shaped p.

    gynecoid p.

    mesatipellic p.

    Nägele's p.

    pithecoid p.

    p. plana

    platypellic p.

    platypelloid p.

    Robert's p.

    rostrate p.

pendulous

Pennington's clamp

Penrose drain

Percy's cautery

Pereyra

    needle

Pereyra *(continued)*
 procedure
perforator
  Blot's p.
  Smellie's p.
pericolpitis
perimetric
perimetrium
perimetrosalpingitis
perinatal
perineal
perineauxesis
perineocele
perineocolporectomyo-
  mectomy
perineometer
perineoplasty
perineorrhaphy
  Emmet-Studdiford p.
perineosynthesis
perineotomy
perineovaginal
perineovaginorectal
perineovulvar
perineum
perioophoritis
perioophorosalpingitis
perioothecitis
perioothecosalpingitis
perisalpingitis
perisalpingo-ovaritis
perisalpinx
peritoneal
peritonealize
peritoneopexy
peritoneum
  parietal p.
peritonitis
periuterine
perivaginal
perivaginitis
per primam

pessary
 cup p.
 diaphragm p.
 doughnut p.
 Emmert-Gellhorn p.
 Gariel's p.
 Gehrung p.
 Gellhorn's p.
 gynefold p.
 Hodge's p.
 lever p.
 Menge's p.
 ring p.
 Smith-Hodge p.
 Smith's p.
 stem p.
 Thomas' p.
 Wylie's p.
 Zwanck's p.
Peterson's operation
Phaneuf's
  forceps
  maneuver
phenomenon
  Arias-Stella's p.
  fern p.
  Strassmann's p.
Phenylstix
phimosis
  p. vaginalis
phlebitis
phlegmasia
  p. alba dolens
  p. alba dolens
   puerperarum
  cellulitic p.
phototherapy
Picot's speculum
PID — pelvic inflammatory
   disease
pielo-. See words beginning
  pyelo-.

Pinard's
  maneuver
  sign
pio-. See words beginning *pyo-*.
Piper's forceps
Piskacek's sign
pithecoid
pitocin drip
pituitary gland
placenta
  accessory p.
  p. accreta
  adherent p.
  annular p.
  battledore p.
  bidiscoidal p.
  bilobate p.
  bilobed p.
  p. bipartita
  bipartite p.
  chorioallantoic p.
  choriovitelline p.
  p. circumvallata
  circumvallate p.
  cirsoid p.
  p. cirsoides
  deciduous p.
  p. diffusa
  p. dimidiata
  dimidiate p.
  discoid p.
  p. discoidea
  duplex p.
  endotheliochorial p.
  epitheliochorial p.
  p. febrilis
  p. fenestrata
  fetal p.
  p. foetalis
  fundal p.
  furcate p.
  hemochorial p.

placenta *(continued)*
  hemoendothelial p.
  horseshoe p.
  incarcerated p.
  p. increta
  labyrinthine p.
  lobed p.
  p. marginalis
  p. marginata
  maternal p.
  p. membranacea
  multilobate p.
  multilobed p.
  p. multipartita
  p. nappiformis
  nondeciduous p.
  p. obsoleta
  panduriform p.
  p. panduriformis
  p. percreta
  p. praevia
  p. praevia centralis
  p. praevia marginalis
  p. praevia partialis
  p. previa
  p. reflexa
  p. reniformis
  retained p.
  Schultze's p.
  p. spuria
  stone p.
  p. succenturiata
  succenturiate p.
  syndesmochorial p.
  p. triloba
  trilobate p.
  p. tripartita
  tripartite p.
  p. triplex
  p. truffée
  p. uterina
  uterine p.

placenta *(continued)*
    velamentous p.
    villous p.
    yolk-sac p.
    zonary p.
    zonular p.
placentae
    ablatio p.
    abruptio p.
    marginalis p.
placental
placentation
placentitis
placentocytotoxin
placentogenesis
placentogram
placentography
placentoid
placentologist
placentology
placentoma
placentopathy
placentotherapy
plaque
platypellic
platypelloid
plethoric
plexus
    Auerbach's p.
    p. cavernosus clitoridis
    cavernous p. of clitoris
    ovarian p.
    p. ovaricus
    pampiniform p.
    p. pampiniformis
    uterine p.
    uterovaginal p.
    p. uterovaginalis
    vaginal p.
    p. venosus vaginalis
    venous p.
plica
    p. rectouterina

plicae
    p. ampullares tubae
      uterinae
    p. isthmicae tubae
      uterinae
    p. palmatae
    p. tubariae tubae
      uterinae
    p. vaginae
plication
PMP — previous menstrual
      period
pneumoamnios
pneumogynecogram
pneumoperitoneum
polycyesis
polycystic
polycystoma
polyhydramnios
polyhypermenorrhea
polyhypomenorrhea
polymenorrhea
polyp
    cervical p.
    endocervical p.
    sessile p.
polypectomy
polypoid
Pomeroy's
    manner
    operation
Porro's
    cesarean section
    hysterectomy
    operation
Porro-Veit operation
portio
    p. supravaginalis cervicis
    p. vaginalis cervicis
position. See *fetal position* and
    General Surgical Terms.
postabortal
postcoital

post coitum
postmenopausal
postmenstrua
postpartum
Potter's version
pouch
    p. of Douglas
    vesicouterine p.
Pozzi's operation
PPA — phenylpyruvic acid
Prague maneuver
Pratt's dilator
preeclampsia
pregnancy
    afetal p.
    bigeminal p.
    cornual p.
    ectopic p.
    entopic p.
    exochorial p.
    extrauterine p.
    gemellary p.
    heterotopic p.
    hydatid p.
    hysteric p.
    interstitial p.
    intraligamentary p.
    intramural p.
    intraperitoneal p.
    intrauterine p.
    mesenteric p.
    molar p.
    mural p.
    ovarioabdominal p.
    oviducal p.
    parietal p.
    sacrofetal p.
    sacrohysteric p.
    spurious p.
    stump p.
    term p.
    tubal p.

pregnancy *(continued)*
    tuboabdominal p.
    tuboligamentary p.
    tubo-ovarian p.
    tubouterine p.
    uteroabdominal p.
    utero-ovarian p.
    uterotubal p.
pregnanediol level
pregnant
Pregnosticon test
premature
premenarchal
premenstrua
premenstrual
premenstruum
prenatal
prepuce
preputial
preputium
    p. clitoridis
presentation. See also *fetal position.*
    breech p.
    brow p.
    cephalic p.
    compound p.
    face p.
    footling breech p.
    footling p.
    frank breech p.
    full breech p.
    funis p.
    knee breech p.
    longitudinal p.
    oblique p.
    parietal p.
    pelvic p.
    placental p.
    polar p.
    shoulder p.
    torso p.

presentation *(continued)*
    transverse p.
    trunk p.
    vertex p.
previable
primigravid
primigravida
primipara
primiparity
primiparous
primitiae
procedure
    Pereyra p.
    Shirodkar p.
    Strap p.
    Temple p.
procidentia
progenital
progestational
progesteroid
progesterone
progestin
progestogen
progestomimetic
progravid
prolactin
prolapse
    p. of uterus
prolapsus
    p. uteri
proliferative
pruritus
Pryor-Pean retractor
pseudocorpus luteum
pseudocyesis
pseudoendometritis
pseudoerosion
pseudomamma
pseudomenstruation
pseudomucin
pseudomucinous
pseudopregnancy

psoas
psychosis
PU — pregnancy urine
pubarche
puberty
pubocervical
pubovesicocervical
pudendal
pudendum
    p. femininum
    p. muliebre
puerpera
puerperal
puerperalism
puerperant
puerperium
punctiform
Puzo's method
pyelitis
    p. gravidarum
pyelocystitis
pylorospasm
pyocolpocele
pyocolpos
pyometra
pyometritis
pyometrium
pyo-ovarium
pyosalpingitis
pyosalpingo-oophoritis
pyosalpingo-oothecitis
pyosalpinx
quadripara
quintipara
rachitic
radium
rakitic. See rachitic.
Ramses' diaphragm
Randall's
    curet
    sign
    stone forceps

Rasch's sign
rating
    Apgar r.
reaction
    depressive r.
Récamier's
    curet
    operation
rectocele
rectolabial
rectouterine
rectovaginal
regime
    Smith & Smith r.
Reichel's cloacal duct
Reich-Nechtow
    curet
    dilator
Reich's clamp
retention
retractor
    Balfour's r.
    Brantley-Turner r.
    Deaver's r.
    DeLee's r.
    Doyen's r.
    Eastman's r.
    Emmet's r.
    Friedman's r.
    Gelpi's r.
    Glenner's r.
    Guttmann's r.
    Heaney-Simon r.
    Heaney's r.
    Jackson's r.
    O'Sullivan-O'Connor r.
    Pryor-Pean r.
    Rigby's r.
    Sims-Kelly r.
    Sims' r.
    Wesson's r.

retrocervical
retrocessed
retrocession
retrodisplacement
retroflexion
retroplacental
retroposition
retrouterine
retroversion
retroverted
Reusner's sign
RFA — right frontoanterior
RFP — right frontoposterior
RFT — right frontotransverse
Rh factor — Rhesus factor
Rh neg. — Rhesus factor
            negative
Rho-Gam test
Rh pos. — Rhesus factor
           positive
Richardson's technique
Ries-Wertheim
    hysterectomy
    operation
Rigby's retractor
ring
    Bandl's r.
    Falope's r.
    hymenal r.
Ringer's lactate stain
Rinman's sign
Ritgen maneuver
Rizzoli's operation
RMA — right mentoanterior
RMP — right mentoposterior
RMT — right mentotransverse
ROA — right occipitoanterior
Robert's pelvis
Rochester-Carmalt forceps
Rochester-Ochsner forceps
Rochester-Pean forceps

Rock-Mulligan hood
Roederer's obliquity
Rohr's stria
rooming-in
ROP — right occipitoposterior
ROT — right occipitotransverse
Rotunda treatment
RSA — right sacroanterior
R. Sc. A. — right scapulo-
           anterior
R. Sc. P. — right scapulo-
           posterior
RSP — right sacroposterior
RST — right sacrotransverse
rubella
Rubin's
        cannula
        operation
        test
ruga
rugae
        r. of vagina
        r. vaginales
rule
        Arey's r.
        Haase's r.
        His' r.
        Nägele's r.
Russell's forceps
Sabin-Feldman test
sacrouterine
sactosalpinx
Saenger's
        macula
        operation
Saf-t-coil
saline
Salmon's sign
salpingectomy
salpingemphraxis
salpingian

salpingitic
salpingitis
        chronic interstitial s.
        chronic vegetating s.
        hemorrhagic s.
        hypertrophic s.
        s. isthmica nodosa
        mural s.
        nodular s.
        parenchymatous s.
        s. profluens
        pseudofollicular s.
        purulent s.
        tuberculous s.
salpingocele
salpingocyesis
salpingogram
salpingography
salpingolithiasis
salpingolysis
salpingo-oophorectomy
salpingo-oophoritis
salpingo-oophorocele
salpingo-oothecitis
salpingo-oothecocele
salpingo-ovariectomy
salpingo-ovariotomy
salpingoperitonitis
salpingopexy
salpingoplasty
salpingorrhaphy
salpingostomatomy
salpingostomatoplasty
salpingostomy
salpingotomy
salpinx
Sampson's cyst
sanguineous
sarcoidosis
        Boeck's s.
sarcoma

Saxtorph's maneuver
Scanzoni's
   maneuver
   operation
Schatz's maneuver
Schauffler's operation
Schaumann's benign
   lymphogranuloma
Schauta-Amreich vaginal
   hysterectomy
Schauta's
   operation
   radical vaginal
     hysterectomy
Schauta-Wertheim operation
Schiller's test
Schröder's operation
Schroeder's
   disease
   forceps
   scissors
   syndrome
   tenaculum
Schubert's forceps
Schuchardt's operation
Schuller's stain
Schultze's
   mechanism
   method
   placenta
Schuman's method
Schwartz's
   forceps
   hook
Schweizer's forceps
scissors
   Braun's s.
   Doyen's s.
   Emmet's s.
   Ferguson's s.
   Kelly's s.

scissors *(continued)*
   Mayo-Harrington s.
   Mayo-Sims s.
   Mayo's s.
   Metzenbaum s.
   Nelson's s.
   Schroeder's s.
   Sims' s.
   umbilical s.
   Waldmann's s.
sclerocystic
sclero-oophoritis
sclero-oothecitis
score
   Apgar s.
   Silverman's s.
Scully's tumor
secretory
section
   cesarean s.
   cesarean s., cervical
   cesarean s., classic
   cesarean s., corporeal
   cesarean s., extra-
     peritoneal
   cesarean s., Kerr's
   cesarean s., Kronig's
   cesarean s., Latzko's
   cesarean s., low
   cesarean s., Porro's
   cesarean s., trans-
     peritoneal
   cesarean s., transverse
   cesarean s., Water's
   frozen s.
secundigravida
secundina
secundinae
secundine
secundipara
secundiparity

secundiparous
sefalo-. See words beginning
    cephalo-.
Segond's
    forceps
    spatula
semen
seminoma
    ovarian s.
Senn forceps
sepsis
    puerperal s.
septate
septicemia
septigravida
septimetritis
septipara
septum
    s. corporum cavernosor-
      um clitoridis
    placental s.
    rectovaginal s.
    s. rectovesicale
serocystoma
serosa
serosal
serosanguineous
serous
Sertoli-Leydig cell tumor
serviko-. See words beginning
    cervico-.
sessile
sextigravida
sextipara
Sheehan's syndrome
shield
    Dacron s.
    Dalkon s.
Shirodkar
    needle
    operation
    procedure

Shorr's stain
sign
    Ahlfeld's s.
    Arnoux's s.
    Beccaria's s.
    Beclard's s.
    Bolt's s.
    Braun-Fernwald s.
    Braxton-Hicks s.
    Chadwick's s.
    Cullen's s.
    Danforth's s.
    Dewees' s.
    Gauss's s.
    Golden's s.
    Goodell's s.
    Halban's s.
    Hegar's s.
    Hicks' s.
    Hoehne's s.
    Jacquemier's s.
    Kanter's s.
    Kergaradec's s.
    Küstner's s.
    Ladin's s.
    Landou's s.
    Mayor's s.
    Olshausen's s.
    Osiander's s.
    Pinard's s.
    Piskacek's s.
    Randall's s.
    Rasch's s.
    Reusner's s.
    Rinman's s.
    Salmon's s.
    Spalding's s.
    Tarnier's s.
    Von Fernwald's s.
Silverman's score
Simmonds' speculum
Simon's operation

Simpson-Luikart forceps
Simpson's
    forceps
    sound
Sims'
    curet
    retractor
    scissors
    sound
    speculum
Sims-Huhner test
Sims-Kelly retractor
sinografin
skeletonized
Skene's
    curet
    duct
    forceps
    gland
smear
    buccal s.
    Nickerson's medium s.
    Pagano-Levin medium s.
    Papanicolaou's s.
smegma
    s. clitoridis
    s. embryonum
Smellie's
    method
    perforator
Smith & Smith regime
Smith-Hodge pessary
Smith's
    forceps
    pessary
sois. See *psoas.*
Somers' forceps
sonogram
Soonawalla uterine elevator
sound
    Simpson's s.

sound *(continued)*
    Sims' s.
    uterine s.
Spalding-Richardson
    hysterectomy
    operation
Spalding's sign
spatula
    Segond's s.
    Tauber's s.
speculum
    Auvard-Remine s.
    Auvard's weighted s.
    Berlind-Auvard s.
    Brewer's s.
    Collin's s.
    Cusco's s.
    Devilbiss' s.
    Devilbiss-Stacey s.
    duck-billed s.
    Fergusson's s.
    Garrigue's s.
    Graves' s.
    Guttmann's s.
    Hardy-Duddy s.
    Henrotin's s.
    Huffman-Graves s.
    Jonas-Graves s.
    Kahn-Graves s.
    Mason-Auvard s.
    Mayer's s.
    Miller's s.
    Nott's s.
    O'Sullivan-O'Connor s.
    Pederson's s.
    Picot's s.
    Simmonds' s.
    Sims' s.
    weighted s.
    Weisman-Graves s.
    wire bivalve s.

sphincter
    s. vaginae
Spinelli's operation
spinnbarkeit
spray
    dermoplast s.
squamocolumnar
stain
    Feulgen s.
    Lugol's s.
    Papanicolaou's s.
    Ringer's lactate s.
    Schuller's s.
    Shorr's s.
Starlinger's dilator
Staude-Moore forceps
Staude's forceps
Stein-Leventhal syndrome
stellate
stenosis
stent
    foam rubber vaginal s.
sterility
sterilization
Steri-strips
stick
    sponge s.
stillbirth
stillborn
Stockholm box
strap
    Montgomery s.
Strap procedure
Strassman-Jones operation
Strassmann's phenomenon
stria
    Langhans' s.
    Rohr's s.
striae
    s. gravidarum
stricture

Stroganoff's (Stroganov's)
    treatment
stroma
    ovarian s.
    s. ovarii
    s. of ovary
stromal
study
    air s.
    cytogenetic s.
Sturmdorf's operation
stylet
subinvolution
submucous
subperitoneal
subserous
subumbilical
subvesical
suction D & C
sudo-. See words beginning
    pseudo-.
suit
    Fletcher's s.
sulcus
Sulkowich's test
supernumerary
suprapubic
supravaginal
surgical procedures. See
    operation.
suspension
suture. See *General Surgical*
    Terms.
Swiss-cheese endometrium
symphysis
    s. pubica
    s. pubis
synchondrosis
syncopal
syncytial
syncytioma

synctiotoxin
syndrome
    Achard-Thiers s.
    Ahumada-Del Castillo s.
    Allen-Masters s.
    Asherman's s.
    Brentano's s.
    Chiari-Frommel s.
    Curtius' s.
    Down's s.
    Dubovitz's s.
    Fitz-Hugh's s.
    Fritsch-Asherman s.
    Gordan-Overstreet s.
    Klinefelter's s.
    Klotz's s.
    Mayer-Rokitansky-
      Küster s.
    Meigs-Cass s.
    Meigs' s.
    Schroeder's s.
    Sheehan's s.
    Stein-Leventhal s.
    Turner's s.
    Young's s.
    Youssef's s.
synechia
    s. vulvae
synechiae
syo-. See words beginning *cyo-*.
syphilis
tampon
    Dührssen's t.
    Genupak t.
tandem
Tarnier's
    forceps
    sign
Tauber's spatula
Taussig-Morton operation
Taussig's operation
Teale's forceps

technique
    Brandt's t.
    Richardson's t.
telangiectatic
telangiecteric
Te Linde operation
Temple procedure
tenaculum
    Adair's t.
    Barrett's t.
    Braun's t.
    DeLee's t.
    Duplay's t.
    Jacobs' t.
    Kahn's t.
    marlex atraumatic t.
    Schroeder's t.
    sharp toothed t.
tent
    Laminaria t.
teratoma
teratome
tertigravida
tertipara
test
    agglutination inhibition t.
    Aschheim-Zondek t.
    AZ t.
    benzidine t.
    Biocept-G t.
    Brouha's t.
    chorionic gonadotropin t.
    Coombs' t.
    Corner-Allen t.
    cross-matching t.
    dexamethasone suppres-
      sion t.
    Dienst's t.
    Farris' t.
    fern t.
    fetal electrocardiogram t.
    fibrindex t.

test *(continued)*
- Friedman-Lapham t.
- Friedman's t.
- frog t.
- Galli-Mainini t.
- gravindex t.
- Hogben's t.
- Huhner's t.
- immunologic t.
- Kapeller-Adler t.
- Kline's flocculation t.
- Kupperman's t.
- Marchetti t.
- nitrazine t.
- norethindrone t.
- norethynodrel t.
- Pap t.
- Pregnosticon t.
- progesterone with-drawal t.
- Rho-Gam t.
- Rubin's t.
- Sabin-Feldman t.
- Schiller's t.
- Sims-Huhner t.
- Sulkowich's t.
- Thorn t.
- thymol turbidity t.
- toad t.
- ultrasound t.
- Visscher-Bowman t.
- von Poehl's t.
- Wampole's t.
- Wilson's t.
- *Xenopus laevis* t.

testiculoma
- t. ovarii

theca
- t. folliculi
- t. lutein

thecoma
thecomatosin
thecosis
thelarche
theleplasty
thelerethism
thelitis
thelorrhagia
thermogram
thermography

Thomas'
- curet
- operation
- pessary

Thoms'
- forceps
- pelvimeter

Thoms-Allis forceps
Thoms-Gaylor forceps
Thorn test
Tischler's forceps

tissue
- endometrial t.
- interstitial t.

titer
- rubella t.

topography
Torpin's operation
torsion
tortuosity
Touhey's needle
towel clamp
- Backhaus t.c.

toxemia
trachelectomy
trachelitis
tracheloplasty
trachelorrhaphy
trachelosyringorrhaphy
trachelotomy
traction handle
- Barton's t.h.
- Bill's t.h.
- Luikart-Bill t.h.

transplacental
transvaginal
treatment
  Brandt's t.
  Elliott's t.
  Rotunda t.
  Stroganoff's
    (Stroganov's) t.
triangle
  Pawlik's t.
Trichomonas vaginalis
trimester
trisomy
trocar
trophoblast
tube
  fallopian t.
  uterine t.
tuboabdominal
tuboadnexopexy
tuboligamentous
tubo-ovarian
tubo-ovariotomy
tubo-ovaritis
tuboperitoneal
tuboplasty
tubouterine
tubovaginal
Tucker-McLean forceps
Tuffier's operation
tumor
  Brenner's t.
  corticoadrenal t.
  Grawitz's t.
  hypernephroid t.
  Krukenberg's t.
  mesenchymal t.
  Scully's t.
  Sertoli-Leydig cell t.
  theca-cell t.
  Wilms' t.

tunica
  t. albuginea
  t. mucosa tubae uterinae
  t. mucosa urethrae
    femininae
  t. mucosa urethrae
    muliebris
  t. mucosa uteri
  t. mucosa vaginae
  t. muscularis cervicis
    uteri
  t. muscularis tubae
    uterinae
  t. muscularis urethrae
    femininae
  t. muscularis urethrae
    muliebris
  t. muscularis uteri
  t. muscularis vaginae
  t. serosa tubae uterinae
  t. serosa uteri
Turner's syndrome
Twombly's operation
Twombly-Ulfelder's operation
UC — uterine contractions
Uchida's operation
ulcus
  u. phagedaenicum
    corrodens
  u. vulvae acutum
ultrasound
umbilical cord
umbilicus
  amniotic u.
  decidual u.
unengaged
unicollis
unicornate
unicornis
unit
  Bovie u.

uremia
> puerperal u.

ureter
ureterouterine
ureterovaginal
urethra
> u. feminina
>
> u. muliebris

urethral
urethrocele
urethrovaginal
urethrovesical
urinary
urogenital
uteralgia
uterectomy
uteri
> fibromyomata u.

uterine
uterismus
uteritis
uteroabdominal
uterocentesis
uterocervical
uterodynia
uterofixation
uterogestation
uterography
uterolith
uteromania
uterometer
uterometry
utero-ovarian
uteropexy
uteroplacental
uteroplasty
uterorectal
uterosacral
uterosalpingography
uteroscope
uterothermometry
uterotomy

uterotonic
uterotropic
uterotubal
uterotubography
uterovaginal
uteroventral
uterovesical
uterus
> u. acollis
>
> arcuate u.
>
> u. arcuatus
>
> u. bicornis
>
> bicornuate u.
>
> u. biforis
>
> u. bilocularis
>
> u. bipartitus
>
> bosselated u.
>
> cochleate u.
>
> u. cordiformis
>
> Couvelaire u.
>
> u. didelphys
>
> duplex u.
>
> u. duplex
>
> fetal u.
>
> gravid u.
>
> u. incudiformis
>
> u. masculinus
>
> u. parvicollis
>
> pubescent u.
>
> u. septus
>
> u. simplex
>
> u. unicornis

utriculoplasty
vagina
vaginae
vaginal
vaginalectomy
vaginalis
> processus v.
>
> *Trichomonas v.*

vaginalitis
vaginapexy

vaginate
vaginectomy
vaginicoline
vaginiperineotomy
vaginismus
vaginitis
    v. adhaesiva
    atrophic v.
    catarrhal v.
    diphtheritic v.
    emphysematous v.
    glandular v.
    granular v.
    monilial v.
    papulous v.
    senile v.
    Trichomonas v.
vaginoabdominal
vaginocele
vaginocutaneous
vaginodynia
vaginofixation
vaginogenic
vaginogram
vaginography
vaginolabial
vaginometer
vaginomycosis
vaginopathy
vaginoperineal
vaginoperineorrhaphy
vaginoperineotomy
vaginoperitoneal
vaginopexy
vaginoplasty
vaginoscope
vaginoscopy
vaginotome
vaginotomy
vaginovesical
vaginovulvar

vagitus
    v. uterinus
    v. vaginalis
Valsuani's disease
Van Doren forceps
Van Hoorn's maneuver
varicocele
    ovarian v.
    utero-ovarian v.
vasa praevia
vasa propria of Jungbluth
vault
    vaginal v.
vectis
vein
    ovarian v.
velamentous
velamentum
ventrofixation
ventrohysteropexy
ventrosuspension
ventrovesicofixation
vernix
Vernon-David operation
Verres' needle
verruca
    v. acuminata
version
    bipolar v.
    Braxton-Hicks v.
    cephalic v.
    Hicks' v.
    podalic v.
    Potter's v.
    Wigand's v.
    Wright's v.
vertex
vesicle
    Baer's v.
    chorionic v.
    graafian v's

vesicle *(continued)*
    Naboth's v's
vesicocervical
vesicouterine
vesicouterovaginal
vesicovaginal
vesicovaginorectal
vesiculae graafianae
vesiculae nabothi
vestibule
    urogenital v.
    v. of vagina
vestibuli vaginae
vestibulourethral
vestibulum
    v. vaginae
viability
viable
vibrio
vibrodilator
villi
villus
Vim-Silverman needle
visceral
Visscher-Bowman test
vitiligo
Von Fernwald's sign
von Poehl's test
Voorhees'
    bag
    needle
vulva
    v. clausa
    v. conivens
    fused v.
    v. hians
vulvae
    kraurosis v.
    noma v.
vulval
vulvar
vulvectomy

vulvismus
vulvitis
    v. blenorrhagica
    creamy v.
    diabetic v.
    diphtheric v.
    diphtheritic v.
    eczematiform v.
    follicular v.
    leukoplakic v.
    monilial v.
    phlegmonous v.
    plasma cell v.
    pseudoleukoplakic v.
    ulcerative v.
vulvocrural
vulvopathy
vulvorectal
vulvouterine
vulvovaginal
vulvovaginitis
Waldmann's scissors
Walthard's cell
Walton-Schubert forceps
Walton's forceps
Wampole's test
Ward-Mayo vaginal
    hysterectomy
Warren's operation
Water's
    cesarean section
    operation
Watkins' operation
Watkins-Wertheim operation
Watson's method
Webster's operation
Weisman-Graves speculum
Weisman's forceps
Wertheim-Cullen forceps
Wertheim's
    forceps
    operation

Wertheim's *(continued)*
    radical hysterectomy
Wertheim-Schauta operation
Wesson's retractor
WF — white female
Wharton's operation
Whitacre's operation
Wigand's
    maneuver
    version
Willett's
    clamp
    forceps
William's
    operation
    pelvimeter
Williams-Richardson operation
Willy Meyer radical
    mastectomy
Wilms' tumor
Wilson's test
Wittner's forceps
wolffian
    w. cyst

wolffian *(continued)*
    w. duct
Wright's version
Wurd's catheter
Wylie's
    dilator
    operation
    pessary
Xenopus laevis test
xerogram
xerography
xeromammogram
xeromammography
xeromenia
Yellan clamp
Yeoman's forceps
yolk sac
Young's syndrome
Youssef's syndrome
zeromeneah. See *xeromenia.*
Zwanck's pessary
Zweifel-DeLee cranioclast
zygosity

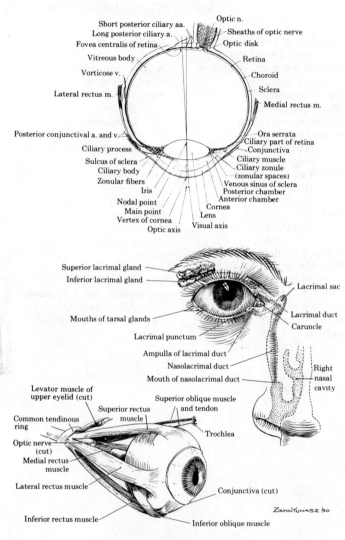

THE EYE AND RELATED STRUCTURES

OPHTHALMOLOGY

Abadie's sign
abducens
abduction
ab externus
abiotrophy
 retinal a.
ablatio
 a. retinae
ablation
ablepharia
ablepharon
ablepharous
ablephary
ablepsia
ablepsy
abrader
 Howard's a.
abrasio
 a. corneae
abrasion
abscess
abscessus
 a. siccus corneae
abscission
 corneal a.
Acc. — accommodation
accommodation
 absolute a.
 binocular a.
 excessive a.

accommodation *(continued)*
 negative a.
 positive a.
 relative a.
 subnormal a.
achlys
achroacytosis
achromatopia
achromatopic
achromatopsia
achromatosis
acne
 a. ciliaris
acorea
acuity
adaptation
 retinal a.
adaptometer
adduction
adenocarcinoma
adenologaditis
adenophthalmia
Adie's
 pupil
 syndrome
aditus
 a. orbitae
adnexa
 a. oculi
Aebli's scissors

463

affakia. See *aphakia.*
Agamodistomum
    A. ophthalmobium
Agnew's
    keratome
    operation
agnosia
    visual a.
Agrikola's retractor
akinesia
    O'Brien a.
    Van-Lint a.
akinesis
akinetic
aklis. See *achlys.*
aknephascopia
akro-. See words beginning
    achro-.
alacrima
albedo
    a. retinae
albinism
albuginea
    a. oculi
albugo
Alcon's cryophake
alexia
    optical a.
Alezzandrini's syndrome
Allen's implant
alopecia
    a. orbicularis
Alpar's implant
Alström-Olsen syndrome
amaurosis
    albuminuric a.
    Burns's a.
    cat's eye a.
    central a.
    a. centralis
    cerebral a.
    congenital a.

amaurosis *(continued)*
    diabetic a.
    a. fugax
    hysteric a.
    intoxication a.
    Leber's a.
    saburral a.
    uremic a.
amaurotic
ambiopia
amblyopia
    a. alcoholica
    arsenic a.
    astigmatic a.
    a. crapulosa
    a. cruciata
    a. ex anopsia
    nocturnal a.
    postmarital a.
    quinine a.
    reflex a.
    strabismic a.
    tobacco a.
    toxic a.
    traumatic a.
    uremic a.
amblyopiatrics
amblyoscope
ametrometer
ametropia
    axial a.
    curvature a.
    index a.
    position a.
    refractive a.
ametropic
Amh. — mixed astigmatism
        with myopia
        predominating
Ammon's operation
Amoils'
    cryoextractor

Amoils' *(continued)*
    cryoprobe
    retractor
amotio
    a. retinae
amphamphoterodiplopia
amplitude
    a. of accommodation
    a. of convergence
ampulla
    a. canaliculi lacrimalis
    a. ductus lacrimalis
ampullae
Amsler's
    grid
    needle
Anagnostakis' operation
anaphoria
Andogsky's syndrome
Anel's operation
anesthesia. See *General
    Surgical Terms.*
Angelucci's syndrome
angiodiathermy
angiography
    fluorescein a.
angioma
angiomatosis
    a. of retina
angiophakomatosis
angle
    alpha a.
    kappa a.
    minimum visual a.
    optic a.
angulus
    a. iridocornealis
    a. oculi lateralis
    a. oculi medialis
anhidrosis
anicteric

aniridia
aniseikonia
aniseikonic
anisoaccommodation
anisocoria
anisometrope
anisometropia
anisometropic
anisophoria
anisopia
ankyloblepharon
    a. filiforme adnatum
annular
    a. plexus
annulus
    a. ciliaris
    a. zinnii
anomalopia
anomaloscope
anomaly
    Peter's a.
anoopsia
anophoria
anophthalmia
anophthalmos
anophthalmus
anopia
anopsia
anorthopia
anotropia
Anthony's compressor
anthrax
Anton-Babinski syndrome
Anton's symptom
anulus
    a. of conjunctiva
    a. conjunctivae
    a. iridis major
    a. iridis minor
    a. tendineus communis
aphakia

aphakic
aphasia
    visual a.
aplasia
    retinal a.
applanation
applanometer
applicator
    Gifford's a.
aqueous
    a. humor
aquocapsulitis
arachnodactyly
arachnoiditis
    optochiasmatic a.
ARC — anomalous retinal
        correspondence
arch
    Salus' a.
arcus
    a. juvenilis
    a. lipoides corneae
    a. palpebralis inferior
    a. palpebralis superior
    a. parieto-occipitalis
    a. senilis
    a. superciliaris
argamblyopia
argema
Argyll-Robertson pupil
argyria
argyrosis
Arlt-Jaesche operation
Arlt's
    disease
    operation
    scoop
    sinus
    trachoma
Arroyo's sign
Arruga's
    expressor

Arruga's *(continued)*
    forceps
    implant
    operation
    protector
    trephine
arteriola
    a. macularis inferior
    a. macularis superior
    a. medialis retinae
    a. nasalis retinae inferior
    a. nasalis retinae superior
    a. temporalis retinae
        inferior
    a. temporalis retinae
        superior
arteriole
    medial a. of retina
    nasal a. of retina
    temporal a. of retina
artery
    cilioretinal a.
    hyaloid a.
    long posterior ciliary a.
    posterior conjunctival a.
    retinal a.
    short posterior ciliary a.
As. H. — hypermetropic
        astigmatism
As. M. — myopic astigmatism
Ast. — astigmatism
asthenocoria
asthenometer
asthenope
asthenopia
    accommodative a.
    muscular a.
    nervous a.
    retinal a.
    tarsal a.
asthenopic
astigmagraph

astigmatic
astigmatism
    a. against the rule
    corneal a.
    hypermetropic a.
    hyperopic a.
    lenticular a.
    myopic a.
    oblique a.
    a. with the rule
astigmatometer
astigmatoscope
astigmatoscopy
astigmia
astigmic
astigmometer
astigmometry
astigmoscope
Atkinson's technique
atresia
    a. iridis
atrophia
    a. choroideae et retinae
    a. dolorosa
    a. gyrata of choroid
atrophy
    Behr's a.
    Fuchs' a.
    Schnabel's a.
    senile a.
atropinism
atropinization
autokeratoplasty
axanthopsia
Axenfeld's syndrome
axis
    optic a.
    visual a.
bacillus
    Koch-Weeks b.
Badal's operation
Baer's nystagmus

Bahn's spud
Ballet's disease
Bamatter's syndrome
band
    silicone b.
Barany's sign
Bardelli's operation
Bard-Parker
    blade
    knife
Barkan's
    knife
    operation
Barraquer-Colibri speculum
Barraquer-DeWecker scissors
Barraquer's
    brush
    erysiphake
    forceps
    knife
    needle holder
    operation
    scissors
    speculum
    trephine
Barrio's operation
Bassen-Kornzweig syndrome
Basterra's operation
Batten-Mayou disease
Beal's
    conjunctivitis
    syndrome
Beaupre's forceps
Beaver's
    blade
    handle
    keratome
    knife
Beer's
    collyrium
    operation
Behçet's syndrome

Behr's
    atrophy
    disease
    pupil
    syndrome
Bekhterev's nystagmus
Bellows' cryoextractor
Bell's
    erysiphake
    palsy
    phenomenon
Benedikt's syndrome
Bennett's forceps
Benson's disease
Berens'
    dilator
    forceps
    implant
    keratome
    operation
    punch
    retractor
    scissors
    spatula
    speculum
Berens-Rosa implant
Bergemeister's papilla
Berke's
    clamp
    forceps
    operation
Berlin's
    disease
    edema
Berneheimer's fibers
Biber-Haab-Dimmer
    degeneration
Bielschowsky-Lutz-Cogan
    syndrome
Bielschowsky's
    disease
    operation

Bielschowsky's *(continued)*
    test
Bietti's
    dystrophy
    syndrome
bifocal
Binkhorst's implant
binocular
binoculus
binophthalmoscope
binoscope
biomicroscopy
    slit lamp b.
biopsy
Birch-Hirschfeld lamp
Bishop-Harmon
    cannula
    forceps
Bitot's spots
Bjerrum's
    scotoma
    scotometer
    screen
blade
    Bard-Parker b.
    Beaver's b.
    McPherson-Wheeler b.
Blair's operation
Blasius' operation
Blaskovics' operation
blastomycosis
Blatt's operation
blef-. See words beginning
    bleph-.
blennorrhea
    b. adultorum
    inclusion b.
    b. neonatorum
blepharadenitis
blepharal
blepharectomy
blepharelosis

blepharism
blepharitis
    b. angularis
    b. ciliaris
    b. marginalis
    nonulcerative b.
    seborrheic b.
    b. squamosa
    b. ulcerosa
blepharoadenitis
blepharoadenoma
blepharoatheroma
blepharochalasis
blepharochromidrosis
blepharoclonus
blepharoconjunctivitis
blepharodiastasis
blepharoncus
blepharopachynsis
blepharophimosis
blepharophryplasty
blepharoplast
blepharoplasty
blepharoplegia
blepharoptosis
blepharopyorrhea
blepharorrhaphy
blepharospasm
blepharosphincterectomy
blepharostat
blepharostenosis
blepharosynechia
blepharotomy
blepharoxysis
Blessig-Iwanoff cysts
Blessig's cysts
blind
    color b.
blindness
    amnesic color b.
    Bright's b.
    color b.

blindness *(continued)*
    cortical psychic b.
    letter b.
    snow b.
    twilight b.
block
    O'Brien b.
    retrobulbar b.
    Van-Lint b.
blow-out fracture
body
    ciliary b.
    cytoid b.
    Landolt's b's
    Prowazek-Greeff b's
Böhm's operation
Bonaccolto-Flieringa operation
Bonaccolto's
    forceps
    scleral ring
Bonnet-Dechaume-Blanc
    syndrome
Bonzel's operation
boosh de tah-per. See *bouche de tapir.*
Borthen's operation
Bossalino's operation
bouche
    b. de tapir
Bourneville's disease
Bovie unit
Bowen's disease
Bowman's
    membrane
    needle
    operation
    probe
Boyd's implant
Boynton's needle holder
Bracken's forceps
Braid's strabismus
Brailey's operation

Brawley's retractor
Briggs' operation
Bright's
    blindness
    eye
Bronson-Turz retractor
Brown-Dohlman implant
Bruch's membrane
Brücke's
    fibers
    lens
    muscle
Bruecke
    tunica nervea of B.
brush
    Barraquer's b.
    Haidinger's b's
Brushfield's spot
B scan ultrasonogram
Budinger's operation
bulbus
    b. oculi
Buller's shield
Bumke's pupil
bundle
    b. of Druault
Bunge's spoon
Bunker's implant
buphthalmia
buphthalmos
buphthalmus
bur
    Burwell's b.
Burch-Greenwood tucker
Burch's
    caliper
    operation
    pick
Burns's amaurosis
Burow's operation
Burwell's bur
Buzzi's operation

byerrum. See *Bjerrum.*
Cairns' operation
calculus
Calhoun-Merz needle
Calhoun's needle
caliculus
    c. ophthalmicus
caligo
    c. corneae
    c. lentis
    c. pupillae
caliper
    Burch's c.
    Castroviejo's c.
    Green's c.
    Jameson's c.
    Thorpe's c.
Callahan's operation
Calmette's ophthalmoreaction
Campbell's retractor
campimeter
campimetry
canal
    Ferrein's c.
    hyaloid c.
    Petit's c.
    c. of Schlemm
    Sondermann's c's
canaliculi
canaliculitis
canaliculodacryocystostomy
canaliculorhinostomy
canaliculus
    c. lacrimalis
cannula
    Bishop-Harmon c.
    Castroviejo's c.
    Goldstein's c.
    Moncrieff's c.
    Randolph's c.
    Roper's c.
    Tenner's c.

Cantelli's sign
canthectomy
canthi
canthitis
cantholysis
canthoplasty
canthorrhaphy
canthotomy
canthus
    inner c.
    outer c.
capsitis
capsula
    c. lentis
capsule
    c. of Tenon
capsulectomy
capsulitis
capsulolenticular
capsulotome
    Darling's c.
capsulotomy
carcinoma
    epidermoid c.
Carter's
    introducer
    operation
caruncle
    lacrimal c.
caruncula
    c. lacrimalis
Casanellas' operation
Caspar's ring opacity
Castallo's retractor
Castroviejo-Arruga forceps
Castroviejo-Kalt needle holder
Castroviejo's
    caliper
    cannula
    dilator
    forceps
    keratome

Castroviejo's *(continued)*
    knife
    needle holder
    operation
    punch
    retractor
    scissors
    spatula
    speculum
    trephine
cataphoria
cataract
    adherent c.
    adolescent c.
    after c.
    arborescent c.
    aridosiliculose c.
    aridosiliquate c.
    axial c.
    black c.
    blood c.
    blue dot c.
    bony c.
    bottlemakers' c.
    brunescent c.
    calcareous c.
    capsular c.
    capsulolenticular c.
    caseous c.
    cerulean c.
    cheesy c.
    choroidal c.
    congenital c.
    contusion c.
    coralliform c.
    coronary c.
    cortical c.
    cupuloform c.
    cystic c.
    diabetic c.
    discission c.
    dry-shelled c.

cataract *(continued)*
    embryonal nuclear c.
    extracapsular c.
    fibroid c.
    floriform c.
    fusiform c.
    glassblowers' c.
    glaucomatous c.
    heat-ray c.
    hedger's c.
    heterochromic c.
    hypermature c.
    immature c.
    incipient c.
    infantile c.
    intracapsular c.
    intumescent c.
    irradiation c.
    juvenile c.
    Koby's c.
    lacteal c.
    lamellar c.
    lenticular c.
    lightning c.
    mature c.
    membranous c.
    morgagnian c.
    myotonic c.
    naphthalinic c.
    nuclear c.
    O'Brien's c.
    overripe c.
    perinuclear c.
    peripheral c.
    polar c.
    primary c.
    progressive c.
    puddler's c.
    punctate c.
    pyramidal c.
    reduplication c.
    ripe c.

cataract *(continued)*
    sanguineous c.
    secondary c.
    sedimentary c.
    senile c.
    siliculose c.
    siliquose c.
    snowflake c.
    snowstorm c.
    spindle c.
    stationary c.
    stellate c.
    subcapsular c.
    subtotal c.
    sunflower c.
    sutural c.
    syphilitic c.
    total c.
    toxic c.
    traumatic c.
    tremulous c.
    unripe c.
    Vogt's c.
    zonular c.
cataracta
    c. accreta
    c. brunescens
    c. cerulea
    c. complicata
    c. congenita
      membranacea
    c. coronaria
    c. electrica
    c. membranacea accreta
    c. neurodermatica
    c. nigra
    c. ossea
    c. syndermotica
cataractous
catarrh
    vernal c.
catheterization

cautery
    Hildreth's c.
    Mueller's c.
    Rommel-Hildreth c.
    Rommel's c.
    Scheie's c.
    von Graefe's c.
    Wadsworth-Todd c.
    wetfield c.
    Ziegler's c.
cecal
cecocentral
Celsus' operation
centrocecal
cerebro-ocular
CF — counting fingers
c. gl. — correction with glasses
chalazia
chalazion
chalcosis
    c. lentis
chamber
    anterior c.
    aqueous c.
    posterior c.
    vitreous c.
Chandler's forceps
chart
    Reuss' color c's
    Snellen's c.
chemosis
Cheyne's nystagmus
chiasma
    c. opticum
    c. syndrome
chiasmal
    c. arachnoiditis
chloropsia
choriocapillaris
choriocele
chorioid
chorioidea

chorioretinal
chorioretinitis
chorioretinopathy
choroid
choroidal
choroidea
choroideremia
choroiditis
    areolar c.
    Doyne's c.
    Förster's c.
    c. guttata senilis
    juxtapapillitic c.
    c. myopica
    c. serosa
    syphilitic c.
    Tay's c.
    toxoplasmic c.
choroidocyclitis
choroidoiritis
choroidopathy
choroidoretinitis
Choyce's implant
Choyce Mark VIII implant
chromatopsia
chromatoptometer
cibisotome
cicatricial
cicatrix
cilia
ciliariscope
ciliarotomy
ciliary
    c. body
    c. muscle
    c. process
    c. vein
    c. zonule
ciliectomy
cilioretinal
    c. artery
    c. vein

cilioscleral
cilium
cillosis
cinching
circle
    Willis' c.
circlet
    Zinn's c.
clamp
    Berke's c.
    serrefine c.
Claude's syndrome
cleft
    corneal c.
clinometer
clinoscope
clip
    tantalum c.
Coats'
    disease
    retinitis
    ring
Cogan's
    dystrophy
    syndrome
Colibri's forceps
collarette
collimator
Collin-Beard operation
collyria
collyrium
    Beer's c.
coloboma
    c. of choroid
    Fuchs' c.
    c. iridis
    c. of iris
    c. lentis
    c. lobuli
    c. of optic nerve
    c. palpebrale
    c. retinae

coloboma *(continued)*
    c. of vitreous
commissura
    c. palpebrarum lateralis
    c. palpebrarum medialis
    c. superior Meynerti
commissurae supraopticae
commissure
    arcuate c.
    Gudden's c.
    interthalamic c.
    Meynert's c.
    optic c.
    palpebral c.
    posterior c., chiasmatic
    supraoptic c's
commotio
    c. retinae
compressor
    Anthony's c.
conclination
cone
    ocular c.
    retinal c.
    twin c's
    visual c.
conformer
    Fox's c.
conjugate
conjunctiva
conjunctival
conjunctiviplasty
conjunctivitis
    acne rosacea c.
    actinic c.
    anaphylactic c.
    arc-flash c.
    atopic c.
    atropine c.
    Beal's c.
    blennorrheal c.
    calcareous c.

conjunctivitis *(continued)*
    catarrhal c.
    chemical c.
    croupous c.
    diphtheritic c.
    diplobacillary c.
    eczematous c.
    Egyptian c.
    Elschnig's c.
    follicular c.
    gonococcal c.
    gonorrheal c.
    granular c.
    inclusion c.
    larval c.
    c. medicamentosa
    membranous c.
    meningococcus c.
    molluscum c.
    Morax-Axenfeld c.
    c. necroticans infectiosus
    Parinaud's c.
    Pascheff's c.
    c. petrificans
    phlyctenular c.
    prairie c.
    pseudomembranous c.
    purulent c.
    Samoan c.
    Sanyal's c.
    scrofular c.
    squirrel plague c.
    trachomatous c.
    c. tularensis
    uratic c.
    vernal c.
    welder's c.
    Widmark's c.
    Wucherer's c.
conjunctivodacryocystostomy
conjunctivoma
conjunctivoplasty

conjunctivorhinostomy
conoid
    Sturm's c.
conophthalmus
consensual
Contino's
    epithelioma
    glaucoma
conus
convergence
convergent
convergiometer
Copeland's
    implant
    retinoscope
copiopia
Coquille plano lens
Corbett's spud
coreclisis
corectasis
corectome
corectomedialysis
corectomy
corectopia
coredialysis
corediastasis
corelysis
coremorphosis
corenclisis
coreometer
coreometry
coreoplasty
corestenoma
coretomedialysis
coretomy
cornea
    conical c.
    c. farinata
    c. globosa
    c. guttata
    c. opaca
    c. plana

cornea *(continued)*
    sugar-loaf c.
    Vogt's c.
corneal
corneal graft
    lamellar c.g.
    mushroom c.g.
    penetrating c.g.
corneitis
corneoblepharon
corneoiritis
corneosclera
corneoscleral
corona
    c. ciliaris
    Zinn's c.
coroparelcysis
coroplasty
coroscopy
corotomy
corpus
    c. adiposum orbitae
    c ciliaris
    c. vitreum
correspondence
    anomalous retinal c.
    harmonious retinal c.
    retinal c.
cortex
    cerebellar c.
    c. lentis
couching
Credé's prophylaxis
crises
    Pel's c's
Critchett's operation
Crookes' lens
Crouzon's disease
cryoextraction
cryoextractor
    Amoils' c.
    Bellows' c.

cryogenic
cryophake
    Alcon's c.
    Keeler's c.
cryopexy
cryoprobe
    Amoils' c.
cryoptor
    Thomas' c.
cryostat
cryosurgery
cryotherapy
cryptoglioma
cryptophthalmia
cryptophthalmos
cryptophthalmus
crystalline
Csapody's operation
cul-de-sac
    conjunctival c.
Curdy's sclerotome
curette
    Gifford's c.
    Green's c.
    Heath's c.
    Meyhoeffer's c.
    Skeele's c.
Custodis' operation
Cutler-Beard operation
Cutler's implant
cyanosis
    c. bulbi
    c. retinae
cyclectomy
cyclicotomy
cyclitis
    heterochromic c.
    purulent c.
    serous c.
cycloanemization
cycloceratitis
cyclochoroiditis

cyclocryopexy
cyclodamia
cyclodialysis
cyclodiathermy
cycloduction
cycloelectrolysis
cyclogram
cyclokeratitis
cyclopentolate
cyclophoria
cyclophorometer
cyclopia
cycloplegia
cycloplegic
cycloscope
cyclotome
cyclotomy
cyclotropia
cyl. — cylindrical lens
cylicotomy
cylindrical
cyst
    Blessig-Iwanoff c's
    Blessig's c's
    meibomian c.
cystitome
cystitomy
cystotome
    von Graefe's c.
    Wheeler's c.
Czermak's operation
D. — diopter
dacryadenalgia
dacryadenitis
dacryadenoscirrhus
dacryagogatresia
dacryagogic
dacryagogue
dacrycystalgia
dacrycystitis
dacryelcosis
dacryoadenalgia

dacryoadenectomy
dacryoadenitis
dacryoblennorrhea
dacryocanaliculitis
dacryocele
dacryocyst
dacryocystalgia
dacryocystectasia
dacryocystectomy
dacryocystis
    phlegmonous d.
    syphilitic d.
    trachomatous d.
    tuberculous d.
dacryocystitis
dacryocystitome
dacryocystoblennorrhea
dacryocystocele
dacryocystoptosis
dacryocystorhinostenosis
dacryocystorhinostomy
dacryocystorhinotomy
dacryocystostenosis
dacryocystostomy
dacryocystosyringotomy
dacryocystotome
dacryocystotomy
dacryogenic
dacryohelcosis
dacryohemorrhea
dacryolin
dacryolith
    Desmarres' d.
dacryolithiasis
dacryoma
dacryon
dacryops
dacryopyorrhea
dacryopyosis
dacryorhinocystotomy
dacryorrhea
dacryosinusitis

dacryosolenitis
dacryostenosis
dacryostomy
dacryosyrinx
Dalrymple's
    disease
    sign
Darling's capsulotome
Daviel's
    operation
    scoop
    spoon
Davis'
    forceps
    knife needle
    spud
debrider
    Sauer's d.
declination
decompression
degeneration
    Biber-Haab-Dimmer d.
    hyaline d.
    Kozlowski's d.
    macular d.
    retinal lattice d.
    Vogt's d.
de Grandmont's operation
dehiscence
    iris d.
Dejean's syndrome
delacrimation
Del Toro's operation
Demours' membrane
deorsumduction
deorsumvergence
deorsumversion
Derf's needle holder
dermolipoma
Descartes' law
Descemet's membrane
descemetitis

descemetocele
Desmarres'
    dacryolith
    forceps
    knife
    law
    lid elevator
    retractor
    scarifier
detachment
    d. of retina
    retinal d.
    rhegmatogenous d.
    d. of vitreous
deutan
deuteranomalopia
deuteranopia
deviation
    primary d.
    secondary d.
    skew d.
Devic's disease
DeVilbiss' irrigator
DeWecker-Pritikin scissors
DeWecker's
    operation
    scissors
dextroclination
dextrocular
dextrocularity
dextrocycloduction
dextrocycloversion
dextroduction
dextrotorsion
dextroversion
dialysis
    d. retinae
diastasis
    iris d.
diathermy
dichromatopsia
diktyoma

dilator
      Berens' d.
      Castroviejo's d.
      Heath's d.
      Jones' d.
      Muldoon's d.
      Nettleship-Wilder d.
Dimitry-Bell erysiphake
Dimitry's erysiphake
Dimitry-Thomas erysiphake
Dimmer's keratitis
dimple
      Fuchs' d's
diopsimeter
diopter
      prism d.
dioptometer
dioptometry
dioptoscopy
dioptre
dioptric
dioptrics
dioptrometer
dioptrometry
dioptroscopy
dioptry
diplopia
      binocular d.
      heteronymous d.
      homonymous d.
      monocular d.
      paradoxical d.
      torsional d.
diplopiometer
diploscope
discission
disclination
disease
      Arlt's d.
      Ballet's d.
      Batten-Mayou d.

disease *(continued)*
      Behr's d.
      Benson's d.
      Berlin's d.
      Bielschowsky's d.
      Bourneville's d.
      Bowen's d.
      Coats' d.
      Crouzon's d.
      Dalrymple's d.
      Devic's d.
      Eales' d.
      Favre's d.
      Franceschetti's d.
      Gaucher's d.
      Graefe's d.
      Graves' d.
      Hand-Schüller-Christian
            d.
      Harada's d.
      Heerfordt's d.
      Hippel's d.
      Jensen's d.
      Kimmelstiel-Wilson d.
      Koeppe's d.
      Kuhnt-Junius d.
      Lauber's d.
      Leber's d.
      Lindau-von Hippel d.
      Masuda-Kitahara d.
      Mikulicz's d.
      Möbius' d.
      Niemann-Pick d.
      Norrie's d.
      Purtscher's d.
      Recklinghausen's d.
      Reis-Bücklers d.
      Reiter's d.
      Schilder's d.
      Sichel's d.
      Sjögren's d.

disease *(continued)*
    Vogt's d.
    Vogt-Spielmeyer d.
    von Hippel-Lindau d.
    von Recklinghausen's d.
    Wagner's d.
    Weil's d.
    Westphal-Strumpell d.
    Wilson's d.
disjugate
disk
    anangioid d.
    ciliary d.
    optic d.
    Placido's d.
    Rekoss' d.
    stroboscopic d.
dissector
    Green's d.
distichia
distichiasis
diurnal
divergence
divergent
Dix's spud
Doherty's implant
Donders'
    glaucoma
    law
dot
    Gunn's d's
    Mittendorf's d.
    Trantas' d's
Dougherty's irrigator
Douvas' rotoextractor
Doyne's
    choroiditis
    iritis
dropper
    Undine's d.
Drualt
    bundle of D.

drugs. See *Drugs and Chemistry* section.
drusen
Duane's syndrome
duct
    lacrimal d.
    lacrimonasal d.
    nasolacrimal d.
    tear d.
duction
ductus
    d. lacrimales
Duke-Elder lamp
Dupuy-Dutemps operation
Durr's operation
Duverger and Velter's operation
DVA — distance visual acuity
dyscoria
dysmegalopsia
dysopia
    d. algera
dysopsia
dystrophy
    Bietti's d.
    Cogan's d.
    corneal d.
    Fehr's d.
    Fleischer's d.
    Franceschetti's d.
    Francois' d.
    Fuchs' d.
    Groenouw's d.
    Maeder-Danis d.
    Meesmann's d.
    Pillat's d.
    Salzmann's d.
    Schlichting's d.
    Schnyder's d.
Eales' disease
Eber's forceps
echinophthalmia

echo-ophthalmography
ectasia
    e. iridis
ectiris
ectochoroidea
ectocornea
ectopia
    e. lentis
    e. pupillae congenita
ectropion
    e. cicatriceum
    cicatricial e.
    flaccid e.
    e. luxurians
    e. paralyticum
    e. sarcomatosum
    e. senilis
    e. spasticum
    e. uveae
ectropium
edema
    Berlin's e.
    Iwanoff's retinal e.
    Stellwag's brawny e.
Edinger-Westphal nucleus
edipism
egilops
Egyptian
    conjunctivitis
    ophthalmia
Ehrhardt's forceps
eikonometer
elastosis
    e. dystrophica
Eldridge-Green lamp
electrode
    Gradle's e.
    Kronfeld's e.
    Pischel's e.
    Weve's e.
electrocoagulation
electronystagmograph

electroparacentesis
electroretinogram
electroretinography
elevator
    Desmarres' lid e.
Elliot's
    operation
    trephine
Ellis' needle holder
Elschnig-O'Brien forceps
Elschnig's
    conjunctivitis
    forceps
    knife
    operation
    retractor
    spatula
    spoon
    spots
    syndrome
Ely's operation
Em. — emmetropia
embolism
    retinal e.
embryotoxon
emmetrope
emmetropia
emmetropic
endophthalmitis
    e. phakoanaphylactica
endothelioma
    Sidler-Huguenin's e.
endothelium
    e. camerae anterioris
      oculi
    corneal e.
ENG — electronystagmograph
enophthalmos
enophthalmus
enstrophe
entophthalmia
entoptic

entoptoscope
entoptoscopy
entoretina
entropion
    e. cicatriceum
    cicatricial e.
    e. spasticum
    e. uveae
entropium
enucleate
enucleation
enzymatic
EOM — extraocular movement
epiblepharon
epibulbar
epicanthal
epicanthus
epicauma
epiphora
episclera
episcleral
episcleritis
    gouty e.
    e. partialis fugax
episclerotitis
epitarsus
epithelioma
    Contino's e.
epitheliosis
    e. desquamativa conjunctivae
epithelium
    e. anterius corneae
    e. corneae
    corneal e.
    e. of lens
    e. lentis
equator
    e. bulbi oculi
    e. of crystalline lens
    e. of eyeball
    e. of lens

equator *(continued)*
    e. lentis
erysipelas
erysiphake
    Barraquer's e.
    Bell's e.
    Dimitry-Bell e.
    Dimitry's e.
    Dimitry-Thomas e.
    Harrington's e.
    Kara's e.
    L'Esperance's e.
    Maumenee's e.
    Nugent-Green-Dimitry e.
    Post-Harrington e.
    Sakler's e.
    Searcy's e.
    Viers' e.
erythropia
erythropsia
esodeviation
esophoria
esophoric
esotropia
esotropic
"E" test
euchromatopsy
euryopia
euthyphoria
Eversbusch's operation
eversion
evisceration
evulsio
    e. nervi optici
Ewald's law
exanthematous
excycloduction
excyclophoria
excyclotropia
exenteration
exodeviation
exophoria

exophoric
exophthalmic
exophthalmogenic
exophthalmometer
    Hertel's e.
    Luedde's e.
exophthalmometric
exophthalmometry
exophthalmos
    endocrine e.
    pulsating e.
exophthalmus
exorbitism
exotropia
exotropic
expressor
    Arruga's e.
    Heath's e.
    Smith's e.
externus
extorsion
extracapsular
extraction
    roto e.
extraocular
eye
    blear e.
    Bright's e.
    cinema e.
    dark-adapted e.
    epiphyseal e.
    exciting e.
    hare's e.
    Klieg e.
    lazy e.
    light-adapted e.
    monochromatic e.
    Nairobi e.
    parietal e.
    pineal e.
    pink e.

eye *(continued)*
    schematic e.
    Snellen's reform e.
    squinting e.
    sympathizing e.
eyeball
eyebrow
eyecup
eyeground
eyelash
eyelid
eyestrain
facies
    Hutchinson's f.
fako-. See words beginning
    phaco-.
farsighted
farsightedness
Fasanella-Servat operation
fascia
    f. bulbi
    Tenon's f.
Favre's disease
FB — foreign body
f.c. — foot candles
Federov's implant
Fehr's dystrophy
Ferree-Rand perimeter
Ferrein's canal
Ferris-Smith retractor
Ferris-Smith-Sewall retractor
fiber
    Berneheimer's f's
    Brücke's f's
    Müller's f's
    optic nerve f.
    Sappey's f's
    von Monakow's f's
fiberoptic
fiberoptics
fiberscope

fibroma
fibroplasia
    retrolental f.
fibrosarcoma
fibrosis
Fick's halo
Filatov-Marzinkowsky
    operation
Filatov's operation
Fink's retractor
Finnoff's transilluminator
Fisher's spud
fissure
    corneal f.
    palpebral f.
fistula
fixation
    binocular f.
Flajani's operation
flare
Fleischer's
    dystrophy
    ring
Flieringa's ring
flikten-. See words beginning
    phlycten-.
floaters
Florentine iris
Flouren's law
fluorescein
focus
Foerster's forceps
Foix's syndrome
fold
    epicanthal f.
    semilunar f. of con-
      junctiva
Foltz's valve
Fontana's space
foot-candle
foramen
    optic f. of sclera

forceps
    Arruga's f.
    Barraquer's f.
    Beaupre's f.
    Bennett's f.
    Berens' f.
    Berke's f.
    Bishop-Harmon f.
    Bonaccolto's f.
    Bonn's f.
    Bracken's f.
    capsule f.
    Castroviejo-Arruga f.
    Castroviejo's f.
    chalazion f.
    Chandler's f.
    Colibri's f.
    Davis' f.
    Desmarres' f.
    Eber's f.
    Ehrhardt's f.
    Elschnig-O'Brien f.
    Elschnig's f.
    fixation f.
    Foerster's f.
    Fuchs' f.
    Gifford's f.
    Green's f.
    Hartman's f.
    Heath's f.
    Hess' f.
    Hess-Barraquer f.
    Hess-Horwitz f.
    Holth's f.
    Hunt's f.
    Jameson's f.
    Judd's f.
    Kalt's f.
    Katzin-Barraquer f.
    Kelman's f.
    Kerrison's f.
    Kirby's f.

forceps *(continued)*
    Knapp's f.
    Kronfeld's f.
    Kuhnt's f.
    Kulvin-Kalt f.
    Lambert's f.
    Lister's f.
    Littauer's f.
    McCullough's f.
    McPherson's f.
    mosquito f.
    Noble's f.
    Noyes' f.
    Nugent's f.
    O'Brien's f.
    Perritt's f.
    Pley's f.
    Prince's f.
    Quevedo's f.
    Reese's f.
    Rolf's f.
    Sauer's f.
    Schweigger's f.
    Shaaf's f.
    Smart's f.
    Spero's f.
    Stevens' f.
    Thorpe's f.
    Verhoeff's f.
    von Graefe's f.
    von Mondak's f.
    Waldeau's f.
    Ziegler's f.
fornix
    inferior f.
foro-. See words beginning
    phoro-.
Forster-Fuchs black spot
Förster's
    choroiditis
    operation
    uveitis

Foster-Kennedy syndrome
fovea
    f. centralis
    f. trochlearis
Foville's syndrome
Foville-Wilson syndrome
Fox's
    conformer
    implant
    irrigator
    operation
    shield
fracture
    blow-out f.
Franceschetti's
    disease
    dystrophy
    operation
    syndrome
Francis' spud
Francois' dystrophy
Franklin glasses
Frey's implant
Fricke's operation
Friede's operation
Friedenwald's
    operation
    ophthalmoscope
    syndrome
Frost-Lang operation
Fuchs'
    atrophy
    coloboma
    dimples
    dystrophy
    forcpes
    heterochromia
    keratitis
    operation
    spot
    syndrome
Fuchs-Kraupa syndrome

Fukala's operation
fundus
    albinotic f.
    f. albipunctatus
    f. flavimaculatus
    f. oculi
    tessellated f.
    f. tigroid
funduscope
funduscopic
funduscopy
fusion
galactosemia
gargoylism
Gaucher's disease
Gaule's spots
Gayet's operation
gaze
    conjugate g.
Georgariou's operation
gerontotoxon, gerontoxon
    g. lentis
Gerstmann's syndrome
Gibson's irrigator
Gifford-Galassi reflex
Gifford's
    applicator
    curette
    forceps
    operation
    reflex
    sign
Gillies' operation
Gill's knife
Girard's operation
Giraud-Teulon law
glabella
gland
    inferior lacrimal g.
    Krause's g.
    lacrimal g.
    Manz's g's

gland *(continued)*
    meibomian g.
    Moll's g.
    Rosenmüller's g.
    superior lacrimal g.
    tarsal g.
    Wolfring's g.
    zeisian g.
glanders
glands of Zeis
glasses
    Franklin g.
    Hallauer's g's
glaucoma
    g. absolutum
    air block g.
    angle-recession g.
    aphakic g.
    apoplectic g.
    auricular g.
    capsular g.
    chronic narrow angle g.
    closed angle g.
    g. consummatum
    Contino's g.
    Donders' g.
    enzyme g.
    fulminant g.
    hemorrhagic g.
    g. imminens
    infantile g.
    inflammatory g.
    juvenile g.
    lenticular g.
    malignant g.
    narrow angle g.
    neovascular g.
    noncongestive g.
    obstructive g.
    open angle g.
    phakogenic g.
    phakolytic g.

glaucoma *(continued)*
 pigmentary g.
 g. simplex
 traumatic g.
 vitreous-block g.
 wide-angle g.
glaucomatous
glaucosis
glioma
 g. endophytum
 g. exophytum
 g. retinae
globe
Goldmann's applanation
 tonometer
Goldstein's
 cannula
 retractor
Gomez-Marquez's operation
Gonin's operation
goniophotography
goniopuncture
gonioscope
gonioscopy
goniosynechia
goniotomy
Gonnin-Amsler marker
gonoblennorrhea
gouge
 Todd's g.
Gowers' sign
Gradenigo's syndrome
Gradle's
 electrode
 operation
 retractor
Graefe's
 disease
 knife
 operation
 sign
 syndrome

graft
 corneal g.
granuloma
 g. iridis
Graves' disease
gray line
Green's
 caliper
 curette
 dissector
 forceps
 hook
 knife
 needle holder
 replacer
Gregg's syndrome
Greig's syndrome
grid
 Amsler's g.
Grieshaber's
 keratome
 needle
 needle holder
 trephine
Groenholm's retractor
Groenouw's dystrophy
Grossmann's operation
Gruning's magnet
Gudden's commissure
Guillain-Barré syndrome
Guist's implant
Gullstrand's
 law
 slit lamp
gumma
Gunn's
 dots
 syndrome
Gutzeit's operation
Guyton-Maumenee speculum
Guyton-Park speculum
Guyton's operation

H. — hypermetropia
Haab's magnet
Haag-Streit slit lamp
Haidinger's brushes
Haik's implant
Hallauer's glasses
Hallermann-Streiff syndrome
halo
    Fick's h.
    h. glaucomatosus
    glaucomatous h.
    h. saturninus
Halpin's operation
Halsey's needle holder
Hand-Schüller-Christian
    disease
handle
    Beaver's h.
Harada's
    disease
    syndrome
Harrington's erysiphake
Harrison's scissors
Hartman's forceps
Hartstein's retractor
Hasner's operation
Hassall-Henle warts
head-tilt test
Heath's
    curette
    dilator
    expressor
    forceps
Heerfordt's disease
Heine's operation
hemangioma
hemangiomatosis
hematoma
hemeralopia
hemianopia
    absolute h.
    altitudinal h.

hemianopia *(continued)*
    binasal h.
    bitemporal h.
    h. bitemporalis fugax
    congruous h.
    equilateral h.
    heteronymous h.
    homonymous h.
    incongruous h.
    nasal h.
    quadrantic h.
    temporal h.
    unilateral h.
    uniocular h.
hemianopic
hemianopsia
hemianoptic
hemianosmia
hemiopalgia
hemiopia
hemiopic
hemorrhage
Hemovac
Herbert's operation
Hering's
    law
    test
    theory
herpes
    h. corneae
    h. iridis
    h. ophthalmicus
    h. simplex
    h. zoster
Hertel's exophthalmometer
Hertwig-Magendie syndrome
Hess'
    forceps
    operation
    spoon
Hess-Barraquer forceps
Hess-Horwitz forceps

heterochromia
    Fuchs' h.
    h. iridis
heterophoralgia
heterophoria
heterophoric
heterophthalmia
heterophthalmos
heteropsia
heteroptics
heteroscopy
heterotropia
hexachromic
Hildreth's cautery
Hillis' retractor
Hippel-Lindau syndrome
Hippel's
    disease
    operation
hippus
Hirschberg's
    magnet
    method
Hm. — manifest hyperopia
Hogan's operation
Hollenhorst's plaque
Holmgren's test
Holth's
    forceps
    operation
    punch
homokeratoplasty
hook
    fixation h.
    Green's h.
    Jameson's h.
    Kirby's h.
    Nugent's h.
    O'Connor's h.
    Smith's h.
    Stevens' h.
    Tyrell's h.

hook *(continued)*
    von Graefe's h.
    Wiener's h.
Horay's operation
hordeolum
Horner-Bernard syndrome
Horner's
    law
    muscle
    ptosis
    pupil
    syndrome
Horner-Trantas spots
horopter
    Vieth-Muller h.
horror
    h. fusionis
Horvath's operation
Hosford's spud
Hotz's operation
Howard's abrader
Ht. — total hyperopia
Hudson's line
Hudson-Stähli line
Huey's scissors
Hughes'
    implant
    operation
humor
    aqueous h.
    h. aquosus
    h. cristallinus
    crystalline h.
    ocular h.
    vitreous h.
    h. vitreus
Hunt's forceps
Hutchinson's
    facies
    pupil
    syndrome
hyaline

hyalinization
hyalitis
    asteroid h.
    h. punctata
    h. suppurativa
hyaloid
    h. canal
    h. membrane
hyalomucoid
hyalonyxis
hydrophthalmia
hydrophthalmos
hydrophthalmus
hyperemia
hyperhidrosis
hyperkeratosis
hypermetropia
hyperopia
    facultative h.
    manifest h.
hyperopic
hyperphoria
hypertelorism
    ocular h.
    orbital h.
hypertonia
    h. oculi
hypertropia
hyphema
hypophoria
hypoplasia
hypopyon
hypotonia
    h. oculi
hypotonus
hypotony
hypotropia
ianthinopsia
ichthyosis
icteric
icterus
Iliff's operation

illusion
    Kuhnt's i.
image
    Purkinje's i.
    Purkinje-Sanson i's
implant
    acorn-shaped i.
    acrylic i.
    Allen's i.
    Alpar's i.
    Arruga's i.
    Berens' i.
    Berens-Rosa i.
    Binkhorst's i.
    Boyd's i.
    Brown-Dohlman i.
    build-up i.
    Bunker's i.
    Choyce's i.
    Choyce Mark VIII i.
    conical i.
    Copeland's i.
    corneal i.
    Cutler's i.
    Doherty's i.
    Federov's i.
    Fox's i.
    Frey's i.
    glass sphere i.
    gold sphere i.
    Guist's i.
    Haik's i.
    hemisphere i.
    Hughes' i.
    Ivalon's i.
    Levitt's i.
    Lincoff's i.
    lucite i.
    magnetic i.
    McGhan's i.
    Mules' i.
    plastic sphere i.

implant *(continued)*
    Plexiglas i.
    polyethylene i.
    Rayner-Choyce i.
    reverse-shape i.
    scleral i.
    scleral buckler i.
    semishell i.
    shelf-type i.
    shell i.
    Silastic i.
    silicone i.
    Snellen's i.
    sphere i.
    spherical i.
    sponge i.
    Stone's i.
    surface i.
    tantalum i.
    Teflon i.
    tire i.
    Troutman's i.
    tunneled i.
    Vitallium i.
    Wheeler's i.
    wire mesh i.
implantation
Imre's
    operation
    treatment
incarceration
incision. See *General Surgical
    Terms.*
incycloduction
incyclophoria
incyclotropia
infarction
infraduction
infraorbital
infraversion
intercilium
interpalpebral

interpupillary
intorsion
intracapsular
intraocular
intraorbital
introducer
        Carter's i.
IOP — intraocular pressure
iridal
iridalgia
iridauxesis
iridectasis
iridectome
iridectomesodialysis
iridectomize
iridectomy
    basal i.
    optic i.
    peripheral i.
    preparatory i.
    sector i.
    stenopeic i.
    therapeutic i.
iridectopia
iridectropium
iridemia
iridencleisis
iridentropium
irideremia
irides
iridesis
iridiagnosis
iridial
iridian
iridic
iridization
iridoavulsion
iridocapsulitis
iridocele
iridochoroiditis
iridocoloboma
iridoconstrictor

iridocorneosclerectomy
iridocyclectomy
iridocyclitis
iridocyclochoroiditis
iridocystectomy
iridodesis
iridodiagnosis
iridodialysis
iridodiastasis
iridodilator
iridodonesis
iridokeratitis
iridokinesia
iridokinesis
iridokinetic
iridoleptynsis
iridology
iridolysis
iridomalacia
iridomesodialysis
iridomotor
iridoncus
iridoparalysis
iridopathy
iridoperiphakitis
iridoplegia
iridoptosis
iridopupillary
iridorhexis
iridoschisis
iridosclerotomy
iridosteresis
iridotasis
iridotomy
iris
      bombé i.
      Florentine i.
      tremulous i.
      umbrella i.
irisopsia
iritic

iritis
    i. blennorrhagique á
      rechutes
    i. catamenialis
    diabetic i.
    Doyne's i.
    follicular i.
    gouty i.
    i. papulosa
    plastic i.
    purulent i.
    i. recidivans staphylo-
      cocco-allergica
    serous i.
    spongy i.
    sympathetic i.
    tuberculous i.
    uratic i.
iritoectomy
iritomy
irrigator
      DeVilbiss' i.
      Dougherty's i.
      Fox's i.
      Gibson's i.
      Rollet's i.
      Sylva's i.
Irvine's scissors
ischemia
    i. retinae
Ishihara's
      plate
      test
isocoria
isophoria
isopia
isopter
isoscope
Ivalon's implant
Iwanoff's retinal edema
Jacob's membrane

Jacobson's retinitis
Jaeger's
    keratome
    lid plate
Jaesche-Arlt operation
Jameson's
    caliper
    forceps
    hook
    operation
jaundice
Javal's ophthalmometer
jaw-winking
Jendrassik's sign
Jensen's
    disease
    retinitis
Jones' dilator
Judd's forceps
junction
    sclerocorneal j.
kahla-. See words beginning
    chala-.
kalko-. See words beginning
    chalco-.
Kalt's
    forceps
    needle holder
kappa angle
Kara's erysiphake
Katzin-Barraquer forceps
Katzin's scissors
Kaufman's vitrector
Kayser-Fleischer ring
Keeler's cryophake
Keith-Wagener retinopathy
Kelman's
    forceps
    operation
kemosis. See *chemosis*.
Kennedy's syndrome
keratalgia

keratectasia
keratectomy
keratic
keratitis
    acne rosacea k.
    actinic k.
    aerosol k.
    alphabet k.
    arborescens k.
    artificial silk k.
    band k .
    k. bandelette
    k. bullosa
    dendriform k.
    dendritic k.
    Dimmer's k.
    k. disciformis
    fascicular k.
    k. filamentosa
    Fuchs' k.
    herpetic k.
    hypopyon k.
    interstitial k.
    lagophthalmic k.
    lattice k.
    marginal k.
    metaherpetic k.
    mycotic k.
    neuroparalytic k.
    neurotrophic k.
    k. nummularis
    oyster shuckers' k.
    parenchymatous k.
    k. petrificans
    phlyctenular k.
    k. profunda
    k. punctata
    k. punctata subepithelialis
    k. pustuliformis profunda
    k. ramificata superficialis
    reaper's k.

keratitis *(continued)*
    reticular k.
    ribbon-like k.
    rosacea k.
    Schmidt's k.
    sclerosing k.
    scrofulus k.
    serpiginous k.
    k. sicca
    striate k.
    suppurative k.
    syphilitic k.
    Thygeson's k.
    trachomatous k.
    trophic k.
    vascular k.
    vasculonebulous k.
    vesicular k.
    xerotic k.
keratocele
keratocentesis
keratoconjunctivitis
    epidemic k.
    epizootic k.
    flash k.
    phlyctenular k.
    k. sicca
    viral k.
    welder's k.
keratoconus
keratocyte
keratoderma
keratoectasia
keratoglobus
keratohelcosis
keratohemia
keratoid
keratoiridocyclitis
keratoiridoscope
keratoiritis
keratoleptynsis
keratoleukoma

keratoma
keratomalacia
keratomata
keratome
    Agnew's k.
    Beaver's k.
    Berens' k.
    Castroviejo's k.
    Grieshaber's k.
    Jaeger's k.
    Kirby's k.
keratometer
keratometric
keratometry
keratomileusis
keratomycosis
keratonosus
keratonyxis
keratopathy
    band k.
keratophakia
keratoplasty
    optic k.
    tectonic k.
keratorhexis
keratoscleritis
keratoscope
keratoscopy
keratotomy
    delimiting k.
keratotorus
kerectasis
kerectomy
keroid
Kerrison's forceps
Key's operation
kias-. See words beginning
    chias-.
Kiloh-Nevin syndrome
Kimmelstiel-Wilson
    disease
    syndrome

kinescope
Kirby's
    forceps
    hook
    keratome
    knife
    operation
    retractor
    scissors
    spoon
Klieg eye
Knapp-Imre operation
Knapp's
    forceps
    knife
    knife needle
    operation
    retractor
    scissors
    scoop
    spatula
    speculum
    spoon
    streaks
    striae
knife
    Bard-Parker k.
    Barkan's k.
    Barraquer's k.
    Beaver's k.
    Castroviejo's k.
    Desmarres' k.
    Elschnig's k.
    Gill's k.
    Graefe's k.
    Green's k.
    Kirby's k.
    Knapp's k.
    Lancaster's k.
    Lundsgaard's k.
    McPherson-Wheeler k.
    McPherson-Ziegler k.

knife *(continued)*
    McReynolds' k.
    Parker's k.
    Scheie's k.
    Smith-Green k.
    Tooke's k.
    von Graefe's k.
    Weber's k.
    Wheeler's k.
    Ziegler's k.
knife needle
    Davis' k.n.
    Knapp's k.n.
    von Graefe's k.n.
Koby's cataract
Koch-Weeks bacillus
Koeppe's
    disease
    nodule
Koerber-Salus-Elschnig
    syndrome
Kofler's operation
kor-. See words beginning
    chor-.
korio-. See words beginning
    chorio-.
Kozlowski's degeneration
KP — keratitic precipitates
Kraupa's operation
Krause's
    gland
    syndrome
Kreiker's operation
Kriebig's operation
Kronfeld's
    electrode
    forceps
    retractor
Krönlein-Berke operation
Krönlein's operation
Krukenberg's spindle
Kuhnt-Junius disease

Kuhnt's
    forceps
    illusion
    operation
Kuhnt-Szymanowski
    operation
Kulvin-Kalt forceps
Kurz's syndrome
L & A — light and accommodation
Lacarrere's operation
lacrima
lacrimal
lacrimalin
lacrimase
lacrimation
lacrimator
lacrimatory
lacrimonasal
lacrimotome
lacrimotomy
lacus
    l. lacrimalis
LaForce's spud
Lagleyze's operation
lagophthalmos
lagophthalmus
Lagrange's
    operation
    scissors
lake
    lacrimal l.
Lambert's forceps
lamella
lamellar
lamina
    l. basalis
    l. basalis choroideae
    l. basalis corporis ciliaris
    l. choriocapillaris
    l. cribrosa sclerae
    l. elastica anterior

lamina *(continued)*
    l. elastica posterior
    episcleral l.
    l. episcleralis
    l. fusca sclerae
    l. limitans anterior
        corneae
    l. limitans posterior
        corneae
    orbital l.
    l. orbitalis ossis ethmoidalis
    l. papyracea
    l. superficialis musculi levatoris palpebrae superioris
    l. suprachorioidea
    suprachoroid l.
    l. suprachoroidea
    l. vasculosa chorioideae
    l. vasculosa choroideae
lamp
    Birch-Hirschfeld l.
    Duke-Elder l.
    Eldridge-Green l.
    Gullstrand's slit l.
    Haag-Streit slit l.
    slit l.
Lancaster's
    knife
    magnet
    speculum
lance
    Rolf's l.
Landolt's
    bodies
    operation
Langenbeck's operation
Lange's speculum
Larcher's sign
laser
    argon l.

laser *(continued)*
>l. photocoagulation
>ruby l.
>xenon arc l.

Lauber's disease

Laurence-Moon-Biedl
>syndrome

law
>Descartes' l.
>Desmarres' l.
>Donders' l.
>Ewald's l.
>Flouren's l.
>Giraud-Teulon l.
>Gullstrand's l.
>Hering's l.
>Horner's l.
>Listing's l.
>Sherrington's l.
>Snell's l.

LE — left eye

Leber's
>amaurosis
>disease

leiomyoma

leiomyosarcoma

lens
>achromatic l.
>acrylic l.
>adherent l.
>aplanatic l.
>apochromatic l.
>biconcave l.
>biconvex l.
>bicylindrical l.
>bifocal l.
>bispherical l.
>Brücke's l.
>cataract l.
>concave l.
>concavoconcave l.

lens *(continued)*
>concavoconvex l.
>contact l.
>converging l.
>convex l.
>convexoconcave l.
>Coquille plano l.
>Crookes' l.
>crystalline l.
>cylindrical l.
>decentered l.
>dispersing l.
>immersion l.
>iseikonic l.
>meniscus l.
>meter l.
>minus l.
>omnifocal l.
>orthoscopic l.
>periscopic l.
>planoconcave l.
>planoconvex l.
>prosthetic l.
>punktal l.
>retroscopic l.
>spherical l.
>Stokes' l.
>toric l.
>trifocal l.

lentectomize

lentectomy

lenticonus

lenticular

lenticulo-optic

lenticulostriate

lenticulothalamic

lentiform

lentiglobus

leptotrichosis
>l. conjunctivae

L'Esperance's erysiphake

leukokoria
leukoma
    l. adhaerens
Levitt's implant
levoclination
levocycloduction
levocycloversion
levoduction
levotorsion
levoversion
Lewis' scoop
lid everter
    Walker's l.e.
lid lag
lid plate
    Jaeger's l.p.
Liebreich's symptom
ligament
    canthal l.
    ciliary l.
    pectinate l.
    suspensory l. of lens
    Zinn's l.
limbal
    l. groove
limbi palpebrales anteriores
limbi palpebrales posteriores
limbus
    l. conjunctivae
    l. corneae
    l. luteus retinae
    l. of cornea
Lincoff's
    implant
    operation
    sponge
Lindau-von Hippel disease
Lindner's
    operation
    spatula
line
    Hudson's l.

line *(continued)*
    Hudson-Stähli l.
    Schwalbe's l.
    Stahli's l.
linea
    l. corneae senilis
lipemia
    l. retinalis
lipoma
liposarcoma
liquor
    l. corneae
    Morgagni's l.
Lister-Burch speculum
Lister's forceps
Listing's law
lithiasis
    l. conjunctivae
Littauer's forceps
Lockwood's tendon
Löhlein's operation
Londermann's operation
loop
    Meyer's l.
Lopez-Enriquez operation
Loring's ophthalmoscope
louchettes
Louis-Bar syndrome
loupe
    corneal l.
Löwenstein's operation
Lowe's
    ring
    syndrome
Luedde's exophthalmometer
Lundsgaard-Burch sclerotome
Lundsgaard's knife
luxation
Lyle's syndrome
lymphangiectasis
lymphangioma
lymphoma

lymphosarcoma
Machek-Blaskovics operation
Machek-Gifford operation
Machek's operation
Mackay-Marg tonometer
macrophthalmia
macrophthalmous
macropsia
macula
    m. corneae
    m. lutea retinae
    m. retinae
macular
    m. degeneration
    m. displacement
Maddox
    prism
    rod
Maeder-Danis dystrophy
Magitot's operation
magnet
    Gruning's m.
    Haab's m.
    Hirschberg's m.
    Lancaster's m.
    Storz' m.
Maier
    sinus of M.
Majewsky's operation
manner
    McLean's m.
Manz's gland
Marcus-Gunn phenomenon
Marfan's syndrome
Mariotte's spot
marker
    Gonnin-Amsler m.
Marlex mesh
Marlow's test
maser
Masselon's spectacles
Masuda-Kitahara disease

Mauksch's operation
Maumenee-Park speculum
Maumenee's erysiphake
Mauthner's test
Maxwell's
    ring
    spot
May's sign
McClure's scissors
McCullough's forceps
McGannon's retractor
McGavic's operation
McGhan's implant
McGuire's
    operation
    scissors
McIntire aspiration-irrigation
    system
McLaughlin's operation
McLean's
    manner
    scissors
    tonometer
McPherson-Castroviejo scissors
McPherson's
    forceps
    needle holder
    scissors
    spatula
    speculum
McPherson-Vannas scissors
McPherson-Wheeler
    blade
    knife
McPherson-Ziegler knife
McReynolds'
    knife
    operation
medications. See *Drugs and
    Chemistry* section.
Meesmann's dystrophy
megalocornea

megalophthalmos
megalophthalmus
megophthalmos
meibomian
    cyst
    gland
meibomianitis
meibomitis
melanoma
melanosis
    m. sclerae
Meller's
    operation
    retractor
Mellinger's speculum
membrana
    m. capsularis lentis
        posterior
    m. epipapillaris
membrane
    Bowman's m.
    Bruch's m.
    cyclitic m.
    Demours' m.
    Descemet's m.
    hyaloid m.
    Jacob's m.
meridian
meridiani bulbi oculi
meridional
mesh
    Marlex m.
    tantalum m.
mesiris
mesoretina
metamorphopsia
    m. varians
method
    Hirschberg's m.
metronoscope
Meyer's loop
Meyhoeffer's curette

Meynerti
    commissura superior of
        m.
Meynert's commissure
microblepharia
microblepharon
microcoria
microcornea
microgonioscope
microphakia
microphthalmia
microphthalmoscope
microphthalmus
micropsia
microptic
microscope
    Zeiss' m.
Mikulicz's
    disease
    syndrome
Millard-Gubler syndrome
Miller's syndrome
Minsky's operation
miosis
    irritative m.
    paralytic m.
    spastic m.
miotic
Mira
    photocoagulator
    unit
Mittendorf's dot
Möbius'
    disease
    sign
    syndrome
Moll's gland
Moncrieff's
    cannula
    operation
monocular
monoculus

Mooren's ulcer
Morax-Axenfeld conjunctivitis
Morax's operation
Morgagni's liquor
Mosher-Toti's operation
Motais's operation
movement
    conjugate m.
Mueller's
    cautery
    retractor
    speculum
Muldoon's dilator
Mules'
    implant
    operation
    scoop
Müller's
    fibers
    muscle
    trigone
Murdock-Wiener speculum
muscae volitantes
muscle
    Brücke's m.
    ciliaris m.
    ciliary m.
    Horner's m.
    inferior oblique m.
    inferior rectus m.
    lateral rectus m.
    levator m.
    levator palpebrae
      superior m.
    medial rectus m.
    Müller's m.
    obliquus inferior m.
    obliquus superior m.
    orbicular m. of eye
    orbital m.
    rectus inferior m.
    rectus lateralis m.

muscle *(continued)*
    rectus medialis m.
    rectus superior m.
    superior oblique m.
    superior rectus m.
My. — myopia
mydriasis
mydriatic
myectomy
myiocephalon
myiodesopsia
myodiopter
myopia
    axial m.
    indicial m.
    pernicious m.
    prodromal m.
myopic
    m. crescent
myotomy
Naffziger's operation
Nairobi eye
nasociliary
nasolacrimal
near-sight
nearsighted
nearsightedness
nebula
needle
    Amsler's n.
    Bowman's n.
    Calhoun-Merz n.
    Calhoun's n.
    Grieshaber's n.
    Stocker's n.
    Weeks' n.
needle holder
    Barraquer's n.h.
    Boynton's n.h.
    Castroviejo-Kalt n.h.
    Castroviejo's n.h.
    Derf's n.h.

needle holder *(continued)*
    Ellis' n.h.
    Green's n.h.
    Grieshaber's n.h.
    Halsey's n.h.
    Kalt's n.h.
    McPherson's n.h.
    Paton's n.h.
neovascularization
nerve
    abducens n.
    infratrochlear n.
    optic n.
Nettleship-Wilder dilator
neurectomy
    opticociliary n.
neurochorioretinitis
neurochoroiditis
neurodeatrophia
neuroepithelioma
neurofibroma
neuroretinitis
neuroretinopathy
    hypertensive n.
neurotomy
    opticociliary n.
nicking
Nida's operation
Niemann-Pick disease
Nizetic's operation
Noble's forceps
nodal
nodule
    Koeppe's n.
Norrie's disease
Noyes' forceps
NPC — near point of conver-
    gence
nucleus
    Edinger-Westphal n.
    Perlia's n.
Nugent-Gradle scissors

Nugent-Green-Dimitry
    erysiphake
Nugent's
    forceps
    hook
Nv. — naked vision
NVA — near visual acuity
nyctalopia
nystagmic
nystagmiform
nystagmograph
nystagmoid
nystagmus
    aural n.
    Baer's n.
    Bekhterev's n.
    Cheyne's n.
    disjunctive n.
    end position n.
    labyrinthine n.
    miner's n.
    optokinetic n.
    oscillating n.
    paretic n.
    pendular n.
    undulatory n.
    vestibular n.
    vibratory n.
nystagmus-myoclonus
nystaxis
O'Brien's
    akinesia
    block
    cataract
    forceps
occlusion
O'Connor-Peter operation
O'Connor's
    hook
    operation
ocular
oculentum

oculi
oculist
oculistics
oculocephalogyric
oculofacial
oculogyration
oculogyria
oculogyric
oculometroscope
oculomotor
oculomotorius
oculomycosis
oculonasal
oculopathy
    pituitarigenic o.
oculopupillary
oculoreaction
oculospinal
oculozygomatic
oculus
OD — oculus dexter — right
    eye
ofthal-. See words beginning
   ophthal-.
opacification
opacity
    Caspar's ring o.
opaque
operation
    Agnew's o.
    Ammon's o.
    Anagnostakis' o.
    Anel's o.
    Arlt-Jaesche o.
    Arlt's o.
    Arruga's o.
    Badal's o.
    Bardelli's o.
    Barkan's o.
    Barraquer's o.
    Barrio's o.
    Basterra's o.

operation *(continued)*
    Beer's o.
    Berens' o.
    Berke's o.
    Bielschowsky's o.
    Blair's o.
    Blasius' o.
    Blaskovics' o.
    Blatt's o.
    Böhm's o.
    Bonaccolto-Flieringa o.
    Bonnett's o.
    Bonzel's o.
    Borthen's o.
    Bossalino's o.
    Bowman's o.
    Brailey's o.
    Briggs' o.
    Budinger's o.
    Burch's o.
    Burow's o.
    Buzzi's o.
    Cairns' o.
    Callahan's o.
    Carter's o.
    Casanellas' o.
    Castroviejo's o.
    Celsus' o.
    Collin-Beard o.
    Critchett's o.
    Csapody's o.
    Custodis' o.
    Cutler-Beard o.
    Czermak's o.
    Daviel's o.
    de Grandmont's o.
    Del Toro's o.
    de Wecker's o.
    Dupuy-Dutemps o.
    Durr's o.
    Duverger and Velter's o.
    Elliot's o.

operation *(continued)*
    Elschnig's o.
    Ely's o.
    equilibrating o.
    Eversbusch's o.
    Fasanella-Servat o.
    Filatov-Marzinkowsky o.
    Filatov's o.
    Flajani's o.
    Förster's o.
    Fox's o.
    Franceschetti's o.
    Fricke's o.
    Friede's o.
    Friedenwald's o.
    Frost-Lang o.
    Fuchs' o.
    Fukala's o.
    Gayet's o.
    Georgariou's o.
    Gifford's o.
    Gillies' o.
    Girard's o.
    Gomez-Marquez's o.
    Gonin's o.
    Gradle's o.
    Graefe's o.
    Grossmann's o.
    Gutzeit's o.
    Guyton's o.
    Halpin's o.
    Hasner's o.
    Heine's o.
    Herbert's o.
    Hess' o.
    Hippel's o.
    Hogan's o.
    Holth's o.
    Horay's o.
    Horvath's o.
    Hotz's o.
    Hughes' o.

operation *(continued)*
    Iliff's o.
    Imre's o.
    Jaesche-Arlt o.
    Jameson's o.
    Kelman's o.
    Key's o.
    Kirby's o.
    Knapp-Imre o.
    Knapp's o.
    Kofler's o.
    Kraupa's o.
    Kreiker's o.
    Kriebig's o.
    Krönlein-Berke o.
    Krönlein's o.
    Kuhnt's o.
    Kuhnt-Szymanowski o.
    Lacarrere's o.
    Lagleyze's o.
    Lagrange's o.
    Landolt's o.
    Langenbeck's o.
    Lincoff's o.
    Lindner's o.
    Löhlein's o.
    Londermann's o.
    Lopez-Enriquez o.
    Löwenstein's o.
    Machek-Blaskovics o.
    Machek-Gifford o.
    Machek's o.
    Magitot's o.
    magnet o.
    Majewsky's o.
    Mauksch's o.
    McGavic's o.
    McGuire's o.
    McLaughlin's o.
    McReynolds' o.
    Meller's o.
    Minsky's o.

operation *(continued)*
  Moncrieff's o.
  Morax's o.
  Mosher-Toti's o.
  Motais's o.
  Mules' o.
  Naffziger's o.
  Nida's o.
  Nizetic's o.
  O'Connor-Peter o.
  O'Connor's o.
  Panas' o.
  Paufique's o.
  Peter's o.
  Physick's o.
  Polyak's o.
  Poulard's o.
  Power's o.
  Quaglino's o.
  Raverdino's o.
  Richet's o.
  Rowinski's o.
  Rubbrecht's o.
  Saemisch's o.
  Scheie's o.
  Schmalz's o.
  Silva-Costa o.
  Smith-Kuhnt-Szyma-
    nowski o.
  Smith's o.
  Snellen's o.
  Soria's o.
  Sourdille's o.
  Spaeth's o.
  Speas' o.
  Spencer-Watson o.
  Stallard's o.
  Stock's o.
  Suarez-Villafranca o.
  Szymanowski-Kuhnt o.
  Szymanowski's o.
  Tansley's o.

operation *(continued)*
  Terson's o.
  Thomas' o.
  Toti-Mosher o.
  Toti's o.
  Trantas' o.
  Troutman's o.
  Verhoeff's o.
  Verwey's o.
  von Graefe's o.
  Waldhauer's o.
  Weekers' o.
  Weeks' o.
  West's o.
  Weve's o.
  Wheeler's o.
  Wicherkiewicz' o.
  Wiener's o.
  Wilmer's o.
  Wolfe's o.
  Worth's o.
  Ziegler's o.
Ophth. — ophthalmology
ophthalmagra
ophthalmalgia
ophthalmatrophia
ophthalmectomy
ophthalmencephalon
ophthalmia
  actinic ray o.
  catarrhal o.
  caterpillar o.
  o. eczematosa
  Egyptian o.
  electric o.
  o. electrica
  flash o.
  gonorrheal o.
  granular o.
  o. hivialis
  jequirity o.
  metastatic o.

ophthalmia *(continued)*
    migratory o.
    mucous o.
    o. neonatorum
    neuroparalytic o.
    o. nodosa
    phlyctenular o.
    purulent o.
    scrofulous o.
    strumous o.
    sympathetic o.
    ultraviolet ray o.
    varicose o.
ophthalmiatrics
ophthalmic
ophthalmin
ophthalmitic
ophthalmitis
ophthalmoblennorrhea
ophthalmocarcinoma
ophthalmocele
ophthalmocopia
ophthalmodesmitis
ophthalmodiagnosis
ophthalmodiaphanoscope
ophthalmodiastimeter
ophthalmodonesis
ophthalmodynamometer
ophthalmodynamometry
ophthalmodynia
ophthalmoeikonometer
ophthalmofunduscope
ophthalmograph
ophthalmography
ophthalmogyric
ophthalmoleukoscope
ophthalmolith
ophthalmologic
ophthalmologist
ophthalmology
ophthalmomalacia

ophthalmometer
    Javal's o.
ophthalmometroscope
ophthalmometry
ophthalmomycosis
ophthalmomyiasis
ophthalmomyitis
ophthalmomyositis
ophthalmomyotomy
ophthalmoneuritis
ophthalmoneuromyelitis
ophthalmopathy
ophthalmophacometer
ophthalmophantom
ophthalmophlebotomy
ophthalmophthisis
ophthalmoplasty
ophthalmoplegia
    basal o.
    exophthalmic o.
    o. externa
    fascicular o.
    o. interna
    internuclear o.
    nuclear o.
    orbital o.
    Parinaud's o.
    o. partialis
    o. progressiva
    Sauvineau's o.
    o. totalis
ophthalmoplegic
ophthalmoptosis
ophthalmoreaction
    Calmette's o.
ophthalmorrhagia
ophthalmorrhea
ophthalmorrhexis
ophthalmoscope
    Friedenwald's o.
    ghost o.

ophthalmoscope *(continued)*
    Loring's o.
ophthalmoscopy
    binocular indirect o.
    direct o.
    medical o.
    metric o.
ophthalmostasis
ophthalmostat
ophthalmostatometer
ophthalmosteresis
ophthalmosynchysis
ophthalmothermometer
ophthalmotomy
ophthalmotonometer
ophthalmotonometry
ophthalmotoxin
ophthalmotrope
ophthalmotropometer
ophthalmovascular
ophthalmoxerosis
ophthalmoxyster
optesthesia
optic
    o. axis
    o. chiasm
    o. disk
    o. nerve
    o. neuritis
    o. tract
optical
optician
opticianry
opticist
opticociliary
opticocinerea
opticokinetic
opticonasion
opticopupillary
optics
optist
optoblast

optogram
optomeninx
optometer
optometrist
optometry
optomyometer
optophone
optostriate
optotype
ora
    o. serrata
    o. serrata retinae
orbicularis
    o. ciliaris
    o. oculi
orbiculus
    o. ciliaris
orbit
orbita
orbitae
orbital
orbitale
orbitalis
orbitonasal
orbitonometer
orbitonometry
orbitostat
orbitotemporal
orbitotomy
orthometer
orthophoria
    asthenic o.
orthophoric
orthoptic
orthoptics
orthoptist
orthoptoscope
orthoscope
orthoscopy
OS — oculus sinister — left eye
ossification
osteoma

OU — oculus unitas — both
    eyes
    oculus uterque — each
    eye
pachyblepharon
pachyblepharosis
palpebra
    tertius p.
palpebrae
palpebral
palpebralis
palpebrate
palpebration
palpebritis
palsy
    Bell's p.
Panas' operation
pannus
    p. carnosus
    p. crassus
    p. degenerativus
    p. eczematosus
    phlyctenular p.
    p. siccus
    p. tenuis
    p. trachomatosus
panophthalmia
panophthalmitis
panoptic
pantankyloblepharon
papilla
    Bergemeister's p.
    lacrimal p.
    optic p.
papillary
papilledema
papillitis
papilloma
papilloretinitis
parenchyma
    p. of lens
paresis

Parinaud's
    conjunctivitis
    ophthalmoplegia
    syndrome
Parker's knife
Park's speculum
parophthalmia
parophthalmoncus
paropsis
pars
    p. caeca retinae
    p. ciliaris retinae
    p. iridica retinae
    p. marginalis musculi
        orbicularis oris
    p. optica retinae
    p. orbitalis glandulae
        lacrimalis
    p. orbitalis musculi
        orbicularis oculi
    p. palpebralis glandulae
        lacrimalis
    p. palpebralis musculi
        orbicularis oculi
    p. plana corporis ciliaris
    p. plicata corporis
        ciliaris
pars planitis
Pascheff's conjunctivitis
patch
Paton's needle holder
Paufique's
    operation
    trephine
PD — interpupillary distance
    prism diopter
pectinate
Pel's crises
pemphigus
perception
    light and color p.
peribulbar

perilenticular
perimeter
    Ferree-Rand p.
periophthalmitis
periorbita
periorbital
periorbititis
periosteum
peripapillary
periphacitis
peripheral
peripheraphose
periscleral
peritectomy
peritomize
peritomy
PERLA — pupils equal, react
           to light and ac-
           commodation
Perlia's nucleus
Perritt's forceps
PERRLA — pupils equal,
         round, regular,
         react to light and
         accommodation
Peter's
    anomaly
    operation
Petit's canal
Petzetakis-Takos syndrome
phacoanaphylaxis
phacocele
phacocyst
phacocystectomy
phacocystitis
phacoemulsification
phacoerysis
phacoglaucoma
phacohymenitis
phacoiditis
phacoidoscope
phacolysis

phacolytic
phacomalacia
phacometachoresis
phacometer
phacopalingenesis
phacoplanesis
phacosclerosis
phacoscope
phacoscopy
phacoscotasmus
phacotoxic
phacozymase
phakitis
phakoma
phakomatosis
phenomenon
    Bell's p.
    Marcus-Gunn p.
phlyctena
phlyctenar
phlyctenoid
phlyctenosis
phlyctenular
phlyctenule
phoria
phoriascope
phorometer
phorometry
phoropter
phoroscope
phorotone
photocoagulation
photocoagulator
    Mira p.
    Zeiss' p.
photography
    fluorescence retinal p.
photo-ophthalmia
photophobia
photophthalmia
photopia
photopic

photopsia
photoptometer
photoptometry
phthiriasis
phthisis
>p. bulbi
>p. corneae
>ocular p.

Physick's operation
pick
>Burch's p.

Pick's
>retinitis
>vision

pigmentation
pigmentum
>p. nigrum

Pillat's dystrophy
pin
>Pischel's p.
>Walker's p.

pinguecula
Pischel's
>electrode
>pin

Placido's disk
pladarosis
plaque
>Hollenhorst's p.

plate
>Ishihara's p.
>tarsal p.

Plexiglas implant
plexus
>annular p.
>intraepithelial p.
>ophthalmic p.
>p. ophthalmicus
>subepithelial p.

Pley's forceps
plica
>p. lacrimalis

plica *(continued)*
>p. palpebronasalis
>p. semilunaris conjunctivae

plicae
>p. ciliares
>p. iridis

poliosis
Polyak's operation
polycoria
>p. spuria
>p. vera

polyopia, polyopsia
>binocular p.
>p. monophthalmica

polyp
Posner-Schlossman syndrome
Post-Harrington erysiphake
Poulard's operation
Power's operation
Pr. — presbyopia
preretinal
presbyope
presbyopia
presbyopic
presenile
>p. melanosis

Prince's forceps
prism
>p. diopter
>Maddox p.
>Risley's p.

Pritikin's punch
probe
>Bowman's p.
>Theobald's p.
>Williams' p.
>Ziegler's p.

prolapse
prophylaxis
>Credé's p.

proptometer

proptosis
prosthesis
protanomalopia
protanomalous
protanomaly
protanopia
protanopic
protanopsia
protector
    Arruga's p.
protrusion
Prowazek-Greeff bodies
PRRE — pupils round, regular,
      and equal
pseudoglioma
pseudoneuritis
pseudonystagmus
pseudopapilledema
pseudophakia
    p. adiposa
    p. fibrosa
pseudopterygium
pseudoptosis
pseudoretinitis pigmentosa
pterion
pterygium
ptosis
    p. adiposa
    Horner's p.
    p. lipomatosis
    p. sympathica
ptotic
punch
    Berens' p.
    Castroviejo's p.
    Holth's p.
    Pritikin's p.
    Rubin-Holth p.
    Walton's p.
puncta
punctum
    p. caecum

punctum *(continued)*
    lacrimal p.
    p. lacrimale
pupil
    Adie's p.
    Argyll-Robertson p.
    Behr's p.
    bounding p.
    Bumke's p.
    cat's eye p.
    cornpicker's p.
    fixed p.
    Horner's p.
    Hutchinson's p.
    keyhole p.
    pinhole p.
    skew p's
    stiff p.
    tonic p.
pupilla
pupillary
pupillatonia
pupillograph
pupillometer
pupillometry
pupillomotor
pupilloplegia
pupilloscope
pupilloscopy
pupillostatometer
pupillotonia
Purkinje's image
Purkinje-Sanson images
Purtscher's
    angiopathic retinopathy
    disease
quadrantanopia
quadrantanopsia
Quaglino's operation
Quevedo's forceps
rabdomiomah. See
    rhabdomyoma.

ramollitio
    r. retinae
Randolph's cannula
Raverdino's operation
Rayner-Choyce implant
recession
Recklinghausen's disease
reclination
Reese's
    forceps
    syndrome
reflex
    Gifford-Galassi r.
    Gifford's r.
    red r.
    tapetal light r.
    Weiss's r.
refract
refraction
    double r.
    dynamic r.
    homatropine r.
    static r.
refractionist
refractive
refractometer
refractometry
refractor
Reis-Bücklers disease
Reiter's
    disease
    syndrome
Rekoss' disk
replacer
    Green's r.
resection
retina
    coarctate r.
    leopard r.
    nasal r.
    physiological r.
    shot silk r.

retina *(continued)*
    temporal r.
    tigroid r.
    watered silk r.
retinal
    r. detachment
retinascope
retinitis
    actinic r.
    r. albuminurica
    apoplectic r.
    central angiospastic r.
    r. centralis serosa
    r. circinata
    circinate r.
    Coats' r.
    diabetic r.
    r. disciformans
    exudative r.
    r. gravidarum
    gravidic r.
    r. haemorrhagica
    hypertensive r.
    Jacobson's r.
    Jensen's r.
    leukemic r.
    metastatic r.
    r. nephritica
    Pick's r.
    r. pigmentosa
    r. proliferans
    r. punctata albescens
    punctate r.
    renal r.
    serous r.
    solar r.
    splenic r.
    r. stellata
    striate r.
    suppurative r.
    r. syphilitica
    uremic r.

retinitis *(continued)*
    Wagener's r.
retinoblastoma
retinochoroid
retinochoroiditis
    r. juxtapapillaris
retinocytoma
retinodialysis
retinograph
retinography
retinoid
retinomalacia
retinopapillitis
retinopathy
    central disk-shaped r.
    circinate r.
    diabetic r.
    exudative r.
    Keith-Wagener r.
    leukemic r.
    pigmentary r.
    Purtscher's angiopathic r.
retinoschisis
retinoscope
    Copeland's r.
retinoscopy
retinosis
retinotopic
retinotoxic
retractor
    Agrikola's r.
    Amoils' r.
    Berens' r.
    Brawley's r.
    Bronson-Turz r.
    Campbell's r.
    Castallo's r.
    Castroviejo's r.
    Desmarres' r.
    Elschnig's r.
    Ferris-Smith r.
    Ferris-Smith-Sewall r.

retractor *(continued)*
    Fink's r.
    Goldstein's r.
    Gradle's r.
    Groenholm's r.
    Hartstein's r.
    Hillis' r.
    Kirby's r.
    Knapp's r.
    Kronfeld's r.
    McGannon's r.
    Meller's r.
    Mueller's r.
    Rizzuti's r.
    Rollet's r.
    Stevenson's r.
retrobulbar
retroiridian
retrolental
retrolenticular
retro-ocular
retro-orbital
retrotarsal
Reuss'
    color charts
    tables
rhabdomyoma
rhinommectomy
rhinoptia
rhytidosis
Richet's operation
Riddoch's syndrome
Rieger's syndrome
Rifkind's sign
Riley-Day syndrome
rima
    r. cornealis
ring
    Bonaccolto's scleral r.
    ciliary r.
    Coats' r.
    common tendinous r.

ring *(continued)*
    conjunctival r.
    Fleischer's r.
    Flieringa's r.
    glaucomatous r.
    Kayser-Fleischer r.
    Lowe's r.
    Maxwell's r.
    Soemmering's r.
    Vossius' lenticular r.
rinommektome. See
    rhinommectomy.
Risley's prism
ritidosis. See *rhytidosis.*
rivus
    r. lacrimalis
Rizzuti's retractor
RLF — retrolental fibroplasia
rod
    Maddox r.
    retinal r's
Rolf's
    forceps
    lance
Rollet's
    irrigator
    retractor
    syndrome
Romana's sign
Rommel-Hildreth cautery
Rommel's cautery
Rönne's nasal step
Roper's cannula
Rosenmüller's gland
Rot-Bielschowsky syndrome
Rothmund's syndrome
Roth's spot
rotoextractor
    Douvas' r.
Rowinski's operation
Rubbrecht's operation

rubeosis
    r. iridis
    r. retinae
Rubin-Holth punch
rupture
Rutherfurd's syndrome
sac
    lacrimal s.
    tear s.
saccade
saccadic
sacculus
    s. lacrimalis
Saemisch's
    operation
    ulcer
Sakler's erysiphake
Salus' arch
Salzmann's dystrophy
Samoan conjunctivitis
Sanyal's conjunctivitis
Sappey's fibers
sarcoma
Sattler's veil
Sauer's
    debrider
    forceps
    speculum
Sauvineau's ophthalmoplegia
scalpel
scarifier
    Desmarres' s.
Scarpa's staphyloma
Schäfer's syndrome
Scheie's
    cautery
    knife
    operation
Schilder's disease
Schiøtz' tonometer
Schirmer's test

Schlemm's canal
Schlichting's dystrophy
Schmalz's operation
Schmidt's keratitis
Schnabel's atrophy
Schnyder's dystrophy
Schöbl's scleritis
Schöler's treatment
Schön's theory
Schwalbe's line
Schweigger's forceps
scirrhoblepharoncus
scirrhophthalmia
scissors
    Aebli's s.
    Barraquer-DeWecker s.
    Barraquer's s.
    Berens' s.
    canalicular s.
    Castroviejo's s.
    corneoscleral s.
    DeWecker-Pritikin s.
    DeWecker's s.
    Harrison's s.
    Huey's s.
    iris s.
    Irvine's s.
    Katzin's s.
    Kirby's s.
    Knapp's s.
    Lagrange's s.
    McClure's s.
    McGuire's s.
    McLean's s.
    McPherson-Castroviejo s.
    McPherson's s.
    McPherson-Vannas s.
    Nugent-Gradle s.
    Smart's s.
    Spencer's s.
    Stevens' s.
    Thorpe-Castroviejo s.

scissors *(continued)*
    Thorpe's s.
    Thorpe-Wescott s.
    Vannas' s.
    Verhoeff's s.
    Walker's s.
    Westcott's s.
    Wilmer's s.
sclera
scleral
    s. crescent
    s. icterus
    s. spur
scleratitis
sclerectasia
sclerectasis
sclerectoiridectomy
sclerectoiridodialysis
sclerectome
sclerectomy
scleriasis
scleriritomy
scleritis
    Schöbl's s.
sclerocataracta
sclerochoroiditis
scleroconjunctival
scleroconjunctivitis
sclerocornea
sclerocorneal
scleroiritis
sclerokeratitis
sclerokeratoiritis
sclerokeratosis
scleromalacia
    s. perforans
scleronyxis
sclero-optic
sclerophthalmia
scleroplasty
sclerostomy
scleroticectomy

scleroticochoroiditis
scleroticonyxis
scleroticopuncture
scleroticotomy
sclerotitis
sclerotome
    Curdy's s.
    Lundsgaard-Burch s.
sclerotomy
scoop
    Arlt's s.
    Daviel's s.
    Knapp's s.
    Lewis' s.
    Mules' s.
    Wilder's s.
scotoma
    arcuate s.
    Bjerrum's s.
    centrocecal s.
    paracentral s.
    peripapillary s.
    scintillating s.
    Seidel's s.
scotomagraph
scotomameter
scotomatous
scotometer
    Bjerrum's s.
scotometry
screen
    Bjerrum's s.
    tangent s.
Searcy's erysiphake
Seidel's scotoma
senile
septum
    orbital s.
    s. orbitale
s. gl. — without correction
Shaaf's forceps
Sherrington's law

shield
    Buller's s.
    Fox's s.
shogrenz. See *Sjögren's.*
Sichel's disease
siderosis
    s. bulbi
    s. conjunctivae
Sidler-Huguenin's endothelioma
Siegrist-Hutchinson syndrome
sign
    Abadie's s.
    Arroyo's s.
    Barany's s.
    Cantelli's s.
    Dalrymple's s.
    Gifford's s.
    Gowers' s.
    Graefe's s.
    Jendrassik's s.
    Larcher's s.
    May's s.
    Möbius' s.
    Rifkind's s.
    Romana's s.
    Stellwag's s.
    von Graefe's s.
    Weber's s.
    Wilder's s.
Silastic implant
siliquose
sillonneur
Silva-Costa operation
sinistrocular
sinistrocularity
sinistrogyration
sinistrotorsion
sinus
    Arlt's s.
    s. of Maier
    s. venosus sclerae

sinus *(continued)*
    venous s. of sclera
Sjögren's
    disease
    syndrome
Skeele's curette
skiametry
skiascopy
Sklar-Schiøtz' tonometer
sleeve
    Watzke's s.
slit lamp
Smart's
    forceps
    scissors
Smith-Green knife
Smith-Kuhnt-Szymanowski
    operation
Smith's
    expressor
    hook
    operation
Snellen's
    chart
    implant
    operation
    reform eye
Snell's law
Soemmering's
    ring
    spot
Sondermann's canals
Soria's operation
Sourdille's operation
space
    Fontana's s.
    periscleral s.
    Tenon's s.
    zonular s's
Spaeth's operation
Spanlang-Tappeiner syndrome
spatia zonularia

spatula
    Berens' s.
    Castroviejo's s.
    Elschnig's s.
    Knapp's s.
    Lindner's s.
    McPherson's s.
    Wheeler's s.
Speas' operation
spectacles
    Masselon's s.
speculum
    Barraquer-Colibri s.
    Barraquer's s.
    Berens' s.
    Castroviejo's s.
    Guyton-Maumenee s.
    Guyton-Park s.
    Knapp's s.
    Lancaster's s.
    Lange's s.
    lid s.
    Lister-Burch s.
    Maumenee-Park s.
    McPherson's s.
    Mellinger's s.
    Mueller's s.
    Murdock-Wiener s.
    Park's s.
    Sauer's s.
    Weeks' s.
    Wiener's s.
    Williams' s.
Spencer's scissors
Spencer-Watson operation
Spero's forceps
sph. — spherical lens
sphere
spherical
sphincter
    s. iridis
    s. oculi

sphincter *(continued)*
    s. oris
    s. pupillae
sphincterectomy
sphincterolysis
spindle
    Krukenberg's s.
sponge
    Lincoff's s.
    Weck-cel s.
spoon
    Bunge's s.
    Daviel's s.
    Elschnig's s.
    Hess' s.
    Kirby's s.
    Knapp's s.
sporotrichosis
spot
    Bitot's s.
    blind s.
    Brushfield's s.
    cherry red s.
    cotton-wool s's
    Elschnig's s's
    Forster-Fuchs black s.
    Fuchs' s.
    Gaule's s's
    Horner-Trantas s's
    Mariotte's s.
    Maxwell's s.
    Roth's s.
    Soemmering's s.
    Tay's s.
spud
    Bahn's s.
    Corbett's s.
    Davis' s.
    Dix's s.
    Fisher's s.
    Francis' s.
    Hosford's s.

spud *(continued)*
    LaForce's s.
    Walter's s.
spur
    scleral s.
squint
    comitant s.
    convergent s.
    divergent s.
    noncomitant s.
    upward and downward s.
Stahli's line
staining
    corneal s.
Stallard's operation
staphyloma
    s. corneae
    s. cornea racemosum
    equatorial s.
    intercalary s.
    s. posticum
    Scarpa's s.
    scleral s.
    uveal s.
staphylomatous
Stargardt's syndrome
Stellwag's
    brawny edema
    sign
stenocoriasis
stenosis
step
    Rönne's nasal s.
stereocampimeter
stereopsis
Stevens'
    forceps
    hook
    scissors
Stevens-Johnson syndrome
Stevenson's retractor
Stilling-Türk-Duane syndrome

Stocker's needle
Stock's operation
Stokes' lens
Stone's implant
Storz' magnet
strabismic
strabismometer
strabismus
    Braid's s.
    s. deorsum vergens
    kinetic s.
    s. sursum vergens
strabometer
strabometry
strabotome
strabotomy
streak
    Knapp's s's
streptotrichosis
striae
    s. ciliares
    Knapp's s.
striascope
striated
stroma
    s. of cornea
    s. iridis
    s. of iris
    vitreous s.
    s. vitreum
Sturge-Weber syndrome
Sturm's conoid
sty
    meibomian s.
    zeisian s.
Suarez-Villafranca operation
subcapsular
subconjunctival
subendothelial
subepithelial
    s. plexus

sublatio
    s. retinae
substantia
    s. propria corneae
sulcus
superblade
superciliary
supercilium
supernumerary
supraduction
supranuclear
supraocular
supraorbital
supratrochlear
surgical procedures. See
    operation.
sursumduction
sursumvergence
sursumversion
suture. See *General Surgical
    Terms.*
Swan's syndrome
Sylva's irrigator
symblepharon
symblepharopterygium
symptom
    Anton's s.
    halo s.
    Liebreich's s.
synathroisis
syncanthus
synchesis
synchysis
    s. scintillans
syndectomy
syndrome
    Adie's s.
    Alezzandrini's s.
    Alström-Olsen s.
    Andogsky's s.
    Angelucci's s.

syndrome *(continued)*
  Anton-Babinski s.
  Axenfeld's s.
  Bamatter's s.
  Bassen-Kornzweig s.
  Beal's s.
  Behçet's s.
  Behr's s.
  Benedikt's s.
  Bielschowsky-Lutz-
    Cogan s.
  Bietti's s.
  Bonnet-Dechaume-
    Blanc s.
  chiasma s.
  Claude's s.
  Cogan's s.
  Dejean's s.
  Duane's s.
  Elschnig's s.
  Foix's s.
  Foster-Kennedy s.
  Foville's s.
  Foville-Wilson s.
  Franceschetti's s.
  Friedenwald's s.
  Fuchs' s.
  Fuchs-Kraupa s.
  Gerstmann's s.
  Gradenigo's s.
  Graefe's s.
  Gregg's s.
  Greig's s.
  Guillain-Barré s.
  Gunn's s.
  Hallermann-Streiff s.
  Harada's s.
  Hertwig-Magendie s.
  Hippel-Lindau s.
  Horner-Bernard s.
  Horner's s.
  Hutchinson's s.

syndrome *(continued)*
  Kennedy's s.
  Kiloh-Nevin s.
  Kimmelstiel-Wilson s.
  Koerber-Salus-Elschnig s.
  Krause's s.
  Kurz's s.
  Laurence-Moon-Biedl s.
  Louis-Bar s.
  Lowe's s.
  Lyle's s.
  Marfan's s.
  Mikulicz's s.
  Millard-Gubler s.
  Miller's s.
  Möbius' s.
  Parinaud's s.
  Petzetakis-Takos s.
  Posner-Schlossman s.
  Reese's s.
  Reiter's s.
  Riddoch's s.
  Rieger's s.
  Riley-Day s.
  Rollet's s.
  Rot-Bielschowsky s.
  Rothmund's s.
  Rutherfurd's s.
  Schäfer's s.
  Siegrist-Hutchinson s.
  Sjögren's s.
  Spanlang-Tappeiner s.
  Stargardt's s.
  Stevens-Johnson s.
  Stilling-Türk-Duane s.
  Sturge-Weber s.
  Swan's s.
  Terry's s.
  Thompson's s.
  Tolosa-Hunt s.
  Touraine's s.
  Uyemura's s.

syndrome *(continued)*
    Vogt-Koyanagi s.
    Vogt's s.
    Weber's s.
    Werner's s.
    Wernicke's s.
    Wolf's s.
synechia
synechotome
synechotomy
synophrys
synophthalmia
synoptophore
synoptoscope
syphilis
    s. of conjunctiva
    s. of iris
system
    McIntire aspiration-
        irrigation s.
Szymanowski-Kuhnt operation
Szymanowski's operation
table
    Reuss' t's
Tansley's operation
tantalum
tapetum
    t. choroideae
    t. lucidum
    t. nigrum
    t. oculi
tarsadenitis
tarsal
tarsectomy
tarsi
tarsitis
tarsocheiloplasty
tarsomalacia
tarsoplasty
tarsorrhaphy
tarsotomy

tarsus
    t. inferior palpebrae
    t. superior palpebrae
tattooing
    t. of cornea
Tay's
    choroiditis
    spot
technique
    Atkinson's t.
    Van Lint t.
Teflon implant
teichopsia
telangiectasia
telangiectasis
telebinocular
tendon
    Lockwood's t.
    superior oblique t.
    Zinn's t.
tendotomy
Tenner's cannula
Tenon's
    capsule
    fascia
    space
tenonitis
tenonometer
tenontotomy
tenotome
tenotomist
tenotomize
tenotomy
tension
    intraocular t.
tereon. See *pterion.*
terijeum. See *pterygium.*
Terry's syndrome
Terson's operation
test
    Bielschowsky's t.

test *(continued)*
    color vision t.
    confrontation field t.
    cover t.
    "E" t.
    head-tilt t.
    Hering's t.
    Holmgren's t.
    Ishihara's t.
    Marlow's t.
    Mauthner's t.
    red glass t.
    Schirmer's t.
    shadow t.
    transillumination t.
tetartanopia
tetartanopic
tetartanopsia
tetrastichiasis
thalamus
Theobald's probe
theory
    Hering's t.
    Schön's t.
    Young-Helmholtz t.
thermosector
thiriahsis. See *phthiriasis.*
Thomas'
    cryoptor
    operation
Thompson's syndrome
Thorpe-Castroviejo scissors
Thorpe's
    caliper
    forceps
    scissors
Thorpe-Wescott scissors
Thygeson's keratitis
tikopseah. See *teichopsia.*
tisis. See *phthisis.*
Todd's gouge

Tolosa-Hunt syndrome
tonogram
tonograph
tonographer
tonography
tonometer
    Goldmann's applanation
        t.
    Mackay-Marg t.
    McLean's t.
    Schiøtz' t.
    Sklar-Schiøtz' t.
tonometry
Tooke's knife
torpor
    t. retinae
torsion
tortuous
tosis. See *ptosis.*
totic. See *ptotic.*
Toti-Mosher operation
Toti's operation
Touraine's syndrome
trabeculectomy
trachoma
    Arlt's t.
    brawny t.
trachomatous
transcorneal
transillumination
transilluminator
    Finnoff's t.
transplant
    corneal t.
transplantation
Trantas'
    dots
    operation
treatment
    Imre's t.
    Schöler's t.

trepanation
    corneal t.
trephination
trephine
    Arruga's t.
    Barraquer's t.
    Castroviejo's t.
    Elliot's t.
    Grieshaber's t.
    Paufique's t.
trichiasis
trichromat
trichromatopsia
trichromic
trifocal
trigone
    Müller's t.
triplokoria
tritanopia
tritanopic
tritanopsia
trochlea
tropometer
Troutman's
    implant
    operation
tucker
    Burch-Greenwood t.
tunica
    t. adnata oculi
    t. conjunctiva
    t. conjunctiva bulbi
    t. conjunctiva bulbi oculi
    t. conjunctiva palpebra-
        rum
    t. fibrosa oculi
    t. interna bulbi
    t. nervea of Bruecke
    t. vasculosa bulbi
    t. vasculosa lentis
    t. vasculosa oculi

tunicary
Tyrell's hook
ulcer
    Mooren's u.
    Saemisch's u.
ulcus
    u. serpens corneae
ulectomy
ultrasonic
ultrasonogram
    B scan u.
Undine's dropper
unit
    Bovie u.
    Mira u.
uvea
uveal
uveitic
uveitis
    Förster's u.
    heterochromic u.
    sympathetic u.
uveoparotid
uveoparotitis
uveoplasty
uveoscleritis
Uyemura's syndrome
VA — visual acuity
vaginae bulbi
valve
    Foltz's v.
Van Lint
    akinesia
    block
    technique
Vannas' scissors
variation
    diurnal v.
varicoblepharon
vasa sanguinea retinae
vascular

vascularization

veil

    Sattler's v.

vein

    ciliary v.

    cilioretinal v.

    posterior conjunctival v.

    retinal v.

    vorticose v.

venae

    v. centralis retinae

    v. vorticosae

venula

    v. macularis inferior

    v. macularis superior

    v. medialis retinae

    v. nasalis retinae inferior

    v. nasalis retinae superior

    v. retinae medialis

    v. temporalis retinae inferior

    v. temporalis retinae superior

venule

    medial v. of retina

    nasal v. of retina, inferior and superior

    temporal v. of retina, inferior and superior

VEP — visual evoked potential

vergence

Verhoeff's

    forceps

    operation

    scissors

version

vertex

Verwey's operation

vesicle

    ocular v.

    ophthalmic v.

    optic v.

vesicula

    v. ophthalmica

VF — visual field

Viers' erysiphake

Vieth-Muller horopter

vision

    achromatic v.

    binocular v.

    chromatic v.

    color v.

    dichromatic v.

    foveal v.

    halo v.

    haploscopic v.

    iridescent v.

    monocular v.

    v. nul

    oscillating v.

    peripheral v.

    photopic v.

    Pick's v.

    pseudoscopic v.

    rod v.

    scoterythrous v.

    scotopic v.

    stereoscopic v.

    tunnel v.

visual

    v. acuity

    v. axis

    v. fields

    v. purple

visual evoked potential

visualization

visualize

visuometer

Vitallium implant

vitrectomy

    pars plana v.

vitrector

    Kaufman's v.

vitreocapsulitis

vitreous
 v. body
 detached v.
 v. floater
 v. humor
 primary persistent hyperplastic v.
 secondary v.
 tertiary v.
vitreum
VOD — visio oculus dextra — vision, right eye
Vogt-Koyanagi syndrome
Vogt's
 cataract
 cornea
 degeneration
 disease
 syndrome
Vogt-Spielmeyer disease
von Graefe's
 cautery
 cystotome
 forceps
 hook
 knife
 knife needle
 operation
 sign
von Hippel-Lindau disease
von Monakow's fibers
von Mondak's forceps
von Recklinghausen's disease
VOS — visio oculus sinister — vision, left eye
Vossius' lenticular ring
VOU — visio oculus uterque — vision of each eye
Wadsworth-Todd cautery
Wagener's retinitis
Wagner's disease
Waldeau's forceps
Waldhauer's operation

Walker's
 lid everter
 pin
 scissors
walleye
Walter's spud
Walton's punch
wart
 Hassall-Henle w's
Watzke's sleeve
Weber's
 knife
 sign
 syndrome
Weck-cel sponge
Weekers' operation
Weeks'
 bacillus
 needle
 operation
 speculum
Weil's disease
Weiss's reflex
Werner's syndrome
Wernicke's syndrome
Westcott's scissors
Westphal-Strumpell disease
West's operation
Weve's
 electrode
 operation
Wheeler's
 cystotome
 implant
 knife
 operation
 spatula
Wicherkiewicz' operation
Widmark's conjunctivitis
Wiener's
 hook
 operation
 speculum

Wilder's
    scoop
    sign
Williams'
    probe
    speculum
Willis' circle
Wilmer's
    operation
    scissors
Wilson's disease
Wolfe's operation
Wolfring's gland
Wolf's syndrome
Worth's operation
Wucherer's conjunctivitis
xanthelasma
    x. palpebrarum
xanthelasmatosis
xanthoma
    x. palpebrarum
xanthomatosis
    x. bulbi
    x. iridis
xanthophane
xanthopia
xanthopsia
xeroma
xerophthalmia
xerophthalmus
xerosis
    x. conjunctivae
    x. superficialis
Young-Helmholtz theory
YS — yellow spot of the retina
zan-. See words beginning *xan-.*

Zeis
    glands of Z.
zeisian gland
Zeiss'
    microscope
    photocoagulator
zero-. See words beginning
    xero-.
zeromah. See *xeroma.*
Ziegler's
    cautery
    forceps
    knife
    operation
    probe
Zinn's
    circlet
    corona
    ligament
    tendon
    zonule
zonula
    z. ciliaris
zonulae
zonular
    z. fibers
    z. space
zonule
    ciliary z.
    z. of Zinn
zonulitis
zonulolysis
    enzymatic z.
zonulotomy
zonulysis

fracture

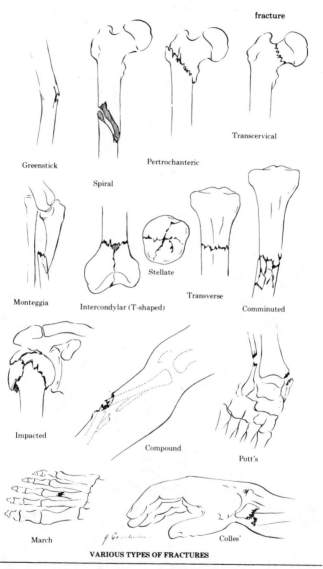

Greenstick

Pertrochanteric

Spiral

Transcervical

Monteggia

Intercondylar (T-shaped)

Stellate

Transverse

Comminuted

Impacted

Compound

Pott's

March

Colles'

VARIOUS TYPES OF FRACTURES

(Courtesy of Dorland's Illustrated Medical Dictionary, 26th ed. Plate XVIII. Philadelphia, W. B. Saunders Company, 1981.)

ORTHOPEDICS

abarticular
abarticulation
Abbott-Lucas operation
Abbott's operation
abduction
abductor
abscess
      Brodie's a.
absconsio
AC — acromioclavicular
acantha
acetabular
acetabulectomy
acetabuloplasty
acetabulum
Achilles
      bursa
      bursitis
      jerk
      tendon
achillobursitis
achillodynia
achillorrhaphy
achillotenotomy
      plastic a.
achondroplasia
aclasia
aclasis
      diaphyseal a.
      tarsoepiphyseal a.

acoustogram
arcocontracture
acromioclavicular
acromiocoracoid
acromiohumeral
acromion
acromionectomy
acromioscapular
acromiothoracic
acromyotonia
acro-osteolysis
acropachy
acropathy
acrostealgia
acrosyndactyly
actinomycosis
Adams'
      operation
      saw
adapter
      McReynolds' a.
adduction
adductor
Adelmann's operation
advancement
adventitious
Agnew's splint
AJ — ankle jerk
AK — above knee
akilez. See *Achilles.*

akilo-. See words beginning
   achillo-.
Akin's bunionectomy
akondroplazea. See
   achondroplasia.
ala
      a. ilii
      a. ossis ilii
      a. ossis ilium
Albee-Delbet operation
Albee's
      operation
      osteotome
Albers-Schönberg
      bone
      disease
Albert's operation
Albright's
      disease
      syndrome
Alexander-Farabeuf periosteo-
   tome
Alexander's
      osteotome
      periosteotome
Allis' sign
Alouette's amputation
ambulation
ambulatory
amphiarthrosis
amputation
      AK (above knee) a.
      Alouette's a.
      aperiosteal a.
      Béclard's a.
      Bier's a.
      Bunge's a.
      Callander's a.
      Carden's a.
      chop a.
      Chopart's a.
      cineplastic a.

amputation (*continued*)
      diaclastic a.
      double flap a.
      Dupuytren's a.
      Farabeuf's a.
      Forbe's a.
      forequarter a.
      Gritti's a.
      Gritti-Stokes a.
      guillotine a.
      Guyon's a.
      Hancock's a.
      Hey's a.
      Kirk's a.
      Larrey's a.
      Le Fort's a.
      Lisfranc's a.
      MacKenzie's a.
      Maisonneuve's a.
      mediotarsal a.
      musculocutaneous a.
      osteoplastic a.
      periosteoplastic a.
      phalangophalangeal a.
      Pirogoff's a.
      Ricard's a.
      Stokes' a.
      subastragalar a.
      Syme's a.
      Teale's a.
      Tripier's a.
      Wladimiroff-Mikulicz a.
amyloid
amyotonia
anapophysis
anarrhexis
anconagra
anconeal
anconitis
Anderson's
      operation
      splint

anesthesia. See *General*
    Surgical Terms.
Anghelescu's sign
Angle's splint
angulation
ankle
    tailors' a.
ankylosis
Annandale's operation
anosteoplasia
anostosis
antebrachium
antecubital
anteversion
anti-inflammatory
anvil
    Bunneli's a.
AP — anteroposterior
apofi-. See words beginning
    apophy-.
aponeurectomy
aponeurorrhaphy
aponeurosis
aponeurotomy
apophyseal
apophysis
apophysitis
    a. tibialis adolescentium
apparatus
    Kirschner's a.
    Sayre's a.
arachnodactyly
arachnoid
arachnoidal
arch
    neural a.
    vertebral a.
areflexia
areten-. See words beginning
    aryten-.
artery
    basilic a.

artery (*continued*)
    brachial a.
    cephalic a.
    femoral a.
    genicular a.
    gluteal a.
    interosseous a.
    obturator a.
    peroneal a.
    popliteal a.
    princeps pollicis a.
    profunda brachii a.
    pudendal a.
    radial a.
    radialis indicis a.
    saphenous a.
    ulnar a.
    vesical a.
    volar a.
arthragra
arthralgia
arthrectomy
arthrempyesis
arthritic
arthritis
    Bekhterev's a.
    chronic villous a.
    degenerative a.
    exudative a.
    gouty a.
    hypertrophic a.
    a. mutilans
    navicular a.
    nonarticular a.
    rheumatoid a.
    rheumatoid a., juvenile
    suppurative a.
    vertebral a.
arthrocentesis
arthrochalasis
arthrochondritis
arthroclasia

arthrodesis
  Charnley's a.
  Moberg's a.
arthrodynia
arthrodysplasia
arthroempyesis
arthroereisis
arthrogram
arthrography
arthrogryposis
arthrokatadysis
arthrokleisis
arthrolithiasis
arthrolysis
arthrometer
arthrometry
arthroncus
arthroneuralgia
arthronosos
arthro-onychodysplasia
arthropathy
arthrophyma
arthroplasty
  Bechtol's a.
  Charnley-Mueller a.
arthropneumoroentgenography
arthropyosis
arthrorheumatism
arthrosclerosis
arthroscope
arthroscopy
arthrosis
  Charcot's a.
  a. deformans
arthrosteitis
arthrostomy
arthrosynovitis
arthrotome
arthrotomy
arthroxerosis
articular
articulated

articulatio
  a. acromioclavicularis
  a. atlantoaxialis mediana
  a. bicondylaris
  a. calcaneocuboidea
  a. capitis costae
  a. carpometacarpea pol-
    licis
  a. costotransversaria
  a. coxae
  a. cricoarytenoidea
  a. cubiti
  a. ellipsoidea
  a. genu
  a. humeri
  a. humeroradialis
  a. ossis pisiformis
  a. radiocarpea
  a. sacroiliaca
  a. sternoclavicularis
  a. tarsi transversa
  a. tibiofibularis
  a. trochoidea
articulation
  acromioclavicular a.
  brachioulnar a.
  calcaneocuboid a.
  carpal a's
  carpometacarpal a's
  chondrosternal a's
  costocentral a.
  costosternal a's
  costotransverse a.
  costovertebral a's
  ellipsoidal a.
  humeroradial a.
  humeroulnar a.
  iliosacral a.
  intermetacarpal a's
  intermetatarsal a's
  interphalangeal a's
  metacarpophalangeal a's

articulation (*continued*)
 metatarsophalangeal a's
 phalangeal a's
 radiocarpal a's
 sacrococcygeal a.
 sacroiliac a.
 sternoclavicular a.
 talocalcaneonavicular a.
 talonavicular a.
 tarsometatarsal a's
 tibiofibular a.
 trochoidal a.
arytenoidectomy
arytenoiditis
arytenoidopexy
Ashhurst's splint
aspiration
astragalar
astragalectomy
astragalocalcanean
astragalocrural
astragaloscaphoid
astragalotibial
astragalus
ataxia
atrophy
 Sudeck's a.
Aufranc-Turner prosthesis
Augustine's nail
Austin-Moore prosthesis
Avila's operation
avulsion
awl
 Wilson's a.
Axer's operation
Baastrup's syndrome
Babinski's sign
Badgley's
 operation
 plate
Baker's cyst
Bakwin-Eiger syndrome

Balkan splint
bandage. See General Surgical
 Terms.
Bankhart's
 operation
 retractor
Bardenheuer's extension
Barker's operation
Barré-Liéou syndrome
Barton's
 fracture
 operation
 tong
Barwell's operation
Basile's screw
Bateman's
 operation
 prosthesis
Baylor's splint
Bechterew-Mendel reflex
Bechterew's reflex
Bechtol's
 arthroplasty
 prosthesis
Beckman-Adson retractor
Béclard's amputation
bed
 CircOlectric b.
Beevor's sign
Bekhterev's
 arthritis
 spondylitis
 test
belly
Bennett's
 elevator
 fracture
 retractor
Bent's operation
Bertin's
 bone
 ligament

Bertolotti's syndrome
Besnier's rheumatism
biceps
    b. brachii
    b. femoris
Bier's amputation
Bigelow's ligament
biopsy
    muscle b.
biparietal
Bishop-Black tendon tucker
Bishop-DeWitt tendon tucker
Bishop-Peter tendon tucker
Bishop's tendon tucker
BK — below knee
Blount's
    disease
    operation
    osteotome
    plate
    retractor
    stapler
Blundell-Jones operation
Bobroff's operation
body
    Schmorl's b.
    vertebral b.
Böhler-Braun splint
Böhler's
    clamp
    splint
Bohlman's pin
bolt
    Webb's b.
    Wilson's b.
Bond's splint
bone
    accessory b.
    acetabular b.
    acromial b.
    alar b.
    Albers-Schönberg b's

bone (*continued*)
    alisphenoid b.
    ankle b.
    astragaloid b.
    astragaloscaphoid b.
    basihyal b.
    basilar b.
    Bertin's b.
    breast b.
    bregmatic b.
    brittle b's
    calcaneal b.
    cancellated b.
    cancellous b.
    capitate b.
    carpal b's
    chalky b's
    coccygeal b.
    collar b.
    compact b.
    cortical b.
    costal b.
    cranial b's
    cuneiform b.
    ectethmoid b's
    ectocuneiform b.
    endochondral b.
    entocuneiform b.
    epactal b's
    ethmoid b.
    exoccipital b.
    femoral b.
    fibular b.
    flank b.
    frontal b.
    hamate b.
    haunch b.
    humeral b.
    hyoid b.
    iliac b.
    incarial b.
    intermaxillary b.

bone (*continued*)
    interparietal b.
    intrachondrial b.
    ischial b.
    ivory b's
    lacrimal b.
    lenticular b.
    lunate b.
    maxillary b.
    mesocuneiform b.
    metacarpal b's
    metatarsal b's
    multangular b.
    nasal b.
    navicular b.
    occipital b.
    orbitosphenoidal b.
    parietal b.
    pelvic b.
    periosteal b.
    petrous b.
    phalangeal b's
    Pirie's b.
    pisiform b.
    pubic b.
    radial b.
    replacement b.
    rider's b.
    sacral b.
    scaphoid b.
    scapular b.
    sesamoid b's
    shin b.
    shoulder b.
    sphenoid b.
    supernumerary b.
    tarsal b's
    temporal b.
    tibia b.
    trapezium b.
    trapezoid b.
    triangular b.

bone (*continued*)
    triquetral b.
    turbinate b.
    ulna b.
    ulnar styloid b.
    unciform b.
    uncinate b.
    vesalian b.
    vomer b.
    whettle b's
    xiphoid b.
    zygomatic b.
bone depression
bone graft
    diamond inlay b.g.
    dual inlay b.g.
    hemicylindrical b.g.
    inlay b.g.
    intramedullary b.g.
    medullary b.g.
    onlay b.g.
    osteoperiosteal b.g.
    peg b.g.
    sliding inlay b.g.
bone head
bone processes
bone wax
Bonnet's sign
bootonyar. See *boutonnière.*
Bosworth's
    operation
    screw
Bouchard's nodes
boutonnière
Bowen-Grover meniscotome
Bowen's osteotome
Bowlby's splint
bowleg
Boyd's operation
Boyes-Goodfellow hook
brace
    drop foot b.

brace (*continued*)
    ischial weight-bearing b.
    Knight's b.
    longleg b.
    Lyman-Smith b.
    Milwaukee b.
    Taylor's b.
    toe drop b.
    weight-bearing b.
brachial
brachiocrural
brachiocubital
brachiocyllosis
brachium
Bradford's frame
Bragard's sign
Brant's splint
Brett's operation
brisement
    b. forcé
Brissaud's scoliosis
Bristow's operation
Brittain's operation
Brockman's operation
Brodie's
    abscess
    disease
    knee
    ligament
Brown's dermatome
Brudzinski's sign
Bryant's
    sign
    traction
Buck's
    extension
    hook
    operation
    splint
    traction
Büdinger-Ludloff-Laewen
    disease

Budin's joint
Bunge's amputation
bunion
bunionectomy
    Akin's b.
    Keller's b.
    Mitchell's b.
    Silver's b.
    Stone's b.
bunionette
Bunnell's
    anvil
    drill
    needle
    operation
    probe
bur
    Jordan-Day b.
    Lempert's b.
Burch-Greenwood tendon
    tucker
bursa
    Achilles b.
    anserine b.
    b. of iliopsoas muscle
    olecranon b.
    patellar b.
    subacromial b.
    subdeltoid b.
bursae
bursectomy
bursitis
    Achilles b.
    Duplay's b.
    prepatellar b.
    radiohumeral b.
    subacromial b.
    subdeltoid b.
bursotomy
Butcher's saw
C-1, C-2, etc. — cervical verte-
    brae

Ca — calcium
Cabot's splint
CAD (computerized assisted
    design) prosthesis
calcaneal
calcaneitis
calcaneoapophysitis
calcaneoastragaloid
calcaneocavus
calcaneocuboid
calcaneodynia
calcaneofibular
calcaneonavicular
calcaneoplantar
calcaneoscaphoid
calcaneotibial
calcaneovalgocavus
calcaneus
calcar
        c. avis
        c. femorale
        c. pedis
calcification
calcinosis
        c. intervertebralis
        tumoral c.
calcium
Callahan's operation
Callander's amputation
Callaway's test
callus
        definitive c.
        ensheathing c.
        intermediate c.
        medullary c.
        myelogenous c.
        permanent c.
        provisional c.
Calvé-Perthes disease
Campbell's
        operation
        osteotome

Canadian crutch
canal
        haversian c.
        Hunter's c.
        neural c.
        tarsal c.
cancellated
cancelli
cancellous
cancellus
capeline
capitellum
capitulum
capsule
        articular c.
        joint c.
capsulectomy
capsulitis
        adhesive c.
capsuloplasty
capsulorrhaphy
capsulotomy
caput
        c. radii
        c. tali
Carden's amputation
Carleton's spots
caro
        c. quadrata manus
        c. quadrata sylvii
carpal
        c. tunnel
carpectomy
carpometacarpal
carpopedal
carpophalangeal
carpoptosis
carpus
        c. curvus
Carrell's operation
Carroll-Legg osteotome
Carroll's osteotome

Carroll-Smith-Petersen
    osteotome
cartilage
    articular c.
    ensiform c.
    falciform c.
    floating c.
    interarticular c.
    interosseous c.
    intervertebral c.
    tendon c.
cartilaginous
cast
    Cotrel's c.
    long-arm c.
    long-leg c.
    Pietrie's c.
    Risser's c.
    short-arm c.
    short-leg c.
Cave-Rowe operation
Cave's operation
cavity
    medullary c.
    synovial c.
cavus
cervical
cervicalis
cervicobrachial
cervicodorsal
cervicodynia
cervico-occipital
cervicoscapular
cervicothoracic
Chaddock's reflex
Chandler's
    disease
    elevator
    splint
Chaput's method
Charcot's
    arthrosis

Charcot's (*continued*)
    joint
charleyhorse
Charnley-Mueller
    arthroplasty
    prosthesis
Charnley's arthrodesis
Charrière's saw
cheirospasm
chemotherapy
Cherry's osteotome
Chiene's
    operation
    test
chisel
    Moore's c.
chondral
chondrectomy
chondritis
    c. intervertebralis
      calcanea
chondroblastoma
chondrocarcinoma
chondrocostal
chondrodynia
chondrodysplasia
chondrodystrophia
chondrodystrophy
    c. malacia
chondroepiphyseal
chondroepiphysitis
chondrolysis
chondroma
chondromalacia
chondromatosis
    Reichel's c.
    synovial c.
chondrometaplasia
    tenosynovial c.
chondronecrosis
chondro-osseous
chondrophyte

chondroplastic
chondroplasty
chondroporosis
chondrosarcoma
chondrosarcomatosis
chondrosternal
chondrosternoplasty
chondrotome
chondrotomy
chondroxiphoid
chonechondrosternon
Chopart's
    amputation
    joint
chordotomy
Chovstek's sign
CircOlectric bed
CK — creatine kinase
clamp
        Böhler's c.
        Forrester's c.
        Humphries' c.
        Jackson's c.
        Lambotte's c.
        Lowman's c.
        Verbrugge's c.
        Wester's c.
        Williams' c.
        Wilman's c.
        Wilson's c.
claudication
clavicle
clavicotomy
clavicula
clavicular
claviculus
clavus
clawfoot
clawhand
Clayton's osteotome
Cleeman's sign
clinodactyly

clonus
Cloward's
    drill
    operation
    osteotome
    rongeur
clubfoot
clubhand
Clutton's joint
coapt
Cobb's
    elevator
    gouge
    osteotome
coccygeal
coccygectomy
coccygerector
coccygeus
coccygodynia
coccygotomy
coccyx
Codivilla's
    extension
    operation
Codman's sign
Cole's operation
collar
    Thomas' c.
Colles'
    fracture
    splint
Collin's osteoclast
Collison's screw
collum
    c. anatomicum humeri
    c. chirurgicum humeri
    c. costae
    c. distortum
    c. femoris
    c. mallei
    c. processus condyloidei
      mandibulae

collum (*continued*)
    c. radii
    c. scapulae
    c. tali
    c. valgum
Colonna's operation
column
    vertebral c.
    spinal c.
comminuted
comminution
Comolli's sign
compact
Compere's
    operation
    pin
compression
concavity
condylar
condyle
condylectomy
condylion
condylotomy
condylus
congenerous
connexus
    c. intertendineus
Conn's operation
contractility
    idiomuscular c.
contraction
contracture
    Dupuytren's c.
    ischemic c.
    Volkmann's c.
contusion
Converse's osteotome
convexity
Conzett's goniometer
Coopernail's sign
coracoacromial
coracoclavicular

coracohumeral
coracoid
coracoiditis
coracoradialis
coracoulnaris
Corbett's forceps
coronoid
corticosteroid
costa
    c. fluctuans
    c. fluctuans decima
costae
    c. spuriae
    c. verae
costal
costalgia
costalis
costectomy
costicartilage
costicervical
costochondral
costochondritis
costoclavicular
costoscapular
costoscapularis
costosternal
costosternoplasty
costotome
costotomy
costotransversectomy
costovertebral
costoxiphoid
Cotrel's cast
Cottle's osteotome
Cotton's fracture
counterextension
countertraction
Coventry's
    osteotomy
    screw
coxa
    c. adducta

coxa (*continued*)
   c. flexa
   c. magna
   c. plana
   c. valga
   c. vara
   c. vara luxans
coxalgia
coxankylometer
coxarthria
coxarthritis
coxarthrocace
coxarthropathy
coxitis
   c. fugax
   senile c.
coxodynia
coxofemoral
coxotomy
coxotuberculosis
Crane's
   mallet
   osteotome
craniotome
craniotomy
Credo's operation
crena
   c. ani
crepitation
crepitus
cricoid
cricoidectomy
cruciate
crutch
   Canadian c.
   jocked stand c.
Crutchfield's
   operation
   tong
Cruveilhier's joint
Cubbins' operation
cubital

cubitocarpal
cubitoradial
cubitus
   c. valgus
   c. varus
cuboid
cuneiform
curet
   Spratt's c.
Curry's splint
CVA — costovertebral angle
cyst
   Baker's c.
Czerny's disease
dactylolysis
Darrach's operation
Davies-Colley operation
Davis' splint
Dawbarn's sign
débridement
decalcification
decapitation
decompression
decubitus
deformity
   boutonnière d.
   buttonhole d.
   Ilfeld-Holder d.
   lobster-claw d.
   Madelung's d.
   recurvatum d.
   seal-fin d.
   silver fork d.
   Sprengel's d.
   swan-neck d.
   ulnar drift d.
   valgus d.
   varus d.
   Velpeau's d.
   Volkmann's d.
degeneration
   Zenker's d.

degenerative
Dejerine's sign
Delore's method
Demianoff's sign
Denis-Browne clubfoot splint
Denuse's operation
DePalma's prosthesis
DePuy's
    prosthesis
    splint
de Quervain's disease
derangement
    Hey's internal d.
dermatome
    Brown's d.
dermatomyositis
Desault's sign
desmotomy
Deutschländer's disease
dextroverted
Deyerle's
    drill
    plate
    punch
diaclasis
diaphyseal
diaphysectomy
diaphysis
diaphysitis
    tuberculous d.
diaplasis
diaplastic
diapophysis
diarthric
diarthrosis
diastasis
Dickson-Diveley operation
Dickson's operation
Dieffenbach's operation
digit
digital
digitation

Dingman's
    forceps
    osteotome
DIP — distal interphalangeal
DIPJ — distal interphalangeal
    joint
diplegia
diploë
diploetic
diploic
dis-. See also words beginning
    dys-.
disarticulation
disc (disk)
discogenic
discoid
discoidectomy
disease
    Albers-Schönberg d.
    Albright's d.
    Blount's d.
    Brodie's d.
    Büdinger-Ludloff-
      Laewen d.
    Calvé-Perthes d.
    Chandler's d.
    Czerny's d.
    degenerative joint d.
    de Quervain's d.
    Deutschländer's d.
    Duplay's d.
    Erb's d.
    Erb-Goldflam d.
    Erichsen's d.
    Freiberg's d.
    Hand-Schüller-
      Christian d.
    Inman's d.
    Jüngling's d.
    Kashin-Bek d.
    Köhler's d.
    Kümmell's d.

disease (*continued*)
    Kümmell-Verneuil d.
    Larsen-Johansson d.
    Legg-Calvé-Waldenström
      d.
    Marie-Strümpell d.
    Marie-Tooth d.
    McArdle's d.
    Morquio's d.
    Ollier's d.
    Osgood-Schlatter d.
    Otto's d.
    Paget's d.
    Pauzat's d.
    Pellegrini-Stieda d.
    Perrin-Ferraton d.
    Perthes' d.
    Pott's d.
    Poulet's d.
    Preiser's d.
    Quervain's d.
    Recklinghausen's d.
    Schanz's d.
    Scheuermann's d.
    Schlatter's d.
    Schmorl's d.
    Sever's d.
    Steinert's d.
    Swediaur's d.
    Talma's d.
    Volkmann's d.
    von Recklinghausen's d.
    Waldenström's d.
disk (disc)
    cartilaginous d's
    herniated d.
    intervertebral d's
diskectomy
diskitis
diskogram
diskography

dislocatio
    d. erecta
dislocation
    divergent d.
    Kienböck's d.
    Monteggia's d.
    Nélaton's d.
    Smith's d.
    subastragalar d.
    subcoracoid d.
    subglenoid d.
dismemberment
dissector
    Lewin's d.
distraction
DJD — degenerative joint
    disease
dolichostenomelia
dorsa
dorsalis
dorsiflexion
dorsispinal
dorsolumbar
dorsoscapular
dorsum
Downing's knife
drain
    Redivac d.
drill
    Bunnell's d.
    Cloward's d.
    Deyerle's d.
    Hall's air d.
    intramedullary d.
    Smedberg's d.
    Vitallium d.
driver
    Küntscher's d.
drugs. See *Drugs and*
    Chemistry section.
DTR — deep tendon reflex

Duchenne's-type muscular
  dystrophy
Dugas' test
Dunn-Brittain operation
Duplay's
    bursitis
    disease
Dupuytren's
    amputation
    contracture
    fracture
    sign
    splint
dura
dura mater
    d.m. spinalis
Durman's operation
Duverney's fracture
dynamometer
    squeeze d.
dysarthrosis
dyschondroplasia
    Ollier's d.
dysesthesia
dysostosis
dysplasia
    diaphyseal d.
    metaphyseal d.
dystrophy
    Duchenne's-type muscu-
      lar d.
    muscular d.
ebonation
eburnation
eccentro-osteochondrodys-
  plasia
ecchondrotome
ectocondyle
ectromelia
ectrometacarpia
ectrometatarsia
ectrophalangia

Eden-Hybbinette operation
Eggers'
    operation
    plate
    screw
    splint
Eicher's prosthesis
elbow
    capped e.
    tennis e.
electromyography
elevator
    Bennett's e.
    Chandler's e.
    Cobb's e.
    Farabeuf's e.
    joker e.
    Lane's e.
    Langenbeck's e.
Elliott's plate
Ellis-Jones operation
Elmslie-Cholmeley operation
Ely's test
eminence
    thenar e.
enarthrosis
enchondroma
enchondromatosis
enchondrosarcoma
endochondral
endoscope
endosteoma
endosteum
Engelmann's splint
enostosis
entepicondyle
epicondylalgia
epicondyle
epicondylitis
epicondylus
epifizee-. See words beginning
    epiphysi-.

epifizeal. See *epiphyseal;*
    epiphysial.
epimysium
epiphyseal
epiphyses
    stippled e.
epiphysial
epiphysiodesis
epiphysioid
epiphysiolysis
epiphysiometer
epiphysiopathy
epiphysis
    e. cerebri
    slipped e.
epiphysitis
    vertebral e.
epipyramis
epirotulian
epistropheus
epitendineum
epitenon
epithesis
epitrochlea
Epstein's osteotome
equinovarus
equinus
erasion
    e. of joint
Erb-Goldflam disease
Erb's disease
ergogram
ergograph
    Mosso's e.
Erichsen's
    disease
    sign
ESR — erythrocyte sedimenta-
        tion rate
Essex-Lopresti method
ethmofrontal
ethmoid

ethmomaxillary
Evans' operation
Ewing's
    sarcoma
    tumor
exarticulation
exercise
    Williams' e.
exostosectomy
exostosis
    e. bursata
    e. cartilaginea
exsanguinate
extension
    Bardenheuer's e.
    Buck's e.
    Codivilla's e.
extensor
extractor
    Jewett's e.
    Moore's e.
extradural
extremities
extremity
Eyler's operation
fabere sign
facet
facetectomy
facial
Fahey's operation
Fajersztajn's sign
falan-. See words beginning
    phalan-.
falanks. See *phalanx.*
falx
    f. inguinalis
    f. ligamentosa
Farabeuf-Lambotte forceps
Farabeuf's
    amputation
    elevator
    forceps

faradization
  galvanic f.
fascia
  f. lata femoris
fascial
fasciatome
  Luck's f.
fasciculation
fasciculus
fasciectomy
fasciitis
  pseudosarcomatous f.
fasciodesis
fascioplasty
fasciorrhaphy
fasciotomy
femora
femoral
femoroiliac
femorotibial
femur
Ferguson's forceps
fiber
  Sharpey's f's
fiberoptic
fibrillation
fibrocartilage
fibrocartilaginous
fibroma
fibromatosis
fibrosarcoma
fibrositis
fibula
fibular
fibularis
fibulocalcaneal
finger
  baseball f.
  mallet f.
  trigger f.
Finkelstein's test
Fink's tendon tucker

fissure
fixation
fizeotherape. See
  physiotherapy.
flatfoot
  spastic f.
flex
flexion
  plantar f.
flexor
  f. retinaculum
fluid
  synovial f.
fontanelle
foramen
  f. magnum
foramina
foraminotomy
Forbe's amputation
forceps
  bayonet f.
  Corbett's f.
  Dingman's f.
  Farabeuf-Lambotte f.
  Farabeuf's f.
  Ferguson's f.
  Hibbs' f.
  Horsley's f.
  Kern's f.
  Lambotte's f.
  Lane's f.
  Liston-Stille f.
  Littauer-Liston f.
  Martin's f.
  Van Buren's f.
forearm
forefoot
Forrester's clamp
fossa
fossae
fovea
  f. capitis femoris

Fowler's operation
Fox's splint
fracture
    agenetic f.
    apophyseal f.
    articular f.
    atrophic f.
    avulsion f.
    Barton's f.
    Bennett's f.
    bimalleolar f.
    boxer's f.
    bucket-handle f.
    bumper f.
    bursting f.
    butterfly f.
    buttonhole f.
    chisel f.
    cleavage f.
    closed f.
    Colles' f.
    comminuted f.
    compound f.
    compression f.
    condylar f.
    Cotton's f.
    depressed f.
    displaced f.
    Dupuytren's f.
    Duverney's f.
    dyscrasic f.
    f. en coin
    endocrine f.
    f. en rave
    epiphysial f.
    Galeazzi's f.
    Gosselin's f.
    greenstick f.
    Guérin's f.
    impacted f.
    intercondylar f.
    intertrochanteric f.

fracture (*continued*)
    lead pipe f.
    LeFort's f.
    linear f.
    march f.
    Monteggia's f.
    Moore's f.
    neoplastic f.
    open f.
    pathologic f.
    pertrochanteric f.
    pillion f.
    Pott's f.
    Quervain's f.
    Shepherd's f.
    silver-fork f.
    Skillern's f.
    Smith's f.
    spiral f.
    splintered f.
    stellate f.
    Stieda's f.
    subcapital f.
    subperiosteal f.
    supracondylar f.
    transcervical f.
    transcondylar f.
    transverse f.
    trimalleolar f.
    Wagstaffe's f.
    willow f.
fracture-dislocation
fragilitas
    f. ossium
frame
    Bradford's f.
    Hibbs' f.
    Stryker's f.
Frankel's sign
Frazier's osteotome
Freiberg's
    disease

Freiberg's (*continued*)
    infraction
    knife
Frejka's splint
Fritz-Lange operation
Froment's sign
funnel chest
fusion
    diaphyseal-epiphyseal f.
    spinal f.
Gaenslen's sign
gait
    antalgic g.
Galeazzi's
    fracture
    sign
galvanic
galvanization
gampsodactylia
ganglion
ganglionectomy
gangrene
    Pott's g.
Gant's operation
Garré's osteomyelitis
Gatellier's operation
Gelfoam packing
Gelpi's retractor
genicular
genu
    g. impressum
    g. recurvatum
    g. valgum
    g. varum
Geomedic prosthesis
Ghormley's operation
gibbosity
gibbous
gibbus
Gibney's perispondylitis
Gibson's operation
Gigli's saw

Giliberty's prosthesis
Gillespie's operation
Gill's operation
Girdlestone's operation
glenohumeral
glenoid
Glisson's sling
gluteal
gluteofemoral
Goldthwait's
    operation
    sign
gonarthritis
gonarthromeningitis
gonarthrotomy
goniometer
    Conzett's g.
gonitis
    fungous g.
    g. tuberculosa
gonocampsis
Gordon's splint
Gosselin's fracture
gouge
    Cobb's g.
    Moore's g.
goundou
gout
Graber-Duvernay operation
graft
    autogenous g.
    heterogenous g.
    homogenous g.
    Russe's bone g.
Grice-Green operation
Gritti's amputation
Gritti-Stokes amputation
Guepar's prosthesis
Guérin's fracture
Guillain-Barré syndrome
Guilland's sign
Guleke-Stookey operation

Guyon's amputation
Haas' operation
Hagie's pin
Hall's air drill
hallux
> h. dolorosa
> h. malleus
> h. rigidus
> h. valgus
> h. varus

hamate
hamatum
Hamilton's test
hammertoe
Hammond's operation
hamulus
Hancock's amputation
hand
> Krukenberg's h.

Hand-Schüller-Christian
disease
Hansen-Street
> nail
> pin

Hark's operation
Harmon's operation
Harrington's
> nail
> rod

Harris-Beath operation
Hart's splint
Hatcher's pin
Hauser's operation
haversian
Heberden's nodes
Hefke-Turner sign
Heifitz's operation
Helbing's sign
hemapophysis
hemarthrosis
hemilaminectomy
hemiphalangectomy

hemiplegia
hemivertebra
Henderson's operation
Hendry's operation
Henry-Geist operation
herniated
herniation
> h. of nucleus pulposus

hetero-osteoplasty
Heuter's operation
Heyman's operation
Hey's
> amputation
> internal derangement

Hibbs'
> forceps
> frame
> operation
> osteotome
> retractor

hip
> snapping h.

Hirschberg's sign
Hodgen's splint
Hoen's plate
Hoffa-Lorenz operation
Hoffa's operation
Hoffmann's sign
Hohmann's
> operation
> retractor

Hoke's osteotome
Holme's operation
Homans' sign
hook
> Boyes-Goodfellow h.
> Buck's h.

Horsley's forceps
Horwitz-Adams operation
Houston's operation
Howorth's
> operation

Howorth's (*continued*)
 osteotome
Hubbard's tank
Hueter's sign
huméral
humeroradial
humeroscapular
humeroulnar
humerus
Humphries' clamp
Hunter's canal
hydrarthrosis
hydrocolator
hypalgesia
hypercalcemia
hyperesthesia
hyperextension
hyperostosis
hypertrophic
hypertrophy
 Marie's h.
hyperuricemia
hypesthesia
hypolemmal
hypoplasia
hypothenar
idiomuscular
iksomeilitis. See *ixomyelitis.*
Ilfeld-Holder deformity
iliac
iliofemoral
iliofemoroplasty
iliopectineal
iliopsoas
iliosacral
iliosciatic
iliospinal
iliotibial
iliotrochanteric
ilioxiphopagus
ilium
IM – intramuscularly

immobilization
incision. See *General Surgical Terms.*
inflammation
inflammatory
infraction
 Freiberg's i.
infrapatellar
Inman's disease
innervation
inochondritis
inotropic
inotropism
instability
 lumbosacral i.
instep
insufficientia
 i. vertebrae
interarticular
intercellular
interdigital
interosseal
interosseous
interphalangeal
interspace
intertrochanteric
intervertebral
intramedullary
ischial
ischialgia
ischiocapsular
ischiococcygeal
ischiococcygeus
ischiofemoral
ischiofibular
ischiohebotomy
ischiopubic
ischiopubiotomy
ischiosacral
ischiovertebral
ischium
iskeal. See *ischial.*

iskealjea. See *ischialgia.*
iskeo-. See words beginning
   ischio-.
iskeum. See *ischium.*
ithyokyphosis
ixomyelitis
jacket
     Kydex body j.
     Minerva's j.
     plaster-of-Paris j.
     Royalite body j.
     Sayre's j.
Jackson's clamp
Jansen's test
jerk
     Achilles j.
     ankle j.
     quadriceps j.
     triceps surae j.
Jewett's
     extractor
     nail
     plate
Jobst's stocking
joint. See also *articulation.*
     amphidiarthrodial j.
     ankle j.
     apophyseal j's
     arthrodial j.
     ball-and-socket j.
     biaxial j.
     bilocular j.
     Budin's j.
     cartilaginous j.
     Charcot's j.
     Chopart's j.
     Clutton's j.
     cochlear j.
     composite j.
     compound j.
     condyloid j.
     Cruveilhier's j.

joint (*continued*)
     diarthrodial j.
     dry j.
     elbow j.
     ellipsoidal j.
     enarthrodial j.
     false j.
     fibrocartilaginous j.
     fibrous j.
     flail j.
     freely movable j.
     fringe j.
     hinge j.
     hip j.
     hysteric j.
     immovable j.
     intercarpal j's
     irritable j.
     knee j.
     ligamentous j.
     Lisfranc's j.
     Luschka's j's
     j. mice
     midcarpal j.
     mixed j.
     multiaxial j.
     pivot j.
     plane j.
     polyaxial j.
     rotary j.
     sacrococcygeal j.
     saddle j.
     scapuloclavicular j.
     shoulder j.
     simple j.
     spheroidal j.
     spiral j.
     stifle j.
     synarthrodial j.
     synovial j.
     tarsal j.
     trochoid j.

joint (*continued*)
    uniaxial j.
    unilocular j.
    von Gies' j.
joint mice
Jones' splint
Joplin's operation
Jordan-Day bur
Judet's prosthesis
Jüngling's disease
Jung's muscle
juxta-articular
juxtaepiphyseal
Kanavel's
    sign
    splint
Kapel's operation
Kashin-Bek disease
Keen's sign
Keith's needle
Keller-Blake splint
Keller's bunionectomy
Kellogg-Speed operation
Kernig's sign
Kern's forceps
Kerrison's rongeur
Kerr's sign
Kessel's plate
Kessler's operation
Kezerian's osteotome
Kidner's operation
Kienböck's dislocation
kifo-. See words beginning
    kypho-.
kineplasty
kinesalgia
King-Richards operation
Kirkaldy-Willis operation
Kirk's amputation
Kirmisson's
    operation
    raspatory

kirospazm. See *cheirospasm*.
Kirschner's
    apparatus
    wire
KJ — knee jerk
KK — knee kick
Klippel-Feil syndrome
knee
    Brodie's k.
knife
    Downing's k.
    Freiberg's k.
    Liston's k.
    Lowe-Breck k.
    Smillie's k.
Knight's brace
Knowles' pin
knuckle
Kocher's operation
Koenig-Wittek operation
Köhler's disease
kokse-. See words beginning
    coccy-.
Kolomnin's operation
kon-. See words beginning
    chon-.
König's operation
Kreuscher's
    operation
    scissors
Kristiansen's screw
Krukenberg's hand
Kümmell's
    disease
    spondylitis
Kümmell-Verneuil disease
Küntscher's
    driver
    nail
    reamer
Kydex body jacket
kyphoscoliosis

kyphosis
    Scheuermann's k.
L-1, L-2, etc. — lumbar verte-
        brae
labrum
    l. acetabulare
    l. glenoidale
Laing's plate
Lambotte-Henderson osteo-
    tome
Lambotte's
    clamp
    forceps
    osteotome
Lambrinudi's operation
lamella
lamellae
lamellar
lamina
laminae
laminectomy
    lumbar l.
    thoracic l.
laminotomy
Lane's
    elevator
    forceps
    plate
Langenbeck's
    elevator
    saw
Lange's operation
Langoria's sign
Larrey's amputation
Larsen-Johansson disease
Lasègue's sign
Laugier's sign
Lawson-Thornton plate
LE — lupus erythematosus
Le Fort's
    amputation
    fracture

Legg-Calvé-Perthes syndrome
Legg-Calvé-Waldenström
    disease
Legg's osteotome
Leichtenstern's sign
Leinbach's
    osteotome
    screw
leiomyoma
leiomyosarcoma
Leksell's rongeur
Lempert's bur
L'Episcopo's operation
Leri's sign
Levine's operation
Lewin's
    dissector
    splint
Lewin-Stern splint
Lhermitte's sign
ligament
    accessory l.
    acromioclavicular l.
    acromiocoracoid l.
    adipose l.
    annular l.
    anterior l.
    arcuate l.
    Bertin's l.
    Bigelow's l.
    Brodie's l.
    calcaneofibular l.
    calcaneonavicular l.
    capsular l.
    carpometacarpal l.
    collateral l.
    coracoacromial l.
    coracoclavicular l.
    coracohumeral l.
    costoclavicular l.
    cruciate l's
    crural l.

ligament (*continued*)
    cuboideonavicular l.
    cuneonavicular l.
    deltoid l.
    dentate l.
    falciform l.
    flaval l.
    hamatometacarpal l.
    iliofemoral l.
    iliotrochanteric l.
    inguinal l.
    laciniate l.
    lateral l.
    medial l.
    olecranon l.
    patellar l.
    pisohamate l.
    pisometacarpal l.
    plantar l.
    popliteal l.
    posterior l.
    pubocapsular l.
    pubofemoral l.
    radiocarpal l.
    rhomboid l.
    sacrospinous l.
    sternoclavicular l.
    sternocostal l.
    talocalcaneal l.
    talofibular l.
    talonavicular l.
    tendinotrochanteric l.
    transverse l.
    trapezoid l.
    ulnar l.
    ulnocarpal l.
    volar l.
    Wrisberg's l.
ligamentous
ligamentum
    l. flavum
    l. teres femoris

Linder's sign
line
    Ogston's l.
    Ullmann's l.
linea
    l. alba cervicalis
    l. arcuata ossis ilii
    l. aspera femoris
    l. epiphysialis
    l. glutea
    l. pectinea femoris
    l. terminalis pelvis
    l. trapezoidea
lipoma
liposarcoma
Lippman's prosthesis
Lisfranc's
    amputation
    joint
Lissauer's zone
Liston's knife
Liston-Stille forceps
Littauer-Liston forceps
Littler's operation
Littlewood's operation
LOM — limitation of motion
    loss of motion
longitudinal
Looser-Milkman syndrome
Looser's zone
lordoscoliosis
lordosis
lordotic
Lorenz's
    osteotomy
    sign
Lottes'
    nail
    operation
Lowe-Breck knife
Lowman's clamp
LS — lumbosacral

Lucae's mallet
Lucas-Cottrell operation
Luck's
>   fasciatome
>   operation
Ludloff's
>   operation
>   sign
lumbago
lumbar
lumbarization
lumbodorsal
lumbodynia
lumboiliac
lumbosacral
Lund's operation
Luschka's joints
luxatio
>   l. coxae congenita
>   l. erecta
>   l. imperfecta
>   l. perinealis
luxation
>   Malgaigne's l.
Lyman-Smith brace
Lytle's splint
MacAusland's operation
Macewen's osteotomy
MacIntosh's prosthesis
MacKenzie's amputation
MacLeod's capsular rheumatism
Madelung's deformity
Magnuson's operation
Magnuson-Stack operation
Mahorner-Mead operation
main
>   m. en crochet
>   m. en griffe
>   m. en lorgnette
>   m. en pince
>   m. fourché

Maisonneuve's
>   amputation
>   sign
Malgaigne's luxation
malleolar
malleoli
malleolus
malleotomy
mallet
>   Crane's m.
>   Lucae's m.
>   Meyerding's m.
>   Rush's m.
malum
>   m. articulorum senilis
>   m. coxae senilis
malunion
mandible
mandibular
manipulation
Marie-Foix sign
Marie's hypertrophy
Marie-Strümpell
>   disease
>   spondylitis
Marie-Tooth disease
marrow
>   yellow bone m.
>   red bone m.
Martin's forceps
Mason-Allen splint
Massie's nail
Matchett-Brown prosthesis
Mauck's operation
maxilla
maxillary
Mayer's reflex
Mayfield's osteotome
Mayo's operation
Mazur's operation
McArdle's disease
McAtee's screw

McBride's operation
McCarroll's operation
McKee-Farrar prosthesis
McKeever's
    operation
    prosthesis
McLaughlin's
    operation
    plate
    screw
McMurray's
    sign
    test
McReynolds' adapter
mediastinum
medications. See *Drugs and Chemistry* section.
medulla
    m. ossium
    m. spinalis
medullary
melorheostosis
membrane
    synovial m.
meningosis
meninx
meniscectomy
    medial m.
menisci
meniscitis
meniscotome
    Bowen-Grover m.
    Smillie's m.
meniscus
    m. of acromioclavicular joint
    m. articularis
    m. articulationis genus, lateralis, medialis
    medial m. of knee joint
    m. of temporomaxillary joint

Mennell's sign
mesh
    Vitallium m.
mesomelic
mesomorphic
mesomorphy
mesotendineum
metacarpal
metacarpectomy
metacarpophalangeal
metacarpus
metaphysis
metaphysitis
metapophysis
metatarsal
metatarsalgia
metatarsectomy
metatarsophalangeal
metatarsus
    m. adductocavus
    m. adductovarus
    m. adductus
    m. atavicus
    m. latus
    m. primus varus
    m. varus
method
    Chaput's m.
    Delore's m.
    Essex-Lopresti m.
methyl
    m. methacrylate
Meyerding's
    mallet
    osteotome
    retractor
Michaelis's rhomboid
Michele's trephine
midcarpal
mielo-. See words beginning *myelo-*.
Mikulicz's operation

Milch's operation
Milkman's syndrome
Mill's test
Milwaukee brace
Miner's osteotome
Minerva's jacket
Minor's sign
Mitchell's
    bunionectomy
    operation
Moberg's arthrodesis
mobilization
Moe's plate
monostotic
Monteggia's
    dislocation
    fracture
Moore's
    chisel
    extractor
    fracture
    gouge
    nail
    osteotome
    pin
    prosthesis
    reamer
    template
Morestin's operation
Morquio's
    disease
    sign
Morton's
    neuralgia
    neuroma
    toe
Mosso's ergograph
MP — metacarpophalangeal
MPJ — metacarpophalangeal
        joint
Mueller's prosthesis
Mumford-Gurd operation

muscle
    abductor digiti quinti m.
    abductor pollicis brevis
        m.
    abductor pollicis longus
        m.
    adductor hallucis m.
    adductor longus m.
    adductor magnus m.
    adductor pollicis m.
    anconeus m.
    appendicular m's
    biceps brachii m.
    biceps femoris m.
    brachialis m.
    brachioradialis m.
    coracobrachialis m.
    deltoid m.
    extensor carpi radialis
        brevis m.
    extensor carpi radialis
        longus m.
    extensor carpi ulnaris m.
    extensor digiti minimi m.
    extensor digiti quinti
        proprius m.
    extensor digitorum brevis
        m.
    extensor digitorum
        communis m.
    extensor digitorum
        longus m.
    extensor hallucis brevis
        m.
    extensor hallucis longus
        m.
    extensor indicis m.
    extensor pollicis brevis
        m.
    extensor pollicis longus
        m.
    flexor carpi radialis m.

muscle (*continued*)
    flexor carpi ulnaris m.
    flexor digitorum brevis m.
    flexor digitorum longus m.
    flexor digitorum profundus m.
    flexor digitorum sublimis m.
    flexor digitorum superficialis m.
    flexor hallucis brevis m.
    flexor hallucis longus m.
    flexor pollicis brevis m.
    flexor pollicis longus m.
    gastrocnemius m.
    gemellus m.
    gluteus maximus m.
    gluteus medius m.
    gluteus minimus m.
    gracilis m.
    greater trochanter m.
    m. iliacus
    iliococcygeal m.
    iliocostalis cervicis m.
    iliocostalis lumborum m.
    iliocostalis thoracis m.
    iliopsoas m.
    interosseous m.
    involuntary m's
    Jung's m.
    lateral malleolus m.
    latissimus dorsi m.
    levator m's
    nonstriated m.
    m. opponens pollicis
    palmaris brevis m.
    palmaris longus m.
    paraspinal m.
    pectineus m.
    pectoralis major m.

muscle (*continued*)
    pectoralis minor m.
    peroneus brevis m.
    peroneus longus m.
    peroneus tertius m.
    piriform m.
    m. piriformis
    plantar m.
    popliteal m.
    pronator quadratus m.
    pronator teres m.
    psoas m.
    quadriceps femoris m.
    rectus m.
    sartorius m.
    scalenus m.
    semimembranosus m.
    semispinalis m.
    semitendinosus m.
    serratus m.
    skeletal m's
    smooth m's
    soleus m.
    spinalis m.
    sternocleidomastoid m.
    striated m's
    subscapular m.
    supinator m.
    tensor fasciae latae m.
    teres m.
    tibialis m.
    transverse m.
    trapezius m.
    triceps brachii m.
    triceps surae m.
    vastus intermedius m.
    vastus lateralis m.
    vastus medialis m.
    visceral m's
    voluntary m's
muscular
muscularis

musculature
musculoskeletal
musculotendinous
musculus
myalgia
myasthenia
myasthenia gravis
myatonia
myectomy
myelitis
myelocele
myelocystomeningocele
myelogram
myelography
myeloid
myeloma
myelomalacia
myelomenia
myelomeningitis
myelomeningocele
myelon
myeloneuritis
myelo-opticoneuropathy
myeloparalysis
myelopathy
myelophthisis
myeloplegia
myelopoiesis
myelopore
myeloradiculitis
myeloradiculodysplasia
myeloradiculopathy
myelorrhagia
myeloschisis
myelosclerosis
myelospasm
myelosyphilis
myelotome
myelotomy
    commissural m.
myesthesia
myoblastoma

myocele
myoclonus
myocrismus
myodemia
myodiastasis
myodynia
myofascitis
myofibril
myofibroma
myofibrosis
myogelosis
myogenic
myohypertrophia
myokerosis
myokinesis
myokymia
myolysis
myoma
myomalacia
myoneurectomy
myopathia
    m. infraspinata
myopathy
myoplasty
myorrhaphy
myorrhexis
myosarcoma
myoscope
myoseism
myositis
    acute progressive m.
    m. fibrosa
    m. ossificans
    progressive ossifying m.
    rheumatoid m.
    m. serosa
    suppurative m.
myospasm
myosteoma
myosthenometer
myotasis
myotatic

myotenositis
myotenotomy
myotome
myotomy
myotonia
    m. acquisita
    m. atrophica
    m. congenita
    m. dystrophica
myotonus
myxoma
Naffziger's syndrome
nail
    Augustine's n.
    Hansen-Street n.
    Harrington's n.
    Jewett's n.
    Küntscher n.
    Lottes' n.
    Massie's n.
    Moore's n.
    Neufeld's n.
    Pugh's n.
    Schneider's n.
    Smillie's n.
    Smith-Petersen n.
    Thornton's n.
    Venable-Stuck n.
    Zickle's n.
nailing
    intramedullary n.
nates
navicula
navicular
nearthrosis
neck
    surgical n.
necrosis
    aseptic n.
    Paget's quiet n.
    Zenker's n.

needle
    Bunnell's n.
    Keith's n.
    Turkel's n.
Neer's prosthesis
Nélaton's
    dislocation
    operation
nerve
    peroneal n.
Neufeld's nail
neuralgia
    Morton's n.
neurofibroma
neurofibromatosis
neurofibrositis
neurolysis
neuroma
    Morton's n.
neuropathy
neurorrhaphy
neuroskeletal
Neviaser's operation
Nicola's operation
node
    Bouchard's n's
    Heberden's n's
nodule
    Schmorl's n.
nonunion
notch
    clavicular n.
    coracoid n.
    interclavicular n.
    intercondylar n.
    intervertebral n.
    semilunar n.
    trochlear n.
    vertebral n.
nucleus
    n. pulposus

Ober's
  operation
  test
Ogston's
  line
  operation
olecranal
olecranarthritis
olecranarthropathy
olecranon
olisthy
Ollier's
  disease
  dyschondroplasia
  operation
operation
  Abbott-Lucas o.
  Abbott's o.
  Adams' o.
  Adelmann's o.
  Albee-Delbet o.
  Albee's o.
  Albert's o.
  Anderson's o.
  Annandale's o.
  Avila's o.
  Axer's o.
  Badgley's o.
  Bankhart's o.
  Barker's o.
  Barton's o.
  Barwell's o.
  Bateman's o.
  Bent's o.
  Blount's o.
  Blundell-Jones o.
  Bobroff's o.
  Bosworth's o.
  Boyd's o.
  Brett's o.
  Bristow's o.
  Brittain's o.

operation (*continued*)
  Brockman's o.
  Buck's o.
  Bunnell's o.
  Callahan's o.
  Campbell's o.
  Carrell's o.
  Cave-Rowe o.
  Cave's o.
  Chiene's o.
  Cloward's o.
  Codivilla's o.
  Cole's o.
  Colonna's o.
  Compere's o.
  Conn's o.
  Credo's o.
  Crutchfield's o.
  Cubbins' o.
  Darrach's o.
  Davies-Colley o.
  Denuse's o.
  Dickson-Diveley o.
  Dickson's o.
  Dieffenbach's o.
  Dunn-Brittain o.
  Durman's o.
  Eden-Hybbinette o.
  Eggers' o.
  Ellis-Jones o.
  Elmslie-Cholmeley o.
  Evans' o.
  Eyler's o.
  Fahey's o.
  Fowler's o.
  Fritz-Lange o.
  Gant's o.
  Gatellier's o.
  Ghormley's o.
  Gibson's o.
  Gillespie's o.
  Gill's o.

operation (*continued*)

Girdlestone's o.
Goldthwait's o.
Graber-Duvernay o.
Grice-Green o.
Guleke-Stookey o.
Haas' o.
Hammond's o.
Hark's o.
Harmon's o.
Harris-Beath o.
Hauser's o.
Heifitz's o.
Henderson's o.
Hendry's o.
Henry-Geist o.
Heuter's o.
Heyman's o.
Hibbs' o.
Hoffa-Lorenz o.
Hoffa's o.
Hohmann's o.
Holme's o.
Horwitz-Adams o.
Houston's o.
Howorth's o.
Joplin's o.
Kapel's o.
Kellogg-Speed o.
Kessler's o.
Kidner's o.
King-Richards o.
Kirkaldy-Willis o.
Kirmisson's o.
Kocher's o.
Koenig-Wittek o.
Kolomnin's o.
König's o.
Kreuscher's o.
Lambrinudi's o.
Lange's o.
L'Episcopo's o.

operation (*continued*)

Levine's o.
Littler's o.
Littlewood's o.
Lottes' o.
Lucas-Cottrell o.
Luck's o.
Ludloff's o.
Lund's o.
MacAusland's o.
Magnuson's o.
Magnuson-Stack o.
Mahorner-Mead o.
Mauck's o.
Mayo's o.
Mazur's o.
McBride's o.
McCarroll's o.
McKeever's o.
McLaughlin's o.
Mikulicz's o.
Milch's o.
Mitchell's o.
Morestin's o.
Mumford-Gurd o.
Nélaton's o.
Neviaser's o.
Nicola's o.
Ober's o.
Ogston's o.
Ollier's o.
Osborne's o.
Osgood's o.
Overholt's o.
Paci's o.
Palmer-Widen o.
Pauwels' o.
Pheasant's o.
Phelps' o.
Phemister's o.
Pollock's o.
Poncet's o.

operation (*continued*)
    Putti-Platt o.
    Puusepp's o.
    Reichenheim-King o.
    Reverdin's o.
    Ridlon's o.
    Routier's o.
    Roux-Goldthwait o.
    Salter's o.
    Sayre's o.
    Schanz's o.
    Schede's o.
    shelf o.
    Slocum's o.
    Smith-Petersen o.
    Sofield's o.
    Speed-Boyd o.
    Stamm's o.
    Steindler's o.
    Swanson's o.
    Thomson's o.
    Turko's o.
    Van Gorder's o.
    Wagoner's o.
    Watson-Jones o.
    Whitman's o.
    Wilson-McKeever o.
    Wladimiroff's o.
    Wyeth's o.
    Yount's o.
    Zahradnicek's o.
    Zancolli's o.
Oppenheim's sign
ortho. — orthopedics
orthopedic
os
    o. calcis
    o. cuboideum
    o. lunatum
    o. magnum
    o. trigonum tarsi
    o. triquetrum

Osborne's operation
osfe-. See words beginning
    osphy-.
Osgood's operation
Osgood-Schlatter disease
osphyarthrosis
osphyomyelitis
osphyotomy
ossature
ossein
osseoaponeurotic
osseocartilaginous
osseofibrous
osseomucin
osseomucoid
osseosonometer
ooseosonometry
osseous
ossicle
ossicula
ossiculum
ossiferous
ossific
ossification
ossifluence
ossifying
ostealgia
ostearthrotomy
ostectomy
osteitis
    o. condensans ilii
    o. deformans
    o. fibrosa cystica
    o. ossificans
ostempyesis
osteoanagenesis
osteoaneurysm
osteoarthritis
osteoarthropathy
osteoarthrosis
osteoarticular
osteoblast

osteoblastic
osteoblastoma
osteocachexia
osteocamp
osteocartilaginous
osteochondral
osteochondritis
    o. deformans
    o. dissecans
osteochondrodystrophy
osteochondroma
osteochondromatosis
    synovial o.
osteochondropathy
osteochondrosarcoma
osteochondrosis
osteochondrous
osteoclasis
osteoclast
    Collin's o.
    Phelps-Gocht o.
    Rizzoli's o.
osteoclastoma
osteocomma
osteocope
osteocystoma
osteocyte
osteodesmosis
osteodiastasis
osteodynia
osteodysplasty
osteodystrophia
    o. cystica
    o. fibrosa
osteodystrophy
osteoepiphysis
osteofibrochondrosarcoma
osteofibroma
osteofibromatosis
osteogenesis
    o. imperfecta
osteogram

osteography
osteohydatidosis
osteoid
osteology
osteolysis
osteoma
    cavalryman's o.
    o. sarcomatosum
    o. spongiosum
osteomalacia
osteometry
osteomiosis
osteomyelitis
    Garré's o.
osteomyelodysplasia
osteomyelography
osteoneuralgia
osteopathy
osteopenia
osteoperiosteal
osteoperiostitis
osteopetrosis
osteophlebitis
osteophore
osteophyma
osteophyte
osteophytosis
osteoplastica
osteoplasty
osteopoikilosis
osteoporosis
osteoporotic
osteopsathyrosis
osteoradionecrosis
osteorrhaphy
osteosarcoma
osteosclerosis
osteoscope
osteosis
osteostixis
osteosynovitis
osteosynthesis

osteothrombosis
osteotome
    Albee's o.
    Alexander's o.
    Blount's o.
    Bowen's o.
    Campbell's o.
    Carroll-Legg o.
    Carroll's o.
    Carroll-Smith-Petersen o.
    Cherry's o.
    Clayton's o.
    Cloward's o.
    Cobb's o.
    Converse's o.
    Cottle's o.
    Crane's o.
    Dingman's o.
    Epstein's o.
    Frazier's o.
    Hibbs' o.
    Hoke's o.
    Howorth's o.
    Kezerian's o.
    Lambotte-Henderson o.
    Lambotte's o.
    Legg's o.
    Leinbach's o.
    Mayfield's o.
    Meyerding's o.
    Miner's o.
    Moore's o.
    Rowland's o.
    Sheehan's o.
    Smith-Petersen o.
    Stille's o.
osteotomoclasis
osteotomy
    block o.
    Coventry's o.
    cuneiform o.
    cup-and-ball o.

osteotomy (*continued*)
    innominate o.
    linear o.
    Lorenz's o.
    Macewen's o.
    subtrochanteric o.
    transtrochanteric o.
osteotribe
osteotylus
Otto's
    disease
    pelvis
Overholt's operation
P – phosphorus
Paci's operation
packing
    Gelfoam p.
Paget's
    disease
    quiet necrosis
palm
palma
    p. manus
palmar
palmaris
Palmer-Widen operation
pannus
panosteitis
parallagma
paralysis
    Pott's p.
paramyoclonus
    p. multiplex
paramyotonia
    ataxia p.
    p. congenita
paramyotonus
paraplegia
paratarsium
paratenon
paravertebral
paresis

paresthesia
Parona's space
paronychia
    p. tendinosa
parosteitis
parosteosis
patella
    p. bipartita
    p. cubiti
    floating p.
    p. partita
    slipping p.
patellapexy
patellar
patellectomy
patellofemoral
patellometer
Patrick's test
Pauwels' operation
Pauzat's disease
pectus
    p. carinatum
    p. excavatum
    p. recurvatum
pedal
pedicle
    p. of vertebral arch
pediculus
    p. arcus vertebrae
Pellegrini-Stieda disease
pelma
pelvic girdle
pelvimetry
pelviotomy
pelvis
    Otto's p.
pelvisacral
pelvisection
pelvitrochanterian
pelvospondylitis
    p. ossificans
periarthritis

periarticular
perichondritis
perichondrium
pericoxitis
peridesmium
perineum
perineuritis
perineurium
periosteal
periosteomyelitis
periosteorrhaphy
periosteotome
    Alexander-Farabeuf p.
    Alexander's p.
periosteotomy
periosteum
periostitis
perispondylitis
    Gibney's p.
peritendineum
peritendinitis
    p. calcarea
    p. crepitans
peritenon
peritenoneum
peritenonitis
peroneal
peroneotibial
Perrin-Ferraton disease
Perthes' disease
pes
    p. abductus
    p. adductus
    p. anserinus
    p. cavus
    p. planus
    p. pronatus
    p. supinatus
    p. valgus
phalangeal
phalangectomy
phalanges

phalangette
phalangophalangeal
phalanx
    distal p.
    proximal p.
Pheasant's operation
Phelps-Gocht osteoclast
Phelps' operation
Phemister's operation
phosphorus
physiotherapy
Pietrie's cast
pillion
pin
    Bohlman's p.
    Compere's p.
    Hagie's p.
    Hansen-Street p.
    Hatcher's p.
    Knowles' p.
    Moore's p.
    Rush's p.
    Steinmann's p.
    Street's p.
    Turner's p.
    von Saal's p.
    Zimmer's p.
Piotrowski's sign
PIP — proximal interphalangeal
PIPJ — proximal interphalan-
       geal joint
Pirie's bone
Pirogoff's amputation
plantar
plantaris
plate
    Badgley's p.
    Blount's p.
    Deyerle's p.
    Eggers' p.
    Elliott's p.
    epiphyseal p.

plate (*continued*)
    Hoen's p.
    Jewett's p.
    Kessel's p.
    Laing's p.
    Lane's p.
    Lawson-Thornton p.
    McLaughlin's p.
    Moe's p.
    Sherman's p.
    Thornton's p.
    Wilson's p.
    Wright's p.
pleurapophysis
plombage
plombierung
poculum
    p. diogenis
podagra
pododynia
Pollock's operation
polyarthric
polyarthritis
polyarticular
polychondritis
polychondropathy
polydactylia
polydactylism
polydactyly
polydysspondylism
polydystrophy
polymyalgia
    p. rheumatica
polymyositis
polyphasic
polytendinitis
polytendinobursitis
Poncet's operation
poples
popliteal
position. See *General Surgical
    Terms.*

Pott's
    disease
    fracture
    gangrene
    paralysis
Poulet's disease
Preiser's disease
prehallux
prepatellar
pretarsal
pretibial
probe
    Bunnell's p.
process
    acromion p.
    articular p.
    capitular p.
    condyloid p.
    conoid p.
    coracoid p.
    intercondylar p.
    mastoid p.
    odontoid p.
    olecranon p.
    spinous p.
    styloid p.
    ungual p.
    xiphoid p.
processus
    p. spinosus vertebrarum
    p. transversus verte-
       brarum
pronation
pronatoflexor
prosthesis
    Aufranc-Turner p.
    Austin-Moore p.
    Bateman's p.
    Bechtol's p.
    CAD (computerized
      assisted design) p.
    Charnley-Mueller p.

prosthesis (*continued*)
    DePalma's p.
    DePuy's p.
    Eicher's p.
    Geomedic p.
    geometric p.
    Giliberty's p.
    Guepar's p.
    Judet's p.
    Lippman's p.
    MacIntosh's p.
    Matchett-Brown p.
    McKee-Farrar p.
    McKeever's p.
    Moore's p.
    Mueller's p.
    Neer's p.
    Shier's p.
    Smith-Petersen p.
    Swanson's p.
    Thompson's p.
    Townley's p.
    Vitallium p.
    Walldius' p.
    Zimaloy's p.
    Zimmer's p.
protractor
    Robinson's p.
protrusion
pseudoarthrosis
pseudohypertrophic
pseudoluxation
psoas muscle
pubetrotomy
pubic
pubioplasty
pubiotomy
pubis
pubofemoral
pubotibial
Pugh's nail
pulvinar

punch
    Deyerle's p.
Putti-Platt operation
Putti's rasp
Puusepp's operation
pyarthrosis
pyknotic
pylon
pyogenic
quadratipronator
quadriceps
quadricepsplasty
quadriplegia
Quervain's
    disease
    fracture
RA — rheumatoid arthritis
rabdo-. See words beginning
    rhabdo-.
rachialgia
rachidial
rachidian
rachigraph
rachilysis
rachiocampsis
rachiocentesis
rachiochysis
rachiodynia
rachiokyphosis
rachiometer
rachiomyelitis
rachiopathy
rachioscoliosis
rachiotome
rachiotomy
rachis
rachisagra
rachischisis
rachitis
rachitomy
radial
radicular

radiculectomy
radiculitis
radiculomedullary
radiculomeningomyelitis
radiculomyelopathy
radiculoneuritis
radiculoneuropathy
radiculopathy
radiobicipital
radiocarpal
radiocarpus
radiohumeral
radiopalmar
radioulnar
radius
rake. See words beginning
    rachi-.
rakealjea. See *rachialgia*.
rakeo-. See words beginning
    rachio-.
rakitis. See *rachitis*.
ramus
    r. of pubis
Raney-Crutchfield tong
rasp
    Putti's r.
raspatory
    Kirmisson's r.
Rauchfuss's sling
ray
    digital r.
reamer
    Küntscher's r.
    Moore's r.
    Rush's r.
Recklinghausen's disease
recurvation
Redivac drain
reduction
    closed r.
    open r.
reef

reflex
> Bechterew-Mendel r.
> Bechterew's r.
> Chaddock's r.
> Mayer's r.
> Stookey r.
> Strümpell's r.

refracture
Reichel's chondromatosis
Reichenheim-King operation
rete
> r. articulare genus
> r. calcaneum
> r. carpi dorsale

retinaculum
retractor
> Bankhart's r.
> Beckman-Adson r.
> Bennett's r.
> Blount's r.
> cobra r.
> Gelpi's r.
> Hibb's r.
> Hohmann's r.
> Meyerding's r.
> Rizzo's r.
> Senn's r.
> Sweet's r.

retropatellar
retropulsion
Reverdin's operation
RF — rheumatoid factor
rhabdomyoma
rhabdomyosarcoma
rheumatism
> Besnier's r.
> MacLeod's capsular r.
> palindromic r.

rheumatoid
rhizomelic
rhomboid
> Michaelis's r.

rib
> bicipital r.
> cervical r.
> false r's
> floating r's
> true r's
> vertebral r's
> vertebrocostal r's
> vertebrosternal r's

Ricard's amputation
Richard's screw
rickets
Ridlon's operation
RIF — right iliac fossa
rigidity
> cogwheel r.

Risser's cast
risomelik. See *rhizomelic*.
Rizzoli's osteoclast
Rizzo's retractor
Robinson's protractor
rod
> Harrington's r.
> Rush's r.

ROM — range of motion
Romberg's sign
romboid. See *rhomboid*.
rongeur
> Cloward's r.
> Kerrison's r.
> Leksell's r.
> Schlesinger's r.

roomatizm. See *rheumatism*.
rotation
Routier's operation
Roux-Goldthwait operation
Rowland's osteotome
Royalite body jacket
Rush's
> mallet
> pin
> reamer

Rush's (*continued*)
    rod
Russell's traction
Russe's bone graft
Ryerson's tenotome
sacral
sacralgia
sacralization
sacrarthrogenic
sacrectomy
sacroanterior
sacrococcygeal
sacrococcyx
sacrocoxalgia
sacrocoxitis
sacrodynia
sacroiliac
sacroiliitis
sacrolisthesis
sacrolumbar
sacroposterior
sacrosciatic
sacrospinal
sacrotomy
sacrovertebral
sacrum
Salter's operation
Sarbó's sign
sarcoidosis
    muscular s.
sarcolemma
sarcoma
    Ewing's s.
    osteogenic s.
    reticulum cell s.
sarcoplasm
sarcoplast
Satterlee's saw
saucerization
saw
    Adams' s.
    Butcher's s.

saw (*continued*)
    Charrière's s.
    Gigli's s.
    Langenbeck's s.
    Satterlee's s.
    Stryker's s.
Sayre's
    apparatus
    jacket
    operation
    splint
scan
    bone s.
scaphoid
scaphoiditis
    tarsal s.
scapula
scapulalgia
scapular
scapulectomy
scapuloclavicular
scapulodynia
scapulohumeral
scapulopexy
scapuloposterior
scapulothoracic
Scarpa's triangle
Schanz's
    disease
    operation
    syndrome
Schede's operation
Scheuermann's
    disease
    kyphosis
Schlatter's disease
Schlesinger's
    rongeur
    sign
Schmorl's
    body
    disease

Schmorl's (*continued*)
    nodule
Schneider's nail
sciatic
sciatica
scissors
    Kreuscher's s.
    Wester's s.
scoliokyphosis
scoliosis
    Brissaud's s.
    cicatricial s.
    coxitic s.
    empyematic s.
    ischiatic s.
    myopathic s.
    ocular s.
    ophthalmic s.
    osteopathic s.
    paralytic s.
    rachitic s.
    rheumatic s.
    sciatic s.
    static s.
scoliosometer
scoliotic
scoliotone
scolopsia
screw
    Basile's s.
    Bosworth's s.
    Collison's s.
    Coventry's s.
    Eggers' s.
    Kristiansen's s.
    Leinbach's s.
    McAtee's s.
    McLaughlin's s.
    Richard's s.
    Sherman's s.
    Thornton's s.
    Vitallium s.

screw (*continued*)
    Zimmer's s.
semilunar
semilunare
Senn's retractor
sequestrectomy
sequestrum
sesamoid
sesamoiditis
Sever's disease
sfirektome. See *sphyrectomy.*
sfirotome. See *sphyrotomy.*
Sharpey's fibers
Sheehan's osteotome
Shepherd's fracture
Sherman's
    plate
    screw
Shier's prosthesis
SI — sacroiliac
siatik. See *sciatic.*
siatika. See *sciatica.*
sign
    Allis' s.
    Anghelescu's s.
    anterior tibial s.
    Babinski's s.
    Beevor's s.
    Bonnet's s.
    Bragard's s.
    Brudzinski's s.
    Bryant's s.
    Chvostek's s.
    Cleeman's s.
    Codman's s.
    Comolli's s.
    Coopernail's s.
    Dawbarn's s.
    Dejerine's s.
    Demianoff's s.
    Desault's s.
    drawer s.

sign (*continued*)
- Dupuytren's s.
- Erichsen's s.
- fabere s.
- Fajersztajn's s.
- Fränkel's s.
- Froment's s.
- Gaenslen's s.
- Galeazzi's s.
- Goldthwait's s.
- Guilland's s.
- Hefke-Turner s.
- Helbing's s.
- Hirschberg's s.
- Hoffmann's s.
- Homans' s.
- Hueter's s.
- Kanavel's s.
- Keen's s.
- Kernig's s.
- Kerr's s.
- Langoria's s.
- Lasègue's s.
- Laugier's s.
- Leichtenstern's s.
- Leri's s.
- Lhermitte's s.
- Linder's s.
- Lorenz's s.
- Ludloff's s.
- Maisonneuve's s.
- Marie-Foix s.
- McMurray's s.
- Mennell's s.
- Minor's s.
- Morquio's s.
- Oppenheim's s.
- Piotrowski's s.
- pronation s.
- radialis s.
- Romberg's s.
- Sarbó's s.
- Schlesinger's s.

sign (*continued*)
- Soto-Hall s.
- Strümpell's s.
- Strunsky's s.
- Thomas' s.
- tibialis s.
- Tinel's s.
- Turyn's s.
- Vanzetti's s.
- Westphal's s.

Silver's bunionectomy
simphysis. See *symphysis.*
sin-. See words beginning *syn-.*
sinew
sino-. See words beginning
   syno-.
sinus
- tarsal s.

skeletal
skeleton
skewfoot
Skillern's fracture
SLE — systemic lupus
       erythematosus
sling
- Glisson's s.
- Rauchfuss's s.
- Teare's s.

Slocum's operation
SLR — straight leg raising
Smedberg's drill
Smillie's
- knife
- meniscotome
- nail

Smith-Petersen
- nail
- operation
- osteotome
- prosthesis

Smith's
- dislocation
- fracture

soas-. See *psoas*.
Sofield's operation
Soto-Hall sign
space
    palmar s.
    Parona's s.
    thenar s.
    web s's
spasmus
    s. nutans
spastic
Speed-Boyd operation
sphyrectomy
sphyrotomy
spica
    hip s.
spina
    s. bifida occulta
spinal
spinalgia
spine
    bamboo s.
    cervical s.
spinogalvanization
spinous
splayfoot
splint
    Agnew's s.
    Anderson's s.
    Angle's s.
    Ashhurst's s.
    Balkan s.
    banjo s.
    Baylor's s.
    Böhler-Braun s.
    Böhler's s.
    Bond's s.
    Bowlby's s.
    Brant's s.
    Buck's s.
    Cabot's s.
    Chandler's s.

splint (*continued*)
    cock-up s.
    Colles' s.
    Curry's s.
    Davis' s.
    Denis-Browne clubfoot s.
    DePuy's s.
    drop-foot s.
    Dupuytren's s.
    Eggers' s.
    Engelmann's s.
    Fox's s.
    Frejka's s.
    Gordon's s.
    Hart's s.
    Hodgen's s.
    Jones' s.
    Kanavel's s.
    Keller-Blake s.
    Lewin's s.
    Lewin-Stern s.
    Lytle's s.
    Mason-Allen s.
    Protecto s.
    Sayre's s.
    Stader's s.
    Taylor's s.
    Thomas' s.
    Valentine's s.
    Volkmann's s.
    Wertheim's s.
    Zimmer's s.
spondylalgia
spondylarthritis
    s. ankylopoietica
spondylarthrocace
spondylexarthrosis
spondylitis
    ankylosing s.
    Bekhterev's s.
    s. deformans
    hypertrophic s.

spondylitis (*continued*)
    s. infectiosa
    Kümmell's s.
    Marie-Strümpell s.
    rheumatoid s.
spondylizema
spondylocace
spondylodesis
spondylodynia
spondylolisthesis
spondylolysis
spondylomalacia
    s. traumatica
spondylopathy
    traumatic s.
spondylopyosis
spondyloschisis
spondylosis
    cervical s.
    s. chronica ankylopoi-
        etica
    rhizomelic s.
    s. uncovertebralis
spondylosyndesis
spondylotherapy
spondylotomy
spot
    Carleton's s's
sprain
    riders' s.
Spratt's curet
Sprengel's deformity
spur
    calcaneal s.
    occipital s.
    olecranon s.
Stader's splint
Stamm's operation
stapler
    Blount's s.
Steindler's operation
Steinert's disease

Steinmann's pin
sternal
sternoclavicular
sternoscapular
sternotomy
sternovertebral
sternum
Stieda's fracture
Stille's osteotome
stockinette
stocking
    Jobst's s.
    thromboembolic s.
Stokes' amputation
Stone's bunionectomy
Stookey reflex
Street's pin
striated
Strümpell's
    reflex
    sign
Strunsky's sign
Stryker's
    frame
    saw
subaponeurotic
subastragalar
subcapsuloperiosteal
subchondral
subluxation
    Volkmann's s.
submaxillary
subparietal
subperiosteal
subscapular
subsultus
    s. tendinum
subvertebral
Sudeck's atrophy
sudoluxation. See *pseudo-*
    luxation.
sulcus

supination
supinator
supraclavicular
supracondylar
sura
sural
surgical procedures. See *operation.*
suture. See *General Surgical Terms.*
Swanson's
      operation
      prosthesis
swayback
Swediaur's disease
Sweet's retractor
Syme's amputation
symphysis
      pubic s.
synarthrophysis
synarthrosis
synchondrectomy
synchondroses
synchondrosis
synchondrotomy
synclonus
syndactyly
syndesis
syndesmectomy
syndesmectopia
syndesmitis
      s. metatarsea
syndesmography
syndesmology
syndesmoma
syndesmo-odontoid
syndesmopexy
syndesmophyte
syndesmoplasty
syndesmorrhaphy
syndesmosis
syndesmotomy

syndrome
      Albright's s.
      Baastrup's s.
      Bakwin-Eiger s.
      Barré-Liéou s.
      Bertolotti's s.
      carpal tunnel s.
      cervical s.
      Guillain-Barré s.
      Klippel-Feil s.
      Legg-Calvé-Perthes s.
      Looser-Milkman s.
      Milkman's s.
      Naffziger's s.
      scalenus anticus s.
      Schanz's s.
      Tietze's s.
synosteology
synosteotomy
synostosis
      radioulnar s.
      tarsal s.
synovectomy
synovia
synovial
synovioma
synoviosarcoma
synovitis
synovium
syntenosis
synthesis
      s. of continuity
synthetism
syntripsis
syringocele
syringomyelitis
systemic lupus erythematosus
T-1, T-2, etc. — thoracic vertebrae
tabatière anatomique
tailbone
taliped

talipes
 t. calcaneovalgus
 t. calcaneovarus
 t. calcaneus
 t. cavovalgus
 t. cavus
 t. equinovalgus
 t. equinovarus
 t. equinus
 t. planovalgus
 t. valgus
 t. varus
talipomanus
Talma's disease
talocalcaneal
talocrural
talofibular
talonavicular
talotibial
talus
tank
 Hubbard's t.
tarsal
tarsectomy
tarsectopia
tarsoclasis
tarsomegaly
tarsometatarsal
tarsophalangeal
tarsoptosis
tarsotarsal
tarsotibial
tarsus
Taylor's
 brace
 splint
Teale's amputation
tear
 bucket-handle t.
Teare's sling
TED — thromboembolic
  disease

teerfo. See *tirefond.*
template
 Moore's t.
tendines
tendinitis
tendinoplasty
tendinosuture
tendinous
tendo
 t. Achillis
 t. calcaneus
tendolysis
tendon
 Achilles t.
 calcaneal t.
 flexor carpi radialis t.
 flexor digitorum pro-
  fundus t.
 flexor digitorum sub-
  limis t.
 palmaris longus t.
 patellar t.
 rider's t.
tendoplasty
tenectomy
tenodesis
tenodynia
tenomyotomy
tenonectomy
tenontitis
 t. prolifera calcarea
tenontodynia
tenontophyma
tenontothecitis
tenophyte
tenoplasty
tenorrhaphy
tenositis
tenostosis
tenosuspension
tenosynovectomy
tenosynovitis

tenotome
      Ryerson's t.
tenotomy
tenovaginitis
Tensilon test
teres
test
      Bekhterev's t.
      Callaway's t.
      Chiene's t.
      Dugas' t.
      Ely's t.
      erythrocyte sedimenta-
         tion rate t.
      fabere (fixation, abduc-
         tion, external rotation,
         extension) t.
      Finklestein's t.
      Hamilton's t.
      Jansen's t.
      latex fixation t.
      lupus erythematosus
         (LE) cell t.
      McMurray's t.
      Mill's t.
      Ober's t.
      Patrick's t.
      rheumatoid factor t.
      serum calcium t.
      serum creatine kinase t.
      serum phosphorus t.
      straight leg raising t.
      Tensilon t.
      Thomas' t.
      thumbnail t.
      Trendelenburg's t.
      uric acid t.
theca
thecitis
thecostegnosis
thenar
thermophore

Thomas'
      collar
      sign
      splint
      test
Thompson's prosthesis
Thomson's operation
thoracic
thoracicohumeral
thoracispinal
thoracolumbar
thorax
Thornton's
      nail
      plate
      screw
thrypsis
thumb
      bidif t.
      tennis t.
      trigger t.
tibia
      saber t.
      t. valga
      t. vara
tibial
tibialgia
tibialis
tibiocalcanean
tibiofemoral
tibiofibular
tibionavicular
tibiotarsal
Tietze's syndrome
Tinel's sign
tirefond
tiring
tissue
      osseous t.
toe
      hammer t.
      Morton's t.

tong
- Barton's t.
- Crutchfield's t.
- Raney-Crutchfield t.

tonus

tophi

tophus

torticollis

tourniquet
- pneumatic t.

Townley's prosthesis

traction
- Bryant's t.
- Buck's t.
- halo-pelvic t.
- Russell's t.
- skeletal t.

transplantation

transposition

transection

transverse

transversectomy

transversotomy

trapeziometacarpal

trapezium

trapezoid

Trendelenburg's test

trephine
- Michele's t.
- Turkel's t.

triangle
- Scarpa's t.

triceps

Tripier's amputation

trochanter

trochanteric

trochanterplasty

trochlea

tubercle

tuberculosis
- t. of bone

tuberositas

tuberosity

tucker
- Bishop-Black tendon t.
- Bishop-DeWitt tendon t.
- Bishop-Peter tendon t.
- Bishop's tendon t.
- Burch-Greenwood tendon t.
- Fink's tendon t.

tumor
- giant cell t.
- Ewing's t.

Turkel's
- needle
- trephine

Turko's operation

Turner's pin

Turyn's sign

Ullmann's line

ulna

ulnar

ulnaris

ulnocarpal

unloradial

ultrasonics

Valentine's splint

Van Buren's forceps

Van Gorder's operation

Vanzetti's sign

vein
- antebrachial cephalic v.
- cephalic v.
- saphenous v.

Velpeau's deformity

Venable-Stuck nail

Verbrugge's clamp

vertebra

vertebrae
- cervical v. (C1–C7)
- coccygeal v.
- lumbar v. (L1–L5)
- sacral v.

vertebrae (*continued*)
    thoracic v. (T1–T12 or
      D1–D12)
vertebral
vertebrectomy
vesalianum
visceral
Vitallium
    drill
    mesh
    prosthesis
    screw
volar
volardorsal
volaris
Volkmann's
    contracture
    deformity
    disease
    splint
    subluxation
vomer
von Gies' joint
von Recklinghausen's disease
von Saal's pin
Wagoner's operation
Wagstaffe's fracture
Waldenström's disease
Walldius' prosthesis
Watson-Jones operation
Webb's bolt
Wertheim's splint
Wester's
    clamp
    scissors
Westphal's
    sign
    zone
Whitman's operation
Williams'
    clamp
    exercise

Wilman's clamp
Wilson-McKeever operation
Wilson's
    awl
    bolt
    clamp
    plate
    wrench
wire
    Kirschner's w.
Wladimiroff-Mikulicz
    amputation
Wladimiroff's operation
wrench
    Wilson's w.
Wright's plate
Wrisberg's ligament
wrist
wristdrop
wryneck
Wyeth's operation
xanthoma
    x. disseminatum
xanthomatosis
xanthosarcoma
xiphisternum
xiphocostal
xiphoid
xiphoiditis
xiphopagotomy
Yount's operation
Zahradnicek's operation
Zancolli's operation
zanthoma. See *xanthoma.*
zanthomatosis. See *xanthoma-*
    tosis.
zanthosarkoma. See *xantho-*
    sarcoma.
Zenker's
    degeneration
    necrosis
Zickle's nail

zifisternum. See *xiphisternum.*
zifo-. See words beginning
    xipho-.
zifoid. See *xiphoid.*
Zimaloy's prosthesis
Zimmer's
    pin
    prosthesis
    screw

Zimmer's (*continued*)
    splint
zone
    cornuradicular z.
    Lissauer's z.
    Looser's z.
    orbicular z. of hip
    Westphal's z.

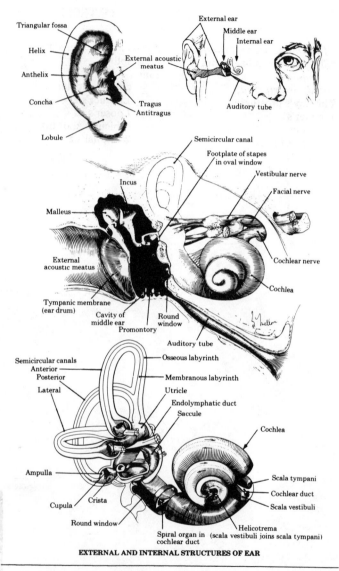

EXTERNAL AND INTERNAL STRUCTURES OF EAR

(Courtesy of Dorland's Illustrated Medical Dictionary, 26th ed. Plate XIV. Philadelphia, W. B. Saunders Company, 1981.)

OTORHINOLARYNGOLOGY

Abelson's adenotome
ablation
Abraham's cannula
abscess
    Bezold's a.
AC — air conduction
achalasia
acouesthesia
acoumeter
acoumetry
acouometer
acouophone
acouophonia
acoustic
acousticon
acoustics
AD — right ear (auris dextra)
Adam's apple
Adams' operation
adaptor
    House's a.
adenocarcinoma
adenofibroma
    a. edematodes
adenoid
adenoidectomy
adenoidism
adenoiditis
adenoma

adenotome
    Abelson's a.
    Kelley's a.
    Laforce-Grieshaber a.
    Laforce's a.
    Shambaugh's a.
    Sluder's a.
adenotomy
adenotonsillectomy
adenovirus
aditus
    a. ad antrum
    a. ad antrum mastoideum
    a. ad antrum tympani-
        cum
    a. laryngis
Adler's punch
Adson's forceps
afagopraksea. See *aphago-*
    praxia.
aftha. See *aphtha.*
aftho-. See words beginning
    aphtho-.
agger
    a. nasi
ala
    a. auris
    a. nasi
alae

Albert-Andrews laryngoscope
Alexander's
    chisel
    gouge
allergy
Allport's
    retractor
    searcher
Almoor's operation
alveolonasal
ama
ampulla
anakusis
anastomosis
    Galen's a.
    Jacobson's a.
Andrews'
    applicator
    gouge
Andrews-Hartmann forceps
anesthesia. See *General
    Surgical Terms.*
angina
    Ludwig's a.
    Plaut-Vincent's a.
angle
    olfactive a.
    olfactory a.
    ophryospinal a.
    orifacial a.
    Topinard's a.
angulus
    a. mastoideus ossis
      parietalis
ankyloglossia
ankylosis
    cricoarytenoid joint a.
ankylotia
ankylotome
ankylotomy
annulus
    a. tracheae

annulus (*continued*)
    tympanic a.
    a. tympanicus
    Vieussen's a.
anosmatic
anosmia
    a. gustatoria
    preferential a.
    a. respiratoria
anosphrasia
anotia
anthelix
Anthony's tube
antihelix
antihistamine
antihistaminic
antitragus
antral
antrectomy
antritis
antroatticotomy
antrocele
antronalgia
antronasal
antroscope
antroscopy
antrostomy
antrotomy
antrotympanic
antrotympanitis
antrum
    attic-aditus a.
    a. auris
    ethmoid a.
    a. ethmoidale
    frontal a.
    a. of Highmore
    a. highmori
    mastoid a.
    a. mastoideum
    a. maxillare
    maxillary a.

antrum (*continued*)
    tympanic a.
    a. tympanicum
anulus tympanicus
anvil
apertura
    a. chordae tympani
    a. externa aqueductus
      vestibuli
    a. sinus frontalis
    a. sinus sphenoidalis
    a. tympanica canaliculi
aperture
    a. of frontal sinus
    a. of larynx
    a. of sphenoid sinus
    tympanic a. of canalicu-
      lus of chorda tympani
apex
    a. auriculae
    a. linguae
    a. nasi
aphagopraxia
aphonia
    a. paralytica
    spastic a.
aphtha
aphthosis
aphthous
aponeurosis
applicator
    Andrews' a.
    Brown's a.
    Dean's a.
    Holinger's a.
    Lathbury's a.
    Lejeune's a.
    Pynchon's a.
    Roberts' a.
aqueduct
    a. of cochlea
    a. of Cotunnius

aqueduct (*continued*)
    fallopian a.
    a. of Fallopius
    a. of the vestibule
aqueductus
    a. endolymphaticus
    a. vestibuli
arachnorhinitis
Arbuckle's probe
arch
    auricular a.
    palatine a.
    a's of Corti
arcus
    a. glossopalatinus
    a. lipoides myringis
    a. palatini
    a. palatoglossus
    a. palatopharyngeus
    a. pharyngopalatinus
area
    Kiesselbach's a.
areepi-. See words beginning
    aryepi-.
aretenoid. See *arytenoid*.
argyria
    a. nasalis
arhinia
ariteno-. See words beginning
    aryteno-.
arjirea. See *argyria*.
Arnold's nerve
Arslan's operation
artery
    carotid a.
    occipital a.
    pharyngeal a.
    thyroid a.
articulation
    a's of auditory ossicles
aryepiglottic
aryepiglotticus

aryepiglottidean
arytenoepiglottic
arytenoid
arytenoidectomy
arytenoideus
arytenoiditis
arytenoidopexy
AS — left ear (auris sinistra)
Asch's
    operation
    splint
aspergillosis
aspiration
aspirator
    Gottschalk's a.
asterion
atelectasis
Atkins-Tucker laryngoscope
atomizer
    Devilbiss' a.
atresia
atrium
    a. glottidis
    a. of glottis
    a. laryngis
    a. of larynx
    a. meatus medii
attic
atticitis
atticoantrotomy
atticomastoid
atticotomy
    transmeatal a.
AU — both ears (aures unitas)
    each ear (auris uterque)
audiogram
audiologist
audiology
audiometer
audiometrician
audiometry
audiosurgery

audiphone
audition
auditive
auditognosis
auditory
    a. canal
Aufricht-Lipsett rasp
Aufricht's
    rasp
    retractor
    speculum
aura
    a. asthmatica
aural
aures
auricle
auricula
auricular
auriculare
auricularis
auriculocranial
auriculotemporal
auriculoventricular
aurilave
aurinarium
aurinasal
auriphone
auripuncture
auris
    a. externa
    a. interna
    a. media
auriscalpium
auriscope
auris dextra
auris sinistra
aurist
auristics
auristilla
auristillae
auris uterque
aurogauge

aurometer
Avellis' syndrome
Baelz's syndrome
bag
    Politzer's b.
Ballenger's
    curet
    elevator
    forceps
    knife
Ballenger-Sluder tonsillectome
Bane's forceps
Bárány's
    symptom
    syndrome
    test
Barlow's forceps
Barnhill's curet
barotitis
    b. media
barotrauma
BC — bone conduction
Bechterew's nucleus
Becker's operation
Beckman-Colver speculum
Beck-Mueller tonsillectome
Beck-Schenck tonsillectome
Beck's knife
Bellocq's cannula
Bell's palsy
Bellucci's scissors
Bermingham's nasal douche
Berne's
    forceps
    rasp
Bespaloff's sign
Beyer's
    forceps
    rongeur
Bezold's
    abscess
    mastoiditis

Bezold's (*continued*)
    perforation
Biederman's sign
Bieg's sign
Billeau's curet
Billroth's operation
binaural
binauricular
Bing's test
binotic
Bizzarri-Guiffrida laryngoscope
Blakemore's tube
Blake's forceps
Blakesley's forceps
blennorrhea
    Stoerk's b.
Boettcher's
    forceps
    hook
    scissors
bone
    b. conduction
    hyoid b.
    petrous b.
    squamosal b.
    temporal b.
    tympanic b.
    zygomatic b.
border
    vermilion b.
Boro's esophagoscope
Bostock's catarrh
Bosworth's snare
Boucheron's speculum
Bouchut's tube
bougie
    Hurst's b.
    Jackson's b.
    Plummer's b.
branchia
branchial
    b. cleft

branchiogenic
branchiogenous
branchioma
branchiomere
branchiomeric
branchiomerism
bronchi
bronchial
bronchiectasis
bronchogram
bronchography
bronchoscope
bronchoscopy
bronchus
Brown's
    applicator
    needle
    retractor
    snare
    tonsillectome
Broyles'
    esophagoscope
    laryngoscope
    nasopharyngoscope
Bruening's
    esophagoscope
    forceps
    otoscope
    snare
Brun's curet
Brunton's otoscope
bucca
    b. cavi oris
buccal
buccoglossopharyngitis
buccomaxillary
buccopharyngeal
Buck's
    curet
    knife
bulla
    b. ethmoidalis cavi nasi

bulla (*continued*)
    b. ethmoidalis ossis eth-
      moidalis
    b. ossea
bur
    diamond b.
    Hall's b.
    Jordan-Day b.
    Lempert's b.
    Wullstein's b.
bursa
    nasopharyngeal b.
    pharyngeal b.
bursitis
    Tornwaldt's b.
button
    polyethylene collar b.
calcification
calculus
    salivary c.
Caldwell-Luc operation
caliculus
    c. gustatorius
canal
    alveolar c's
    auditory c.
    carotid c.
    c. of Corti
    eustachian c.
    Huschke's c.
    palatine c's
    semicircular c.
canaliculus
    c. of chorda tympani
    c. chordae tympani
    c. of cochlea
    c. cochleae
    mastoid c.
    c. mastoideus
    tympanic c.
    c. tympanicus
canaloplasty

cancrum
    c. nasi
    c. oris
Canfield's
    knife
    operation
cannula
    Abraham's c.
    Bellocq's c.
    Coakley's c.
    Day's c.
    Goodfellow's c.
    Kos' c.
    Krause's c.
    Paterson's c.
    Scott's c.
cannulization
capitulum
    c. stapedis
capsule
    articular c.
caput stapedis
carcinoma
    basal cell c.
    epidermoid c.
    schneiderian c.
Carmack's curet
caroticotympanic
carotid
    c. artery
Carpenter's knife
Carpue's
    operation
    rhinoplasty
Carter's
    operation
    splint
cartilage
    alar c.
    arytenoid c.
    corniculate c.
    cricoid c.

cartilage (*continued*)
    cuneiform c.
    epiglottic c.
    hyaline c.
    intrathyroid c.
    laryngeal c. of Luschka
    Santorini's c.
    thyroid c.
    Wrisberg's c.
cartilagines
    c. alares minores
    c. laryngis
    c. nasales accessoriae
    c. nasi
    c. sesamoideae nasi
    c. tracheales
cartilaginous
cartilago
    c. alaris major
    c. arytenoidea
    c. auriculae
    c. corniculata
    c. cricoidea
    c. cuneiformis
    c. epiglottica
    c. meatus acustici
    c. nasi lateralis
    c. santorini
    c. septi nasi
    c. sesamoidea laryngis
    c. sesamoidea ligamenti
        vocalis
    c. thyroidea
    c. triquetra
    c. tubae auditivae
    c. wrisbergi
caruncle
    sublingual c.
caruncula
    c. salivaris
    c. sublingualis
Cassel's operation

Castelli's tube
catarrh
    Bostock's c.
catarrhal
catheter
    Yankauer's c.
catheterization
    laryngeal c.
cauda
    c. helicis
cavity
    tympanic c.
cavum
    c. conchae
    c. infraglotticum
    c. laryngis
    c. nasi
    c. nasi osseum
    c. oris
    c. oris externum
    c. pharyngis
    c. tympani
cecum
    cupular c. of cochlear
      duct
    c. cupulare ductus
      cochlearis
    vestibular c. of cochlear
      duct
    c. vestibulare ductus
      cochlearis
cellulae
    c. ethmoidales osseae
    c. mastoideae
    c. pneumaticae tubae
      auditivae
    c. pneumaticae tubariae
    c. tympanicae
cephalalgia
    histamine c.
    pharyngotympanic c.
cephalgia

cerumen
    inspissated c.
ceruminal
ceruminolysis
ceruminolytic
ceruminosis
ceruminous
cervical
chain
    ossicular c.
Cheever's operation
cheilectropion
cheilitis
cheilognathoprosoposchisis
cheilognathoschisis
cheilognathouranoschisis
cheiloplasty
cheiloschisis
cheilosis
chemodectoma
Chevalier Jackson
    esophagoscope
    laryngoscope
    operation
    speculum
    tube
chisel
    Alexander's c.
    Converse's c.
    Derlacki's c.
    Derlacki-Shambaugh c.
    Fomon's c.
    Freer's c.
    guarded c.
    Hajek's c.
    House's c.
    Killian's c.
    Sewall's c.
    Shambaugh-Derlacki c.
    Sheehan's c.
    Troutman's c.
choana

choanae
    c. osseae
choanal
choanoid
cholesteatoma
    c. tympani
chondroma
chorda
    c. tympani
chordectomy
chorditis
    c. cantorum
    c. fibrinosa
    c. nodosa
    c. tuberosa
    c. vocalis
chromorhinorrhea
cicatricial
cicatrix
    manometric c.
Cicherelli's forceps
cilia
Citelli-Meltzer punch
clamp
    Cottle's c.
    Jesberg's c.
Clerf's
    laryngoscope
    saw
Cloquet's ganglion
Coakley's
    cannula
    curet
    forceps
    operation
    speculum
    trocar
cochlea
cochleae
cochlear
cochleariform
cochleitis

cochleovestibular
cochlitis
Cody's operation
cog-tooth
Cohen's forceps
collum
collunarium
columella
    c. cochleae
    c. nasi
columna
    c. nasi
columnae
Colver's
    forceps
    knife
Commando's operation
commissure
    laryngeal c.
commissurorrhaphy
concha
    c. of auricle
    c. auriculae
    c. bullosa
    ethmoidal c.
    c. nasalis inferior ossea
    c. nasalis media ossea
    c. nasalis superior ossea
    c. nasalis suprema ossea
    nasoturbinal c.
    sphenoidal c.
    c. sphenoidalis
conchae
conchitis
conchoscope
conchotome
conchotomy
conduction
    air c.
    bone c.
conjunctivorhinostomy
constriction

conus
    c. elasticus laryngis
Converse's
    chisel
    rongeur
    speculum
cord
    vocal c.
cordal
cordectomy
Cordes-New forceps
cordopexy
cordotomy
corniculate
cornu
    ethmoid c.
    c. majus ossis hyoidei
    c. minus ossis hyoidei
cornua
corona
coronae
coronal
coronale
coronalis
corone
coronion
coronoid
Corti's
    arches
    canal
    organ
    rods
    tunnel
Corwin's hemostat
coryza
    allergic c.
    c. oedematosa
cosmesis
Costen's syndrome
Cottle-Arruga forceps
Cottle-Jansen forceps
Cottle-Kazanjian forceps

Cottle-Neivert retractor
Cottle's
    clamp
    elevator
    forceps
    knife
    osteotome
    rasp
    retractor
    saw
    scissors
    speculum
    tenaculum
Cotunnius
    aqueduct of C.
Craig's forceps
cranioaural
craniopharyngeal
cribriform
cricoarytenoid
cricoid
cricoidectomy
cricoidynia
cricopharyngeal
cricopharyngeus
cricothyreotomy
cricothyroid
cricothyroidotomy
cricotomy
cricotracheotomy
crista
    c. ampullaris
    c. arcuata cartilaginis
        arytenoideae
    c. conchalis maxillae
    c. conchalis ossis palatini
    c. ethmoidalis maxillae
    c. ethmoidalis ossis
        palatini
    c. fenestrae cochleae
    c. frontalis
    c. galli

cristae
>c. nasalis maxillae
>c. tympanica

croup

crura
>c. anthelicis
>c. of anthelix

crus
>anterior c. of stapes
>c. anterius stapedis
>c. breve incudis
>c. helicis
>c. of helix
>posterior c. of stapes
>c. posterius stapedis

cryosurgery

cuneiform

cupula
>c. of cochlea
>c. cochleae
>c. cristae ampullaris

cupulae

curet
>Ballenger's c.
>Barnhill's c.
>Billeau's c.
>Brun's c.
>Buck's c.
>Carmack's c.
>Coakley's c.
>Derlacki's c.
>Faulkner's c.
>Freimuth's c.
>Gross' c.
>Halle's c.
>Hartmann's c.
>Hayden's c.
>Hotz's c.
>House's c.
>Ingersoll's c.
>Jones' c.
>Lempert's c.

curet (*continued*)
>McCaskey's c.
>Middleton's c.
>Mosher's c.
>Myles' c.
>Pratt's c.
>Richards' c.
>Ridpath's c.
>Rosenmüller's c.
>Schaeffer's c.
>Shapleigh's c.
>Shea's c.
>Spratt's c.
>St. Clair-Thompson's c.
>Stubbs' c.
>Tabb's c.
>Vogel's c.
>Weisman's c.
>Whiting's c.
>Yankauer's c.

Cushing's forceps

cymba
>c. conchae auriculae

dacryocystorhinostenosis

dacryocystorhinostomy

Daniels' tonsillectome

Davis-Crowe mouth gag

Davis' retractor

Day's
>cannula
>operation

deafness
>acoustic trauma d.
>apoplectiform d.
>cerebral d.
>ceruminous d.
>conduction d.
>cortical d.
>labyrinthine d.
>neural d.
>paradoxic d.
>perceptive d.

deafness (*continued*)
 sensorineural d.
 toxic d.
 vascular d.
Dean's
 applicator
 forceps
 knife
 periosteotome
 scissors
decibel
decongestant
Dedo-Pilling laryngoscope
Dedo's laryngoscope
degeneration
deglutition
Deiters' nucleus
Demarquay's sign
Denhardt-Dingman mouth gag
Denhardt's mouth gag
Denker's operation
Denonvilliers' operation
Derlacki's
 chisel
 curet
 gouge
 knife
 mobilizer
 operation
Derlacki-Shambaugh chisel
desensitization
Devilbiss' atomizer
diapason
diastolization
dilation
dilator
 Maloney's d.
Dingman's
 elevator
 forceps
 osteotome
 retractor

diplacusis
 binaural d.
 d. binauralis dysharmon-
  ica
 d. binauralis echoica
 disharmonic d.
 echo d.
 monaural d.
disease
 attic d.
 Hunt's d.
 Legal's d.
 Ménière's d.
 Mikulicz's d.
 Ramsey-Hunt d.
dissector
 Fisher's d.
 Holinger's d.
 Hurd's d.
 McWhinnie's d.
 Pierce's d.
 Rogers' d.
 Walker's d.
diverticula
diverticulum
Donaldson's tube
dorsum
 d. nasi
Dott's operation
douche
 Bermingham's nasal d.
Douglas' knife
drill
 Jordan-Day d.
 Shea's d.
drugs. See *Drugs and
 Chemistry* section.
drumhead
duct
 cochlear d.
 endolymphatic d.
 lacrimal d.

duct (*continued*)
    d's of Rivinus
    Stensen's d.
    Walther's d's
    Wharton's d.
ductus
    d. cochlearis
    d. endolymphaticus
    d. reuniens
Duf,urmentel's
    forceps
    rongeur
Duplay-Lynch speculum
Duplay's speculum
dura
dysacousia
dysaudia
dysosmia
dysphagia
dysphonia
    d. plicae ventricularis
    d. spastica
dyspnea
EAC — external auditory canal
EAM — external auditory meatus
eardrum
Eaton's speculum
ecchymosis
edentulous
Eder-Hufford esophagoscope
EENT — eyes, ears, nose, and throat
electrocoagulation
electropneumatotherapy
elevator
    Ballenger's e.
    Cottle's e.
    Dingman's e.
    Freer's e.
    Hajek-Ballenger e.
    Hamrick's e.

elevator (*continued*)
    House's e.
    Hurd's e.
    Killian's e.
    Lamont's e.
    Lempert's e.
    Mackenty's e.
    Pennington's e.
    periosteal e.
    Pierce's e.
    Proctor's e.
    Ray-Parsons-Sunday e.
    Shambaugh-Derlacki e.
    Shambaugh's e.
    Sunday's e.
eminence
    arytenoid e.
    nasal e.
    pyramidal e.
eminentia
    e. articularis ossis temporalis
    e. conchae
    e. fallopii
    e. fossae triangularis auriculae
emissarium
    e. mastoideum
enanthema
enchondroma
endolabyrinthitis
endolaryngeal
endolarynx
endolymph
endolympha
endolymphatic
endomastoiditis
endonasal
endoscope
endoscopy
    peroral e.
endotoscope

English rhinoplasty
ENT — ear, nose, and throat
entacoustic
entotic
entotympanic
enucleation
eparterial
epiglottectomy
epiglottic
epiglottidean
epiglottidectomy
epiglottiditis
epiglottis
epiglottitis
epiotic
epipharyngeal
epipharyngitis
epipharynx
epistaxis
epiturbinate
epitympanic
epitympanum
Equen-Neuffer knife
equilibrium
Erhard's test
Erhardt's speculum
Erich's
    forceps
    splint
errhine
erysipelas
esophageal
esophagectomy
esophagogram
esophagolaryngectomy
esophagopharynx
esophagoscope
    Boros' e.
    Broyles' e.
    Bruening's e.
    Chevalier Jackson e.
    Eder-Hufford e.

esophagoscope (*continued*)
    fiberoptic e.
    full-lumen e.
    Haslinger's e.
    Holinger's e.
    Jackson's e.
    Jesberg's e.
    Lell's e.
    Moersch's e.
    Mosher's e.
    Moure's e.
    optical e.
    oval e.
    Roberts' e.
    Schindler's e.
    Tucker's e.
    Yankauer's e.
esophagoscopy
esophagostomy
esophagotomy
esophagus
espundia
esthesioneuroblastoma
ETF — eustachian tube function
ethmofrontal
ethmoid
ethmoidal
ethmoidectomy
ethmoideomaxillary
ethmoiditis
ethmoidotomy
ethmolacrimal
ethmomaxillary
ethmonasal
ethmopalatal
ethmosphenoid
ethmoturbinal
ethmovomerine
ethmyphitis
eustachian
    e. tube

eustachitis
eustachium
Eves' snare
Ewing's sign
excavator
    Schuknecht's e.
excernent
excochleation
exostosis
expectorant
expectoration
explorer
    Rosen's e.
exudate
facial
fahringo-. See words beginning
    pharyngo-.
Fallopius
    aqueduct of F.
farin-. See words beginning
    pharyn-.
Farrington's forceps
Farrior's speculum
fauces
faucial
faucitis
Faulkner's curet
Fauvel's forceps
fenestra
        f. cochleae
        f. of cochlea
        f. novovalis
        f. ovalis
        f. rotunda
        f vestibuli
fenestrae
fenestrated
fenestrater
    Rosen's f.
fenestration
Fergusson's operation
Ferris-Robb knife

Ferris-Smith
        forceps
        operation
Ferris-Smith-Kerrison forceps
Ferris-Smith-Sewall retractor
fibers
        Prussak's f's
fibroangioma
fibroma
fibrosarcoma
Fick's operation
Fink's laryngoscope
Fisher's
        dissector
        knife
Fish's forceps
fissure
        entorbital f.
        ethmoid f.
        glaserian f.
        petrotympanic f.
fistula
Flagg's laryngoscope
Flannery's speculum
flap
        tympanomeatal f.
flebektazea. See *phlebectasia*.
flem. See *phlegm*.
Fletcher's knife
fold
        aryepiglottic f.
        salpingopharyngeal f.
folium
        lingual f.
folliculitis
Fomon's
        chisel
        knife
        periosteotome
        rasp
        scissors
footplate

foramen
- Huschke's f.
- f. incisivum
- f. mastoideum
- rivinian f.
- Scarpa's f.
- f. sphenopalatinum
- Stensen's f.
- f. stylomastoideum

forceps
- Adson's f.
- Andrews-Hartmann f.
- Ballenger's f.
- Bane's f.
- Barlow's f.
- Berne's f.
- Beyer's f.
- Blake's f.
- Blakesley's f.
- Boettcher's f.
- Bruening's f.
- Cicherelli's f.
- Coakley's f.
- Cohen's f.
- Colver's f.
- Cordes-New f.
- Cottle-Arruga f.
- Cottle-Jansen f.
- Cottle-Kazanjian f.
- Cottle's f.
- Craig's f.
- Cushing's f.
- Dean's f.
- Dingman's f.
- Dufourmentel's f.
- Erich's f.
- Farrington's f.
- Fauvel's f.
- Ferris-Smith f.
- Ferris-Smith-Kerrison f.
- Fish's f.
- Fraenkel's f.

forceps (*continued*)
- Goldman-Kazanjian f.
- Goodhill's f.
- Gruenwald-Bryant f.
- Gruenwald's f.
- Guggenheim's f.
- Hajek-Koffler f.
- Hartmann-Citelli f.
- Hartmann-Gruenwald f.
- Hartmann's f.
- Hoffmann's f.
- House's f.
- Howard's f.
- Hurd's f.
- Imperatori's f.
- Jackson's f.
- Jansen-Middleton f.
- Jansen's f.
- Jansen-Struycken f.
- Juers-Lempert f.
- Jurasz's f.
- Kazanjian's f.
- Knight's f.
- Knight-Sluder f.
- Koffler-Lillie f.
- Koffler's f.
- Krause's f.
- Lempert's f.
- Lillie's f.
- Littauer's f.
- Lucae's f.
- Luc's f.
- Lutz's f.
- Lynch's f.
- Marshik's f.
- Martin's f.
- McHenry's f.
- McKay's f.
- Metzenbaum's f.
- Moritz-Schmidt f.
- Museholdt's f.
- Myerson's f.

forceps (*continued*)
- Myles' f.
- Noyes' f.
- Pang's f.
- Paterson's f.
- Reiner-Knight f.
- Robb's f.
- Robertson's f.
- Rowland's f.
- Ruskin's f.
- Sawtell's f.
- Scheinmann's f.
- Seiffert's f.
- Semken's f.
- Shearer's f.
- Struempel's f.
- Struyken's f.
- Takahashi's f.
- Tivnen's f.
- Tobold's f.
- Tydings' f.
- Tydings-Lakeside f.
- Van Struycken f.
- Walsham's f.
- Watson-Williams f.
- Weil's f.
- Weingartner's f.
- White-Lillie f.
- White's f.
- Wilde's f.
- Wullstein-House f.
- Wullstein's f.
- Yankauer-Little f.
- Yankauer's f.

Foregger's laryngoscope
formula
- Seiler's f.

fossa
- f. incudis
- f. ovalis
- pharyngomaxillary f.
- Rosenmüller's f.

fossa (*continued*)
- triangular f.

fovea
Fraenkel's forceps
Frazier's tube
Freer's
- chisel
- elevator
- knife
Freimuth's curet
frenotomy
frenulum
frenum
Friesner's knife
frontoethmoidal
frontolacrimal
frontomaxillary
frontonasal
fronto-occipital
frontoparietal
frontotemporal
frontozygomatic
Fröschel's symptom
fundus
- f. meatus acustica interni
- f. tympani
furcula
furuncular
furunculosis
galea
- g. aponeurotica
- tendinous g
Galen's anastomosis
Gandhi's knife
ganglion
- Cloquet's g.
- geniculate g.
- g. geniculi nervi facialis
- nodose g.
- otic g.
gangosa
Garfield-Holinger laryngoscope

Gault's test
Gellé's test
geniohyoid
genyantralgia
genyantritis
genyantrum
genycheiloplasty
genyplasty
Gerzog's speculum
Gifford's retractor
Gillies'
    hook
    operation
Gillies-Dingman hook
glabella
glabellad
glabellum
gland
    Rivinus' g.
    salivary g.
glomangioma
glomus
    g. jugulare
glossa
glossagra
glossal
glossalgia
glossanthrax
glossectomy
glossitis
glossocele
glossocoma
glossodynamometer
glossodynia
glossoepiglottidean
glossoncus
glossopathy
glossopexy
glossopharyngeal
glossopharyngeum
glossoplasty

glossoplegia
glossopyrosis
glossorrhaphy
glossoscopy
glossotomy
glottic
glottides
glottis
Goldman-Kazanjian forceps
Goodfellow's cannula
Goodhill's forceps
Good's rasp
Goodyear's knife
Gottschalk's
    aspirator
    saw
gouge
    Alexander's g.
    Andrews' g.
    Derlacki's g.
    Holmes' g.
    Troutman's g.
goundou
Gradenigo's syndrome
graft
granulation
granuloma
groove
    Verga's lacrimal g.
Gross'
    curet
    spoon
    spud
Gruber's speculum
Gruenwald-Bryant forceps
Gruenwald's forceps
Guedel's laryngoscope
Guggenheim's forceps
Guilford's stapedectomy
guillotine
    Sluder's g.

guillotine (*continued*)
  Sluder-Sauer g.
Gundelach's punch
Hajek-Ballenger elevator
Hajek-Koffler forceps
Hajek-Skillern punch
Hajek's
  chisel
  retractor
Halle's
  curet
  speculum
Halle-Tieck speculum
Hall's bur
hammer
  Quisling's h.
Hamrick's elevator
Harrison's knife
Hartmann-Citelli forceps
Hartmann-Dewaxer speculum
Hartmann-Gruenwald forceps
Hartmann-Herzfeld rongeur
Hartmann's
  curet
  forceps
  punch
  rongeur
  speculum
  tuning fork
Haslinger's
  esophagoscope
  laryngoscope
  retractor
Haverhill's operation
Hayden's curet
HD — hearing distance
headrest
  Shambaugh's h.
Heath's operation
HEENT — head, eyes, ears,
          nose and throat
Heerman's operation

Heffernan's speculum
helicotrema
helix
hemangioma
hematoma
  h. auris
hemiglossal
hemiglossectomy
hemiglossitis
hemilaryngectomy
hemostat
  Corwin's h.
Henle's spine
Henner's retractor
herpes
  h. catarrhalis
  h. febrilis
  h. labialis
  h. oticus
  h. simplex
Hertz unit
hiatus
  h. semilunaris
Highmore's antrum
highmori
  sinus maxillaris h.
highmoritis
Hilger's operation
hircus
histamine
hoarseness
hoe
  Hough's h.
Hoffmann's
  forceps
  punch
  rongeur
Holinger's
  applicator
  dissector
  esophagoscope
  laryngoscope

Holmes'
  gouge
  nasopharyngoscope
hook
  Boettcher's h.
  Gillies' h.
  Gillies-Dingman h.
  House's h.
  Lillie's h.
  Schuknecht's h.
  Shambaugh's h.
  Shea's h.
Hopmann's polyp
Hopp's laryngoscope
Horgan's operation
Hotz's curet
Hough's
  hoe
  stapedectomy
Hourin's needle
House-Barbara needle
House-Rosen needle
House's
  adaptor
  chisel
  curet
  elevator
  forceps
  hook
  irrigator
  knife
  needle
  prosthesis
  rod
  scissors
  separator
  stapedectomy
  tube
House-Urban retractor
Howard's forceps
Howorth's operation
Huguier's sinus

Hunt's disease
Hurd's
  dissector
  elevator
  forceps
Hurst's bougie
Huschke's
  canal
  foramen
  valve
Husks' rongeur
hydrocephalus
  otitic h.
hydrorrhea
  nasal h.
hydrotis
hydrotympanum
hyothyroid
hypacusis
hyperacusis
hyperemic
hyperkeratosis
  h. lacunaris
hyperptyalism
hyperrhinoplasty
hypertrophy
hypoglossal
hypoglottis
hypopharyngoscope
hypopharyngoscopy
hypopharynx
hypoplasia
hypotympanotomy
hypotympanum
Hz — Hertz
IA — internal auditory
IAC — internal auditory canal
Imperatori's forceps
incision. See *General Surgical Terms.*
incisura
  i. anterior auris

incisura (*continued*)
    i. intertragica
    i. mastoidea ossis
      temporalis
    Santorini's i.
    i. terminalis auris
    i. tympanica
incisure
    Rivinus' i.
incostapedial
incudal
incudectomy
incudomalleal
incudostapedial
incus
Indian
    operation
    rhinoplasty
infection
    Vincent's i.
infundibulum
    ethmoidal i.
    i. nasi
Ingals' speculum
Ingersoll's curet
interarytenoid
intercricothyrotomy
intermaxillary
internarial
internasal
intralaryngeal
intramastoiditis
intranarial
intranasal
intubation
irrigator
    House's i.
    Shambaugh's i.
    Shea's i.
isthmus
Italian
    operation

Italian (*continued*)
    rhinoplasty
iter
Ivy's rongeur
Jackson's
    bougie
    esophagoscope
    forceps
    laryngoscope
    scissors
Jacobson's
    anastomosis
    nerve
Jako's laryngoscope
Jansen-Middleton forceps
Jansen-Newhart probe
Jansen's
    forceps
    operation
    retractor
Jansen-Struycken forceps
Jarvis' operation
Jennings' mouth gag
Jesberg's
    clamp
    esophagoscope
joint
    incudostapedial j.
Jones'
    curet
    splint
Jordan-Day
    bur
    drill
Joseph-Maltz saw
Joseph's
    knife
    periosteotome
    saw
    scissors
Juers-Lempert forceps
jugomaxillary

jugular
Jurasz's forceps
Kartagener's
    syndrome
    triad
Kazanjian's
    forceps
    splint
Keegan's operation
Kelley's adenotome
keratosis
    k. pharyngeus
Kerrison's rongeur
kHz - kilohertz
Kiesselbach's
    area
    plexus
Killian's
    chisel
    elevator
    knife
    operation
    speculum
kilo-. See words beginning
    cheilo-.
Knapp's scissors
knife
    Ballenger's k.
    Beck's k.
    Buck's k.
    Canfield's k.
    Carpenter's k.
    Colver's k.
    Cottle's k.
    Dean's k.
    Derlacki's k.
    Douglas' k.
    Equen-Neuffer k.
    Ferris-Robb k.
    Fisher's k.
    Fletcher's k.
    Fomon's k.

knife (*continued*)
    Freer's k.
    Friesner's k.
    Gandhi's k.
    Goodyear's k.
    Harrison's k.
    House's k.
    Joseph's k.
    Killian's k.
    Leland's k.
    Lempert's k.
    Lothrop's k.
    Lynch's k.
    Maltz's k.
    McHugh's k.
    Robertson's k.
    Rosen's k.
    Schuknecht's k.
    Seiler's k.
    Sexton's k.
    Shambaugh-Lempert k.
    Shea's k.
    Sheehy's k.
    Tobold's k.
    Tydings' k.
    Wullstein's k.
Knight's
    forceps
    scissors
Knight-Sluder forceps
koanah. See *choana.*
Koffler-Lillie forceps
Koffler's forceps
kokle-. See words beginning
    cochle-.
koklea. See *cochlea.*
Koplik's spots
Kos' cannula
Kramer's speculum
Krause's
    cannula
    forceps

Krause's (*continued*)
    snare
Kuhnt's operation
Kuster's operation
Kyle's speculum
labial
labium
    anterius ostii pharyngei
        tubae auditivae
labyrinth
    acoustic l.
    ethmoidal l.
    membranous l.
    nonacoustic l.
    osseous l.
labyrinthectomy
labyrinthine
labyrinthitis
labyrinthosis
labyrinthotomy
lacrimation
lacrimoconchal
lacrimomaxillary
lacrimonasal
Laforce-Grieshaber adenotome
Laforce's
    adenotome
    tonsillectome
lahringo-. See words beginning
    laryngo-.
lamina
    l. spiralis ossea
    l. spiralis secundaria
Lamont's
    elevator
    saw
Lane's mouth gag
LaRocca's tube
laryngalgia
laryngeal
laryngect
laryngectomee

laryngectomy
laryngemphraxis
laryngendoscope
laryngismal
laryngismus
    l. paralyticus
    l. stridulus
laryngitic
laryngitis
    catarrhal l.
    croupous l.
    diphtheritic l.
    membranous l.
    phlegmonous l.
    l. sicca
    l. stridulosa
    subglottic l.
    syphilitic l.
    tuberculous l.
    vestibular l.
laryngocele
laryngocentesis
laryngofission
laryngofissure
laryngogram
laryngograph
laryngography
laryngohypopharynx
laryngology
laryngomalacia
laryngometry
laryngoparalysis
laryngopathy
laryngophantom
laryngopharyngeal
laryngopharyngectomy
laryngopharyngeus
laryngopharyngitis
laryngopharynx
laryngophony
laryngophthisis
laryngoplasty

laryngoplegia
laryngoptosis
laryngopyocele
laryngorhinology
laryngorrhagia
laryngorrhaphy
laryngorrhea
laryngoscleroma
laryngoscope
    Albert-Andrews l.
    Atkins-Tucker l.
    Bizzarri-Guiffrida l.
    Broyles' l.
    Chevalier Jackson l.
    Clerf's l.
    commissure l.
    Dedo-Pilling l.
    Dedo's l.
    fiberoptic l.
    Fink's l.
    Flagg's l.
    Foregger's l.
    Garfield-Holinger l.
    Guedel's l.
    Haslinger's l.
    Holinger's l.
    Hopp's l.
    Jackson's l.
    Jako's l.
    Lewy's l.
    Lundy's l.
    Lynch's l.
    MacIntosh's l.
    Magill's l.
    Miller's l.
    reverse-bevel l.
    Roberts' l.
    rotating l.
    Rusch's l.
    Sanders' l.
    self-retaining l.
    Siker's l.

laryngoscope (*continued*)
    slotted l.
    suspension l.
    Tucker's l.
    Welch-Allyn l.
    Wis-Foregger's l.
    Wis-Hipple's l.
    Yankauer's l.
laryngoscopic
laryngoscopist
laryngoscopy
laryngospasm
laryngostasis
laryngostat
laryngostenosis
laryngostomy
laryngostroboscope
laryngotome
laryngotomy
    subhyoid l.
    thyrohyoid l.
laryngotracheal
laryngotracheitis
laryngotracheobronchitis
laryngotracheobronchoscopy
laryngotracheoscopy
laryngotracheotomy
laryngotyphoid
laryngovestibulitis
laryngoxerosis
larynx
    artificial l.
Lathbury's applicator
Latrobe's retractor
Lauren's operation
Legal's disease
Lejeune's
    applicator
    scissors
Leland's knife
Lell's esophagoscope
Lempert-Colver speculum

Lempert's
    bur
    curet
    elevator
    forceps
    knife
    operation
    perforator
    retractor
Lermoyez's
    punch
    syndrome
leukoplakia
Lewis'
    rasp
    snare
    tube
Lewy's laryngoscope
ligament
    annular l.
    axis l.
    cricoarytenoid l.
    cricopharyngeal l.
    cricothyroarytenoid l.
    cricothyroid l.
    cricotracheal l.
    hyoepiglottic l.
    posterior l.
    superior l.
    thyroepiglottic l.
    thyrohyoid l.
Lillie's
    forceps
    hook
    scissors
    speculum
limen
    l. nasi
Lindeman-Silverstein tube
line
    cricoclavicular l.
    Topinard's l.

lingua
    l. dissecta
    l. fraenata
    l. geographica
    l. nigra
    l. plicata
    l. villosa nigra
lingual
linguale
lingualis
lingually
lingula
lingulectomy
lipoma
Littauer's forceps
lobule
lobulus
    l. auriculae
Lombard-Boies rongeur
Lombard's test
Lothrop's
    knife
    retractor
loupe
Love's
    retractor
    splint
Lucae's forceps
Luc's forceps
Ludwig's angina
Luer's retractor
Lundy's laryngoscope
Luongo's retractor
Luschka's
    laryngeal cartilage
    tonsil
Lutz's forceps
lymphadenectomy
lymphadenitis
lymphadenoid
lymphangioma
lymphatic

lymphoblastoma
lymphoepithelioma
lymphosarcoma
lymphotism
lymphotome
Lynch's
    forceps
    knife
    laryngoscope
    scissors
MacFee neck flap
MacIntosh's laryngoscope
Mackenty's
    choanal plug
    elevator
    tube
Mack's tonsillectome
Maclay's scissors
macrocephalia
macrocheilia
macroglossia
macrognathia
macrostomia
macrotia
macula
    m. acustica sacculi
    m. acustica utriculi
    m. sacculi
    m. utriculi
Magill's laryngoscope
Mahoney's speculum
malar
malleoincudal
malleolar
malleotomy
malleus
Maloney's dilator
Maltz-Lipsett rasp
Maltz's
    knife
    rasp
    saw

mandible
mandibula
mandibulae
mandibular
mandibulopharyngeal
Mandl's paint
manubria
    m. of malleus
manubrium
    m. mallei
    m. of malleus
Marshik's forceps
Martin's forceps
mastoid
mastoidal
mastoidale
mastoidalgia
mastoidea
mastoidectomy
    radical m.
    simple m.
mastoideocentesis
mastoideum
mastoiditis
    Bezold's m.
    m. externa
    m. interna
    sclerosing m.
    silent m.
mastoidotomy
mastoidotympanectomy
maxilla
maxillary
maxillofacial
Mayer's splint
McCaskey's curet
McCurdy's needle
McGee's operation
McHenry's forceps
McHugh's
    knife
    speculum

McIvor's mouth gag
McKay's forceps
McWhinnie's dissector
meatoantrotomy
meatus
       auditory m.
       external acoustic m.
       m. conchae ethmotur-
          binalis minoris
       m. nasi communis osseus
       m. nasopharyngeus
          osseus
medications. See *Drugs and*
    Chemistry section.
Meltzer's
       nasopharyngoscope
       punch
membrana
       m. basilaris ductus
          cochlearis
       m. elastica laryngis
       m. fibroelastica laryngis
       m. mucosa nasi
       m. spiralis ductus coch-
          learis
       m. stapedis
       m. tympani secundaria
membrane
       buccopharyngeal m.
       hyothyroid m.
       hypoglossal m.
       mucous m.
       Reissner's m.
       Rivinus' m.
       Scarpa's m.
       Shrapnell's m.
       tectorial m.
       tympanic m.
membranous
Ménière's disease
meningitis
mesocephalic

mesoturbinal
mesoturbinate
metopantralgia
metopantritis
Metzenbaum-Lipsett scissors
Metzenbaum's
       forceps
       scissors
Meyeri sinus
Meyer's sinus
microglossia
micrognathia
microlaryngoscopy
microrhinia
microscope
       Zeiss' m.
microstomia
microtia
Middleton's curet
Mikulicz's
       disease
       syndrome
Miller's laryngoscope
mobilization
       stapes m.
mobilizer
       Derlacki's m.
modiolus
Moeller's reaction
Moersch's esophagoscope
Moltz-Storz tonsillectome
Morch's tube
Morgagni's
       sacculus
       sinus
       ventricle
Moritz-Schmidt forceps
Mosher's
       curet
       esophagoscope
       punch
       speculum

Moure's esophagoscope
mouth gag
    Davis-Crowe m.g.
    Denhardt-Dingman m.g.
    Denhardt's m.g.
    Jennings' m.g.
    Lane's m.g.
    McIvor's m.g.
    Roser's m.g.
    Sluder-Jansen m.g.
mucocele
mucoid
mucoperichondrium
mucoperiosteal
mucoperiosteum
mucopurulent
mucosa
mucus
muscle
    arytenoid m.
    cricoarytenoid m.
    cricopharyngeus m.
    cricothyroid m.
    depressor septi nasi m.
    genioglossus m.
    geniohyoideus m.
    glossopalatinus m.
    glossopharyngeus m.
    helicis m.
    interarytenoid m.
    levator veli palatini m.
    longissimus m.
    palatoglossus m.
    palatopharyngeus m.
    pharyngeal constrictor m.
    pharyngopalatinus m.
    salpingopharyngeal m.
    splenius m.
    stapedius m.
    sternocleidomastoid m.
    strap m.
    stylopharyngeus m.

muscle (*continued*)
    temporalis m.
    tensor m. of tympanic
      membrane
    tensor m. of tympanum
    tensor veli palatini m.
    thyroarytenoid m.
    thyrohyoid m.
    vocal m.
musculoplasty
musculus
    m. temporalis
    m. tensor tympani
Museholdt's forceps
Mustarde otoplasty
myasthenia
    m. gravis
    m. laryngis
mycosis
    m. leptothrica
Myerson's
    forceps
    saw
Myles'
    curet
    forceps
    punch
    snare
    speculum
    tonsillectome
mylohyoid
myringa
myringectomy
myringitis
    bullous m.
    m. bullosa
myringodectomy
myringodermatitis
myringomycosis
    m. aspergillina
myringoplasty
myringorupture

myringoscope
myringostapediopexy
myringotome
myringotomy
myrinx
nares
naris
nasal
nasalis
nasion
nasitis
nasoantral
nasoantritis
nasobronchial
nasociliary
nasofrontal
nasograph
nasolabial
nasolacrimal
nasomanometer
nasomaxillary
nasonnement
naso-oral
nasopalatine
nasopharyngeal
nasopharyngitis
nasopharyngoscope
    Broyles' n.
    Holmes' n.
    Meltzer's n.
nasopharynx
nasorostral
nasoscope
nasoseptal
nasoseptitis
nasosinusitis
nasospinale
nasotracheal
nasoturbinal
nasus
    n. externus
Nebinger-Praun operation

neck flap
    MacFee n.f.
necrosis
needle
    Brown's n.
    Hourin's n.
    House-Barbara n.
    House-Rosen n.
    House's n.
    McCurdy's n.
    Rosen's n.
    Shambaugh's n.
    Updegraff's n.
Neivert's retractor
nerve
    abducens n.
    acoustic n.
    alveolar n.
    Arnold's n.
    chorda tympani n.
    cochlear n.
    ethmoidal n.
    facial n.
    glossopharyngeal n.
    hypoglossal n.
    infraorbital n.
    infratrochlear n.
    Jacobson's n.
    laryngeal n.
    nasopalatine n.
    olfactory n's
    palatine n.
    petrosal n.
    n. of pterygoid canal
    pterygopalatine n's
    n. of tensor tympani
    trigeminal n.
    vagus n.
    vestibular n.
neuralgia
    glossopharyngeal n.
    retrobulbar n.

neuralgia (*continued*)
    trigeminal n.
neurofibroma
neuroma
    acoustic n.
New-Lambotte osteotome
niche
nodular
nodule
noma
nose
    cleft n.
    potato n.
    saddle-back n.
    swayback n.
nostril
notch
    n. of Rivinus
    rivinian n.
Noyes' forceps
Noyes-Shambaugh scissors
NP — nasopharyngeal
    nasopharynx
NT — nasotracheal
nucha
nuchal
nucleus
    Bechterew's n.
    Deiters' n.
numatizashun. See *pneumatization.*
numo-. See words beginning *pneumo-.*
nystagmus
    aural n.
    caloric n.
    labyrinthine n.
    vestibular n.
occipital
occipitofrontal
occipitomastoid
occipitomental

occiput
odynophagia
ogo
Ogston-Luc operation
olfaction
olfactory
operation
    Adams' o.
    Almoor's o.
    Arslan's o.
    Asch's o.
    Becker's o.
    Billroth's o.
    Caldwell-Luc o.
    Canfield's o.
    Carpue's o.
    Carter's o.
    Cassel's o.
    Cheever's o.
    Chevalier Jackson o.
    Coakley's o.
    Cody's o.
    Commando's o.
    Day's o.
    Denker's o.
    Denonvilliers' o.
    Derlacki's o.
    Dott's o.
    Fergusson's o.
    Ferris-Smith o.
    Fick's o.
    Gillies' o.
    Haverhill's o.
    Heath's o.
    Heerman's o.
    Hilger's o.
    Horgan's o.
    Howorth's o.
    Indian o.
    Italian o.
    Jansen's o.
    Jarvis' o.

operation (*continued*)

    Keegan's o.
    Killian's o.
    Kuhnt's o.
    Kuster's o.
    Lauren's o.
    Lempert's o.
    McGee's o.
    Nebinger-Praun o.
    Ogston-Luc o.
    radical antrum o.
    Ridell's o.
    Roberts' o.
    Rosen's o.
    Rouge's o.
    Schonbein's o.
    Schuknecht's o.
    Schwartze's o.
    Shambaugh's o.
    Sistrunk's o.
    Sluder's o.
    Sonneberg's o.
    Sourdille's o.
    Stacke's o.
    Stallard's o.
    tagliacotian o.
    Vicq d'Azyr's o.
    West's o.
    Wood's o.
    Wullstein's o.
    Yankauer's o.

opisthogenia
opisthognathism
opisthotic
orbit
orbital
orbitonasal
organ
    o. of Corti
organum
    o. spirale
    o. vestibulocochleare

orifice
    tympanic o.
oroantral
oronasal
oropharynx
os
    o. epitympanicum
    o. ethmoidale
    o. frontale
    o. hyoideum
    o. interparietale
    o. lacrimale
    o. mastoideum
    o. nasale
    o. occipitale
    o. orbiculare
    o. palatinum
    o. parietale
    o. sphenoidale
    o. temporale
    o. unguis
    o. zygomaticum
osseosonometry
osseous
ossicle
    auditory o's
ossicula
    o. auditus
ossiculectomy
ossiculotomy
ossiculum
osteotome
    Cottle's o.
    Dingman's o.
    New-Lambotte o.
    Rowland's o.
    Silver's o.
ostium
    o. pharyngeum tubae auditivae
    o. tympanicum tubae auditivae

otacoustic
otagra
otalgia
    o. dentalis
    o. intermittens
    reflex o.
otalgic
otectomy
othelcosis
othematoma
othemorrhea
othygroma
otiatrics
otic
oticodinia
otitic
    o. barotrauma
otitis
    o. crouposa
    o. desquamativa
    o. diphtheritica
    o. externa cricumscripta
    o. externa diffusa
    o. externa furunculosa
    o. externa hemorrhagica
    o. externa mycotica
    furuncular o.
    o. haemorrhagica
    o. labyrinthica
    o. mastoidea
    o. media catarrhalis acuta
    o. media catarrhalis
      chronica
    o. media purulenta acuta
    o. media purulenta
      chronica
    o. media sclerotica
    o. media serosa
    o. media suppurativa
    o. media vasomotorica
    mucosis o.
    mucosus o.

otitis (*continued*)
    o. mycotica
    o. sclerotica
Oto. − otolaryngology
    otology
otoantritis
otoblennorrhea
otocatarrh
otocephalus
otocerebritis
otocleisis
otoconia
otoconium
otocranial
otocranium
otodynia
otoencephalitis
otoganglion
otogenic
otogenous
otography
otohemineurasthenia
Otol. − otology
Otolar. − otolaryngology
otolaryngology
otolith
otolithiasis
otologic
otologist
otology
otomassage
otomastoiditis
otomicroscope
otomicroscopy
otomucormycosis
otomyasthenia
Otomyces
otomycosis
    o. aspergillina
otomyiasis
otoncus
otonecrectomy

otoneuralgia
otoneurasthenia
otoneurology
otopathy
otopharyngeal
otophone
otopiesis
otoplasty
    Mustarde o.
otopolypus
otopyorrhea
otopyosis
otor
otorhinolaryngologist
otorhinolaryngology
otorhinology
otorrhagia
otorrhea
otosalpinx
otosclerectomy
otoscleronectomy
otosclerosis
otoscope
    Bruening's o.
    Brunton's o.
    Siegle's o.
    Toynbee's o.
    Welch-Allyn o.
otoscopy
    pneumatic o.
otosis
otospongiosis
otosteal
otosteon
ototomy
ototoxic
ototoxicity
ozena
    o. laryngis
paint
    Mandl's p.
palata

palatal
palate
    cleft p.
palateoethmoidal
palatine
palatitis
palatoglossal
palatognathous
palatograph
palatography
palatomaxillary
palatomyograph
palatonasal
palatopharyngeal
palatoplasty
palatoplegia
palatoschisis
palatostaphylinus
palatouvularis
palatum
palsy
    Bell's p.
Pang's forceps
panotitis
panseptum
pansinuitis
pansinusectomy
pansinusitis
panturbinate
Paparella's tube
papilla
    acoustic p.
    p. parotidea
papillae
    filliform p.
    p. filiformes
    p. foliatae
    foliate p.
    fungiform p.
    p. fungiformes
    lingual p.
    p. linguales

papilloma
paracusia
    p. acris
    p. duplicata
    p. loci
    p. willisiana
paracusis of Willis
paraglossa
paraglossia
paraglossitis
paries
    p. externus ductus
      cochlearis
    p. jugularis cavi tympani
    p. labyrinthicus cavi
      tympani
    p. mastoideus cavi
      tympani
    p. medialis orbitae
    p. membranaceus cavi
      tympani
    p. membranaceus
      tracheae
    p. tegmentalis cavi
      tympani
    p. tympanicus ductus
      cochlearis
    p. vestibularis ductus
      cochlearis
parietal
parietofrontal
parietomastoid
parieto-occipital
parietosphenoid
parietosquamosal
parietotemporal
parosmia
parotid
parotidean
parotidectomy
parotitis

pars
    p. flaccida membranae
      tympani
    p. tensa membranae
      tympani
patch
    Silastic p.
Paterson's
    cannula
    forceps
peenash
Pennington's elevator
perforation
    Bezold's p.
perforator
    Lempert's p.
    Royce's p.
    Thornwald's p.
    Wellaminski's p.
periauricular
perichondritis
perichondrium
perilabyrinth
perilabyrinthitis
perilaryngeal
perilaryngitis
perilymph
perilymphatic
periorbital
periosteotome
    Dean's p.
    Fomon's p.
    Joseph's p.
periosteum
periotic
perirhinal
perisinuitis
perisinuous
perisinusitis
peritonsillar
peritonsillitis

Per-Lee tube
perpendicular plate
petiolus
    p. epiglottidis
petromastoid
petro-occipital
petropharyngeus
petrosal
petrosectomy
petrositis
petrosphenoid
petrosquamosal
petrous
PE tube — ventilating tube
          placed in the ear-
          drum
pharyngalgia
pharyngeal
pharyngectasia
pharyngectomy
pharyngemphraxis
pharyngeus
pharyngism
pharyngismus
pharyngitic
pharyngitid
pharyngitis
    atrophic p.
    catarrhal p.
    croupous p.
    diphtheric p.
    follicular p.
    gangrenous p.
    glandular p.
    granular p.
    p. herpetica
    hypertrophic p.
    p. keratosa
    membranous p.
    phlegmonous p.
    p. sicca

pharyngitis (*continued*)
    p. ulcerosa
pharyngoamygdalitis
pharyngocele
pharyngoconjunctivitis
pharyngodynia
pharyngoepiglottic
pharyngoesophageal
pharyngoglossal
pharyngoglossus
pharyngokeratosis
pharyngolaryngeal
pharyngolaryngitis
pharyngolith
pharyngolysis
pharyngomaxillary
pharyngomycosis
pharyngonasal
pharyngo-oral
pharyngopalatine
pharyngoparalysis
pharyngopathy
pharyngoperistole
pharyngoplasty
pharyngoplegia
pharyngorhinitis
pharyngorhinoscopy
pharyngorrhagia
pharyngorrhea
pharyngosalpingitis
pharyngoscleroma
pharyngoscope
pharyngoscopy
pharyngospasm
pharyngostenosis
pharyngostomy
pharyngotherapy
pharyngotome
pharyngotomy
pharyngotonsillitis
pharyngotyphoid

pharynx
philtrum
phlebectasia
    p. laryngis
phlegm
phonation
photophore
Pierce's
    dissector
    elevator
    retractor
Pierre Robin syndrome
pillar
pinna
pinnal
piriform
platinectomy
Plaut-Vincent's angina
pledget
plegaphonia
plexus
    Kieselbach's p.
    laryngeal p.
    pharyngeal p.
    tympanic p.
plica
    p. nervi laryngei
    p. salpingopharyngea
    p. stapedis
    p. supratonsillaris
    p. triangularis
    p. vocalis
plicotomy
plug
    Mackenty's choanal p.
Plummer's bougie
Plummer-Vinson syndrome
PND — postnasal drainage
    postnasal drip
pneumatization
pneumothorax

pocket
    Rathke's p.
politzerization
Politzer's
    bag
    speculum
    test
    treatment
pollinosis
polyp
    Hopmann's p.
polypectomy
polypoid
ponticulus
    p. auriculae
    p. promontorii
position. See *General Surgical Terms.*
postaurale
postauricular
pouch
    Prussak's p.
    Rathke's p.
Pratt's curet
preauricular
presbycusis
Prince's scissors
probe
    Arbuckle's p.
    Jansen-Newhart p.
    Rosen's p.
    Spencer's p.
    Theobald's p.
    Welch-Allyn p.
    Yankauer's p.
procedure
    Valsalva's p.
process
    clinoid p.
    hamular p.
    mastoid p.

process (*continued*)
    styloid p.
    zygomatic p.
Proctor's
    elevator
    retractor
Proetz's treatment
prognathism
prognathous
prominentia
    p. laryngea
    p. styloidea
promontorium
    p. faciei
    p. tympani
promontory
prosthesis
    House's p.
    Sheehy-House p.
    Teflon p.
    TORP (total ossicular
      replacement p.)
Prussak's
    fibers
    pouch
    space
pseudocholesteatoma
pseudoglottis
Pseudomonas
    P. aeruginosa
pterygomandibular
pterygomaxillary
pterygopalatine
ptyalectasis
ptyalism
ptyalith
ptyalize
ptyalocele
ptyalolithiasis
ptyalorrhea
punch
    Adler's p.

punch (*continued*)
    Citelli-Meltzer p.
    Gundelach's p.
    Hajek-Skillern p.
    Hartmann's p.
    Hoffmann's p.
    Lermoyez's p.
    Meltzer's p.
    Mosher's p.
    Myles' p.
    Schmeden's p.
    Spencer's p.
    Spies' p.
    Takahashi's p.
    Van Struycken's p.
    Wagner's p.
    Watson-Williams p.
    Wilde's p.
    Yankauer's p.
purulent
pyemia
    otogenous p.
pyknosis
Pynchon's
    applicator
    speculum
pyothorax
pyramid
    petrous p.
    p. of tympanum
quinsy
    lingual q.
Quisling's hammer
Ramsey-Hunt disease
ramus
ranula
raphe
    r. pharyngis
rasp
    Aufricht-Lipsett r.
    Aufricht's r.
    Berne's r.

rasp (*continued*)
    Cottle's r.
    Fomon's r.
    Good's r.
    Lewis' r.
    Maltz-Lipsett r.
    Maltz's r.
    Wiener-Pierce r.
Rathke's
    pocket
    pouch
    tumor
Ray-Parsons-Sunday elevator
Ray's speculum
reaction
    Moeller's r.
recess
    Tröltsch's r's
recessus
    r. cochlearis vestibuli
    r. ellipticus vestibuli
    r. epitympanicus
    r. membranae tympani
        anterior
    r. membranae tympani
        posterior
    r. membranae tympani
        superior
    r. pharyngeus
    r. piriformis
    r. pro utriculo
    r. sphenoethmoidalis
    r. sphenoethmoidalis
        osseus
    r. sphericus vestibuli
Reiner-Beck snare
Reiner-Knight forceps
Reissner's membrane
resection
    submucous r.
retractor
    Allport's r.

retractor (*continued*)
    Aufricht's r.
    Brown's r.
    Cottle-Neivert r.
    Cottle's r.
    Davis' r.
    Dingman's r.
    Ferris-Smith-Sewall r.
    Gifford's r.
    Hajek's r.
    Haslinger's r.
    Henner's r.
    House-Urban r.
    Jansen's r.
    Latrobe's r.
    Lempert's r.
    Lothrop's r.
    Love's r.
    Luer's r.
    Luongo's r.
    Neivert's r.
    Pierce's r.
    Proctor's r.
    Schuknecht's r.
    Senn-Dingman r.
    Shambaugh's r.
    Snitman's r.
    Weitlaner's r.
    White-Proud r.
    Wullstein's r.
retroauricular
retrolabyrinthine
retromandibular
retromastoid
retronasal
retropharyngeal
retropharyngitis
retropharynx
Reuter's tube
rhinal
rhinalgia
rhinallergosis

rhinedema
rhinenchysis
rhinesthesia
rhineurynter
rhinion
rhinism
rhinitis
    allergic r.
    anaphylactic r.
    atrophic r.
    r. caseosa
    catarrhal r.
    croupous r.
    dyscrinic r.
    fibrinous r.
    gangrenous r.
    hypertrophic r.
    membranous r.
    perennial r.
    pseudomembranous r.
    purulent r.
    scrofulous r.
    r. sicca
    syphilitic r.
    tuberculous r.
    vasomotor r.
rhinoanemometer
rhinoantritis
rhinobyon
rhinocephalia
rhinocephalus
rhinocheiloplasty
rhinocleisis
rhinocoele
rhinodacryolith
rhinodynia
rhinogenous
rhinokyphectomy
rhinokyphosis
rhinolalia
    r. aperta
    r. clausa

rhinolaryngitis
rhinolaryngology
rhinolith
rhinolithiasis
rhinologist
rhinology
rhinomanometer
rhinometer
rhinomiosis
rhinomycosis
rhinonecrosis
rhinonemmeter
rhinoneurosis
rhinopathia
    r. vasomotoria
rhinopathy
rhinopharyngeal
rhinopharyngitis
    r. mutilans
rhinopharyngocele
rhinopharyngolith
rhinopharynx
rhinophonia
rhinophore
rhinophycomycosis
rhinophyma
rhinoplastic
rhinoplasty
    Carpue's r.
    dactylocostal r.
    English r.
    Indian r.
    Italian r.
    tagliacotian r.
rhinopneumonitis
rhinopolypus
rhinoreaction
rhinorrhagia
rhinorrhaphy
rhinorrhea
    cerebrospinal r.
rhinosalpingitis

rhinoscleroma
rhinoscope
rhinoscopic
rhinoscopy
rhinosporidiosis
rhinostegnosis
rhinostenosis
rhinotomy
rhinotracheitis
rhinovaccination
rhinovirus
rhonchal
rhonchial
rhonchus
Richards' curet
Ridell's operation
Ridley's sinus
Ridpath's curet
rima
    r. glottidis
    r. glottidis cartilaginea
    r. glottidis membranacea
    intercartilaginous r.
    intermembranous r.
    r. oris
    r. vestibuli
    r. vocalis
ring
    Waldeyer's r.
Ringer's solution
Rinne's test
Rivinus'
    ducts
    gland
    incisure
    membrane
    notch
Robb's forceps
Roberts'
    applicator
    esophagoscope
    laryngoscope

Roberts' (*continued*)
    operation
Robertson's
    forceps
    knife
rod
    Corti's r's
    House's r.
Roeder's treatment
Rogers' dissector
rongeur
    Beyer's r.
    Converse's r.
    duckbill r.
    Dufourmentel's r.
    Hartmann-Herzfeld r.
    Hartmann's r.
    Hoffmann's r.
    Husks' r.
    Ivy's r.
    Kerrison's r.
    Lombard-Boies r.
    Rowland's r.
    Ruskin's r.
    Tobey's r.
    Whiting's r.
Rosenmüller's
    curet
    fossa
Rosen's
    explorer
    fenestrater
    knife
    needle
    operation
    probe
    separator
    tube
Roser's mouth gag
Rouge's operation
Rowland's
    forceps

Rowland's (*continued*)
    osteotome
    rongeur
Royce's perforator
ruga
    r. palatina
Rusch's laryngoscope
Ruskin's
    forceps
    rongeur
Ruysch's tube
sacculation
saccule
    laryngeal s.
    s. of larynx
sacculi
sacculocochlear
sacculus
    s. communis
    s. lacrimalis
    s. laryngis
    s. morgagnii
    s. proprius
    s. rotundus
    s. sphaericus
    s. ventricularis
    s. vestibularis
sagittal
saliva
salivant
salivary
salivation
salpingitis
    eustachian s.
salpingocatheterism
salpingopharyngeal
salpingoscope
salpingoscopy
salpingostaphyline
Salvatore-Maloney tracheotome
Sanders' laryngoscope

Santorini's
    cartilage
    incisura
sarcoma
Sauer's tonsillectome
Sauer-Sluder tonsillectome
saw
    Clerf's s.
    Cottle's s.
    Gottschalk's s.
    Joseph-Maltz s.
    Joseph's s.
    Lamont's s.
    Maltz's s.
    Myerson's s.
    Slaughter's s.
    Woakes' s.
Sawtell's forceps
scala
    s. media
    s. tympani
    s. vestibuli
scapha
Scarpa's
    foramen
    membrane
Schaeffer's curet
Schall's tube
Scheinmann's forceps
Schindler's esophagoscope
Schmeden's punch
Schmincke's tumor
Schonbein's operation
Schuknecht's
    excavator
    hook
    knife
    operation
    retractor
    speculum
    stapedectomy

Schwabach's test
Schwartze's
    operation
    sign
scissors
        Bellucci's s.
        Boettcher's s.
        Cottle's s.
        Dean's s.
        Fomon's s.
        House's s.
        Jackson's s.
        Joseph's s.
        Knapp's s.
        Knight's s.
        Lejeune's s.
        Lillie's s.
        Lynch's s.
        Maclay's s.
        Metzenbaum-Lipsett s.
        Metzenbaum's s.
        Noyes-Shambaugh s.
        Prince's s.
        Seiler's s.
        Stevens' s.
Scott's
    cannula
    speculum
scute
    tympanic s.
SD — septal defect
searcher
        Allport's s.
Searcy's tonsillectome
Seiffert's forceps
Seiler's
    formula
    knife
    scissors
sella
    s. turcica
sellar

semicanal
    s. of auditory tube
    s. of tensor tympani
        muscle
semicanales
semicanalis
        s. musculi tensoris
            tympani
        s. tubae auditivae
Semken's forceps
Sengstaken-Blakemore tube
Sengstaken's tube
Senn-Dingman retractor
sensorineural
Senturia's speculum
separator
        House's s.
        Rosen's s.
septal
septectomy
septonasal
septoplasty
septotome
septotomy
septum
        s. canalis musculotubarii
        s. cartilagineum nasi
        s. mobile nasi
        s. nasi osseum
        s. sinuum frontalium
        s. sinuum sphenoidalium
        s. of sphenoidal sinuses
Sewall's chisel
Sexton's knife
sfeno-. See words beginning
        spheno-.
Shambaugh-Derlacki
        chisel
        elevator
Shambaugh-Lempert knife
Shambaugh's
        adenotome

Shambaugh's (*continued*)
    elevator
    headrest
    hook
    irrigator
    needle
    operation
    retractor
Shapleigh's curet
Shearer's forceps
Shea's
    curet
    drill
    hook
    irrigator
    knife
    stapedectomy
    tube
Sheehan's chisel
Sheehy-House prosthesis
Sheehy's
    knife
    tube
Shepard's tube
Shiley's tube
Shrapnell's membrane
siagantritis
siagonagra
siagonantritis
sialaden
sialadenitis
sialadenography
sialadenoncus
sialagogic
sialagogue
sialaporia
sialectasia
sialectasis
sialitis
sialoadenectomy
sialoadenitis
sialoadenotomy

sialocele
sialodochiectasis
sialodochitis
sialodochoplasty
sialogram
sialography
sialolith
sialolithiasis
sialolithotomy
sialoma
sialorrhea
sialosis
sialostenosis
sialosyrinx
sialozemia
Siegle's otoscope
Sierra-Sheldon tracheotome
sign
    Bespaloff's s.
    Biederman's s.
    Bieg's s.
    Demarquay's s.
    Ewing's s.
    Schwartze's s.
    Wreden's s.
    Zaufal's s.
Siker's laryngoscope
Silastic patch
Silver's osteotome
sinistraural
sinobronchitis
sinodural
sinography
sinus
    s. cochleae
    ethmoidal s.
    s. ethmoidalis
    frontal s.
    s. frontalis osseus
    Huguier's s.
    laryngeal s.
    mastoid s.

sinus (*continued*)
    s. maxillaris highmori
    s. maxillaris osseus
    maxillary s.
    s. meyeri
    Meyer's s.
    s. of Morgagni
    occipital s.
    s. occipitalis
    paranasal s's
    s. paranasales
    s. posterior cavi tympani
    pyriform s.
    Ridley's s.
    sigmoid s.
    sphenoidal s.
    s. sphenoidalis
    s. sphenoidalis osseus
    s. tympani
    tympanic s.
sinusitis
sinusotomy
SISI — short increment sensitivity index
Sistrunk's operation
Sjögren's syndrome
Slaughter's saw
Sluder-Demarest tonsillectome
Sluder-Jansen mouth gag
Sluder-Sauer
    guillotine
    tonsillectome
Sluder's
    adenotome
    guillotine
    operation
    tonsillectome
SMR — submucous resection
SMRR — submucous resection and rhinoplasty
SMR speculum

snare
    Bosworth's s.
    Brown's s.
    Bruening's s.
    Eves' s.
    Krause's s.
    Lewis' s.
    Myles' s.
    Reiner-Beck s.
    Storz-Beck s.
    Stutsman's s.
    Tydings' s.
    Wilde-Bruening s.
    Wright's s.
Snitman's retractor
solution
    Ringer's s.
SOM — secretory otitis media
       serous otitis media
Sonneberg's operation
Sonnenschein's speculum
Sourdille's operation
space
    poststyloid s.
    prestyloid s.
    Prussak's s.
    retropharyngeal s.
speculum
    Aufricht's s.
    Beckman-Colver s.
    Boucheron's s.
    Chevalier Jackson s.
    Coakley's s.
    Converse's s.
    Cottle's s.
    Duplay-Lynch s.
    Duplay's s.
    Eaton's s.
    Erhardt's s.
    Farrior's s.
    Flannery's s.

speculum (*continued*)
    Gerzog's s.
    Gruber's s.
    Halle's s.
    Halle-Tieck s.
    Hartmann-Dewaxer s.
    Hartmann's s.
    Heffernan's s.
    Ingals' s.
    Killian's s.
    Kramer's s.
    Kyle's s.
    Lempert-Colver s.
    Lillie's s.
    Mahoney's s.
    McHugh's s.
    Mosher's s.
    Myles' s.
    Politzer's s.
    Pynchon's s.
    Ray's s.
    Schuknecht's s.
    Scott's s.
    Senturia's s.
    SMR s.
    Sonnenschein's s.
    Toynbee's s.
    Tröltsch's s.
    Vienna s.
    Welch-Allyn s.
    Yankauer's s.
Spencer's
    probe
    punch
sphenoethmoid
sphenofrontal
sphenoid
sphenoidal
sphenoidectomy
    frontoethmoid s.
sphenoiditis
sphenoidostomy

sphenoidotomy
sphenomaxillary
sphenopalatine
sphenoparietal
sphenosquamous
sphenozygomatic
Spies' punch
spine
    s. of Henle
    suprameatal s.
splint
    Asch's s.
    Carter's s.
    Erich's s.
    Jones' s.
    Kazanjian's s.
    Love's s.
    Mayer's s.
spoon
    Gross' s.
spot
    Koplik's s's
Spratt's curet
spud
    Gross' s.
squama
squamomastoid
SRT — speech reception test
    speech reception
    threshold
Stacke's operation
Stallard's operation
stapedectomy
    Guilford's s.
    Hough's s.
    House's s.
    Schuknecht's s.
    Shea's s.
stapedial
stapediolysis
stapedioplasty
stapediotenotomy

stapediovestibular
stapes
staphylagra
saphylectomy
staphyledema
staphylematoma
staphyline
staphylinus
staphylion
staphylitis
staphyloangina
staphyloncus
staphylopharyngorrhaphy
staphyloplasty
staphyloptosia
staphyloptosis
staphylorrhaphy
staphyloschisis
staphylotome
staphylotomy
St. Clair-Thompson's curet
Stenger's test
stenosis
Stensen's
    duct
    foramen
stent
sternohyoid
sternomastoid
sternothyroid
sternotracheal
Stevens' scissors
Stoerk's blennorrhea
stomatitides
stomatitis
stomatomycosis
stomatoplasty
Storz-Beck snare
Straight's tenaculum
stria
    s. vascularis ductus
      cochlearis

stricture
stridor
Struempel's forceps
struma
Struyken's forceps
Stubbs' curet
stump
    tracheal s.
Stutsman's snare
stylohyal
stylohyoid
styloid
stylomandibular
stylomastoid
subarachnoid
subglossitis
subglottic
sublingual
submandibular
submaxillary
submental
submucous
sudo-. See words beginning
    pseudo-.
sudokolesteatoma. See
    pseudocholesteatoma.
sulcus
    tympanic s.
summit
    s. of nose
Sunday's elevator
suppuration
suppurative
supraclavicular
supraglottic
suprahyoid
supramandibular
supramastoid
supramaxillary
supramental
supranasal
supraorbital

suprastapedial
suprasternal
supratemporal
surgical procedures. See *operation.*
suture. See *General Surgical Terms.*
symptom
    Bárány's s.
    esophagosalivary s.
    Fröschel's s.
    labyrinthine s's
synchondrosis
syndrome
    Avellis' s.
    Baelz's s.
    Bárány's s.
    Costen's s.
    Gradenigo's s.
    Kartagener's s.
    Lermoyez's s.
    Mikulicz's s.
    Pierre Robin s.
    Plummer-Vinson s.
    Sjögren's s.
synechia
Tabb's curet
Takahashi's
    forceps
    punch
tampon
    nasal t.
tantalum
technique
    guillotine t.
Teflon
    prosthesis
    tube
tegmen
    t. antri
    t. cellulae

tegmen (*continued*)
    t. mastoideotympanicum
    t. mastoideum
    t. tympani
tegmental
tegmentum
    t. auris
temple
tempora
temporal
temporalis
temporoauricular
temporofacial
temporofrontal
temporohyoid
temporomandibular
temporomaxillary
temporo-occipital
temporoparietal
temporosphenoid
temporozygomatic
tenaculum
    Cottle's t.
    Straight's t.
tendon
    stapedius t.
tentorial
tentorium
terigo-. See words beginning *pterygo-.*
test
    Bárány's t.
    Bing's t.
    caloric t.
    clivogram t.
    Erhard's t.
    Gault's t.
    Gellé's t.
    Lombard's t.
    Politzer's t.
    Rinne's t.

test (*continued*)
    Schwabach's t.
    short increment sensitivity index (SISI) t.
    Stenger's t.
    Tobey-Ayer t.
    torsion t.
    tuning fork t.
    watch t.
    Weber's t.
    whisper t.
    whistle t.
Theobald's probe
Thornwald's perforator
thrush
thyrochondrotomy
thyrocricotomy
thyroglossal
thyrohyoid
thyroid
thyromegaly
thyrotomy
tia-. See words beginning *ptya-*.
tialektasis. See *ptyalectasis*.
tializm. See *ptyalism*.
tic
    t. douloureux (doo-loo-roo)
tinnitus
Tivnen's forceps
TM — tympanic membrane
TMJ — temporomandibular joint
Tobey-Ayer test
Tobey's rongeur
Tobold's
    forceps
    knife
tonguetie
tonsil
    buried t.
    eustachian t.

tonsil (*continued*)
    faucial t.
    lingual t.
    Luschka's t.
    palatine t.
    pharyngeal t.
    submerged t.
tonsilla
    t. lingualis
    t. palatina
    t. pharyngea
    t. tubaria
tonsillar
tonsillectome
    Ballenger-Sluder t.
    Beck-Mueller t.
    Beck-Schenck t.
    Brown's t.
    Daniels' t.
    Laforce's t.
    Mack's t.
    Moltz-Storz t.
    Myles' t.
    Sauer's t.
    Sauer-Sluder t.
    Searcy's t.
    Sluder-Demarest t.
    Sluder-Sauer t.
    Sluder's t.
    Tydings' t.
    Van Osdel's t.
    Whiting's t.
tonsillectomy
tonsillitis
    caseous t.
    catarrhal t.
    diphtherial t.
    erythematous t.
    follicular t.
    herpetic t.
    lacunar t.
    t. lenta

tonsillitis (*continued*)
    lingual t.
    mycotic t.
    parenchymatous t.
    preglottic t.
    pustular t.
    streptococcal t.
    Vincent's t.
tonsilloadenoidectomy
tonsillolith
tonsilloscope
tonsilloscopy
tonsillotome
tonsillotomy
Topinard's
    angle
    line
Tornwaldt's bursitis
TORP — total ossicular replace-
        ment prosthesis
torticollis
torus
    t. frontalis
    t. levatorius
    t. occipitalis
    t. palatinus
    t. tubarius
Toynbee's
    otoscope
    speculum
trachea
tracheal
tracheitis
tracheobronchial
tracheobronchitis
tracheobronchoscopy
tracheocele
tracheoesophageal
tracheofissure
tracheofistulization
tracheolaryngeal

tracheolaryngotomy
tracheomalacia
tracheopharyngeal
tracheoplasty
tracheorrhaphy
tracheoscopy
    peroral t.
tracheostenosis
tracheostomy
tracheotome
    Salvatore-Maloney t.
    Sierra-Sheldon t.
tracheotomy
tragus
transillumination
transnasal
Trautmann's triangle
treatment
    Politzer's t.
    Proetz's t.
    Roeder's t.
trephine
triad
    Kartagener's t.
triangle
    Trautmann's t.
trismus
trocar
    Coakley's t.
Tröltsch's
    recesses
    speculum
Troutman's
    chisel
    gouge
tube
    Anthony's t.
    auditory t.
    Blakemore's t.
    Bouchut's t.
    Castelli's t.

tube (*continued*)
    Chevalier Jackson t.
    Donaldson's t.
    eustachian t.
    Frazier's t.
    House's t.
    intubation t.
    LaRocca's t.
    Lewis' t.
    Lindeman-Silverstein t.
    Mackenty's t.
    Morch's t.
    nasopharyngeal t.
    otopharyngeal t.
    Paparella's t.
    Per-Lee t.
    Reuter's t.
    Rosen's t.
    Ruysch's t.
    Schall's t.
    Sengstaken-Blakemore t.
    Sengstaken's t.
    Shea's t.
    Sheehy's t.
    Shepard's t.
    Shiley's t.
    Teflon t.
    Voltolini's t.
    Welch-Allyn t.
    Yankauer's t.
tubercle
    darwinian t.
tuberculosis
    t. of larynx
    tracheobronchial t.
tuborrhea
tubotorsion
tubotympanal
Tucker's
    esophagoscope
    laryngoscope
tumefaction

tumor
    Rathke's t.
    Schmincke's t.
tuning fork
    Hartmann's t.f.
tunnel
    t. of Corti
turbinate
    sphenoid t.
turbinectomy
turbinotome
turbinotomy
Tydings'
    forceps
    knife
    snare
    tonsillectome
Tydings-Lakeside forceps
tympanal
tympanectomy
tympanic
tympanichord
tympanichordal
tympanicity
tympanion
tympanitic
tympanitis
tympanoacryloplasty
tympanoeustachian
tympanolabyrinthopexy
tympanomalleal
tympanomandibular
tympanomastoiditis
tympanomeatal
tympanometry
tympanophonia
tympanoplasty
tympanosclerosis
tympanosquamosal
tympanostapedial
tympanosympathectomy
tympanotemporal

tympanotomy
tympanum
tympany
uloglossitis
uloncus
ultrasonogram
ultrasonography
ultrasound
umbo
    u. of tympanic mem-
        brane
unit
    Hertz u.
Updegraff's needle
uraniscochasma
uraniscolalia
uranisconitis
uranoplasty
utricle
uvula
    u. palatina
    palatine u.
uvulectomy
uvulitis
uvuloptosis
uvulotome
uvulotomy
vallecula
    v. epiglottica
Valsalva's procedure
valve
    Huschke's v.
Van Osdel's tonsillectome
Van Struycken
    forceps
    punch
varix
vas
vasa
    v. auris internae
vault
    cartilaginous v.

velum
    v. palatinum
ventricle
    Morgagni's v.
ventricular
ventriculocordectomy
Verga's lacrimal groove
vermilion border
vermilionectomy
vertiginous
vertigo
vestibular
vestibule
vestibulotomy
vestibulum
    v. auris
    v. glottidis
    v. laryngis
    v. nasi
    v. oris
vibrissa
vibrissae
vibromasseur
vibrometer
Vicq d'Azyr's operation
Vienna speculum
Vieussens' annulus
Vincent's
    infection
    tonsillitis
vocal
Vogel's curet
Voltolini's tube
vomer
vomeronasal
Wagner's punch
Waldeyer's ring
Walker's dissector
Walsham's forceps
Walther's ducts
Watson-Williams
    forceps

Watson-Williams (*continued*)
    punch
Weber's test
Weil's forceps
Weingartner's forceps
Weisman's curet
Weitlaner's retractor
Welch-Allyn
    laryngoscope
    otoscope
    probe
    speculum
    tube
Wellaminski's perforator
West's operation
Wharton's duct
White-Lillie forceps
White-Proud retractor
White's forceps
Whiting's
    curet
    rongeur
    tonsillectome
Wiener-Pierce rasp
Wilde-Bruening snare
Wilde's
    forceps
    punch
Willis' paracusis
window
    oval w.
    round w.
windowing
Wis-Foregger's laryngoscope
Wis-Hipple's laryngoscope
Woakes' saw

Wood's operation
Wreden's sign
Wright's snare
Wrisberg's cartilage
Wullstein-House forceps
Wullstein's
    bur
    forceps
    knife
    operation
    retractor
xanthosis
    x. of septum nasi
xeromycteria
xerostomia
Yankauer-Little forceps
Yankauer's
    catheter
    curet
    esophagoscope
    forceps
    laryngoscope
    operation
    probe
    punch
    speculum
    tube
Zaufal's sign
Zeiss' microscope
zygoma
zygomatic
zygomaticofacial
zygomaticofrontal
zygomaticomaxillary
zygomaxillary

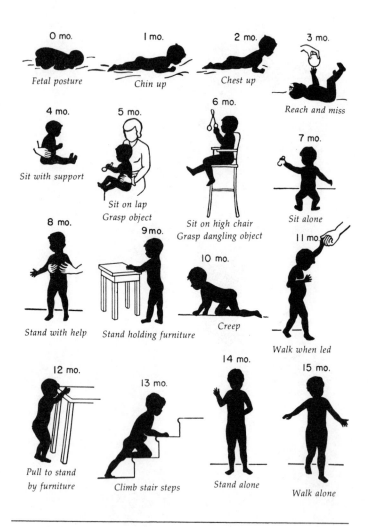

0 mo.
Fetal posture

1 mo.
Chin up

2 mo.
Chest up

3 mo.
Reach and miss

4 mo.
Sit with support

5 mo.
Sit on lap
Grasp object

6 mo.
Sit on high chair
Grasp dangling object

7 mo.
Sit alone

8 mo.
Stand with help

9 mo.
Stand holding furniture

10 mo.
Creep

11 mo.
Walk when led

12 mo.
Pull to stand
by furniture

13 mo.
Climb stair steps

14 mo.
Stand alone

15 mo.
Walk alone

(Courtesy of Shirley, M. M.: The First Two Years: A Study of Twenty-Five Babies. [Child Welfare Monograph No. 7, Vol. II.] Minneapolis, University of Minnesota Press, copyright 1933 by the University of Minnesota.)

PEDIATRICS

Abderhalden-Fanconi
   syndrome
abetalipoproteinemia
ABO incompatibility
abscess
      amebic a.
      perinephric a.
      pyogenic a.
      retropharyngeal a.
      subphrenic a.
Abt-Letterer-Siwe syndrome
acantholysis
      a. bullosa
achalasia
achondroplasia
acidosis
      diabetic a.
      hyperchloremic renal a.
      metabolic a.
aciduria
      β-aminoisobutyric a.
aclasis
      diaphyseal a.
acne
      a. neonatorum
acrania
acrobrachycephaly
acrocephalosyndactylia
acrocyanosis

acrodermatitis
      a. enteropathica
acrodynia
acromegaly
Actinomyces
actinomycosis
Addison's disease
adenitis
      cervical a.
      mesenteric a.
adenocarcinoma
adenoiditis
adenoma
      a. sebaceum
adenopathy
      cervical a.
adhesions
Adie's syndrome
adiponecrosis
      a. subcutanea
         neonatorum
adnexa
adolescence
adrenarche
adrenocortical
aerophore
aftha. See *aphtha.*
agammaglobulinemia
aganglionosis

agenesia
    a. corticalis
agenesis
    callosal a.
    gonadal a.
    nuclear a.
    ovarian a.
    renal a.
agglutinin
agranulocytosis
akalazea. See *achalasia.*
akinesia
    a. algera
akondroplazea. See *achondro-*
    plasia.
akrobrakesefale. See *acro-*
    brachycephaly.
Albers-Schönberg's syndrome
albinism
Albright's syndrome
albuminuria
aldosteronism
    juvenile a.
Aldrich's syndrome
aleukia
    congenital a.
Alexander's disease
alkalosis
allergic
allergy
Alper's disease
Alport's syndrome
alymphocytosis
alymphoplasia
amaurotic familial idiocy
ambient
amebiasis
amelia
amenorrhea
aminoacidemia
aminoaciduria

aminoaciduriasis
amnionitis
amyloidosis
amylopectinosis
amyoplasia
    a. congenita
amyotonia
    a. congenita
anaphylaxis
anasarca
ancylostomiasis
Andersen's disease
Andogsky's syndrome
anemia
    aplastic a.
    breast a.
    congenital a. of new-
      born
    congenital nonsphero-
      cytic hemolytic a.
    Cooley's a.
    Czerny's a.
    erythroblastic a. of child-
      hood
    familial erythroblastic a.
    Fanconi's a.
    globe-cell a.
    glucose-6-phosphate
      dehydrogenase
      deficiency a.
    hemolytic a.
    a. hypochromica sidero-
      chrestica hereditaria
    hypoplastic a., congenital
    Jaksch's a.
    Larzel's a.
    Mediterranean a.
    megaloblastic a.
    a. neonatorum
    ovalocvtary a.
    pernicious a., juvenile

anemia (*continued*)
    physiologic a.
    a. pseudoleukemica infantum
    pyridoxine-responsive a.
    sickle cell a.
    von Jaksch's a.
anemic
anencephaly
aneurysm
    aortic a.
angiitis
angiocardiography
anorchia
anorchism
anorexia
    a. nervosa
anoxia
ansilostomiasis. See *ancylostomiasis*.
antigen
    Australia a.
antrum
anuria
anus
    imperforate a.
aorta
aortitis
Apgar
    rating
    score
aphtha
    Bednar's a.
aplasia
    a. axialis extracorticalis congenita
    a. cutis congenita
    gonadal a.
    nuclear a.
    retinal a.
    thymic a.
    thymic-parathyroid a.

apnea
    initial a.
    late a.
    a. neonatorum
appendicitis
arachnidism
arachnodactyly
arachnoiditis
arak-. See words beginning *arach-*.
Aran-Duchenne disease
areflexia
arginosuccinicaciduria
Arnold-Chiari syndrome
arrhythmia
    sinus a.
arteriosclerosis
    infantile a.
arteritis
    a. umbilicalis
arthritis
    rheumatoid a.
arthrogryposis
    a. multiplex congenita
ascariasis
Ascaris
    A. lumbricoides
ascites
    chylous a.
ASD — atrial septal defect
asphyxia
    a. neonatorum
asplenia
asthma
    thymic a.
astigmatism
astrocytoma
ataxia
    cerebellar a.
    Friedreich's a.
atelectasis
    congenital a.

atelectasis (*continued*)
    primary a.
athetoid
athetosis
    congenital a.
atopic
atopy
atresia
    biliary a.
    esophageal a.
    ileal a.
    pyloric a.
    tricuspid a.
atrial septal defect
atrophia bulborum hereditaria
atrophy
    Déjerine-Sottas a.
    Fazio-Londe a.
    Parrot's a. of the new-
        born
Australia antigen
autism
autistic
autoprothrombin I
bacteroidosis
Ballantyne-Runge syndrome
Banti's syndrome
Barlow's disease
Bartter's syndrome
Batten-Mayou disease
Beck's disease
Beckwith's syndrome
Bednar's aphtha
Berger's paresthesia
beriberi
Best's disease
bezoar
bilirubin
Blalock-Hanlon operation
Blalock-Taussig operation
blefaritis. See *blepharitis.*

blefarospasm. See *blepharo-*
    spasm.
blennorrhea
blepharitis
blepharospasm
Bloch-Sulzberger syndrome
blood
    cord b.
Bloom's syndrome
Bochdalek
    foramen of B. hernia
    B. hernia
Bonnevie-Ullrich syndrome
Bornholm's disease
botulism
Bouchut's respiration
Bourneville's syndrome
Brachmann-de Lange syndrome
brachycephalic
brachydactyly
bradycardia
Brandt's syndrome
brash
    weaning b.
bronchiectasis
bronchiolitis
bronchitis
    acute laryngotracheal b.
    arachidic b.
    chronic obstructive b.
    epidemic capillary b.
bronchopneumonia
bronchus
    esophageal b.
Brown-Symmers disease
brucella
brucellosis
Brudzinski's sign
bruit
    carotid b.
Brushfield's spots

bruxism
brwe. See *bruit.*
Buhl's disease
Byrd-Dew method
Caffey's disease
Caffey-Silverman syndrome
Caffey-Smyth-Roske syndrome
calculus
    urate c.
Calvé-Legg-Perthes syndrome
Camurati-Engelmann syndrome
Canavan's disease
cancer
cancerous
Candida
    C. albicans
candidiasis
canker
caput
    c. medusae
    c. succedaneum
cardiospasm
cataplexy
cataract
catarrhal
catheter
    arterial c.
    umbilical c.
    venous c.
catheterization
celiaca
cellulitis
cephalhematoma
cerebellar
cerebral
cerebrospinal
cerebrovascular
Chagas' disease
chalasia
chalazion
Chapple's syndrome

Charcot-Marie-Tooth-Hoff-
    mann syndrome
Cheadle's disease
Chédiak-Higashi syndrome
chickenpox
Chilaiditi's syndrome
cholangitis
cholecystitis
    acute acalculous c.
cholera
    c. infantum
chondrodystrophia
    c. calcificans congenita
    c. fetalis calcificans
chondrodystrophy
chondro-osteodystrophy
chorea
    Sydenham's c.
chorioepithelioma
choriomeningitis
    lymphocytic c.
chorioretinitis
Christ-Siemens-Touraine
    syndrome
chromaffinoma
circumcision
cirrhonosus
cirrhosis
    biliary c.
citrullinuria
Clark-Hadfield syndrome
clinodactyly
cloaca
    congenital c.
clonus
    ankle c.
clostridia
clubfoot
CNS — central nervous system
coarctation
    c. of the aorta

Coat's disease
coccidioidomycosis
Cockayne's syndrome
colic
colicky
colitis
    amoebic c.
    granulomatous c.
    infectious c.
    tuberculous c.
    ulcerative c.
coloboma
colonization
    stool c.
Colorado tick fever
colostration
colostrum
coma
    diabetic c.
    hyperosmolar c.
Comby's sign
communicable
complex
    Eisenmenger's c.
    Ghon c.
concussion
congenital
conjunctivitis
Conradi's disease
constipation
contusion
conversion
    hysterical c.
convulsion
    febrile c.
Cooley's anemia
Coombs' test
cor
    c. biloculare
    c. triloculare biatriatum
Cori's disease
Cornelia de Lange's syndrome

corpora
    c. quadrigemina
Corrigan's pulse
cortex
    adrenal c.
Corynebacterium
    C. diphtheriae
coryza
coxa
    c. vara
Coxsackie virus
cradle cap
craniopharyngioma
craniostenosis
craniosynostosis
craniotabes
crease
    simian c.
    sole c.
creatinine
crepitation
cretinism
cri-du-chat syndrome
Crigler-Najjar syndrome
crisis
    adrenal c.
croup
Crouzon's disease
crusta
    c. lactea
cryoprecipitate
cryptococcosis
cryptorchidism
culture
    sputum c.
    tracheal-aspirate c.
curse
    Ondine's c.
Cushing's syndrome
cutis
    c. elastica
    c. hyperelastica

CVP – central venous pressure
cyanosis
cyst
     choledochal c.
     colloid c.
     dermoid c.
     hydatid c.
     omental c.
     porencephalic c's
     urachal c.
     vitelline duct c.
cystathioninuria
cystic fibrosis
cystinosis
cystinuria
Czerny's anemia
dacryocystostenosis
dance
     St. Vitus' d.
dandruff
Dandy-Walker
     deformity
     syndrome
Darrow-Gamble syndrome
Dawson's encephalitis
defect
     atrial septal d.
     ventricular septal d.
deficiency
     disaccharidase d.
     erythrocyte glutathione
       peroxidase d.
     Factor VIII d.
     fibrinogen d.
     glucose-6-phosphate de-
       hydrogenase d.
     IgA d.
     IgM d.
     immunoglobulin d.
     riboflavin d.
deformity
     Dandy-Walker d.

deformity (*continued*)
     Sprengel's d.
     Volkmann's d.
degeneration
     cerebellar d.
     cerebromacular d.
     congenital macular d.
dehydration
Déjerine's disease
Déjerine-Sottas
     atrophy
     disease
de Lange's syndrome
delinquency
delirium
dengue
Dennett's diet
Dennie-Marfan syndrome
depigmentation
dermatitis
     atopic d.
     d. excoriativa infantum
     d. exfoliativa infantum
     d. gangrenosa infantum
     Jacquet's d.
     seborrheic d.
     d. venenata
dermatomyositis
dermatophytosis
DeSanctis-Cacchione syndrome
desensitization
determination
     sweat chloride d.
de Toni-Fanconi-Debre
     syndrome
dextrocardia
Dextrostix
diabetes
     d. insipidus
     d. mellitus
diabetic
Diamond-Blackfan syndrome

diarrhea
diastematomyelia
diencephalic syndrome
diet
    Dennett's d.
    Moro-Heisler d.
difenilthiourea. See *diphenyl-
    thiourea.*
difilobothriasis. See *diphyl-
    lobothriasis.*
diftherea. See *diphtheria.*
DiGeorge's syndrome
dilatation
    esophageal d.
diphenylthiourea
diphtheria
diphyllobothriasis
diplegia
    atonic-astatic d.
    facial d., congenital
    infantile d.
    spastic d.
Diplococcus
    D. pneumoniae
dis-. See also words beginning
    dys-.
disease
    Addison's d.
    Alexander's d.
    Alper's d.
    Andersen's d.
    Aran-Duchenne d.
    Barlow's d.
    Batten-Mayou d.
    Beck's d.
    Best's d.
    Bornholm's d.
    Brown-Symmers d.
    Buhl's d.
    Caffey's d.
    Canavan's d.
    celiac d.

disease (*continued*)
    central nervous system d.
    Chagas' d.
    Cheadle's d.
    Coat's d.
    communicable d.
    Conradi's d.
    Cori's d.
    Crouzon's d.
    cytomegalic inclusion d.
     of the newborn
    cytomegalovirus d.
    Déjerine's d.
    Déjerine-Sottas d.
    Duke's d.
    Duroziez's d.
    Factor X deficiency d.
    Feer's d.
    fibrocystic d.
    fifth d.
    Fölling's d.
    Gaucher's d.
    Gee-Herter-Heubner d.
    genetotrophic d.
    glycogen storage d.
    Goldstein's d.
    Hartnup's d.
    helminthic d.
    hemoglobin C-thalas-
     semia d.
    hemoglobin E-thalas-
     semia d.
    hemolytic d. of the new-
     born
    hemorrhagic d. of new-
     born
    Henoch's d.
    hereditary d.
    heredoconstitutional d.
    heredodegenerative d.
    Hers' d.
    Hirschsprung's d.

disease (*continued*)
Hodgkin's d.
Hutinel's d.
hyaline membrane d.
hydrocephaloid d.
infantile celiac d.
Kashin-Beck d.
Köhler's d.
Krabbe's d.
Kufs' d.
Kugelberg-Welander d.
Leber's d.
Leigh's d.
Leiner's d.
Letterer-Siwe d.
Little's d.
maple syrup urine d.
Marion's d.
McArdle's d.
Milroy's d.
Minot's d.
Möller-Barlow d.
Morquio's d.
Niemann-Pick d.
Norrie's d.
Oppenheim's d.
Osler-Weber-Rendu d.
Paas's d.
Pelizaeus-Merzbacher d.
pink d.
Pompe's d.
Potter's d.
Recklinghausen's d.
Refsum's d.
renal cystic d.
Ritter's d.
Saunders' d.
Scheuermann's d.
Schilder's d.
Scholz's d.
sickle cell d.

disease (*continued*)
sickle cell–hemoglobin
C d.
sickle cell–hemoglobin
D d.
sickle cell–thalassemia d.
spinocerebellar degenerative d.
Sticker's d.
Still's d.
Stuart-Prower factor deficiency d.
Tangier d.
Tay-Sachs d.
Thiemann's d.
Thomsen's d.
Thomson's d.
Underwood's d.
Unverricht's d.
Vogt-Spielmeyer d.
Volkmann's d.
von Gierke's d.
von Hippel-Lindau d.
von Recklinghausen's d.
Weil's d.
Wilkins' d.
Wilson's d.
Winckel's d.
Wolman's d.
disfagia. See *dysphagia.*
disjenisis. See *dysgenesis.*
distress
idiopathic respiratory d.
of newborn
diverticula
diverticulosis
diverticulum
Meckel's d.
pharyngeal d.
Down's syndrome
drooling

drugs. See *Drugs and Chemistry* section.
Dubin-Johnson syndrome
Dubovitz's syndrome
Duchenne's dystrophy
duct
    omphalomesenteric d.
    Stensen's d.
    vitelline d.
ductus
    d. arteriosus
Duke's disease
duplication
    d. of colon
    d. of duodenum
    d. of esophagus
    d. of ileum
    d. of rectum
    d. of stomach
Duroziez's disease
dwarfism
    pituitary d.
dysautonomia
    familial d.
dyschondroplasia
dysentery
    amebic d.
    bacillary d.
dysfibrinogenemia
dysfunction
    placental d.
dysgammaglobulinemia
dysgenesis
    gonadal d.
dysgerminoma
dyshepatia
    lipogenic d.
dysmaturity
dysmenorrhea
dysostosis
    cleidocranial d.

dysostosis (*continued*)
    craniofacial d.
    mandibulofacial d.
    d. multiplex
    orodigitofacial d.
dysphagia
dysplasia
    anhidrotic ectodermal d.
    bronchopulmonary d.
    chondroectodermal d.
    congenital alveolar d.
    craniodiaphyseal d.
    cretinoid d.
    diaphyseal d.
    ectodermal d.
    d. epiphysealis punctata
    hereditary bone d.
    hidrotic ectodermal d.
    oculoauriculovertebral (OAV) d.
    oculodentodigital (ODD) d.
    ophthalmomandibulo-melic d.
    polyostotic fibrous d.
    spondyloepiphyseal d.
    thymic d.
dyspnea
dysrhythmia
dystaxia
    d. cerebralis infantilis
dystonia
dystrophy
    Duchenne's d.
    Meesmann's d.
    muscular d.
EBV — Epstein-Barr virus
eccentrochondroplasia
eccentro-osteochondrodys-plasia
ecchymosis

Echinococcus
ECHO — enteric cytopatho-
        genic human
        orphan (virus)
echoencephalography
echovirus
ecthyma
eczema
    e. herpeticum
    infantile e.
    e. marginatum
    e. neonatorum
    e. vaccinatum
edema
    angioneurotic e.,
      hereditary
    e. neonatorum
eelworm
efeb-. See words beginning
    epheb-.
efelidez. See *ephelides.*
efelis. See *ephelis.*
effusion
Ehlers-Danlos syndrome
Eisenmenger's complex
ekimosis. See *ecchymosis.*
ekinokokus. See *Echinococcus.*
eksanthem. See *exanthem.*
ekthima. See *ecthyma.*
ekzema. See *eczema.*
electrocardiography
electrodesiccation
electroencephalogram
electrolyte
electrophoresis
elephantiasis
    congenital e.
elliptocytosis
Ellis–van Creveld syndrome
embolus
embryoma
emesis

emphysema
    lobar e., infantile
empyema
emulsion
    Pusey's e.
encephalitis
    Dawson's e.
    e. neonatorum
    Schilder's e.
    St. Louis e.
    viral e.
encephalocele
encephalomyelitis
encephalopathy
    demyelinating e.
enchondroma
encopresis
endocarditis
    subacute bacterial e.
enteritis
    bacterial e.
    regional e.
enterobiasis
Enterobius
    E. vermicularis
enterocolitis
    necrotizing e.
enteropathy
enuresis
eosinophilia
ependymoma
ephebiatrics
ephebic
ephebogenesis
ephebogenic
ephebology
ephelides
ephelis
epicanthus
epidermolysis
    e. bullosa
epidermophytosis

epididymis
epifisis. See *epiphysis.*
epilepsy
    abdominal e.
    focal e.
    grand mal e.
    jacksonian e.
    myoclonus e.
    nocturnal e.
    petit mal e.
    psychomotor e.
epileptic
epileptiform
epiloia
epiphysis
epistaxis
epituberculosis
Epstein-Barr virus
Epstein's
    pearls
    symptom
Erb-Duchenne paralysis
erithema. See *erythema.*
erithro-. See words beginning
    erythro-.
Erlacher-Blount syndrome
eruption
    Kaposi's varicelliform e.
Erysipelothrix
erythema
    e. infectiosum
    Jacquet's e.
    e. neonatorum toxicum
    e. streptogenes
erythredema polyneuropathy
erythroblastosis
    e. fetalis
    e. neonatorum
erythroderma
    atopic e.
    e. desquamativum
erythroleukoblastosis

Escherichia
    E. coli
esophagitis
    infectious e.
    monilia e.
    reflux e.
eventration
Ewing's
    sarcoma
    tumor
exanthem
exostosis
exstrophy
Factor VII
Factor VIII
    deficiency
    inhibitor
Factor X deficiency disease
Fallot's tetralogy
familial
    f. osteochondrodys-
        trophy
Fanconi-Albertini-Zellweger
    syndrome
Fanconi-Petrassi syndrome
Fanconi's
    anemia
    syndrome
Farber's test
farinjitis. See *pharyngitis.*
Fazio-Londe atrophy
fecalith
    appendiceal f.
feces
Feer's disease
fenilketonurea. See *phenyl-
    ketonuria.*
feochromocytoma. See *pheo-
    chromocytoma.*
fever
    cat scratch f.
    Colorado tick f.

fever (*continued*)
    Haverhill f.
    hay f.
    paratyphoid f.
    Q f.
    relapsing f.
    rheumatic f.
    Rocky Mountain spotted f.
    scarlet f.
    South African tick f.
    spotted f.
    tick f.
    typhoid f.
    undulant f.
    valley f.
    yellow f.
fibrillation
    atrial f.
    ventricular f.
fibroelastosis
    endocardial f.
fibroma
    histiocytic f.
fibroplasia
    retrolental f.
fibrosis
    cystic f.
fissure
fistula
    tracheoesophageal f.
fitobezor. See *phytobezoar.*
FJN – familial juvenile nephrophthisis
flaccid
flaring
    alar f.
    nasal f.
fobia. See *phobia.*
fokomelea. See *phocomelia.*
folliculitis
Fölling's disease

fontanelle
fonticulus
foramen
    f. of Bochdalek hernia
    f. of Morgagni hernia
    pleuroperitoneal f.
    f. primum
    f. secundum
formiminoglutamicaciduria
fragilitas
    f. ossium
Franceschetti's syndrome
Frei test
Freiberg's infraction
Friedreich's ataxia
fungi
furuncle
furunculosis
galactosemia
gallbladder
gamma globulin
ganglioneuroma
gangrene
Gardner's syndrome
gargoylism
Gasser's syndrome
gastritis
gastroenteritis
    eosinophilic g.
gastrointestinal
Gaucher's disease
Gee-Herter-Heubner disease
genitalia
geophagia
German measles
gestation
gestational
Ghon
    complex
    tubercle
giardiasis
    intestinal g.

gigantism
    cerebral g.
    eunuchoid g.
    fetal g.
    hyperpituitary g.
    pituitary g.
Gilbert-Dreyfus' syndrome
Gilbert-Lereboullet syndrome
Gilles de la Tourette's
    syndrome
gingivitis
    herpetic g.
gingivostomatitis
    herpetic g.
gland
    parotid g.
    Philip's g's
    salivary g.
    sublingual g.
    submaxillary g.
Glanzmann's syndrome
glaucoma
glioblastoma
glioma
globulin
glomerulonephritis
glycinuria
glycogen
glycosuria
goiter
Goldstein's disease
Goltz-Gorlin syndrome
Goltz's syndrome
gonad
gonorrhea
Goodpasture's syndrome
Gowers' sign
G6PD — glucose-6-phosphate
    dehydrogenase
grand mal
Granger's sign
granuloma

granulomatosis
Grünfelder's reflex
grunting
Hallermann-Streiff syndrome
Hallervorden-Spatz syndrome
hammer toe
Hand-Schüller-Christian
    syndrome
Hanhart's syndrome
Hartnup's
    disease
    syndrome
Hart's syndrome
Haverhill fever
HDN — hemolytic disease of
    the newborn
heart block
    Wenckebach h.b.
hebetic
hemangioblastoma
hemangioma
    cavernous h.
hemangiomatosis
hemarthrosis
hematemesis
hematoma
    extradural h.
    subdural h.
    sublingual h.
    submental h.
hematopoiesis
hematuria
hemiatrophy
hemiplegia
hemivertebra
hemochromatosis
hemoglobinopathy
hemolysis
hemolytic
hemophilia
hemophiliac
hemophilus

hemorrhage
    sternocleidomastoid h.
    subarachnoid h.
hemosiderosis
Henoch's disease
hepatic
hepatitis
    neonatal h.
hepatocellular
hepatolenticular
hepatoma
hepatomegaly
hepatosplenomegaly
hereditary
heredity
    autosomal h.
    sex-linked h.
heredoataxia
heredobiologic
heredodegeneration
heredodiathesis
heredofamilial
heredoimmunity
heredolues
heredopathia
    h. atactica polyneuriti-
       formis
heredosyphilis
heritability
heritable
hernia
    Bochdalek h.
    congenital h.
    diaphragmatic h.
    hiatus h.
    incarcerated h.
    inguinal h.
    Morgagni h.
    paraduodenal h.
    peritoneopericardial h.
    pleuroperitoneal h.
    retrocecal h.

hernia (*continued*)
    retrosternal h.
    transmesenteric h.
    umbilical h.
herniation
herniorrhaphy
herpangina
herpes
    visceral h. simplex
Hers' disease
hipsarithmea. See *hypsarrhyth-mia.*
Hirschsprung's disease
histidinemia
histiocytosis
    h. X
histoplasmosis
Hodgkin's disease
Holt-Oram syndrome
homocystinuria
hookworm
hordeolum
Hunter's syndrome
Hurler's syndrome
Hutchinson-Gilford syndrome
Hutchinson's syndrome
Hutinel's disease
hydranencephaly
hydroa
    h. puerorum
    h. vacciniforme
hydrocele
hydrocelectomy
hydrocephalic
hydrocephalocele
hydrocephaloid
hydrocephalus
hydrocolpos
hydrometrocolpos
hydronephrosis
hydrops
    h. fetalis

hydroxyprolinemia
hygroma
hyperacidity
hyperaldosteronism
hyperbilirubinemia
hyperbilirubinemic
hypercalcemia
    idiopathic h.
hyperemesis
    h. lactentium
hyperglycemia
hyperglycinemia
hyperinsulinism
hyperkalemia
hyperkeratosis
hyperlipidemia
hypernatremia
hyperopia
hyperostosis
    infantile cortical h.
hyperparathyroidism
hyperplasia
    lymphoid h.
hyperprolinemia
hyperpyrexia
hypersensitization
hypersplenism
hypertelorism
hypertension
hyperthyroidism
hyperthyroxinemia
hyperuricemia
hypervalinemia
hyperventilation
hypervitaminosis
hypoadrenalism
hypocalcemia
hypocalcemic
hypocapnia
hypochondriasis
hypodermoclysis

hypogammaglobulinemia
    acquired h.
    congenital h.
    physiologic h.
    transient h.
hypogenesis
hypoglycemia
hypoglycemic
hypokalemia
hypomagnesemia
hyponatremia
hyponatremic
hypoparathyroidism
hypopharynx
hypophosphatasia
hypopituitarism
hypopotassemia
hypoproteinemia
hypospadias
hypothermia
hypothyroidism
hypotonia
hypovitaminosis
hypovolemia
hypovolemic
hypoxemic
hypoxia
hypsarrhythmia
ichthyosis
icterus
    i. gravis neonatorum
    Liouville's i.
    i. melas
    i. neonatorum
idiocy
    amaurotic familial i.
    mongolian i.
idiopathic
IDM − infant of diabetic
        mother
IgA deficiency

IgM deficiency
iktheosis. See *ichthyosis.*
ileitis
    terminal i.
ileus
    adynamic i.
    meconium i.
imbecile
immunity
immunization
immunoelectrophoresis
impaction
    fecal i.
impetigo
    i. neonatorum
incarceration
incompatibility
    ABO i.
    Rh i.
incompetence
    gastroesophageal i.
incontinentia
    i. pigmenti
incubation
incubator
infancy
infant
infantile
infarct
    bilirubin i's
    uric acid i.
influenza
infraction
    Freiberg's i.
inhibitor
    Factor VIII i.
insufficiency
    adrenocortical i.
    aortic i.
intertrigo
intussusception
    cecocolic i.

intussusception (*continued*)
    colocolic i.
    ileocolic i.
    ileoileal i.
IRDS — idiopathic respiratory
        distress syndrome
iritis
irritability
isohemagglutinin
isoimmunization
Isolette
isovalericacidemia
Ivemark's syndrome
jacksonian epilepsy
Jacquet's
    dermatitis
    erythema
Jaksch's anemia
Jansen's syndrome
jaundice
    physiologic j.
jitteriness
jittery
Joseph's syndrome
kala-azar
kalazea. See *chalasia.*
Kaposi's varicelliform
    eruption
karnikterus. See *kernicterus.*
Kartagener's syndrome
Kasabach-Merritt syndrome
Kashin-Beck disease
Kaufman's pneumonia
keratitis
    interstitial k.
keratoconjunctivitis
keratolysis
    k. neonatorum
keratopathy
    band k.
keratosis
    k. pilaris

kerion
kernicterus
Kernig's sign
ketoacidosis
        diabetic k.
ketosis
Klebsiella
        K. pneumoniae
Klinefelter's syndrome
Klippel-Feil syndrome
Kloepfer's syndrome
Klumpke's paralysis
Köhler's disease
kolanjitis. See cholangitis.
kolera. See cholera.
kondro-. See words beginning
        chondro-.
Koplik's spots
korea. See chorea.
korio-. See words beginning
        chorio-.
koriza. See coryza.
Krabbe's disease
Kufs' disease
Kugelberg-Welander disease
Kussmaul's respiration
kwashiorkor
kyphosis
        k. dorsalis juvenilis
lactobezoar
Landau's
        reflex
        test
Landry-Guillain-Barré
        syndrome
lanugo
laringoskope. See laryngo-
        scope.
larinks. See larynx.
Larsen's syndrome
larva
        l. migrans

laryngoscopy
larynx
Larzel's anemia
Launois' syndrome
Laurence-Moon syndrome
Laurence-Moon-Biedl
        syndrome
lavage
        gastric l.
LBW — low birth weight
LBWI — low birth weight
        infant
LE — lupus erythematosus
Leber's disease
Leigh's disease
Leiner's disease
Lennox's syndrome
leptomeningitis
Leptospira
        L. icterohaemorrhagiae
leptospirosis
Leptothrix
leptotrichosis
lethargic
Letterer-Siwe disease
leukemia
        aplastic l.
        basophilic l.
        eosinophilic l.
        granulocytic l.
        hemoblastic l.
        leukopenic l.
        lymphocytic l.
        lymphosarcoma cell l.
        mast cell l.
        megakaryocytic l.
        micromyeloblastic l.
        myeloblastic l.
        myelogenous l.
leukocytosis
leukodystrophy
        globoid cell l.

leukodystrophy (*continued*)
    sudanophilic l.
LeVeen shunt
lichen
    l. striatus
Lightwood-Albright syndrome
Liouville's icterus
lipidosis
lipochondrodystrophy
lipogranulomatosis
Little's disease
lupus
    l. erythematosus dissem-
      inatus
Lutembacher's syndrome
luteoma
lymphadenitis
    mesenteric l.
lymphadenopathy
lymphangiectasis
    congenital pulmonary l.
lymphangitis
lymphangioma
    l. circumscriptum
    l. cysticum
lymphocytosis
lymphogranuloma
    l. venereum
lymphoma
lymphoreticulosis
lymphosarcoma
Macewen's sign
macrocephaly
macrogenitosomia
    m. praecox
macroglobulinemia
    Waldenström's m.
Magnus and de Kleijn neck
    reflexes
malaise
malaria

malformation
    bronchopulmonary fore-
      gut m.
    vascular m.
malnutrition
malrotation
marasmus
Marfan's syndrome
Marie's syndrome
Marinesco-Sjögren syndrome
Marion's disease
Marmo's method
Maroteaux-Lamy syndrome
mastoiditis
masturbation
McArdle's disease
McCune-Albright syndrome
measles
    German m.
Meckel's diverticulum
meconium
mediastinitis
medications. See *Drugs and
    Chemistry* section.
Mediterranean anemia
medulloblastoma
Meesmann's dystrophy
megacolon
    congenital m.
megalencephaly
melena
    m. neonatorum
Melkersson-Rosenthal syn-
    drome
menarche
meningioma
meningismus
meningitis
    aseptic m.
    tuberculous m.
meningocele

meningococcemia
meningococcus
meningomyelocele
menstruation
mesenteric
metastasis
metatarsus
    m. varus
methemoglobinemia
methemoglobinuria
method
    Byrd-Dew m.
    Marmo's m.
Metopirone test
micrencephaly
microangiopathy
    thrombotic m.
microcephaly
microcytosis
microgastria
Microsporum
    M. audouini
    M. furfur
    M. lanosum
mielitis. See *myelitis.*
mielo-. See words beginning *myelo-.*
migraine
miksedema. See *myxedema.*
milium
Milroy's disease
Minkowski-Chauffard syndrome
Minot's disease
mio-. See words beginning *myo-.*
Möbius' syndrome
Möller-Barlow disease
molluscum
mongolian
mongolism
    double-trisomy m.

mongolism (*continued*)
    translocation m.
mongoloid
moniliasis
mononucleosis
    infectious m.
monosomy
morbilliform
Morgagni hernia
Moro embrace reflex
Moro-Heisler diet
Moro's reflex
Morquio's
    disease
    syndrome
Morquio-Ullrich syndrome
mucoid
mucopolysaccharidosis
    m. I; m. II; m. III; m. IV; m. V; m. VI
mucoviscidosis
mumps
murmur
    diastolic m.
    functional m.
    holosystolic m.
    pansystolic m.
    Still's m.
    systolic ejection m.
myalgia
myasthenia
    m. gravis
Mycobacterium
    M. leprae
    M. tuberculosis
Mycoplasma
mycosis
myelitis
    transverse m.
myelodysplasia
myelofibrosis
myelomeningocele

myelophthisis
myeloproliferative
myocardial
myocarditis
myocardium
myoclonic
myoclonus
myopia
myotonia
    m. congenita
    m. neonatorum
myxedema
    infantile m.
narcolepsy
nares
naris
nasopharyngeal
nausea
nefritis. See *nephritis.*
nefrosis. See *nephrosis.*
neogaster. See *pneogaster.*
neonatal
neonate
neoplasm
nephritis
nephrophthisis
nephrosis
nepiology
Nettleship's syndrome
neuritis
neuroblastoma
neurofibromatosis
neutropenia
nevi
nevoxanthoendothelioma
nevus
    n. flammeus
    n. pilosus
    n. spilus
    n. verrucosus
Nezelof's syndrome
Niemann-Pick disease

Nocardia
noma
    n. pudendi
    n. vulvae
normocephalic
Norrie's disease
numo-. See words beginning
    pneumo-.
obesity
obstipation
ofthalmea. See *ophthalmia.*
oksesefale. See *oxycephaly.*
okseuriasis. See *oxyuriasis.*
oliguria
Ollier's syndrome
omphalocele
Ondine's curse
operation. See *General Surgical*
    Terms.
ophthalmia
    o. neonatorum
opisthotonos
    o. fetalis
Oppenheim's disease
orchitis
organomegaly
orkitis. See *orchitis.*
oropharynx
Ortolani's test
Osgood-Schlatter syndrome
Osler-Weber-Rendu disease
osteitis
    o. condensans
        generalisata
osteochondritis
    o. deformans juvenilis
    o. dissecans
    o. ischiopubica
osteochondrodystrophia
    deformans
osteochondrodystrophy
osteochondroma

osteochondrosis
    o. deformans tibiae
osteodystrophia
    o. juvenilis
osteogenesis
      o. imperfecta
      o. imperfecta cystica
osteoma
    osteoid o.
osteomalacia
    juvenile o.
osteomyelitis
osteopetrosis
osteoporosis
osteopsathyrosis
osteotabes
otitis
    o. media
oxycephaly
oxygen
oxyuriasis
Paas's disease
palsy
    brachial plexus p.
    cerebral p.
pancreas
    annular p.
pancreatitis
panencephalitis
papilledema
papilloma
paracentesis
parainfluenza
paralysis
    congenital abducens-facial p.
    congenital oculofacial p.
    Erb-Duchenne p.
    Klumpke's p.
    spastic p.
    Werdnig-Hoffmann p.

parapertussis
paraplegia
parathyroid
paresthesia
    Berger's p.
paroksizmal. See *paroxysmal.*
paronychia
parotitis
paroxysmal
Parrot's atrophy of the new-born
Pastia's sign
Patau's syndrome
patent ductus arteriosus
pavor
    p. diurnus
    p. nocturnus
PDA — patent ductus arteri-osus
pearl
    Epstein's p's
pedarthrocace
pediatric
pediatrician
pedicterus
pediculosis
pedobaromacrometer
pedobarometer
pedologist
pedometer
Pelizaeus-Merzbacher disease
pellagra
Pellizzi's syndrome
Pendred's syndrome
Perez's sign
periarteritis
    p. nodosa
pericarditis
perinephritis
peritonitis
    meconium p.

pertussis
petechia
petit mal
Peutz-Jeghers syndrome
pharyngitis
    lymphonodular p.
    purulent p.
    streptococcal p.
    viral p.
phenomenon
    Rumpel-Leede p.
phenylketonuria
pheochromocytoma
Philip's glands
phobia
phocomelia
phonocardiography
phytobezoar
pica
Pierre Robin syndrome
pigeon toe
piknocytosis. See *pyknocytosis.*
pilitis. See *pyelitis.*
pilonephritis. See *pyelonephritis.*
pinealoma
pink disease
pink-eye
pinna
pinworm
pityriasis
PKU — phenylketonuria
placentitis
plague
pleurisy
pleurodynia
pneogaster
pneumatosis cystoides intestinalis
pneumococcus

Pneumocystis
    P. carinii
pneumomediastinum
pneumonia
    p. alba
    aspiration p.
    Kaufman's p.
    lobar p.
pneumonitis
pneumopericardium
pneumoperitoneum
pneumothorax
poisoning
    barbiturate p.
    lead p.
    petroleum distillate p.
    phenothiazine p.
    salicylate p.
    scopolamine p.
    strychnine p.
    thallium p.
polioencephalitis
    bulbar p.
poliomyelitis
polyarteritis
polyarthritis
polycythemia
    p. vera
polydactylia
polydactyly
polydipsia
polydysplasia
    hereditary ectodermal p.
polydysspondylism
polydystrophic
polydystrophy
    pseudo-Hurler p.
polyneuropathy
polyp
    inflammatory p.
    intestinal p.

polyp (*continued*)
    pedunculated juvenile p.
polyposis
    colonic p.
polyserositis
    idiopathic p.
Pompe's disease
porencephalia
porphyria
port wine mark
Potter's disease
precocity
premature
prematurity
prepubertal
progeria
projectile
pronate
prostration
proteinuria
    orthostatic p.
    postural p.
prothrombokinase
prurigo
pruritus
    p. ani
pseudocyst
pseudohermaphroditism
pseudohypoparathyroidism
pseudoleukemia
pseudomenstruation
Pseudomonas
    P. aeruginosa
pseudoparalysis
pseudotumor
    p. cerebri
psittacosis
psoriasis
psychosis
    symbiotic p.
PTA — plasma thromboplastin
    antecedent

pterygium
    p. coli
ptosis
pubarche
pubertas
    p. praecox
puberty
pubescent
Pudenz'
    reservoir
    shunt
pulse
    Corrigan's p.
puncture
    bone marrow p.
    cisternal p.
    lumbar p.
    pericardial p.
    subdural p.
purpura
    anaphylactoid p.
    p. fulminans
    p. hemorrhagica
    Schönlein-Henoch p.
    thrombocytopenic p.
    thrombotic p.
Pusey's emulsion
pustulosis
    p. vacciniformis acuta
pyelitis
pyelonephritis
pyknocytosis
pylorospasm
pyuria
Q fever
quarantine
rabies
ragadez. See *rhagades.*
rales
rating
    Apgar r.
Recklinghausen's disease

reflex
    grasp r.
    Grünfelder's r.
    Landau's r.
    Magnus and de Kleijn
      neck r's
    Moro embrace r.
    Moro's r.
    rooting r.
    sucking r.
reflux
    gastroesophageal r.
Refsum's disease
regurgitation
reservoir
    Pudenz' r.
respiration
    Bouchut's r.
    Kussmaul's r.
respirator
    negative pressure r.
respiratory
resuscitation
retardation
    mental r.
reticuloendotheliosis
retinitis
    r. pigmentosa
Reye's syndrome
rhagades
Rh incompatibility
rheumatic fever
rheumaticosis
rhinitis
Rhus
    R. diversiloba
    R. toxicodendron
    R. venenata
rickets
Rickettsia
rickettsiae
rickettsial

rickettsialpox
Riley-Day syndrome
Riley-Shwachman syndrome
ringworm
Ritter's disease
Rocky Mountain spotted fever
Romaña's sign
roomatikosis. See *rheumatico-*
    sis.
roseola
    r. infantum
Rothmund's syndrome
roundworm
Roussy-Lévy syndrome
RS virus
rubella
    r. scarlatinosa
rubeola
    r. scarlatinosa
Rubinstein-Taybi syndrome
rubor
Rud's syndrome
Rumpel-Leede phenomenon
rus. See *Rhus.*
Russell's syndrome
salicylism
salmonella
salmonellosis
Sanfilippo's syndrome
sarcoidosis
sarcoma
    embryonal s.
    Ewing s.
sarcosinemia
Saunders' disease
scabies
scaphocephaly
scarlatina
Scheie's syndrome
Scheuermann's disease
Scheuthauer-Marie-Sainton
    syndrome

Schick's
    sign
    test
Schilder's
    disease
    encephalitis
schizophrenia
Scholz's disease
Schönlein-Henoch purpura
scissoring
scleredema
    s. neonatorum
sclerema
    s. neonatorum
scleroderma
sclerosis
    tuberous s.
scoliosis
score
    Apgar s.
    Silverman's s.
scrofula
scurvy
    hemorrhagic s.
    infantile s.
seborrhea
sefalhematoma. See *cephal-*
    hematoma.
seizure
seminoma
sepsis
septal
septicemia
serum prothrombin conversion
    accelerator
sferositosis. See *spherocytosis.*
shigella
shigellosis
shock
    anaphylactic s.
    bacteremic s.

shock (*continued*)
    cardiogenic s.
    endotoxic s.
    hypovolemic s.
shunt
    LeVeen s.
    parietal s.
    Pudenz' s.
    ventricular atrial s.
    ventriculoperitoneal s.
shunting
    left-to-right ductus s.
SID — sudden infant death
SIDS — sudden infant death
    syndrome
sifilis. See *syphilis.*
sign
    Brudzinski's s.
    Comby's s.
    Gowers' s.
    Granger's s.
    Kernig's s.
    Macewen's s.
    Pastia's s.
    Perez's s.
    Romaña's s.
    Schick's s.
    Wreden's s.
sikosis. See *psychosis.*
silicosis
Silverman's score
Silver's syndrome
Similac
sinobronchitis
sinus
    pilonidal s.
sinusitis
sirronosus. See *cirrhonosus.*
sirrosis. See *cirrhosis.*
sitakosis. See *psittacosis.*
situs inversus

skafosefale. See *scaphocephaly.*
skizofrenea. See *schizophrenia.*
SLE — systemic lupus
    erythematosus
smallpox
soriasis. See *psoriasis.*
South African tick fever
spasm
spastic
spasticity
SPCA — serum prothrombin
    conversion acceler-
    ator
spherocytosis
spina
    s. bifida
spirillum
spirochetal
spirochete
splenic flexure
splenomegaly
spondylitis
    ankylosing s.
spongioblastoma
spot
    Brushfield's s's
    Koplik's s's
Sprengel's deformity
sprue
squint
St. Louis encephalitis
St. Vitus' dance
stafilokokkis. See *Staphylo-*
    coccus.
stammering
Staphylococcus
    S. aureus
starvation
status
    s. asthmaticus
    s. dysmyelinatus
    s. dysmyelinisatus

status (*continued*)
    s. epilepticus
steatorrhea
    idiopathic s.
stenosis
    anorectal s.
    antral s.
    aortic s.
    esophageal s.
    hypertrophic s.
    mitral s.
    postischemic s.
    pulmonic s.
    pyloric s.
    valvular pulmonic s.
Stensen's duct
Stevens-Johnson syndrome
Sticker's disease
Stilling-Türk-Duane syndrome
Still's
    disease
    murmur
Stock-Spielmeyer-Vogt
    syndrome
stomatitis
    herpetic s.
strabismus
strawberry mark
streptococci
streptococcus
    beta-hemolytic s.
Streptothrix
stricture
    esophageal s.
stridor
strophulus
Stuart-Prower factor deficiency
    disease
Sturge-Weber syndrome
stuttering
sty
sucking

sudo-. See words beginning
   pseudo-.
Sydenham's chorea
symptom
   Epstein's s.
syncope
syndactyly
syndrome
   Abderhalden-Fanconi s.
   Abt-Letterer-Siwe s.
   Adie's s.
   adrenogenital s.
   Albers-Schönberg's s.
   Albright's s.
   Aldrich's s.
   Alport's s.
   Andogsky's s.
   Arnold-Chiari s.
   asplenia s.
   Ballantyne-Runge s.
   Banti's s.
   Bartter's s.
   battered child s.
   Beckwith's s.
   blind loop s.
   Bloch-Sulzberger s.
   Bloom's s.
   Bonnevie-Ullrich s.
   Bourneville's s.
   Brachmann-de Lange s.
   Brandt's s.
   Caffey-Silverman s.
   Caffey-Smyth-Roske s.
   Calvé-Legg-Perthes s.
   Camurati-Engelmann s.
   Chapple's s.
   Charcot-Marie-Tooth-
     Hoffmann s.
   Chédiak-Higashi s.
   Chilaiditi's s.
   Christ-Siemens-Touraine
     s.
   Clarke-Hadfield s.

syndrome (*continued*)
   Cockayne's s.
   concussion s.
   Cornelia de Lange's s.
   cri-du-chat s.
   Crigler-Najjar s.
   cryptophthalmos s.
   Cushing's s.
   Dandy-Walker s.
   Darrow-Gamble s.
   de Lange's s.
   Dennie-Marfan s.
   De Sanctis–Cacchione s.
   de Toni-Fanconi-Debre s.
   Diamond-Blackfan s.
   diencephalic s.
   DiGeorge's s.
   Down's s.
   Dubin-Johnson s.
   Dubovitz's s.
   Ehlers-Danlos s.
   Ellis-van Creveld s.
   epiphyseal s.
   Erlacher-Blount s.
   Fanconi-Albertini-
     Zellweger s.
   Fanconi-Petrassi s.
   Fanconi's s.
   floppy infant s.
   focal dermal hypoplasia
     s.
   Franceschetti's s.
   Gardner's s.
   Gasser's s.
   Gilbert-Dreyfus' s.
   Gilbert-Lereboullet s.
   Gilles de la Tourette's s.
   Glanzmann's s.
   Goltz-Gorlin s.
   Goltz's s.
   Goodpasture's s.
   Hallermann-Streiff s.
   Hallervorden-Spatz s.

syndrome (*continued*)
- Hand-Schüller-Christian s.
- Hanhart's s.
- Hartnup's s.
- Hart's s.
- hemolytic-uremic s.
- hereditary benign intra-epithelial dyskeratosis s.
- Holt-Oram s.
- Hunter's s.
- Hurler's s.
- Hutchinson-Gilford s.
- Hutchinson's s.
- 17-hydroxylase deficiency s.
- hypoplastic left heart s.
- idiopathic respiratory distress s.
- inspissated milk s.
- Ivemark's s.
- Jansen's s.
- Joseph's s.
- Kartagener's s.
- Kasabach-Merritt s.
- Klinefelter's s.
- Klippel-Feil s.
- Kloepfer's s.
- Landry-Guillain-Barré s.
- Larsen's s.
- Launois' s.
- Laurence-Moon s.
- Laurence-Moon-Biedl s.
- Lennox's s.
- leopard s.
- Lightwood-Albright s.
- Lutembacher's s.
- malabsorption s.
- Marfan's s.
- Marie's s.
- Marinesco-Sjögren s.

syndrome (*continued*)
- Maroteaux-Lamy s.
- McCune-Albright s.
- meconium plug s.
- Melkersson-Rosenthal s.
- methionine malabsorption s.
- Minkowski-Chauffard s.
- Möbius' s.
- Morquio's s.
- Morquio-Ullrich s.
- multiple lentigines s.
- nephrotic s.
- Nettleship's s.
- Nezelof's s.
- Ollier's s.
- Osgood-Schlatter s.
- pancreatic insufficiency s.
- Patau's s.
- Pellizzi's s.
- Pendred's s.
- Peutz-Jeghers s.
- Pierre Robin s.
- placental dysfunction s.
- postperfusion s.
- Reye's s.
- Riley-Day s.
- Riley-Shwachman s.
- Rothmund's s.
- Roussy-Lévy s.
- Rubinstein-Taybi s.
- Rud's s.
- Russell's s.
- Sanfilippo's s.
- Scheie's s.
- Scheuthauer-Marie-Sainton s.
- Silver's s.
- slick-gut s.
- small left colon s.
- Stevens-Johnson s.

syndrome (*continued*)
    Stilling-Türk-Duane s.
    Stock-Spielmeyer-Vogt s.
    Sturge-Weber s.
    sudden infant death s.
    testicular feminizing s.
    Treacher Collins s.
    trisomy 13-15 s.
    trisomy 16-18 s.
    trisomy 18 s.
    trisomy 21 s.
    Turner's s.
    Vogt's s.
    Waardenburg's s.
    Weill-Marchesani s.
    Werdnig-Hoffmann s.
    Wiedemann's s.
    Willebrand-Jürgens s.
    Wilson-Mikity s.
    Wiskott-Aldrich s.
    Wolff-Parkinson-White s.
synostosis
    tribasilar s.
synovitis
syphilis
tabes
    hereditary t.
    t. infantum
    t. mesaraica
    t. mesenterica
tachycardia
    paroxysmal t.
tachypnea
taeniasis
takekardea. See *tachycardia.*
takipnea. See *tachypnea.*
talipes
    t. calcaneovalgus
    t. cavus
    t. equinovarus
tamponade
    cardiac t.

Tangier disease
tapeworm
Tay-Sachs disease
telangiectasia
teratoma
terijeum. See *pterygium.*
test. See also *Laboratory Terminology* section.
    Coombs' t.
    Farber's t.
    Frei t.
    Landau's t.
    Metopirone t.
    Ortolani's t.
    Schick's t.
    tine t.
testes
    undescended t.
testicle
testicular
tetanus
tetany
tetralogy
    t. of Fallot
thalassemia
thelarche
therapy
    aerosol t.
    hyperbaric oxygen t.
Thiemann's disease
Thomsen's disease
Thomson's disease
thoracentesis
thorax
thrombasthenia
thrombin
thrombocytopenia
    idiopathic t.
thrombosis
thrombus
thrush
thumbsucking

thyroid
thyroiditis
thyrotoxicosis
tic
tinea
    t. capitis
    t. corporis
    t. cruris
    t. versicolor
tissue factor
titer
    antistreptolysin t.
tonsillitis
    white t.
torticollis
torulosis
tosis. See *ptosis.*
Toxocara
toxocariasis
toxoid
Toxoplasma
toxoplasmosis
trachea
tracheostomy
tracheotomy
trachoma
transfusion
    exchange t.
transillumination
transposition
    t. of great vessels
Treacher Collins syndrome
tremulous
trichinosis
trichobezoar
trismus
    t. nascentium
    t. neonatorum
trisomy
tryptophanuria
tubercle
    Ghon t.

tuberculoma
tuberculosis
    t. papulonecrotica
tularemia
tumor
    Ewing's t.
    granulosa cell t.
    pineal t.
    pontine t.
    theca cell t.
    Wilms' t.
Turner's syndrome
tympanites
typhlitis
typhoid
typhus
    t. degenerativus am-
       stelodamensis
tyrosinosis
ulcer
    duodenal u.
    peptic u.
umbilical
umbilicus
Underwood's disease
Unverricht's disease
urachus
    patent u.
uremia
URI – upper respiratory infec-
       tion
urinalysis
urticaria
    u. pigmentosa
uveitis
vaccine
valve
    mitral v.
valvotomy
varicella
    v. gangrenosa
    v. inoculata

varicella (*continued*)
  pustular v.
  v. pustulosa
  vaccination v.
  v.-zoster immune globulin (VZIG)
varicelliform
varices
variola
varioliform
varix
vasospasm
venipuncture
ventricular septal defect
ventriculogram
ventriculography
vernix
  v. caseosa
verruca
  v. plana juvenilis
vertebra
  v. plana
virus
  Coxsackie v.
  ECHO v.
  Epstein-Barr v.
  herpes simplex v.
  RS v.
visceromegaly
vitiligo
VMA — vanillylmandelic acid
Vogt-Spielmeyer disease
Vogt's syndrome
Volkmann's
  deformity
  disease
volvulus
  gastric v.
  v. neonatorum
vomiting
  projectile v.

von Gierke's disease
von Hippel–Lindau disease
von Jaksch's anemia
von Recklinghausen's disease
VSD — ventricular septal defect
vulvovaginitis
VZIG — varicella-zoster immune globulin
Waardenburg's syndrome
Waldenström's macroglobulinemia
weaning
Weill-Marchesani syndrome
Weil's disease
Wenckebach heart block
Werdnig-Hoffmann
  paralysis
  syndrome
whipworm
whooping cough
Wiedemann's syndrome
Wilkins' disease
Willebrand-Jürgens syndrome
Wilms' tumor
Wilson-Mikity syndrome
Wilson's disease
Winckel's disease
Wiskott-Aldrich syndrome
Wolff-Parkinson-White syndrome
Wolman's disease
Wreden's sign
wryneck
xanthomatosis
xerophthalmia
zanthomatosis. See *xanthomatosis.*
zerofthalmea. See *xerophthalmia.*
zygodactyly

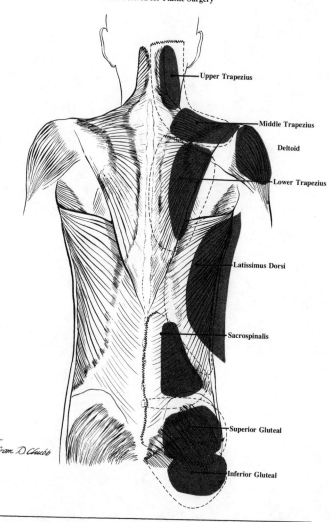

Secondary Myocutaneous and Cutaneous Areas
from Which Arterialized Flaps
Can Be Derived for Plastic Surgery

Upper Trapezius

Middle Trapezius

Deltoid

Lower Trapezius

Latissimus Dorsi

Sacrospinalis

Superior Gluteal

Inferior Gluteal

K. D. Barker
Adapted from D. Chubb

(Courtesy of Converse, J. M.: Reconstructive Plastic Surgery, 2nd ed.
Vol. I, Fig. 6-71, p. 220. Philadelphia, W. B. Saunders Company, 1977.)

PLASTIC SURGERY

Abbé-Estlander operation
Abbe's operation
Adams' operation
akinesia
> O'Brien a.
> Van Lint a.

ala
> a. nasi

alae
alanasi
alar
Alexander's operation
allograft
alloplasty
allotransplantation
allotriodontia
Allport's operation
Alsus-Knapp operation
alveolar
> a. arch
> a. ridge

alveololingual
alveolus
Alvis' operation
Ammon's operation
anaplasty
anaplerosis
anesthesia. See *General Surgical Terms*.
Angelucci's operation

angkilo-. See words beginning *ankylo-*.
angle
> cheilar a.
> conchal mastoid a.
> scaphoconchal a.

ankyloblepharon
ankylochilia
anthelix
Antia-Busch chondrocutaneous flap
antitragus
aperture
> pharyngeal a.

aponeurosis
arch
> palatine a.
> zygomatic a.

area
> Kiesselbach's a.

areolar
Argamaso-Lewin composite flap
Aries-Pitanguy mammaplasty
Arlt's operation
Asch's forceps
Ashley's breast prosthesis
ATL — antitension line
atrium
auricle

671

auricula
auricular
Austin's knife
autocystoplasty
autograft
autografting
Bakamjian flap
Baker's velum
bandage. See *General Surgical Terms.*
bar
    Erich's arch b.
    Passavant's b.
Bard-Parker blade
Barsky's
    elevator
    operation
Battle's operation
B-B graft
Beard-Cutler operation
Becker's operation
Bell's operation
Berke-Motais operation
Berke's operation
Bernard-Burrows operation
Biesenberger's operation
Binnie's operation
bistoury
    Brophy's b.
blade
    Bard-Parker b.
Blair-Brown
    graft
    knife
    operation
Blair's
    knife
    operation
    serrefine
Blaskovics' operation
blef-. See words beginning *bleph-.*

blepharal
blepharectomy
blepharelosis
blepharism
blepharitis
blepharoatheroma
blepharochalasis
blepharophryplasty
blepharoplasty
blepharoptosis
blepharorrhaphy
blepharostat
bone
    malar b.
    maxillary b.
    sesamoid b's
Boo-Chai craniofacial cleft
border
    mucocutaneous b.
    vermilion b.
Borges and Alexander line
bow
    Logan's b.
Brauer's operation
Braun's
    graft
    operation
Braun-Wangensteen
    graft
    operation
Brent's eyebrow reconstruction
bridge
Brophy's
    bistoury
    knife
    operation
    plate
Brown-Blair operation
Browne's needle
Brown's
    dermatome
    knife

Brown's (*continued*)
    operation
    splint
Bruner's line
B's graft
buccal
bulla
    b. ethmoidalis cava nasi
    b. ethmoidalis ossis eth-
        moidalis
bullae
bundle
    neurovascular b.
Bunnell's flap
Burow's operation
bursa
    pharyngeal b.
B-W graft
caliper
    Ladd's c.
Caltagirone's knife
canal
    pterygopalatine c.
canthus
    lateral c.
cartilage
    alar c.
    septal c.
    sesamoid c.
    vomeronasal c.
cartilaginous
caruncula
catheter
    Hickman c.
cauda
    c. helicis
cavum
    c. conchae
cephaloauricular angle
cephalocaudad
cervicoplasty
chalinoplasty

Charretera's flap
cheilectomy
cheilectropion
cheilitis
cheilognathoprosoposchisis
cheilognathoschisis
cheilognathouranoschisis
cheiloplasty
cheilorrhaphy
cheiloschisis
cheilostomatoplasty
cheiroplasty
chemosurgery
choana
choanae
Chopart's operation
chordee
ciliary
clamp
    Hunt's c.
cleft
    lip
    palate
clinoid process
columella
    c. cochleae
    c. nasi
columna
comminuted
comminution
concha
    c. auriculae
    c. sphenoidalis
conchae
conjunctiva
conjunctivoplasty
contracture
Converse's
    line
    operation
cosmesis
cosmetic

Cox's line
Crane's flap
craniofacial cleft
    Boo-Chai c.c.
    Karfik's c.c.
    Tessier's c.c.
Crawford's operation
cribriform
Crile's knife
crista
    c. galli
    c. nasalis maxillae
    c. nasalis ossis palatini
Cronin-Matthews eave flap
Cronin's operation
crura
    c. anthelicis
crus
    c. laterale
    c. mediale
cushion
    Passavant's c.
Cutler's operation
cymba
    c. conchae auriculae
Davis and Kitlowski operation
Davis'
    graft
    line
debridement
de Grandmont's operation
Demel and Ruttin operation
Denhardt-Dingman mouth gag
Denis-Browne needle
Denonvillier's operation
Derby's operation
dermabraded
dermabrader
    Iverson's d.
dermabrasion
dermanaplasty
dermatochalasis

dermatome
    Brown's d.
    Hall's d.
    Padgett's d.
    Reese's d.
dermatoplasty
dermolipectomy
Dieffenbach's operation
Dieffenbach-Warren operation
Dingman's
    elevator
    forceps
    osteotome
    retractor
Dorrance's operation
dorsum nasi
Dott's mouth gag
double lip
Douglas'
    graft
    operation
Dragstedt's
    graft
    operation
drain
    Penrose d.
dressing. See *General Surgical Terms.*
drugs. See *Drugs and Chemistry* section.
duct
    lacrimal d.
    nasolacrimal d.
Duke-Elder operation
Duplay's operation
Dupuy-Dutemps operation
durum
    palatine d.
Eckstein-Kleinschmidt operation
ectropion
Edgerton's line

Eitner's operation
electrocoagulation
elevator
      Barsky's e.
      Dingman's e.
      Freer's e.
      McIndoe's e.
      Veau's e.
ellipse
elliptical
Elschnig's operation
Ely's operation
eminence
      malar e.
eminentia
      e. conchae
      e. triangularis
entropion
epicanthus
epidermatoplasty
epispadias
Erich's
      arch bar
      operation
eschar
Esmarch's operation
esophagoplasty
Esser's
      graft
      operation
esthetic
Estlander's
      operation
ethmofrontal
ethmoid
ethmoidal
Everbusch's operation
facial
facioplasty
faringoplasty. See *pharyngo-*
      plasty.
farinjeal. See *pharyngeal.*

fascia
      f. lata femoris
fasciaplasty
fascioplasty
fauces
Fergus' operation
Fernandez' operation
filtrum. See *philtrum.*
fissura antitragohelicina
fissure
      antitragohelicine f.
      palpebral f.
fixation
      intermaxillary f.
flap
      Antia-Busch chondro-
        cutaneous f.
      Argamaso-Lewin f.
      artery island f.
      Bakamjian f.
      bilobed f.
      bipedicle f.
      Bunnell's f.
      Charretera's f.
      compound f.
      Crane's f.
      Cronin-Matthews eave f.
      delayed f.
      double pedicle f.
      French sliding f.
      Frickle's f.
      Gillies' up-and-down f.
      Hodgson-Tuksu tumble f.
      Hueston spiral f.
      Indian rotation f.
      island leg f.
      Italian distant f.
      jump abdominal f.
      MacFee neck f.
      marsupial f.
      McGregor's forehead f.
      Millard's island f.

flap (*continued*)
  Monks-Esser island f.
  Moore and Chong sandwich f.
  New's sickle f.
  over-and-out cheek f.
  skin f.
  Stein-Abbé lip f.
  Stein-Kazanjian lower lip f.
  Stenstrom foot f.
  Tagliacozzi's f.
  tumbler f.
  Wookey's neck f.
  Zimany's f.
  Zovickian's f.
fold
  salpingopalatine f.
  salpingopharyngeal f.
  semilunar f.
Fomon's operation
foramen
  greater palatine f.
  Scarpa's f.
foramina
  lesser palatine f.
forceps
  Asch's f.
  Dingman's f.
  Walsham's f.
fornix
  f. conjunctivae
  superior f.
fossa
  conchal f.
  hypophyseal f.
  Rosenmüller's f.
  scaphoid f.
  f. triangularis auriculae
Fox's operation
fracture
  blow-out f.

fracture (*continued*)
  comminuted f.
  nasomaxillary f.
  zygomaticomaxillary f.
Freer's elevator
French
  method
  sliding flap
frenulum
frenum labiorum
Fricke's operation
Frickle's flap
Friedenwald-Guyton operation
frontal
FSR — fusiform skin revision
furrow
  palpebral f.
Gabarro's
  graft
  operation
Gaillard's operation
ganglion
Gavello's operation
Gayet's operation
genioplasty
genitoplasty
genycheiloplasty
genyplasty
Gersuny's operation
Gibson-Stark and Kenedi line
Gifford's operation
Gigli's saw
Gillies-Dingman hook
Gillies'
  graft
  hook
  operation
  up-and-down flap
Gillies-Fry operation
Giralde's operation
gland
  meibomian g.

gland (*continued*)
    tarsal g.
glossoplasty
gnathodynia
gnathoplasty
gnathoschisis
graft
    B-B g.
    Blair-Brown g.
    bolus tie-over g.
    Braun's g.
    Braun-Wangensteen g.
    B's g.
    B-W g.
    chessboard g.
    Davis' g.
    Douglas' g.
    Dragstedt's g.
    Esser's g.
    fascia lata g.
    free g.
    full-thickness skin g.
    Gabarro's g.
    Gillies' g.
    Kebab's g.
    Konig's g.
    Ollier-Thiersch g.
    Padgett's g.
    patch g.
    pedicle g.
    pinch g.
    Reverdin's g.
    Seddon's nerve g.
    split-thickness skin g.
    stent g.
    Tanner-Vanderput g.
    Thiersch's g.
    Van Millingen's g.
    Wolfe-Krause g.
    Wolfe's g.
Grant's operation
Grimsdale's operation

groove
    sinus g.
gustatory
Guyton's operation
Hagedorn-LeMesurier
    operation
Hagedorn's operation
Hagerty's operation
Hall's dermatome
hamular
hamulus
harelip
Harman's operation
helix
hemisection
hemisphincter
    pharyngeal h.
Hess' operation
heterograft
hiatus
    h. semilunaris
Hickman catheter
Hodgson-Tuksu tumble flap
Holmes' operation
homeotransplant
homograft
homoplastic
homoplasty
hook
    Gillies-Dingman h.
    Gillies' h.
Hotchkiss' operation
Hotz' operation
Hueston spiral flap
Hughes' operation
Hunt's clamp
Hutchinson and Koop line
hyperpigmentation
hypognathous
hypospadias
Illiff's operation
immunosuppressive

implant
    Silastic i.
incision. See *General Surgical Terms*.
incisive
incisura
    i. intertragica
Indian
    method
    rotation flap
infraorbital
infratrochlear
infundibulum
    ethmoidal i.
injection
    Silastic i.
intercartilaginous
isograft
isthmus
    i. faucium
Italian
    distant flap
    method
Iverson's dermabrader
Jaesche's operation
jenekiloplaste. See *genycheiloplasty*.
jeneplaste. See *genyplasty*.
Johnson's operation
Jones' operation
Joseph's operation
Kanavel's line
Karfik's craniofacial cleft
Kazanjian and Converse line
Kazanjian's line
Kebab's graft
Keith's needle
keloid
keloplasty
Kiesselbach's
    area
    plexus

Kilner's operation
kilo-. See words beginning *cheilo-*.
kiroplaste. See *cheiroplasty*.
Kirschner's wire
Kitlowski's operation
knife
    Austin's k.
    Blair-Brown k.
    Blair's k.
    Brophy's k.
    Brown's k.
    Caltagirone's k.
    Crile's k.
    MacKenty's k.
    Virchow's k.
koana-. See *choana*.
Kocher's line
Kolle-Lexer operation
Konig's
    graft
    operation
Kowalzig's operation
Krause-Wolfe operation
Krimer's operation
Krönlein's operation
Kuhnt-Szymanowski operation
labial
    inferior l.
    superior l.
lacus
    l. lacrimalis
Ladd's caliper
Lagleyze's operation
lamina
    posterior l.
Lancaster's operation
Landolt's eyelid reconstruction
Langenbeck's operation
Langer's line
Larsen's syndrome
Latrobe's retractor

Lauren's operation
Leahey's operation
LeMesurier's operation
leukoplakia
Lewis' line
Lexer's operation
ligament
    medial palpebral l.
line
    Borges and Alexander l.
    Bruner's l.
    cleavage l.
    contour l.
    Converse's l.
    Cox's l.
    crease l.
    crinkle l.
    Davis' l.
    dependency l.
    division l.
    dominant l.
    dynamic facial l.
    Edgerton's l.
    elastic l.
    election l.
    expression folds l.
    flexion l.
    flexure l.
    force l.
    Gibson-Stark and Kenedi l.
    grain l.
    gravitational l.
    Hutchinson and Koop l.
    increased tension l.
    junction l.
    Kanavel's l.
    Kazanjian and Converse l.
    Kazanjian's l.
    Kocher's l.
    Langer's l.
    Lewis' l.

line (*continued*)
    maximal tension l.
    minimal tension l.
    minimum extensibility l.
    natural l.
    orthostatic l.
    relaxed skin tension l.
    Stark's l.
    tension l.
    Terry's l.
    Webster's l.
    wrinkle l.
lip
    cleft l.
lipectomy
lobule
lobulus
    l. auriculae
Logan's bow
Luckett's operation
MacFee neck flap
Machek's operation
MacKenty's knife
macrocheilia
macrostomia
macrostructural
macrotia
Magnus' operation
Malbec's operation
Malbran's operation
maloplasty
mammaplasty
    Aries-Pitanguy m.
    augmentation m.
mammoplasty
    augmentation m.
mandible
Marcks' operation
margin
    orbital m.
Martin's retractor
mastoid

mastopexy
mastoplasty
mastoptosis
maxilla
maxillae
    frontal processes of m.
maxillary
maxillectomy
McCash-Randall operation
McDowell's operation
McGregor's forehead flap
McIndoe's elevator
meatus
    acoustic m.
    inferior m.
    middle m.
    superior m.
medications. See *Drugs and Chemistry* section.
meloncus
meloplasty
membrane
    mucous m.
mental
mentalis
mentolabial
method
    French m.
    Indian m.
    Italian m.
    triangle m.
metopoplasty
micrognathia
micrognathism
microstomia
Millard's
    island flap
    operation
Minsky's operation
Mirault-Brown-Blair operation
Mirault's operation
Mladick ear reconstruction

Monks-Esser island flap
Monks' operation
Moore and Chong sandwich flap
Morestin's operation
Motais' operation
mouth gag
    Denhardt-Dingman m.g.
    Dott's m.g.
mucomembranous
mucoperichondrium
mucoperiosteal
mucoperiosteum
mucosa
    buccal m.
Mueller's operation
Mules' operation
Müller's muscle
muscle
    frontalis m.
    glossopalatine m.
    levator m. of palatine velum
    Müller's m.
    pharyngopalatine m.
    platysma m.
    Riolan's m.
    superior constrictor m.
    tarsal m.
    temporalis m.
musculi
    m. levator veli palatini
    m. temporoparietalis
    m. tensor veli palatini
musculus
    m. adductor pollicis
    m. extensor pollicis brevis
    m. extensor pollicis longus
    m. flexor pollicis brevis
    m. flexor pollicis longus

musculus (*continued*)
    m. levator palpebrae
      superioris
    m. orbicularis oculi
    m. pectoralis major
    m. pectoralis minor
    m. salpingopharyngeus
    m. uvulae
myoplasty
nares
naris
nasal
nasion
nasoantral
nasoantritis
nasociliary
nasofrontal
nasograph
nasolabial
nasolacrimal
naso-oral
nasopalatine
nasopharyngeal
nasorostral
nasoseptal
nasoturbinal
nasus
    n. externus
natho-. See words beginning
  gnatho-.
needle
    Browne's n.
    Denis-Browne n.
    Keith's n.
    Reverdin's n.
Nelaton's operation
neoplasty
New's sickle flap
nostril
notch
    intertragic n.
O'Brien akinesia

oculi
    orbicularis o.
olfactory
Ollier-Thiersch
    graft
    operation
Ombrédanne's operation
operation
    Abbé-Estlander o.
    Abbe's o.
    Adams' o.
    Alexander's o.
    Allport's o.
    Alsus-Knapp o.
    Alvis' o.
    Ammon's o.
    Angelucci's o.
    Arlt's o.
    Barsky's o.
    Battle's o.
    Beard-Cutler o.
    Becker's o.
    Bell's o.
    Berke-Motais o.
    Berke's o.
    Bernard-Burrows o.
    Biesenberger's o.
    Binnie's o.
    Blair-Brown o.
    Blair's o.
    Blaskovics' o.
    Brauer's o.
    Braun's o.
    Braun-Wangensteen o.
    Brophy's o.
    Brown-Blair o.
    Brown's o.
    Burow's o.
    Chopart's o.
    Converse's o.
    cosmetic o.
    Crawford's o.

operation (*continued*)
- Cronin's o.
- Cutler's o.
- Davis and Kitlowski o.
- de Grandmont's o.
- Demel and Ruttin o.
- Denonvillier's o.
- Derby's o.
- Dieffenbach's o.
- Dieffenbach-Warren o.
- Dorrance's o.
- Douglas' o.
- Dragstedt's o.
- Duke-Elder o.
- Duplay's o.
- Dupuy-Dutemps o.
- Eckstein-Kleinschmidt o.
- Eitner's o.
- Elschnig's o.
- Ely's o.
- Erich's o.
- Esmarch's o.
- Esser's o.
- Estlander's o.
- Everbusch's o.
- Fergus' o.
- Fernandez' o.
- Fomon's o.
- Fox's o.
- Fricke's o.
- Friedenwald-Guyton o.
- Gabarro's o.
- Gaillard's o.
- Gavello's o.
- Gayet's o.
- Gersuny's o.
- Gifford's o.
- Gillies' o.
- Gillies-Fry o.
- Giralde's o.
- Grant's o.
- Grimsdale's o.

operation (*continued*)
- Guyton's o.
- Hagedorn-LeMesurier o.
- Hagedorn's o.
- Hagerty's o.
- Harman's o.
- Hess' o.
- Holmes' o.
- Hotchkiss' o.
- Hotz' o.
- Hughes' o.
- Illiff's o.
- Jaesche's o.
- Johnson's o.
- Jones' o.
- Joseph's o.
- Kilner's o.
- Kitlowski's o.
- Kolle-Lexer o.
- Konig's o.
- Kowalzig's o.
- Krause-Wolfe o.
- Krimer's o.
- Krönlein's o.
- Kuhnt-Szymanowski o.
- Lagleyze's o.
- Lancaster's o.
- Langenbeck's o.
- Lauren's o.
- Leahey's o.
- LeMesurier's o.
- Lexer's o.
- Luckett's o.
- Machek's o.
- Magnus' o.
- Malbec's o.
- Malbran's o.
- Marcks' o.
- McCash-Randall o.
- McDowell's o.
- Millard's o.
- Minsky's o.

operation (*continued*)
- Mirault-Brown-Blair o.
- Mirault's o.
- Monks' o.
- Morestin's o.
- Motais' o.
- Mueller's o.
- Mules' o.
- Nelaton's o.
- Ollier-Thiersch o.
- Ombrédanne's o.
- Owens' o.
- Pagenstecher's o.
- Panas' o.
- Parkhill's o.
- Pfeifer's o.
- Pierce-O'Connor o.
- plastic o.
- Randall's o.
- Reese's o.
- Reverdin's o.
- Rosenburg's o.
- Rose's o.
- Savin's o.
- Sayoc's o.
- Schimek's o.
- Schuchardt-Pfeifer o.
- Sédillot's o.
- Serre's o.
- Simon's o.
- Smith's o.
- Snellen's o.
- Sourdille's o.
- Spaeth's o.
- Stallard's o.
- Stein's o.
- Straith's o.
- Swenson's o.
- Szymanowski's o.
- tagliacotian o.
- Tansley's o.
- Teale's o.

operation (*continued*)
- Tennison's o.
- Textor's o.
- Thiersch's o.
- Thompson's o.
- Trainor-Nida o.
- Tripier's o.
- Truc's o.
- Ulloa's o.
- Van Millingen's o.
- Veau-Axhausen o.
- Veau's o.
- Verhoeff's o.
- Verweys' o.
- Vogel's o.
- von Blaskovics-Doyen o.
- von Langenbeck's o.
- V-Y o.
- Wardill-Kilner o.
- Webster's o.
- Wheeler's o.
- Wicherkiewicz' o.
- Wiener's o.
- Wies' o.
- Wolfe's o.
- Wolff's o.
- Worth's o.
- Wright's o.
- W-Y o.
- Young's o.

orbicular
orbicularis oculi
orbital
osteoplastic
osteoplasty
osteoseptum
osteotome
- Dingman's o.

osteotomy
ostium maxillare
otoplasty
Owens' operation

Padgett's
    dermatome
    graft
Pagenstecher's operation
palatal
palate
    cleft p.
palatine
palatognathous
palatomaxillary
palatonasal
palatoplasty
palatum
    p. durum
    p. durum osseum
    p. fissum
    p. molle
    p. ogivale
    p. osseum
palpebra
palpebral
palpebralis
Panas' operation
Parkhill's operation
Passavant's
    bar
    cushion
peau d'orange
pectus
    p. excavatum
pedicle
pedunculated
Penrose drain
periosteum
Pfeifer's operation
pharyngeal
pharyngoplasty
philtrum
Pierce-O'Connor operation
pillar of fauces
piriform

plate
    Brophy's p.
    perpendicular p. of
        ethmoid
    tarsal p.
plexus
    Kiesselbach's p.
plica
    p. nasi
    p. semilunaris
po dorahnj. See *peau d'orange.*
polydactylism
ponticulus
    p. auriculae
position. See *General Surgical
    Terms.*
preauricular
procedure
    four-flap p.
    push-back p.
process
    hamular p.
    mastoid p.
    palatine p.
    sphenoidal p.
    uncinate p.
prognathism
prognathous
prosopoanoschisis
prosopodiplegia
prosopodysmorphia
prosoponeuralgia
prosopoplegia
prosopoplegic
prosoposchisis
prosopospasm
prosthesis
    Ashley's breast p.
pterygium
    p. colli
pterygoid

pterygomandibular
pterygomaxillary
pterygopalatine
ptosis
rafe. See *raphe.*
Randall's operation
raphe
    linear r.
    palatine r.
    palpebral r.
    pterygomandibular r.
reaction
    antigen-antibody r.
    immunity r.
reconstruction
    Brent's eyebrow r.
    Landolt's eyelid r.
    Mladick ear r.
    Steffanoff's ear r.
    Tagliacozzi's nasal r.
    Tanzer's auricle r.
    Wookey's pharyngo-
      esophageal r.
Reese's
    dermatome
    operation
repair
    Rose-Thompson r.
resection
    submucous r.
retractor
    Dingman's r.
    Latrobe's r.
    Martin's r.
    Senn-Dingman r.
    Sluder's r.
retrenchment
retroauricular
retrusion
Reverdin's
    graft
    needle

Reverdin's (*continued*)
    operation
revision
    W-plasty r.
    Z-plasty r.
rhinocheiloplasty
rhinokyphectomy
rhinokyphosis
rhinoplasty
rhytidectomy
rhytidoplasty
rhytidosis
rino-. See words beginning
    rhino-.
Riolan's muscle
Ritchie's tenaculum
ritidektome. See *rhytidectomy.*
ritido-. See words beginning
    rhytido-.
Rosenburg's operation
Rosenmüller's fossa
Rose's operation
Rose-Thompson repair
rostrum of sphenoid
RSTL — relaxed skin tension
    lines
ruga
    r. palatina
rugae
sac
    lacrimal s.
salpingopharyngeal
Savin's operation
saw
    Gigli's s.
Sayoc's operation
scapha
scarification
Scarpa's foramen
Schimek's operation
Schuchardt-Pfeifer operation
Seddon's nerve graft

Sédillot's operation
sefalo-. See words beginning
    cephalo-.
Senn-Dingman retractor
septal
septonasal
septoplasty
septotomy
septum
        deviated nasal s.
        s. mobile nasi
        nasal s.
        orbital s.
        tarsus orbital s.
sera
        antilymphocytic s.
serrefine
        Blair's s.
Serre's operation
sfeno-. See words beginning
    spheno-.
sfenoid. See sphenoid.
sfenoidal. See sphenoidal.
shelf
        palatal s.
Silastic
        implant
        injection
Simon's operation
sinus
        paranasal s.
skafa. See scapha.
Sluder's retractor
Smith's operation
Snellen's operation
Sourdille's operation
Spaeth's operation
sphenoethmoid
sphenoethmoidal
sphenofrontal
sphenoid
sphenoidal

sphenopalatine
sphincter oris
splint
        Brown's s.
        volar s.
Stallard's operation
staphylectomy
staphyloplasty
staphylorrhaphy
staphylotomy
Stark's line
Steffanoff's ear reconstruction
Stein-Abbé lip flap
Stein-Kazanjian lower lip flap
Stein's operation
Stenstrom foot flap
stomatoplasty
Straith's operation
submental
sulci
        gingivolabial s.
sulcus
        s. anthelicis transversus
        s. nasolabialis
        retroauricular s.
        tympanic s.
supra-auricular
surgical procedures. See
    operation.
suture. See General Surgical
    Terms.
Swenson's operation
syndrome
        Larsen's s.
        Treacher-Collins s.
Szymanowski's operation
tagliacotian operation
Tagliacozzi's
        flap
        nasal reconstruction
Tanner-Vanderput graft
Tansley's operation

Tanzer's auricle reconstruction
tarsal
tarsoplasty
tarsorrhaphy
tarsus
    t. inferior palpebrae
    t. superior palpebrae
Teale's operation
tectonic
temporal
temporomandibular
tenaculum
    Ritchie's t.
Tennison's operation
tenomyoplasty
tenoplastic
tenoplasty
terigo-. See words beginning
    pterygo-.
terigoid. See *pterygoid*.
terijeum. See *pterygium*.
Terry's line
Tessier's craniofacial cleft
Textor's operation
Thiersch's
    graft
    operation
Thompson's operation
tonsil
    palatine t.
    pharyngeal t.
torus
    t. frontalis
    t. levatorius
    t. mandibularis
    t. occipitalis
    t. palatinus
tosis. See *ptosis*.
tracheostomy
tragus
Trainor-Nida operation

transplant
    autogenous t.
    homogenous t.
transplantation
Treacher-Collins syndrome
Tripier's operation
Truc's operation
tube
    orotracheal t.
tunica
    t. conjunctiva palpe-
        brarum
turbinate
Ulloa's operation
unciform
uncinate
uraniscochasma
uraniscoplasty
uraniscorrhaphy
uranoplastic
uranoplasty
uranorrhaphy
uranoschisis
uranoschism
uranostaphyloplasty
uranostaphylorrhaphy
uranostaphyloschisis
uranosteoplasty
urethroplasty
uvula
    u. palatina
Van Lint akinesia
Van Millingen's
    graft
    operation
vault
    cartilaginous v.
Veau-Axhausen operation
Veau's
    elevator
    operation

velopharyngeal
velopharynx
velum
    Baker's v.
    palatine v.
Verhoeff's operation
vermilion
vermilionectomy
Verweys' operation
vestibule
Virchow's knife
Vogel's operation
vomer
vomeronasal
von Blaskovics-Doyen
   operation
von Langenbeck's operation
V-Y operation
Walsham's forceps
Wardill-Kilner operation
Webster's
    line
    operation
Wheeler's operation
Wicherkiewicz' operation
Wiener's operation
Wies' operation
wire
    interdental w.
    Kirschner's w.

Wolfe-Krause graft
Wolfe's
    graft
    operation
Wolff's operation
Wookey's
    neck flap
    pharyngoesophageal
     reconstruction
Worth's operation
W-plasty revision
Wright's operation
W-Y operation
xenograft
xenotransplantation
Young's operation
zeno-. See words beginning
    xeno-.
Zimany's flap
zoograft
zoografting
zooplasty
Zovickian's flap
Z-plasty revision
zygomatic
zygomaticofrontal
zygomaticomaxillary
zygomaticotemporal

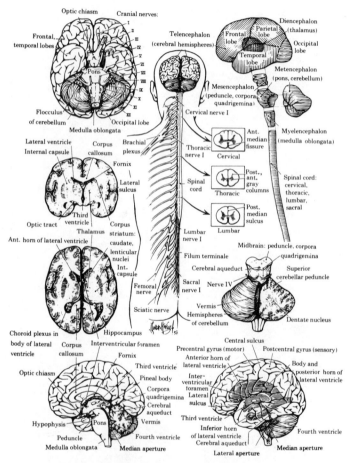

VARIOUS ASPECTS AND SECTIONS OF BRAIN AND SPINAL CORD

(Courtesy of Dorland's Illustrated Medical Dictionary, 26th ed. Plate IX. Philadelphia, W. B. Saunders Company, 1981.)

PSYCHIATRY, NEUROLOGY, AND NEUROSURGERY

AA — achievement age
    Alcoholics Anonymous
abalienated
abalienatio
    a. mentis
abalienation
abasia
    a. atactica
    choreic a.
    paralytic a.
    paroxysmal trepidant a.
    spastic a.
    trembling a.
    a. trepidans
abasic
abducens
abducent
aberration
ablutomania
abreaction
abscess
    Dubois' a.
absentia
    a. epileptica
abstinence
abulia
    cyclic a.
abulic

abulomania
acalculia
acarophobia
acatamathesia
acataphasia
accident prone
acervulus
acetylcholine
ACh — acetylcholine
Achilles tendon reflex
acousma
acousmatagnosis
acousmatamnesia
acrobrachycephaly
acrocephalosyndactylia
acrodynia
acromania
acroneuropathy
acroneurosis
acroparalysis
acroparesthesia
acrophobia
acting out
adaptation
addict
addiction
    polysurgical a.
addictologist

addictology
adenocarcinoma
adhesio
    a. interthalamica
adhesion
adiadochokinesia
adiadochokinesis
Adie's syndrome
adiposis
    a. cerebralis
    a. dolorosa
    a. orchalis
    a. orchica
    a. tuberosa simplex
adipositas
    a. cerebralis
adiposity
    cerebral a.
Adler's theory
adolescence
adolescent
adoyomanea. See *aidoiomania.*
adrenergic
Adson's
    bur
    cannula
    chisel
    clip
    conductor
    drill
    elevator
    forceps
    hook
    knife
    maneuver
    needle
    retractor
    scissors
    suction tube
adventitial

adventitious
adynamia
    a. episodica hereditaria
aero-asthenia
aerodromophobia
aeroneurosis
aerophagia
aerophagy
aerophobia
afazea. See *aphasia.*
afefobea. See *aphephobia.*
afemea. See *aphemia.*
affect
affection
affective
affectivity
affectomotor
affektepilepsie
afferent
afonea. See *aphonia.*
African meningitis
agenesia
    a. corticalis
agenesis
    callosal a.
aggression
agitated
agitation
agitographia
agitolalia
agitophasia
agnosia
agoraphobia
agrammatica
agrammatism
agrammatologia
agraphia
    absolute a.
    acoustic a.
    a. amnemonica

agraphia (*continued*)
    a. atactica
    cerebral a.
    jargon a.
    literal a.
    mental a.
    motor a.
    optic a.
    verbal a.
agraphic
agromania
agyria
ahmiel-. See words beginning
    amyel-.
ahmio-. See words beginning
    amyo-.
ahservulus. See *acervulus*.
aichmophobia
aidoiomania
ailurophilia
ailurophobia
AJ − ankle jerk
akatamathesia
akatanoesis
akathisia
akinesia
akinesis
akinesthesia
akinetic
akmofobea. See *aichmophobia*.
ala
    a. cerebelli
    a. cinerea
alalia
    a. cophica
    a. organica
    a. physiologica
    a. prolongata
alalic
alcoholic
alcoholism
alcoholomania

alcoholophilia
alexanderism
Alexander's operation
alexia
alexic
algophilia
algophily
algophobia
algopsychalia
alienation
alienism
alienist
allochiria
alteregoism
alurofilea. See *ailurophilia*.
alurofobea. See *ailurophobia*.
Alzheimer's
    dementia
    disease
    sclerosis
    syndrome
amathophobia
amaurosis
    a. centralis
    a. cerebral
amaxophobia
ambiguous
ambivalence
ambivalent
ambiversion
ambivert
amenomania
ament
amentia
    a. agitata
    a. attonita
    nevoid a.
    a. occulta
    a. paranoides
    phenylpyruvic a.
    Stearn's alcoholic a.
amential

amerisia
ametamorphosis
amimia
    amnesic a.
    ataxic a.
amine
Ammon's horn
amnemonic
amnesia
    anterograde a.
    auditory a.
    Broca's a.
    infantile a.
    lacunar a.
    localized a.
    olfactory a.
    patchy a.
    posthypnotic a.
    psychogenic a.
    retroactive a.
    retrograde a.
    tactile a.
amnesiac
amnesic
amnestic
amok
amoral
amoralia
amoralis
amphetamine
amychophobia
amyelia
amyelineuria
amyelotrophy
amygdala
    a. of cerebellum
amyostasia
amyostatic
amyosthenia
amyosthenic
amyotonia
    a. congenita

amyotrophia
    neuralgic a.
    a. spinalis progressiva
amyotrophic
amyotrophy
    diabetic a.
    neuralgic a.
anaclitic
analgesia
analysand
analysis
analysor
analytic
anamnesis
anamnestic
anancastic
anarithmia
anarthria
    a. literalis
Anders' disease
André-Thomas sign
anencephalia
anencephalic
anencephalohemia
anencephalous
anencephaly
anesthesia. See *General
    Surgical Terms.*
aneurysm
    arteriovenous a.
    berry a.
    cirsoid a.
    innominate a.
    intracranial a.
    miliary a.
    mycotic a.
    PICA a.
    racemose a.
aneurysmal
aneurysmectomy
angioblastoma
angiography

angioma
a. arteriale racemosum
a. cavernosum
cavernous a.
encephalic a.
a. venosum racemosum
angioneurosis
angioneurotic
angiospasm
angophrasia
angzietas. See *anxietas.*
anhedonia
anima
animus
anisocoria
anomia
anorexia
a. nervosa
anosmic
ansa
a. cervicalis
a. hypoglossi
a. of lenticular nucleus
a. lenticularis
a. subclavia
a. of Vieussens
ansae
a. nervorum spinalium
ansotomy
antianxiety
anticonvulsant
anticonvulsive
antidepressant
antihallucinatory
antiphlogistic
antisocial
antisocialism
anurizm. See *aneurysm.*
anxietas
a. presenilis
a. tibiarum

anxiety
free floating a.
apandria
apanthropia
apanthropy
apastia
apastic
apathetic
apathic
apathism
apathy
Apert's syndrome
aphasia
ageusic a.
amnemonic a.
amnesic a.
amnestic a.
anosmic a.
associative a.
Broca's a.
aphemia
aphephobia
aphonia
hysteric a.
a. paranoica
apicotomy
aplasia
a. axialis extracorticalis
congenita
apnea
apocarteresis
apophyseal
apophysis
cerebral a.
a. cerebri
genial a.
apoplexy
Broadbent's a.
cerebellar a.
cerebral a.
fulminating a.

apoplexy (*continued*)
    ingravescent a.
    meningeal a.
    pontile a.
    Raymond's a.
    thrombotic a.
apperception
apperceptive
appersonification
apractic
apraxia
    akinetic a.
    a. algera
    amnestic a.
    cortical a.
    ideational a.
    ideokinetic a.
    ideomotor a.
    innervation a.
    limb-kinetic a.
    motor a.
    sensory a.
    transcortical a.
apraxic
aprophoria
aprosexia
apselaphesia
apsithyria
apsychia
apsychosis
aqueduct
    cerebral a.
    a. of midbrain
    a. of Sylvius
    a. of vestibule
aqueductus
    a. cerebri
arachnitis
arachnoid
arachnoidea
    a. encephali
    a. spinalis

arachnoideae
arachnoiditis
arachnophobia
Aran-Duchenne
    disease
    muscular atrophy
Arantius
    ventricle of A.
arbor
    a. medullaris vermis
    a. vitae cerebelli
archipallial
archipallium
area
    Broca's a.
    Brodmann's a.
    Flechsig's a.
    Obersteiner-Redlich a.
    postcentral a.
    a. postpterygoidea
    a. postrema
    prefrontal a.
    premotor a.
    a. pterygoidea
    silent a.
    somatosensory a.
    vagus a.
    Wernicke's a.
areflexia
arhinencephalia
arithmomania
Arnold-Chiari
    deformity
    syndrome
arteriogram
arteriography
arteriosclerosis
artery
    basilar a.
    callosomarginal a.
    carotid a.
    cerebellar a.

artery (*continued*)
    cerebral a.
    choroidal a.
    communicating a.
    pericallosal a.
    vertebral a.
asaphia
asemasia
asemia
    a. graphica
    a. mimica
    a. verbalis
assaultive
association
astasia
    a. abasia
astatic
astereocognosy
astereognosis
asterixis
asthenia
asthenic
asthenophobia
astrapophobia
astrocyte
astrocytoma
astroglia
astroid
asynchronism
asynergia
asynergy
    appendicular a.
    axial a.
    axioappendicular a.
    truncal a.
ataractic
ataraxia
ataraxic
ataraxy
ataxia
    autonomic a.
    Briquet's a.

ataxia (*continued*)
    Broca's a.
    central a.
    cerebellar a.
    cerebral a.
    Fergusson and Critchley's
      a.
    Friedreich's a.
    frontal a.
    hereditary cerebellar a.
    hysteric a.
    intrapsychic a.
    kinetic a.
    labyrinthic a.
    Leyden's a.
    Marie's a.
    motor a.
    noothymopsychic a.
    Sanger-Brown's a.
    spinal a.
    spinocerebellar a.
    static a.
    a. telangiectasia
    thermal a.
    vasomotor a.
ataxiagram
ataxiagraph
ataxiamnesic
ataxiaphasia
atelencephalia
atelomyelia
athetoid
athetosis
atonia
atremia
atrophy
    Aran-Duchenne muscular
      a.
    Charcot-Marie-Tooth a.
    circumscribed a. of brain
    convolutional a.
    Cruveilhier's a.

atrophy (*continued*)
    degenerative a.
    Dejerine-Sottas a.
    denervated muscle a.
    Duchenne-Aran muscular
      a.
    Erb's a.
    facioscapulohumeral a.
    Fazio-Londe a.
    Hoffmann's a.
    Hunt's a.
    idiopathic muscular a.
    Landouzy-Dejerine a.
    lobar a.
    myelopathic muscular a.
    neural a.
    neuritic muscular a.
    neuropathic a.
    neurotic a.
    neurotrophic a.
    olivopontocerebellar a.
    Parrot's a. of the new-
      born
    peroneal a.
    Pick's convolutional a.
    pseudohypertrophic
      muscular a.
    spinoneural a.
    trophoneurotic a.
    Vulpian's a.
    Werdnig-Hoffmann a.
ATS — anxiety tension state
attack
    vasovagal a.
atypical
aula
aulatela
aulic
auliplexus
aura
autism
autistic

autocerebrospinal
autoerotic
autoeroticism
autoerotism
autognosis
autognostic
autokinesis
autokinetic
automatism
autonomic
autonomy
autopunition
autotopagnosia
aversive
awla. See *aula.*
awlatela. See *aulatela.*
awlepleksus. See *auliplexus.*
awlik. See *aulic.*
axon
Aztec idiocy
Baastrup's syndrome
Babcock's needle
Babès' tubercles
Babinski-Nageotte syndrome
Babinski's
    law
    phenomenon
    reflex
    sign
    syndrome
Bacon's forceps
Bailey's
    conductor
    leukotome
Balint's syndrome
Ballet's
    disease
    sign
ballismus
band
    Meckel's b.
Bane's forceps

Bárány's
    pointing test
    syndrome
barbiturate
Barré-Liéou syndrome
Barré's pyramidal sign
Barrett-Adson retractor
Barton-Cone tongs
Bärtschi-Rochain's syndrome
basicranial
basilar
basilaris
    b. cranii
basioccipital
basion
basophobia
basophobiac
Batten-Mayou disease
Beard's syndrome
Beckman-Adson retractor
Beckman-Eaton retractor
Beckman's retractor
Beck's syndrome
behavior
behaviorism
Bell-Magendie law
Bell's
    law
    mania
    nerve
    palsy
    phenomenon
Bender-Gestalt test
Berger rhythm
Bergeron's chorea
bestiality
bifrontal
Binswanger's
    dementia
    disease
biodynamics

Biot's respiraton
Birtcher's cautery
bisexual
bisexuality
bistoury
bitemporal
biventer
    b. cervicis
bizarre
Blackfan-Diamond syndrome
Blair's saw guide
blepharoptosis
block
    spinal subarachnoid b.
    stellate b.
    sympathetic b.
    ventricular b.
body
    pacchionian b's
    pineal b.
    Schmorl's b.
Bonhoeffer's symptom
Bonnet's syndrome
boopia
Bourneville's disease
brace
    Hudson's b.
brachial plexus
brachium
    b. cerebelli
    b. cerebri
    b. of colliculus
    b. conjunctivum
    b. copulativum
    b. of mesencephalon
    b. opticum
    b. pontis
    b. quadrigeminum
brachybasia
brachycephalic
brachycephaly

brachycranic
bradwemaw. See
   bredouillement.
bradylalia
bradylexia
bradylogia
bradyphasia
bradyphrasia
bradyphrenia
bradypsychia
bradyteleokinesis
Bragard's sign
Bragg peak
brain scan
Brain's reflex
Bravais-jacksonian epilepsy
bredouillement
bregma
Briquet's
   ataxia
   syndrome
Brissaud's reflex
Brissaud-Sicard syndrome
Bristowe's syndrome
Broadbent's apoplexy
Broca's
   amnesia
   aphasia
   area
   ataxia
   center
   convolution
   fissure
   gyrus
   space
Brodmann's area
Brown-Séquard syndrome
Brudzinski's sign
Bruns' syndrome
Brushfield-Wyatt disease
BSAP − brief short-action
   potential

Bucy-Frazier cannula
Bucy's
   knife
   retractor
bulbonuclear
bulbopontine
bulimia
bundle
   Helweg's b.
   Meynert's b.
bur
   Adson's b.
   D'Errico's b.
   Hudson's b.
   McKenzie's b.
Burdach's tract
CA − chronological age
cacergasia
cacesthenic
cacesthesia
cachinnation
cacodemonomania
cafard
Cairns' forceps
callomania
callosal
calvaria
calvarium
Campbell's elevator
camptocormia
camptocormy
canalicular
canaliculus
canalization
cannabis
cannabism
cannula
   Adson's c.
   Bucy-Frazier c.
   Cone's c.
   Cooper's c.
   Frazier's c.

cannula (*continued*)
    Haynes' c.
    Kanavel's c.
    Sachs' c.
    Scott's c.
    Seletz's c.
cannulation
Capgras's syndrome
captation
carcinophobia
carfol-. See words beginning
    carphol-.
carnal
carnophobia
carotid
carphologia
carphology
castration
CAT — computed axial
    tomography
catalepsy
cataleptic
cataleptiform
cataleptoid
cataphasia
cataphora
cataphoric
cataphrenia
cataplectic
cataplexie
    c. du reveil
cataplexis
cataplexy
catapophysis
catathymic
catatonia
catatonic
catatony
catecholamine
catharsis
cathectic

catheter
    red Robinson c.
cathexis
cathisophobia
CAT scan
cauda
    c. cerebelli
    c. equina
causalgia
cautery
    bipolar c.
    Birtcher's c.
    Mils' c.
cautionary
cavity
    Meckel's c.
cavum
    c. epidurale
    c. septi pellucidi
    c. subarachnoideale
    c. subdurale
    c. vergae
cell
    glitter c.
    Golgi c's
    Hortega's c.
    microglial c.
cella
    c. lateralis ventriculi
        lateralis
    c. media ventriculi
        lateralis
cell body
censor
    freudian c.
    psychic c.
center
    Broca's c.
    Setchenow's c's
centrencephalic
centriciput

centripetal
cephalalgia
cephalhematocele
　　　Stromeyer's c.
cephalhematoma
　　　c. deformans
cephalhydrocele
cephalic
cephalocentesis
cephalogyric
cephalomeningitis
cephalometry
cephalomotor
cephaloplegia
cephalorhachidian
cerebellar
cerebellifugal
cerebellipetal
cerebellitis
cerebellofugal
cerebello-olivary
cerebellopontile
cerebellopontine
cerebellorubral
cerebellorubrospinal
cerebellospinal
cerebellum
cerebral
cerebralgia
cerebrasthenia
cerebration
　　　unconscious c.
cerebriform
cerebrifugal
cerebripetal
cerebritis
　　　saturnine c.
cerebrocardiac
cerebrocentric
cerebrogalactose
cerebrohyphoid
cerebroid

cerebrol
cerebrolein
cerebrology
cerebroma
cerebromalacia
cerebromedullary
cerebromeningeal
cerebromeningitis
cerebrometer
cerebron
cerebro-ocular
cerebropathia
　　　c. psychica toxemica
cerebropathy
cerebrophysiology
cerebropontile
cerebropsychosis
cerebrorachidian
cerebrosclerosis
cerebroscope
cerebroscopy
cerebrose
cerebroside
cerebrosis
cerebrospinal
cerebrospinant
cerebrospinase
cerebrostimulin
cerebrostomy
cerebrotomy
cerebrotonia
cerebrovascular
cerebrum
ceroid
cervical plexus
Céstan-Chenais syndrome
Chaddock's
　　　reflex
　　　sign
Chandler's
　　　forceps
　　　retractor

Charcot-Marie-Tooth
    atrophy
    disease
Charcot's
    disease
    gait
chemopallidectomy
chemopallidothalamectomy
cheromania
Cherry-Kerrison forceps
Cherry's
    osteotome
    retractor
    tongs
Cheyne-Stokes psychosis
chiasma
chiasmatic
chisel
    Adson's c.
cholesteatoma
cholinergic
chondroma
chordotomy
chorea
    automatic c.
    Bergeron's c.
    button-makers' c.
    chronic c.
    c. cordis
    dancing c.
    diaphragmatic c.
    c. dimidiata
    Dubini's c.
    electric c.
    epidemic c.
    c. festinans
    fibrillary c.
    c. gravidarum
    habit c.
    hemilateral c.
    Henoch's c.
    hereditary c.

chorea (*continued*)
    Huntington's c.
    hyoscine c.
    hysterical c.
    imitative c.
    c. insaniens
    juvenile c.
    laryngeal c.
    limp c.
    local c.
    c. major
    malleatory c.
    maniacal c.
    methodic c.
    mimetic c.
    c. minor
    c. mollis
    Morvan's c.
    c. nocturna
    c. nutans
    one-sided c.
    paralytic c.
    posthemiplegic c.
    prehemiplegic c.
    procursive c.
    rhythmic c.
    rotary c.
    saltatory c.
    school-made c.
    Schrötter's c.
    c. scriptorum
    senile c.
    simple c.
    Sydenham's c.
    tetanoid c.
    tic c.
choreal
choreiform
choreoathetoid
choreoathetosis
choreoid
choreomania

choreophrasia
choriomeningitis
 lymphocytic c.
 pseudolymphocytic c.
choroid
choroidectomy
chromosomes
Chvostek's sign
cinerea
cingula
cingulectomy
cingulum
cingulumotomy
circle
 c. of Willis
circumstantiality
cistern
 cerebellomedullary c.
 c. of fossa of Sylvius
 c. of lateral fossa of
  cerebrum
 c. of Pecquet
 subarachnoidal c's
 c. of Sylvius
cisterna
 c. ambiens
 c. basalis
 c. cerebellomedullaris
 c. chiasmatica
 c. chiasmatis
 c. fossae lateralis cerebri
 c. fossae Sylvii
 c. intercruralis profunda
 c. interpeduncularis
 c. magna
 c. sulci lateralis
 c. Sylvii
 c. venae magnae cerebri
cisternae
 c. subarachnoidales
 c. subarachnoideales
cisternal

cisternography
 metrizamide c.
clairaudience
clairsentience
clairvoyance
clamp
 bulldog c.
 Crutchfield's c.
 Gandy's c.
 Salibi's c.
 Wertheim's c.
classification
 Kraepelin's c.
Claude's
 hyperkinesis sign
 syndrome
claudication
 intermittent c.
 venous c.
claustra
claustrophilia
claustrophobia
claustrum
clava
climacteric
clinoid
clip
 Adson's c.
 Cushing's c.
 Heifitz' c.
 Mayfield's c.
 McKenzie's c.
 Michel's c.
 Olivecrona's c.
 Raney's c.
 Schutz's c.
 Schwartz' c.
 Scoville-Lewis c.
 Scoville's c.
 Smith's c.
 Sugar's c.
 tantalum c.

clip (*continued*)
    Weck's c.
    Yasargil's c.
clivus
clonic
clonism
clonus
    ankle c.
Cloward-Hoen retractor
Cloward's
    drill
    operation
CNS — central nervous system
coagulator
    Malis' c.
cobalt-60
cocaine
coccyx
coconscious
coconsciousness
cognition
cognitive
cognizant
colliculus
    facial c.
collimator
column
    Gowers' c.
coma
comatose
commissura
    c. alba medulae spinalis
    c. anterior cerebri
    c. cerebelli
    c. habenularum
commissure
    Meynert's c.
commitment
commotio
    c. cerebri
    c. spinalis
compensation

complex
    castration c.
    Electra c.
    inferiority c.
    Oedipus c.
compression
compulsion
compulsive
computed tomography
conamen
conarium
conation
conative
concept
conception
conconscious
concretism
concussion
condensation
conditioning
conduction
    bone c.
conductor
    Adson's c.
    Bailey's c.
    Davis' c.
    Kanavel's c.
Cone's
    cannula
    needle
    retractor
confabulation
confidentiality
configuration
conflict
confluens
    c. sinuum
confusion
congenital
connector
    Rochester's c.
Conolly's system

conscience
conscious
consciousness
constellation
constitution
    ideo-obsessional c.
    psychopathic c.
content
    latent c.
Contour's retractor
contraction
    Gowers' c.
contrecoup
conus
    c. medullaris
conversion
convexobasia
convolution
    Broca's c.
    c's of cerebrum
    Heschl's c.
    occipitotemporal c.
    Zuckerkandl's c.
convulsant
convulsibility
convulsion
    choreic c.
    clonic c.
    coordinate c.
    epileptiform c.
    hysteroid c.
    mimetic c.
    mimic c.
    puerperal c.
    salaam c.
    static c.
    tetanic c.
    tonic c.
    uremic c.
convulsive
Cooper's cannula
coprolagnia

coprolalomania
coprophagia
coprophagy
coprophilia
coprophiliac
coprophobia
Corning's puncture
cornu
    c. anterius ventriculi
      lateralis
    c. inferius ventriculi
      lateralis
    c. medullae spinalis
corona
    c. radiata
corpora
    c. amylacea
    c. arenacea
    c. bigemina
    c. flava
    c. quadrigemina
    c. restiformis
corporeal
corpus
    c. amygdaloideum
    c. callosum
    c. fornicis
    c. medullare cerebelli
    c. medullare vermis
    c. nuclei caudati
    c. ossis sphenoidalis
    c. pineale
    c. pyramidale medullae
    c. rhomboidale
    c. striatum
    c. trapezoideum
correlation
cortex
    cerebral c.
cortical
corticectomy
cortices

corticoafferent
corticoautonomic
corticobulbar
corticocerebral
corticodiencephalic
corticoefferent
corticomesencephalic
corticopeduncular
corticopontine
corticospinal
corticothalamic
costotransversectomy
costovertebral
Cotard's syndrome
Cotte's operation
counterphobia
countertransference
Craig's scissors
Crane's mallet
cranial
cranialis
craniamphitomy
craniectomy
cranioacromial
cranioaural
craniocele
craniocerebral
craniomalacia
craniomeningocele
craniopharyngioma
cranioplasty
craniopuncture
craniorachischisis
cranioschisis
craniosclerosis
cranioscopy
craniospinal
craniostenosis
craniostosis
craniosynostosis
craniotabes
craniotome

craniotomy
craniotonoscopy
craniotopography
craniotympanic
cranitis
cranium
crescent
crescentic
cretin
cretinism
cretinistic
cretinoid
cretinous
cribriform
Crile's
    forceps
    knife
criminaloid
criminosis
crisis
    Lundvall's blood c.
crista
    c. galli
cross-tolerance
Crouzon's disease
crura
crus
    c. cerebelli ad pontem
    c. cerebri
crusta
Crutchfield-Raney tongs
Crutchfield's
    clamp
    drill
    tongs
Cruveilhier's atrophy
cryptomnesia
cryptomnesic
cryptoneurous
cryptopsychic
cryptopsychism
CSF — cerebrospinal fluid

CSM — cerebrospinal meningitis
CST — convulsive shock therapy
CT — computed tomography
CT scan
culmen monticuli
cuneate
cuneus
cunnilingus
curet
    Govons' c.
    Hibbs' c.
    Meyerding's c.
    Pratt's c.
    Raney's c.
    Volkman's c.
cushingoid
Cushing's
    clip
    depressor
    disease
    drill
    forceps
    law
    medulloblastoma
    reaction
    retractor
    spatula
    spoon
    syndrome
    tumor
CVA — cerebrovascular accident
CVOD — cerebrovascular obstructive disease
cybernetics
cyclothymia
cyclothymiac
cyclothymic
cyclothymosis
daler. See *délire.*

Dana's operation
dance
    St. Vitus' d.
Dandy's
    hemostat
    hook
    scissors
Dandy-Walker syndrome
Darkschewitsch's
    fibers
    nucleus
Davidoff's retractor
Davidson's retractor
Davis'
    conductor
    forceps
    retractor
    spatula
dazhah aproova. See *déjà éprouvé.*
dazhah fa. See *déjà fait.*
dazhah ontondoo. See *déjà entendu.*
dazhah ponsa. See *déjà pensé.*
dazhah rakonta. See *déjà raconté.*
dazhah vakoo. See *déjà vécu.*
dazhah voo. See *déjà vu.*
dazhah vooloo. See *déjà voulu.*
dazhanara. See *degénéré.*
decerebellation
decerebrate
decerebration
decerebrize
decision
    Durham's d.
declinator
declive
    d. monticuli cerebelli
decompression
    cerebral d.
    subtemporal d.

decortication
decursus
    d. fibrarum cerebralium
decussation
    Forel's d.
    fountain d. of Meynert
defecalgesiophobia
defense mechanism
deflection
deformity
    Arnold-Chiari d.
degeneration
    Holmes' d.
    wallerian d.
degénéré
degenitalize
dehumanization
déjà entendu
déjà éprouvé
déjà fait
déjà pensé
déjà raconté
déjà vécu
déjà voulu
déjà vu
dejection
Dejerine-Roussy syndrome
Dejerine's
    sign
    syndrome
Dejerine-Sottas atrophy
de la Camp's sign
delinquent
deliquium
    d. animi
délire
    d. de toucher
deliria
deliriant
delirifacient
delirious

delirium
    d. mussitans
    d. schizophrenoides
    d. sine delirio
    d. tremens
de lunatico inquirendo
delusion
delusional
dement
demented
dementia
    Alzheimer's d.
    Binswanger's d.
    epileptic d.
    d. myoclonica
    paralytic d.
    d. paralytica
    d. paranoides
    paretic d.
    d. praecox
    d. praesenilis
    d. pugilistica
    semantic d.
    senile d.
    terminal d.
    toxic d.
demonomania
demyelinate
dendrite
Dennie-Marfan syndrome
dependence
dependency
depersonalization
depraved
deprementia
depressant
depressed
depression
    agitated d.
    involutional d.
    pacchionian d's

depression (*continued*)
    postdormital d.
depressive
depressor
    Cushing's d.
deprivation
deranencephalia
Dercum's disease
dereism
dereistic
derencephalocele
D'Errico-Adson retractor
D'Errico's
    bur
    drill
    forceps
    retractor
De Sanctis-Cacchione
    syndrome
desensitization
deterioration
determinism
    psychic d.
Devic's syndrome
DeVilbiss'
    forceps
    rongeur
    trephine
diachesis
diadochokinesia
diadochokinesis
diadochokinetic
diakesis. See *diachesis*.
diaphragma
    d. sellae
diastematocrania
diastematomyelia
diatela
diaterma
dichotomy
diencephalic
diencephalohypophysial

diencephalon
dilemma
Dimitri's disease
dinomania
diocoele
diplegia
    atonic-astatic d.
    spastic d.
diploë
diplopia
diplopiaphobia
dipsomania
dipsopathy
dipsosis
dis-. See also words beginning
    dys-.
disc. See *disk*.
disciplinary
disease
    Alzheimer's d.
    Anders' d.
    Aran-Duchenne d.
    Ballet's d.
    Batten-Mayou d.
    Binswanger's d.
    Bourneville's d.
    Brushfield-Wyatt d.
    Charcot-Marie-Tooth d.
    Charcot's d.
    Crouzon's d.
    Cushing's d.
    Dercum's d.
    Dimitri's d.
    Down's d.
    Dubini's d.
    Dubois' d.
    Duchenne-Aran d.
    Duchenne's d.
    Economo's d.
    Erb-Charcot d.
    Erb-Goldflam d.
    Erb-Landouzy d.

disease (*continued*)
Erb's d.
Frankl-Hochwart's d.
Friedreich's d.
Fürstner's d.
Gerlier's d.
Gilles de la Tourette's d.
Goldflam's d.
Gowers' d.
Huntington's d.
Hunt's d.
Janet's d.
Kalischer's d.
Koshevnikoff's d.
Krabbe's d.
Lasègue's d.
Little's d.
Merzbacher-Pelizaeus d.
Mills' d.
Morel-Kraepelin d.
Niemann-Pick d.
Parkinson's d.
Pick's d.
Rendu-Osler-Weber d.
Romberg's d.
Roth-Bernhardt d.
Roth's d.
Schilder's d.
Schmorl's d.
Scholz's d.
Simmonds' d.
Spielmeyer-Vogt d.
Steiner's d.
Sturge's d.
Sturge-Weber-Dimitri d.
Tay-Sachs d.
Thomsen's d.
Tourette's d.
Unverricht's d.
Vogt's d.
von Hippel-Lindau d.
von Recklinghausen's d.

disease (*continued*)
Weber's d.
Wernicke's d.
Winkelman's d.
Ziehen-Oppenheim d.
disfajea. See dysphagia.
disfazea. See dysphasia.
disfemia. See dysphemia.
disfonia. See dysphonia.
disfor-. See words beginning
dysphor-.
disfrasia. See dysphrasia.
disfrenia. See dysphrenia.
disk
intervertebral d.
diskectomy
diskogram
disorder
affective d.
anxiety d.
bipolar d.
conversion d.
cyclothymic d.
dissociative d.
dysthymic d.
obsessive-compulsive d.
panic d.
paranoid d.
personality d.
psychosexual d.
schizophrenic d.
somatoform d.
disorientation
displacement
dissector
Hurd's d.
Oldberg's d.
Sheldon-Pudenz' d.
dissociation
distaxia
cerebral d.
distortion

distractibility
disvolution
divagation
DNA — deoxyribonucleic acid
dolichocephalic
dolichocephalism
domatophobia
dominance
Down's
    disease
    syndrome
dramatism
dramatization
drapetomania
dream
    clairvoyant d.
    d. interpretation
    veridical d.
dressing. See *General Surgical Terms.*
drill
    Adson's d.
    Cloward's d.
    Crutchfield's d.
    Cushing's d.
    D'Errico's d.
    Hall's d.
    Hudson's d.
    McKenzie's d.
    Raney's d.
    Stille's d.
dromomania
dromophobia
drugs. See *Drugs and Chemistry* section.
DT — delirium tremens
DTP — distal tingling on percussion
DTR — deep tendon reflex
Dubini's
    chorea
    disease

Dubois'
    abscess
    disease
    method
Duchenne-Aran
    disease
    muscular atrophy
Duchenne-Erb paralysis
Duchenne's disease
ductus
    d. perilymphatici
Duncan's ventricle
dura
dural
dura mater
    d. m. of brain
    d. m. encephali
    d. m. of spinal cord
    d. m. spinalis
duramatral
duraplasty
durematoma
Durham's decision
duroarachnitis
durosarcoma
dysarthria
    d. literalis
    d. syllabaris spasmodica
dysarthric
dysautonomia
dysbasia
    d. angiosclerotica
    d. angiospastica
    d. intermittens angiosclerotica
    d. lordotica progressiva
    d. neurasthenica intermittens
dysbulia
dysbulic
dyscalculia
dyscephaly

dyschiria
dysdiadochokinesia
dysergasia
dysergastic
dysergia
dysesthesia
dysgraphia
dyskinesia
    d. algera
dyskinetic
dyslalia
dyslexia
dyslogia
dysmetria
dysnomia
dyspareunia
dysphagia
dysphasia
dysphemia
dysphonia
dysphoretic
dysphoria
dysphoriant
dysphoric
dysphrasia
dysphrenia
dyspraxia
dysrhythmia
dyssocial
dyssymbolia
dyssymboly
dyssynergia
    d. cerebellaris myo-
      clonica
    d. cerebellaris progressiva
dystaxia
    d. agitans
dystectia
dysthymia
dysthymic

dystonia
    d. musculorum de-
      formans
dystrophia
    d. myotonica
dystrophoneurosis
dystrophy
    Erb's d.
    Landouzy-Dejerine d.
    muscular d.
    thyroneural d.
dystropic
dystropy
Ebbinghaus' test
eccentric
ecchordosis physaliphora
ecdemomania
echoencephalography
echogram
echographia
echokinesis
echolalia
echolalus
echomimia
echomotism
echopathy
echophrasia
echopraxia
echopraxis
eclampsia
eclysis
ecmnesia
ecomania
Economo's disease
ecophobia
ecphoria
ecphorize
ecphory
ECT — electroconvulsive
    therapy

ectocinerea
edema
    Huguenin's e.
edipism
edipus. See Oedipus.
EEE — eastern equine en-
    cephalomyelitis
EEG — electroencephalogram
efferent
ego
egocentric
egodystonic
egomania
egosyntonic
egotistical
egotropic
eidetic
ejaculation
    premature e.
eko-. See words beginning
    echo-.
elaboration
elation
Electra complex
electroconvulsive
electrocorticography
electroencephalogram
electroencephalograph
electroencephalography
electroencephaloscope
electromyogram
electromyography
electronarcosis
electroneuromyography
electroplexy
electroshock
electrospectrography
electrospinogram
electrostimulation
elevator
    Adson's e.
    Campbell's e.

elevator (*continued*)
    Frazier's c.
    Freer's e.
    Hajek-Ballenger e.
    Hibbs' e.
    Killian's e.
    Langenbeck's e.
    Love-Adson e.
    Rochester's e.
    Woodson's e.
ellipsis
emasculate
emasculation
embolism
    cerebral e.
embolalia
embolus
EMG — electromyogram
EMI — Electric and Musical
    Industries (brain
    scanner)
EMI scan
emotion
emotional
empathize
empathy
emprosthotonos
encephalalgia
encephalatrophy
encephalemia
encephalic
encephalitis
encephaloarteriography
encephalocele
encephalocoele
encephalocystocele
encephalogram
encephalolith
encephaloma
encephalomalacia
encephalomeningitis
encephalomeningocele

encephalomeningopathy
encephalomyelitis
encephalomyelocele
encephalomyeloneuropathy
encephalomyelopathy
encephalomyeloradiculitis
encephalomyeloradiculo-
    neuritis
encephalomyeloradiculopathy
encephalomyocarditis
encephalon
encephalonarcosis
encephalopathia
        e. alcoholica
encephalopathy
        Wernicke's e.
encephalophyma
encephalopsy
encephalopsychosis
encephalopuncture
encephalopyosis
encephaloradiculitis
encephalorrhagia
encephalosclerosis
encephaloscope
encephaloscopy
encephalosepsis
encephalosis
encephalospinal
encephalothlipsis
encephalotome
encephalotomy
encopresis
endarterectomy
endarteritis
endocrinasthenia
endomorph
endomorphic
endomorphy
endothelioma
        dural e.
engram

enomania
enosimania
ensef-. See words beginning
    enceph-.
entropy
enuresis
environment
EOM — extraocular movements
epencephalic
epencephalon
ependopathy
ependyma
ependymal
ependymitis
ependymoblast
ependymoblastoma
ependymocyte
ependymocytoma
ependymoma
ependymopathy
epicoele
epidemiology
epidermoid
epidermoidoma
epidural
epilepsia
        e. gravior
        e. major
        e. minor
        e. mitior
        e. nutans
        e. partialis continua
        e. procursiva
        e. rotatoria
        e. tarda
epilepsy
        abdominal e.
        Bravais-jacksonian e.
        cortical e.
        cryptogenic e.
        diurnal e.
        focal e.

epilepsy (*continued*)
    grand mal e.
    hysterical e.
    idiopathic e.
    jacksonian e.
    larval e.
    latent e.
    matutinal e.
    menstrual e.
    musicogenic e.
    myoclonus e.
    nocturnal e.
    petit mal e.
    physiologic e.
    procursive e.
    psychic e.
    psychomotor e.
    reflex e.
    rolandic e.
    sensory e.
    serial e.
    symptomatic e.
    tardy e.
    tonic e.
    traumatic e.
    uncinate e.
epileptic
    e. equivalent
    e. seizure
epileptiform
epileptogenic
epileptogenous
epileptoid
epileptologist
epileptology
epileptosis
epiloia
episode
    psycholeptic e.
episthotonos
epithalamus

epithelioma
    e. myxomatodes psam-
        mosum
epithelium
    mesenchymal e.
Erb-Charcot disease
Erb-Goldflam disease
Erb-Landouzy disease
Erb's
    atrophy
    disease
    dystrophy
    sclerosis
    syndrome
eremophobia
erethism
erethisophrenia
erethistic
erethitic
ergasia
ergasiatrics
ergasiatry
ergasiology
ergasiomania
ergasiophobia
ergasthenia
ergomania
ergomaniac
ergometer
erithredema. See *erythredema.*
erithro-. See words beginning
    erythro-.
erogenous
erotic
eroticism
eroticomania
erotism
    anal e.
    muscle e.
    oral e.
erotogenesis

erotogenic
erotographomania
erotomania
erotomaniac
erotopath
erotopathy
erotophobia
erotopsychic
erotosexual
erratic
erythredema polyneuropathy
erythromelalgia
erythrophobia
eschar
    neuropathic e.
ESP — extrasensory perception
EST — electroshock therapy
estheticokinetic
eunoia
euphoretic
euphoria
euphoriant
euphoric
euphorigenic
excitability
excitable
excitation
excitomotor
exencephalia
exhibitionism
exhilarant
existential
existentialism
exteroceptive
exterofection
exterofective
extradural
extrapsychic
extrapyramidal
extraversion

extrovert
facetectomy
facies
    Parkinson's f.
factitious
Fajersztajn's sign
falik. See *phallic.*
falx
    f. cerebelli
    f. cerebri
fan-. See words beginning
    phan-.
Fañana
    glia of F.
fantasy. See *phantasy.*
fascia
    dentate f.
fasciculation
fasciculus
    f. aberrans of Monokow
    f. cuneatus
    f. of Foville
    f. of Gowers
    f. gracilis
    f. lenticularis
    f. of Rolando
fastigium
Fazio-Londe atrophy
feeblemindedness
fellatio
felo-de-se
fenil-. See words beginning
    phenyl-.
fenomenon. See *phenomenon.*
fenotype. See *phenotype.*
Ferguson's forceps
Fergusson and Critchley's
    ataxia
Ferris-Smith forceps
fetish

fetishism
fiber
        Darkschewitsch's f's
fibrae
     f. arcuatae cerebri
     f. arcuatae externae
     f. arcuatae internae
     f. cerebello-olivares
     f. corticonucleares
     f. corticospinales
     f. pyramidales medullae
fibroblastoma
    meningeal f.
fibroma
fibrosarcoma
figure
    fortification f's
fila
    f. olfactoria
    f. radicularia nervorum
      spinalium
filum
    f. durae matris spinalis
    f. of spinal dura mater
    f. terminale
fissure
    Broca's f.
    calcarine f.
    dentate f.
    Pansch's f.
    f. of Sylvius
fistula
fixation
    freudian f.
fizeo-. See words beginning
   physio-.
flagellantism
Flatau's law
Flechsig's area
flegmatik. See *phlegmatic.*
flexibilitas
    f. cerea

flight
    f. of ideas
floccillation
flocculus
fluid
    cerebrospinal f.
    xanthochromic f.
fobia. See *phobia.*
fobic. See *phobic.*
fobofobia. See *phobophobia.*
Foix-Alajouanine syndrome
fold
    Veraguth's f.
folee. See *folie.*
folia cerebelli
folie
    f. à deux
    f. circulaire
    f. du doute
    f. du pourquoi
    f. gemellaire
    f. musculaire
    f. raisonnante
folium
    f. cacuminis
    f. vermis
fontanel
fontanelle
foramen
    f. caecum medullae
      oblongatae
    f. cecum ossis frontalis
    interventricular f.
    Luschka's f.
    Magendie's f.
    f. magnum
    f. of Monro
    f. occipitale magnum
    f. ovale ossis sphenoidalis
    f. rotundum ossis
      sphenoidalis
    f. spinosum

foramina
foraminotomy
forceps
    Adson's f.
    Bacon's f.
    Bane's f.
    bayonet f.
    Cairns' f.
    Chandler's f.
    Cherry-Kerrison f.
    Crile's f.
    Cushing's f.
    Davis' f.
    D'Errico's f.
    DeVilbiss' f.
    Ferguson's f.
    Ferris-Smith f.
    Gerald's f.
    Gruenwald's f.
    Hudson's f.
    Hurd's f.
    Leksell's f.
    Lewin's f.
    Love-Gruenwald f.
    Love-Kerrison f.
    Luer's f.
    McKenzie's f.
    Oldberg's f.
    Raney's f.
    Ruskin's f.
    Schlesinger's f.
    Schutz's f.
    Scoville's f.
    Sewall's f.
    Smithwick's f.
    Spence-Adson f.
    Spence's f.
    Spurling's f.
    Stevenson's f.
    Stille-Liston f.
    Stille-Luer f.

forceps (*continued*)
    Sweet's f.
    Wilde's f.
forebrain
foreconscious
Forel's decussation
forensic
formatio
    f. alba
    f. grisea
    f. reticularis pontis
    f. vermicularis
formication
fornix
    f. cerebri
Förster-Penfield operation
fossa
    cerebellar f.
    cerebral f.
    cranial f.
    f. cranii anterior
    f. cranii media
    f. cranii posterior
    posterior f.
Fothergill's neuralgia
fovea
Foville
    fasciculus of F.
Foville's
    syndrome
    tract
frame
    Stryker's f.
Francke's striae
Frankl-Hochwart's disease
Frazier-Spiller operation
Frazier's
    cannula
    elevator
    hook
    retractor

Frazier's (*continued*)
    suction tube
free association
Freer's elevator
fren-. See words beginning
    phren-.
French s-shaped retractor
frenetic
freno-. See words beginning
    phreno-.
frenzy
freudian
Freud's
    cathartic method
    theory
Friderichsen-Waterhouse syndrome
Friedmann's vasomotor syndrome
Friedreich's
    ataxia
    disease
    tabes
frigidity
Fröhlich's syndrome
Froin's syndrome
frons
    f. cranii
frontal
fronto-occipital
frontotemporal
frustration
fugue
    epileptic f.
    psychogenic f.
functional
fundus
funduscope
funicular
funiculitis
funiculus
    f. cuneatus

funiculus (*continued*)
    f. cuneatus medullae
      oblongatae
    f. gracilis medullae
      oblongatae
    f. medullae spinalis
    f. solitarius
    f. teres
    f. ventralis
furibund
furor
    f. epilepticus
furrow
Fürstner's disease
gait
    ataxic g.
    cerebellar g.
    Charcot's g.
    double-step g.
    drag-to g.
    equine g.
    festinating g.
    Oppenheim's g.
    scissor g.
    staggering g.
    steppage g.
    swing-to g.
    tabetic g.
galea
    g. aponeurotica
    tendinous g.
Galt's trephine
galvanism
galvanopalpation
gamophobia
Gandy's clamp
ganglia
ganglion
    gasserian g.
    Meckel's g.
    trigeminal g.
ganglionectomy

ganglioneure
ganglioneuroblastoma
ganglioneuroma
gangliosympathectomy
Ganser's
    symptom
    syndrome
Garcin's syndrome
Gardner's
    needle
    operation
gargoylism
gegenhalten
gelasmus
Gélineau's syndrome
Gelpi's retractor
gene
genetic
geniculate
geniculum
genotype
genu
    g. corporis callosi
    g. nervi facialis
geophagia
geophagist
gephyrophobia
Gerald's forceps
geriatric
geriatrics
geriopsychosis
Gerlier's disease
Gerstmann's syndrome
gestaltism
Gestalt theory
Gifford's retractor
Gigli's saw
Gilles de la Tourette's
    disease
    syndrome
Gill's operation
glabella

gland
    pituitary g.
glia
    cytoplasmic g.
    g. of Fañana
    fibrillary g.
glial
glioblast
glioblastoma
    g. multiforme
gliocytoma
gliofibrillary
gliogenous
glioma
    astrocytic g.
    ependymal g.
    ganglionic g.
    g. multiforme
    g. sarcomatosum
gliomatosis
gliomatous
gliomyoma
gliomyxoma
glioneuroma
gliophagia
gliopil
gliosa
gliosarcoma
gliosis
    basilar g.
    cerebellar g.
    diffuse g.
    hemispheric g.
    hypertrophic nodular g.
    isomorphic g.
    lobar g.
    perivascular g.
    spinal g.
    unilateral g.
gliosome
globus
    g. hystericus

glossolalia
glycorrhachia
Goldflam's disease
Golgi cells
Goll's tract
gouge
    Hibbs' g.
    Meyerding's g.
Govons' curet
Gowers
    fasciculus of G.
Gowers'
    column
    contraction
    disease
    sign
    syndrome
    tract
Gradenigo's syndrome
Graham's hook
grandiosity
grand mal
graphesthesia
gratification
"gray matter"
Gruenwald's forceps
GSR — galvanic skin response
guard
    Sachs' g.
guide
    Blair's saw g.
Guillain-Barré syndrome
gumma
gustatory
gyri
    g. annectentes
    g. breves insulae
    g. cerebri
    g. insulae
    g. occipitales
    g. operti
    g. orbitales

gyri (*continued*)
    g. profundi cerebri
    g. transitivi cerebri
gyrus
    g. angularis
    Broca's g.
    g. callosus
    cingulate g.
    g. cinguli
    dentate g.
    g. dentatus
    g. fasciolaris
    g. fornicatus
    fusiform g.
    g. fusiformis
    hippocampal g.
    g. hippocampi
    g. infracalcarinus
    g. limbicus
    g. lingualis
    marginal g.
    g. marginalis
    g. olfactorius
    g. parahippocampalis
    g. paraterminalis
    g. precentralis
    g. rectus
    g. temporalis
    g. uncinatus
habenula
habitual
habituation
habromania
Haenel's symptom
Hajek-Ballenger elevator
Hallervorden-Spatz syndrome
Hall's
    drill
    neurotome
hallucination
    auditory h.
    depressive h.

hallucination (*continued*)
    gustatory h.
    haptic h.
    hypnagogic h.
    lilliputian h.
    olfactory h.
    reflex h.
    stump h.
    tactile h.
    visual h.
hallucinative
hallucinatory
hallucinogen
hallucinogenesis
hallucinogenetic
hallucinogenic
hallucinosis
hallucinotic
Halstead-Reitan test
hamartoma
Hamby's retractor
Harris' migrainous neuralgia
haut-mal
Haynes'
    cannula
    operation
headrest
    Light-Veley h.
hebephrenia
hebephreniac
hebetude
heboid
heboidophrenia
hedonia
hedonic
hedonism
hedonophobia
Heifitz' clip
Helweg's
    bundle
    tract
hemangioblastoma

hemangioendothelioma
hemangioma
hemangiomatosis
hemangiosarcoma
hematoma
    subdural h.
hematomyelia
hemianencephaly
hemianesthesia
hemianopia
hemiballismus
hemicraniectomy
hemihypesthesia
hemihypoplasia
hemilaminectomy
hemiparesis
hemiplegia
hemisection
hemisphere
    cerebellar h.
    cerebral h.
hemispherectomy
hemispherium
    h. cerebelli
hemorrhage
hemostat
    Dandy's h.
    Kolodny's h.
Henoch's chorea
hereditary
heredity
heredoataxia
hermaphrodite
herniation
    h. of intervertebral disk
    h. of nucleus pulposus
    tonsillar h.
    transtentorial h.
    uncal h.
heroin
herpes
    h. zoster

hertz
Heschl's convolution
heteroerotism
heterosexual
heterosexuality
heterosuggestion
heterotonic
heterotopia
Hibbs'
    curet
    elevator
    gouge
hindbrain
hipnagojik. See *hypnagogic.*
hipno-. See words beginning
    hypno-.
hipo-. See words beginning
    hypo-.
hippocampus
    h. leonis
    h. nudus
Hirschberg's reflex
histrionic
hodology
Hoen's skull plate
Hoffmann's
    atrophy
    sign
holergasia
holergastic
holism
holistic
Holmes'
    sign
    degeneration
holorachischisis
Holter's shunt
Homén's syndrome
homicidal
homicidomania
homilophobia
homonymous

homosexual
homosexuality
homunculus
hook
    Adson's h.
    Dandy's h.
    Frazier's h.
    Graham's h.
horn
    Ammon's h.
Horsley's separator
Hortega's cell
Horton's syndrome
hostility
H-reflex
Hudson's
    brace
    bur
    drill
    forceps
Huguenin's edema
Huntington's
    chorea
    disease
Hunt's
    atrophy
    disease
    neuralgia
    paradoxical phenomenon
    striatal syndrome
    tremor
Hurd's
    dissector
    forceps
Hurler's syndrome
hydranencephaly
hydrargyromania
hydrencephalocele
hydrencephalomeningocele
hydrocephalic
hydrocephalocele
hydrocephaloid

hydrocephalus
> communicating h.
> h. ex vacuo
> noncommunicating h.
> obstructive h.
> otitic h.

hydrocephaly
hydromeningitis
hydromeningocele
hydromicrocephaly
hydromyelia
hydromyelocele
hydromyelomeningocele
hygroma
> subdural h.

hyla
hypalgesia
hypencephalon
hyperalgesia
hyperesthesia
hypergeusesthesia
hypergeusia
hyperkinesia
hyperkinesis
hyperkinetic
hypernea
hypernoia
hyperostosis
> h. cranii
> h. frontalis interna
> Morgagni's h.

hyperpathia
hyperphrenia
hyperplasia
hyperreflexia
hypertarachia
hyperthymergasia
hyperthymia
hyperventilation
hypesthesia
hypnagogic
hypnoanalysis

hypnoanesthesia
hypnobatia
hypnogenic
hypnolepsy
hypnonarcoanalysis
hypnonarcosis
hypnopompic
hypnosia
hypnosis
hypnotherapy
hypnotic
hypnotism
hypnotize
hypoactive
hypochondria
hypochondriac
hypochondriacal
hypochondriasis
hypoesthesia
hypoglycorrhachia
hypokinesia
hypomania
hypomaniac
hypomanic
hypophrenosis
hypophyseal
hypophysectomy
hypophysis
> h. cerebri

hypophysitis
hypophysoma
hypoplasia
hyporeflexia
hypotelorism
> orbital h.

hypothalamotomy
hypothalamus
hypothermia
hypotonia
hypotonic
hysteria
> anxiety h.

hysteria (*continued*)
    canine h.
    conversion h.
    fixation h.
    h. libidinosa
    monosymptomatic h.
hysteric
hysterical
hystericism
hystericoneuralgic
hysteriform
hysteroepilepsy
hysteroepileptogenic
hysteroerotic
hysterogenic
hysteroid
hysteromania
hysteronarcolepsy
hysteroneurasthenia
hysteroneurosis
hysteropia
hysteropsychosis
iatrogenic
ICA — internal carotid artery
ICAO — internal carotid artery
        occlusion
ICT — insulin coma therapy
ictal
ictus
    i. epilepticus
    i. paralyticus
    i. sanguinis
id
ideal
    ego i.
idealization
ideation
    incoherent i.
ideational
idée
    i. fixe
identification

ideodynamism
ideogenetic
idetik. See *eidetic.*
idiocy
    absolute i.
    amaurotic familial i.
    athetosic i.
    Aztec i.
    cretinoid i.
    developmental i.
    diplegic i.
    eclamptic i.
    epileptic i.
    erethistic i.
    genetous i.
    hemiplegic i.
    hydrocephalic i.
    intrasocial i.
    Kulmuk i.
    microcephalic i.
    mongolian i.
    paralytic i.
    paraplegic i.
    plagiocephalic i.
    profound i.
    scaphocephalic i.
    sensorial i.
    spastic amaurotic axonal
      i.
    torpid i.
    traumatic i.
    xerodermic i.
idioglossia
idioglottic
idiohypnotism
idioimbecile
idioneural
idioneurosis
idiopathic
idiophrenic
idiopsychologic
idiosyncrasy

idiosyncratic
idiot
    erethistic i.
    mongolian i.
    pithecoid i.
    profound i.
    i.-savant
    superficial i.
    torpid i.
idiotropic
illusion
illusional
image
imagines
imago
imbecile
imbecility
immature
impotence
impoverishment
imprinting
impulse
    irresistible i.
impulsion
    wandering i.
inadequacy
inadequate
incallosal
incest
incision. See *General Surgical Terms.*
incisura
    i. cerebelli
    i. clavicularis sterni
    i. frontalis
    i. temporalis
    i. tentorii cerebelli
incoherent
incompetent
incoordination
incorrigible
incubus

indifference
    belle i.
indifferent
Indoklon therapy
indole
indusium griseum
ineon. See *inion.*
infantile
infantilism
infarction
    cerebral i.
infundibulum
    i. hypothalami
inhibition
iniencephaly
inion
insane
insanity
    adolescent i.
    affective i.
    alcoholic i.
    alternating i.
    anticipatory i.
    choreic i.
    circular i.
    climacteric i.
    communicated i.
    compound i.
    compulsive i.
    consecutive i.
    cyclic i.
    doubting i.
    emotional i.
    hereditary i.
    homicidal i.
    homochronous i.
    hysteric i.
    idiophrenic i.
    impulsive i.
    manic-depressive i.
    moral i.
    perceptional i.

insanity (*continued*)
  periodic i.
  polyneuritic i.
  primary i.
  puerperal i.
  recurrent i.
  senile i.
  simultaneous i.
  toxic i.
insanoid
insensible
insight
insolation
  hyperpyrexial i.
insomnia
insomniac
insomnic
inspectionism
instinct
  death i.
  ego i.
  herd i.
instinctive
insula
insultus
  i. hystericus
integration
intellect
intellection
intellectualization
intelligence
interneuron
interpediculate
interpeduncular
interpretation
interstitial
interventricular
intervertebral
intracephalic
intracerebellar
intracerebral
intracisternal

intracranial
intralobar
intramedullary
intraparietal
intrapsychic
intraspinal
intrathecal
intraventricular
introjection
introspection
introversion
introvert
inversion
  sexual i.
invert
involuntary
involutional
iodoventriculography
IQ — intelligence quotient
irascibility
irreversible
irritability
irritation
  cerebral i.
  spinal i.
ischogyria
island of Reil
ismus. See *isthmus.*
isolation
IST — insulin shock therapy
isthmus
  i. of cingulate gyrus
jacksonian epilepsy
Jackson's
  law
  rule
  syndrome
Jakob-Creutzfeldt syndrome
Janet's
  disease
  test
Jansen's retractor

Javid's shunt
jefirofobea. See *gephyrophobia.*
Joffroy's reflex
Jolly's reaction
Jung's method
juvenile
kakergasea. See *cacergasia.*
kakesthenik. See *cacesthenic.*
kakesthezea. See *cacesthesia.*
kakinashun. See *cachinnation.*
kakodemonomanea. See
   cacodemonomania.
Kalischer's disease
Kanavel's
    cannula
    conductor
Kanner's syndrome
karnshvoont. See
   kernschwund.
kemo-. See words beginning
   chemo-.
kenophobia
keraunoneurosis
kernicterus
Kernig's sign
kernschwund
keromanea. See *cheromania.*
Kerrison's rongeur
Killian's elevator
Kiloh-Nevin syndrome
kinanesthesia
kinesiesthesiometer
kinesiology
kinesioneurosis
kinesis
kinesodic
kinesthesia
kinesthetic
kinetic
KJ — knee jerk
KK — knee kick
Klemme's retractor

kleptolagnia
kleptomania
kleptomaniac
kleptophobia
Klippel-Feil syndrome
Klippel-Feldstein syndrome
Klüver-Bucy syndrome
knife
    Adson's k.
    Bucy's k.
    Crile's k.
kolesteatoma. See
   cholesteatoma.
kolinerjik. See *cholinergic.*
Kolodny's hemostat
kooroo. See *kuru.*
kor-. See words beginning
   chor-.
koro
Korsakoff's
    psychosis
    syndrome
Koshevnikoff's disease
Krabbe's
    disease
    sclerosis
Kraepelin's classification
Krause's
    operation
    ventricle
Kretschmer types
Kulmuk idiocy
kuru
labile
lability
labiochorea
Lafora's sign
laliophobia
laloneurosis
lalophobia
lambda
Lambotte's osteotome

lamella
lamina
    inferior l. of sphenoid
      bone
    l. medullaris lateralis
      corporis striati
    l. medullaris medialis
      corporis striati
    l. ossium cranii
laminae
    l. albae cerebelli
    l. medullares cerebelli
    l. medullares thalami
laminagram
laminagraph
laminectomy
laminotomy
Landouzy-Dejerine
    atrophy
    dystrophy
Landry's paralysis
Langenbeck's elevator
lapsus
    l. linguae
    l. memoriae
Laségue's
    disease
    sign
latah
latency
latent
laterality
lateropulsion
law
    Babinski's l.
    Bell-Magendie l.
    Bell's l.
    Cushing's l.
    Flatau's l.
    Jackson's l.
    Magendie's l.
    wallerian l.

Leichtenstern's sign
Leksell's
    forceps
    rongeur
lemniscus
Lennox's syndrome
lenticular
lenticulo-optic
leptocephalia
leptomeninges
leptomeningioma
leptomeningitis
    l. interna
    sarcomatous l.
leptomeningopathy
leptomeninx
Leriche's operation
Leri's sign
lesbian
lesbianism
lethargy
    hysteric l.
    induced l.
    lucid l.
lethe
letheomania
lethologica
leukodystrophy
leukoencephalitis
leukoencephalopathy
    metachromatic l.
    progressive multifocal l.
    subacute sclerosing l.
leukoerythroblastosis
leukomyelitis
leukomyelopathy
leukotome
    Bailey's l.
    Love's l.
leukotomy
Lewin's forceps
Leyden's ataxia

Lhermitte's sign
libidinal
libidinous
libido
	bisexual l.
	ego l.
Lichtheim's
	plaques
	sign
ligamenta
	l. flava
ligamentum
	l. denticulatum
	l. flavum
Light-Veley headrest
likenshadel. See *lückenschädel.*
limbic
lingula
	l. cerebelli
Lissauer's
	paralysis
	tract
lithium
Little's disease
lobe
	caudate l. of cerebrum
	crescentic l. of cerebel-
		lum
	flocculonodular l.
	limbic l.
	occipital l.
	quadrangular l. of cere-
		bellum
	quadrate l. of cerebral
		hemisphere
	temporal l.
	temporosphenoidal l. of
		cerebral hemisphere
lobectomy
lobotomy
	frontal l.
	prefrontal l.

lobotomy (*continued*)
	transorbital l.
lobule
	l. of cerebellum
	posteromedian l.
lobulus
	l. centralis cerebelli
	l. paracentralis
	l. parietalis
	l. quadrangularis
		cerebelli
	l. semilunaris
lobus
	l. frontalis
	l. occipitalis
	l. olfactorius
	l. parietalis
	l. temporalis
locus
	l. ceruleus
	l. ferrugineus
logagnosia
logagraphia
logamnesia
logaphasia
logasthenia
logoklony
logokophosis
logomania
logoneurosis
logopathy
logoplegia
logorrhea
logospasm
lordosis
Love-Adson elevator
Love-Gruenwald
	forceps
	rongeur
Love-Kerrison forceps
Love's
	leukotome

Love's (*continued*)
    retractor
LP — lumbar puncture
LSD — lysergic acid diethyla-
    mide
Lucae's mallet
lucid
lückenschädel
Luer's forceps
luko-. See words beginning
    leuko-.
lumbar puncture
lumbosacral
lunacy
lunatic
lunatism
Lundvall's blood crisis
lura
lural
Luschka's foramen
Lust's reflex
lymphosarcoma
MA — mental age
macrencephalia
macrocrania
macrogyria
macromania
macromelia
    m. paraesthetica
maculocerebral
Magendie's
    foramen
    law
    spaces
maladjustment
malingerer
malingering
Malis' coagulator
malleation
mallet
    Crane's m.
    Lucae's m.

mallet (*continued*)
    Meyerding's m.
maneuver
    Adson's m.
    Valsalva's m.
mania
    acute hallucinatory m.
    akinetic m.
    m. à potu
    Bell's m.
    dancing m.
    doubting m.
    epileptic m.
    hysterical m.
    m. mitis
    periodical m.
    puerperal m.
    Ray's m.
    reasoning m.
    religious m.
    m. secandi
    transitory m.
    unproductive m.
maniac
maniaphobia
manic
manic-depressive
manifest
mannerism
MAOI — monoamine oxidase
    inhibitor
Marchiafava-Bignami syndrome
Marie's
    ataxia
    sclerosis
marihuana, marijuana
marital
marrowbrain
masochism
masochist
Mayfield's clip
MCA — middle cerebral artery

McCarthy's reflex
McKenzie's
    bur
    clip
    drill
    forceps
MD — muscular dystrophy
mechanism
    defense m.
    neutralizing m.
Meckel's
    band
    cavity
    ganglion
mecocephalic
medications. See *Drugs and Chemistry* section.
medicerebellar
medicerebral
medulla
    m. oblongata
    m. spinalis
medullary
medullispinal
medullitis
medulloblast
medulloblastoma
    Cushing's m.
medulloencephalic
medulloepithelioma
megalomania
megalomaniac
melancholia
    affective m.
    m. agitata
    agitated m.
    m. attonita
    m. with delirium
    flatuous m.
    m. hypochondriaca
    involution m.
    m. religiosa

melancholia (*continued*)
    m. simplex
    stuporous m.
melancholiac
melanoma
melomania
melyuh. See *milieu.*
membrane
    arachnoid m.
memory
    affect m.
    anterograde m.
menarche
Mendel-Bekhterew reflex
Ménière's syndrome
meningeal
meningematoma
meningeocortical
meningeoma
meningeorrhaphy
meninges
meninghematoma
meningina
meninginitis
meningioma
    angioblastic m.
    olfactory groove m.
meningiomatosis
meningism
meningismus
meningitic
meningitides
meningitis
    acute aseptic m.
    African m.
    aseptic m.
    benign lymphocytic m.
    cerebral m.
    cerebrospinal m.
    gummatous m.
    lymphocytic m.
    meningococcic m.

meningitis (*continued*)
   metastatic m.
   m. necrotoxica reactiva
   occlusive m.
   m. ossificans
   otitic m.
   parameningococcus m.
   purulent m.
   Quincke's m.
   septicemic m.
   m. serosa
   m. serosa circumscripta
   m. serosa circumscripta
     cystica
   serous m.
   m. sympathica
   torula m.
   torular m.
   tubercular m.
   tuberculous m.
meningitophobia
meningoarteritis
meningoblastoma
meningocele
meningocephalitis
meningocerebritis
meningococcemia
   acute fulminating m.
meningococci
meningococcidal
meningococcin
meningococcosis
meningococcus
meningocortical
meningocyte
meningoencephalitis
meningoencephalocele
meningoencephalomyelitis
meningoencephalomyelopathy
meningoencephalopathy
meningoexothelioma
meningofibroblastoma

meningogenic
meningoma
meningomalacia
meningomyelitis
meningomyelocele
meningomyeloencephalitis
meningoencephalopathy
meningoexothelioma
meningofibroblastoma
meningoma
meningomalacia
meningomyelitis
meningomyelocele
meningomyeloradiculitis
meningomyelorrhaphy
meningo-osteophlebitis
meningopathy
meningopneumonitis
meningorachidian
meningoradicular
meningoradiculitis
meningorecurrence
meningorrhagia
meningorrhea
meningothelioma
meningotyphoid
meningovascular
meninguria
meninx
   m. fibrosa
   m. serosa
   m. tenuis
   m. vasculosa
mentalia
meralgia
   m. paresthetica
merergastic
merorachischisis
Merzbacher-Pelizaeus disease
mesencephalon
mesencephalotomy
mesmerism

mesoglia
metacoele
metaphrenia
metaplexus
metapsyche
metapsychics
metapsychology
metatela
metathalamus
metencephal
metencephalic
metencephalon
metencephalospinal
method
    Dubois' m.
    Freud's cathartic m.
    Jung's m.
    Pavlov's m.
methomania
metonymy
Meyerding's
    curet
    gouge
    mallet
    osteotome
    retractor
Meyer's theory
Meynert's
    bundle
    commissure
    decussation
    tract
Michel's clip
microcephaly
microcrania
microglia
microglial
microgliocyte
microglioma
microgliomatosis
microgyri
microgyrus

micromania
microneurosurgery
microsurgery
midbrain
miel-. See words beginning
    myel-.
mielo-. See words beginning
    myelo-.
migraine
    fulgurating m.
    ophthalmic m.
    ophthalmoplegic m.
migrateur
milieu
Millard-Gubler syndrome
Mills' disease
Mils' cautery
Minnesota Multiphasic
    Personality Inventory test
mio-. See words beginning
    myo-.
misaction
misandria
misanthropia
miso-. See also words beginning
    myso-.
misocainia
misogamy
misogyn
misogyny
misologia
misoneism
misopedia
mitho-. See words beginning
    mytho-.
MMPI — Minnesota Multiphasic
    Personality Inven-
    tory
M'Naghten rule
Möbius' syndrome
Mönckeberg's sclerosis
mongolian idiot

mongolism
mongoloid
Monokow
    fasciculus aberrans of M.
monomania
monomoria
monoplegia
monorecidive
Monro
    foramen of M.
monticulus
    m. cerebelli
Morel-Kraepelin disease
Morgagni's hyperostosis
moria
moron
moronity
morphinomania
Morquio's sign
Morvan's chorea
motor
motorium
    m. commune
MS — multiple sclerosis
Munchausen's syndrome
muscle
    digastric m.
    frontalis m.
    gluteus maximus m.
    intercostal m.
    latissimus dorsi m.
    occipitalis m.
    orbicularis oculi m.
    rhomboid major m.
    rhomboid minor m.
    sartorius m.
    scalenus m.
    sternocleidomastoid m.
    temporalis m.
    teres major m.
    teres minor m.
    trapezius m.

mutation
mute
mutism
    akinetic m.
    hysterical m.
myalgia
myasthenia
    m. gravis pseudopara-
      lytica
myatonia
mydriasis
    spinal m.
myelalgia
myelanalosis
myelapoplexy
myelasthenia
myelatelia
myelatrophy
myelauxe
myelencephalitis
myelencephalon
myelencephalospinal
myelencephalous
myeleterosis
myelic
myelin
myelinated
myelinization
myelinoclasis
    acute perivascular m.
    central pontine m.
    postinfection perivenous
      m.
myelinogeny
myelinolysin
myelinolysis
myelinopathy
myelinosis
myelitis
myeloarchitecture
myelobrachium
myelocele

myelocoele
myelocone
myelocyst
myelocystic
myelocystocele
myelocystomeningocele
myelocyte
myelodysplasia
myeloencephalic
myeloencephalitis
myelofibrosis
myelogenesis
myelogeny
myelogram
myelography
myeloid
myeloma
myelomalacia
myelomeningitis
myelomeningocele
myelon
myeloneuritis
myelo-opticoneuropathy
myeloparalysis
myelopathy
myelophthisis
myeloplegia
myeloradiculitis
myeloradiculodysplasia
myeloradiculopathy
myelorrhagia
myelorrhaphy
myelosarcoma
myeloschisis
myeloscintogram
myelosclerosis
myelosis
myelospasm
myelospongium
myelosyphilis
myelosyphilosis
myelotome

myelotomy
    commissural m.
Myerson's sign
myoclonia
    m. epileptica
myoclonic
myoclonus
myohypertrophia
    m. kymoparalytica
myokymia
myoneural
mysophilia
mysophobia
mythomania
mythophobia
mythoplasty
Naffziger's syndrome
napex
narcism
narcissism
narcissistic
narcoanalysis
narcodiagnosis
narcohypnosis
narcolepsy
narcoleptic
narcolysis
narcomania
narcosis
narcosomania
narcosynthesis
narcotic
nasion
necrencephalus
necromania
necrophilia
necrophilism
necrophobia
necrosadism
necrosis
needle
    Adson's n.

needle (*continued*)
    Babcock's n.
    Cone's n.
    Gardner's n.
    New's n.
    Sachs' n.
    Ward-French n.
neencephalon
negativism
neocerebellum
neokinetic
neolallia
neolallism
neologism
neopallium
neophilism
neophobia
neophrenia
neoplasm
neostriatum
neothalamus
nerve
    abducens n.
    accessory n.
    acoustic n.
    afferent n.
    autonomic n.
    Bell's n.
    cranial n.
    efferent n.
    facial n.
    glossopharyngeal n.
    hypoglossal n.
    intermediate n.
    mandibular n.
    maxillary n.
    oculomotor n.
    olfactory n.
    ophthalmic n.
    optic n.
    parasympathetic n.
    spinal n.

nerve (*continued*)
    sympathetic n.
    trigeminal n.
    trochlear n.
    vagus n.
neuradynamia
neuragmia
neural
neuralgia
    cervicobrachial n.
    cranial n.
    Fothergill's n.
    hallucinatory n.
    Harris' migrainous n.
    Hunt's n.
    migrainous n.
    trigeminal n.
    vidian n.
neuranagenesis
neurangiosis
neurapophysis
neurapraxia
neurarchy
neurasthenia
neurastheniac
neurasthenic
neurataxia
neurataxy
neuratrophia
neuratrophic
neuratrophy
neuraxial
neuraxis
neuraxitis
neuraxon
neure
neurectasia
neurectomy
    presacral n.
neurectopia
neurenteric
neurergic

neurexeresis
neuriatry
neuridine
neurilemma
neurilemmitis
neurilemmoma
neurilemoma
neurinoma
    acoustic
neuritic
neuritis
neuroallergy
neuroamebiasis
neuroanastomosis
neuroanatomy
anuroarthropathy
neuroastrocytoma
neurobehavioral
neuroblast
neuroblastoma
neurobrucellosis
neurocanal
neurocardiac
neurocentrum
neuroceptor
neurochemistry
neurochitin
neurocirculatory
neurocladism
neuroclonic
neurocommunications
neurocranial
neurocranium
neurocrine
neurocrinia
neurocyte
neurocytology
neurocytoma
neurodegenerative
neurodendrite
neurodiagnosis
neurodynia

neuroelectricity
neuroelectrotherapeutics
neuroencephalomyelopathy
neuroendocrine
neuroendocrinology
neuroepithelium
neurofibril
neurofibrilla
neurofibrillae
neurofibroma
neurofibromatosis
neurofilament
neurofixation
neurogangliitis
neuroganglion
neurogen
neurogenesis
neurogenic
neurogenous
neuroglia
    fascicular n.
    peripheral n.
neurogliocytoma
neuroglioma
neurogliosis
neuroglycopenia
neurogram
neurography
neurohumoralism
neurohypophysis
neuroimmunology
neuroinduction
neurokeratin
neurolemma
neuroleptic
neurolipomatosis
neurologia
neurological
neurologist
neurology
neurolymph
neurolysis

neuroma
    acoustic n.
    medullated n.
    myelinic n.
    plexiform n.
    Verneuil's n.
neuromalacia
neuromatosis
neuromere
neuromittor
neuromotor
neuromyasthenia
neuromyelitis
neuron
neuronal
neuronitis
neuroparalysis
neuroparalytic
neuropath
neuropathic
neuropathogenesis
neuropathology
neuropathy
neurophonia
neuroplasty
neuropsychiatrist
neuropsychiatry
neuropsychic
neuropsychopathy
neuropsychosis
neuropyra
neuropyretic
neuroradiology
neurorecidive
neurorecurrence
neuroregulation
neurorelapse
neuroretinopathy
    hypertensive n.
neurorrhaphy
neurorrheuma
neurosarcokleisis

neurosarcoma
neurosclerosis
neurosecretion
neurosegmental
neurosensory
neuroses
neurosis
    anxiety n.
    association n.
    cardiac n.
    compensation n.
    compulsion n.
    conversion n.
    depersonalization n.
    depressive n.
    expectation n.
    fatigue n.
    fixation n.
    gastric n.
    homosexual n.
    hypochondriacal n.
    hysterical n.
    intestinal n.
    obsessional n.
    obsessive-compulsive n.
    occupational n.
    pension n.
    phobic n.
    professional n.
    rectal n.
    regression n.
    sexual n.
    torsion n.
    transference n.
    traumatic n.
    vegetative n.
    war n.
neurosism
neuroskeletal
neuroskeleton
neurosome
neurospasm

neurosplanchnic
neurospongioma
neurospongium
neurostatus
neurosthenia
neurosurgeon
neurosurgery
    microvascular n.
    stereotaxic n.
neurosyphilis
    ectodermogenic n.
    meningeal n.
    meningovascular n.
    mesodermogenic n.
    paretic n.
    tabetic n.
neurosystemitis
    n. epidemica
neurotabes
    n. diabetica
neurotagma
neurotherapy
neurothlipsis
neurotic
neurotica
neuroticism
neurotization
neurotmesis
neurotome
    Hall's n.
neurotomography
neurotomy
    retrogasserian n.
neurotoxin
neurotransducer
neurotransmitter
neurotripsy
neurotrophasthenia
neurotubule
neurovirulence
neurovirulent
New's needle

Niemann-Pick disease
nihilism
nimfo-. See words beginning
    nympho-.
nistagmus. See *nystagmus.*
noctiphobia
nodule
    Schmorl's n.
non compos mentis
non sequitur
notencephalocele
Nothnagel's
    sign
    syndrome
notomyelitis
nuclei
    n. arcuati
nucleus
    n. ambiguus
    cuneate n.
    Darkschewitsch's n.
    n. gracilis
    n. lateralis medullae
      oblongatae
    n. pulposus
numo-. See words beginning
    pneumo-.
nura-. See words beginning
    neura-.
nuro-. See words beginning
    neuro-.
nympholepsy
nymphomania
nymphomaniac
nystagmus
nystagmus-myoclonus
OA — occipital artery
Obersteiner-Redlich area
obex
obliteration
    cortical o.
obnubilation

OBS — organic brain syndrome
obsession
obsessive
obsessive-compulsive
obtund
occipital
occipitalis
occipitalization
occipito-atloid
occipito-axoid
occipitobasilar
occipitobregmatic
occipitocervical
occipitofacial
occipitofrontal
occipitomastoid
occipitomental
occipitoparietal
occipitotemporal
occipitothalamic
occiput
occlusion
oedipism
Oedipus complex
Oehler's symptom
ofthal-. See words beginning
ophthal-.
oksesefale. See *oxycephaly*.
Oldberg's
    dissector
    forceps
    retractor
olfactory
oligergasia
oligergastic
oligodendroglia
oligodendroglioma
oligomania
oligophrenia
    phenylpyruvic o.
    o. phenylpyruvica
oligopsychia

oligoria
oliva
olivary
olive
    inferior o.
    spurge o.
    superior o.
Olivecrona's clip
olivifugal
olivipetal
olivopontocerebellar
omahl. See *haut-mal*.
Ommaya's reservoir
onanism
oneiric
oneirism
oneiroanalysis
oneirodynia
oneirogenic
oneirophrenia
oneiroscopy
onikotilomanea. See
    onychotillomania.
oniomania
onirik. See *oneiric*.
onirizm. See *oneirism*.
oniro-. See words beginning
    oneiro-.
onomatomania
onomatopoiesis
onychotillomania
operation
    Alexander's o.
    Cloward's o.
    Cotte's o.
    Dana's o.
    Förster-Penfield o.
    Frazier-Spiller o.
    Gardner's o.
    Gill's o.
    Haynes' o.
    Krause's o.

operation (*continued*)
    Leriche's o.
    Pancoast's o.
    Puusepp's o.
    Smithwick's o.
    Sonneberg's o.
    Torkildsen's o.
opercula
operculum
ophthalmencephalon
ophthalmoplegia
opiate
opioid
opisthion
opisthotonos
Oppenheim's
    gait
    sign
orientation
oriented
orthopsychiatry
oscillopsia
osteogenic
osteoma
osteoplastic
osteoplasty
osteotome
    Cherry's o.
    Lambotte's o.
    Meyerding's o.
    Stille's o.
osteotomy
otohemineurasthenia
overcompensation
overdetermination
overlay
    emotional o.
    psychogenic o.
overt
overtone
    psychic o.

oxycephaly
pacchionian
pachycephalia
pachyleptomeningitis
pachymeningitis
pakeonean. See *pacchionian.*
paleencephalon
paleocerebellar
paleocerebellum
paleocortex
paleophrenia
paleothalamus
palikinesia
palilalia
palinphrasia
pallidal
pallidectomy
pallidoansection
pallidoansotomy
pallidofugal
pallidotomy
pallidum
pallium
palsy
    Bell's p.
Pancoast's operation
Pandy's test
panic
panophobia
Pansch's fissure
pantaphobia
pantophobia
pantophobic
papilledema
papilloma
    p. neuroticum
paracoele
paraganglioma
paraganglion
paragrammatism
paragraphia

paralexia
paralogia
    thematic p.
paralogism
paralysis
    p. agitans
    bulbar p.
    conjugate p.
    cortical p.
    Duchenne-Erb p.
    Landry's p.
    Lissauer's p.
    Todd's p.
    Werdnig-Hoffmann p.
paramyoclonus
paramyotonia
paranoia
    p. hallucinatoria
    heboid p.
    litigious p.
    p. originaria
    querulous p.
    p. simplex
paranoiac
paranoic
paranoid
paranoidism
paranomia
paranormal
paranosic
paranosis
paraparesis
parapathia
paraphasia
paraphasic
paraphasis
paraphemia
paraphia
paraphilia
paraphiliac
paraphobia
paraphora

paraphrasia
paraphrenia
    p. confabulans
    p. expansiva
    p. phantastica
    p. systematica
paraphrenic
paraphronia
paraplegia
paraplegic
parapraxia
parapsychology
parapsychosis
parareaction
parasympathetic
parasympathin
parasympatholytic
parasympathomimetic
parataxic
    p. distortion
paratonia
paratrophy
parenchymal
parergasia
parergastic
paresis
paresthesia
parietal
parietofrontal
parieto-occipital
parietotemporal
Parinaud's syndrome
Parkinson's
    disease
    facies
    syndrome
parkinsonian
parkinsonism
    postencephalitis p.
paroksizmal. See *paroxysmal.*
parorexia
paroxysmal

Parrot's
  atrophy of the newborn
  sign
Parry-Romberg syndrome
pars
  p. centralis ventriculi
    lateralis cerebri
  p. cervicalis medullae
    spinalis
  p. frontalis radiationis
    corporis callosi
  p. inferior fossae
    rhomboideae
  p. inferior gyri frontalis
    medii
  p. intermedia fossae
    rhomboideae
  p. lumbalis medullae
    spinalis
  p. marginalis sulci cinguli
  p. occipitalis radiationis
    corporis callosi
  p. opercularis gyri
    frontalis inferioris
  p. orbitalis gyri frontalis
    inferioris
  p. parasympathica
    systematis nervosi
    autonomici
  p. parietalis operculi
  p. parietalis radiationis
    corporis callosi
  p. petrosa ossis
    temporalis
  p. posterior commissurae
    anterioris cerebri
  p. posterior rhinencephali
  p. subfrontalis sulci
    cinguli
  p. superior fossae
    rhomboideae

pars (*continued*)
  p. superior gyri frontalis
    medii
  p. sympathica systematis
    nervosi autonomici
passive-aggressive
pathergasia
pathognomonic
pathognomy
pathophobia
Patrick's test
Pavlov's method
pavor
  p. diurnus
  p. nocturnus
peak
  Bragg p.
Pecquet's
  cistern
  reservoir
pederasty
pederosis
pedophilia
pedophilic
pedophobia
peduncle
  cerebellar p.
  cerebral p.
  p. of flocculus
  p. of hypophysis
  olfactory p.
  olivary p. of Schwalbe
  pineal p.
  p. of pineal body
  p. of thalamus, inferior
pedunculotomy
pedunculus
  p. cerebellaris, inferior,
    medius, superior
  p. cerebri
  p. corporis callosi

pedunculus (*continued*)
    p. corporis pinealis
    p. flocculi
    p. thalami inferior
PEG — pneumoencephalography
    raphy
pellagra
perception
    extrasensory p.
perceptorium
perceptual
Perez's sign
pericranitis
pericranium
periosteal
periosteum
peripheral nervous system
peronarthrosis
perseveration
persona
personality
    affective p.
    alternating p.
    anankastic p.
    antisocial p.
    asthenic p.
    compulsive p.
    cycloid p.
    cyclothymic p.
    disordered p.
    double p.
    dual p.
    dyssocial p.
    explosive p.
    hysterical p.
    inadequate p.
    multiple p.
    obsessive-compulsive p.
    paranoid p.
    passive-aggressive p.
    passive-dependent p.
    psychopathic p.

personality (*continued*)
    schizoid p.
    seclusive p.
    shut-in p.
    sociopathic p.
    split p.
perversion
pervert
pessimism
petit mal
petroclinoid
petrosal
petrosphenoid
pfropfhebephrenia
pfropfschizophrenia
phallic
phaneromania
phantasm
phantasmatomoria
phantasmoscopia
phantasy
pharmacomania
pharmacophilia
pharmacophobia
pharmacopsychosis
phenomenology
phenomenon
    Babinski's p.
    Bell's p.
    Hunt's paradoxical p.
    Trousseau's p.
phenothiazine
phenotype
phenylketonuria
phenylpyruvic
    p. oligophrenia
pheochromocytoma
phlebitis
phlegmatic
phobia
phobic
phobophobia

phrenemphraxis
phrenic
phrenicectomy
phreniclasia
phrenicoexeresis
phreniconeurectomy
phrenicotomy
phrenicotripsy
phrenology
phrenopathic
phrenopathy
phrenoplegia
phthisiomania
phthisiophobia
physiopathic
physiopsychic
pia
    p. mater
pia-arachnitis
pia-arachnoid
piaglia
pial
pia mater
    p. m. encephali
    p. m. spinalis
piamatral
piarachnitis
piarachnoid
pica
PICA — posterior inferior
      cerebellar artery
PICA aneurysm
Pick's
    convolutional atrophy
    disease
piknic. See *pyknic.*
pikno-. See words beginning
    pykno-.
pileum
pileus
pineal
pinealectomy

pinealoma
Pinel's system
Piotrowski's sign
pira-. See words beginning
    pyra-.
piro-. See words beginning
    pyro-.
pituitary
pituitectomy
PKU — phenylketonuria
plagiocephalic
plagiocephaly
plaque
    Lichtheim's p's
    Redlich-Fisher miliary
      p's
    senile p's
plate
    Hoen's skull p.
platybasia
pleocytosis
plexus
    brachial p.
    carotid p.
    cervical p.
    p. cervicobrachialis
    choroid p.
    p. choroideus ventriculi
      lateralis
    p. choroideus ventriculi
      quarti
    p. choroideus ventriculi
      tertii
    lumbosacral p.
    p. vertebralis
pneumocephalon
    p. artificiale
pneumocephalus
pneumoencephalogram
pneumoencephalography
pneumoencephalomyelogram
pneumoencephalomyelography

pneumoencephalos
pneumomyelography
poliencephalomyelitis
polioclastic
poliodystrophy
polioencephalitis
polioencephalomeningo-
    myelitis
polioencephalomyelitis
polioencephalopathy
poliomyelencephalitis
poliomyelitis
    bulbar p.
    cerebral p.
    spinal paralytic p.
poliomyelopathy
polioneuromere
polyclonia
polymerization
polyneural
polyneuralgia
polyneuritic
polyneuritis
polyneuromyositis
polyneuropathy
polyneuroradiculitis
polynuclear
polyparesis
polyphagia
polytomography
polyvinyl
pons
    p. cerebelli
    p. varolii
pons-oblongata
pontibrachium
ponticulus
pontile
pontine
pontobulbia
pontocerebellar
porencephalia

porencephalic
porencephalitis
porencephaly
poriomania
pornographomania
pornolagnia
porphyria
position. See *General Surgical
    Terms.*
postictal
potency
pouch
    Rathke's p.
Pratt's curet
precocious
precocity
precognition
preconscious
preconvulsant
preconvulsive
precuneus
predilection
predisposition
prefrontal
pregenital
preoblongata
priapism
processus
    p. clinoideus anterior
    p. clinoideus medius
    p. clinoideus posterior
projection
pronation
propons
proprioceptive
proprioceptor
prosencephalon
proton beam (Bragg peak)
protuberance
    occipital p.
psalis
psalterium

pseudocoele
pseudologia
    p. fantastica
pseudosclerosis
    p. spastica
pseudotabes
psychalgalia
psychalgia
psychalgic
psychalia
psychanalysis
psychanopsia
psychasthene
psychasthenia
psychasthenic
psychataxia
psyche
psycheclampsia
psychedelic
psychiater
psychiatric
psychiatrist
psychiatry
psychic
psychinosis
psychlampsia
psychoalgalia
psychoallergy
psychoanaleptic
psychoanalysis
psychoanalyst
psychoanalytic
psychoanalyze
psychoasthenics
psychoauditory
psychobacillosis
psychobiological
psychobiology
psychocatharsis
psychocentric
psychochemistry
psychochrome

psychochromesthesia
psychocoma
psychocortical
psychodelic
psychodiagnosis
psychodiagnostics
psychodometer
psychodometry
psychodrama
psychodynamics
psychodysleptic
psychoepilepsy
psychogalvanometer
psychogenesis
psychogenia
psychogenic
psychogenous
psychogeriatrics
psychognosis
psychognostic
psychogogic
psychogram
psychograph
psychokinesia
psychokinesis
psychokym
psycholagny
psycholepsy
psycholeptic
psycholinguistics
psychologic
psychological
psychologist
psychology
psychomathematics
psychometer
psychometrics
psychometry
psychomotor
psychoneuroses
psychoneurosis
    p. maidica

psychoneurosis (*continued*)
    paranoid p.
psychonomy
psychonosema
psychonosis
psychoparesis
psychopath
psychopathia
    p. martialis
    p. sexualis
psychopathic
psychopathist
psychopathology
psychopathosis
psychopathy
psychopharmacology
psychophonasthenia
psychophylaxis
psychophysical
psychophysics
psychophysiology
psychoplegia
psychoplegic
psychopneumatology
psychoprophylactic
psychoprophylaxis
psychoreaction
psychorhythmia
psychorrhagia
psychorrhea
psychorrhexis
psychosensorial
psychosensory
psychoses
psychosexual
psychosis
    bipolar p.
    Cheyne-Stokes p.
    gestational p.
    idiophrenic p.
    involutional p.

psychosis (*continued*)
    Korsakoff's p.
    manic p.
    manic-depressive p.
    paranoiac p.
    paranoid p.
    polyneuritic p.
    p. polyneuritica
    postpartum p.
    puerperal p.
    schizoaffective p.
    senile p.
    situational p.
    toxic p.
    unipolar p.
    zoophil p.
psychosolytic
psychosomatic
psychosomaticist
psychosomimetic
psychosurgery
psychotechnics
psychotherapeutics
psychotherapy
psychotic
psychotogenic
psychotomimetic
psychotonic
psychotropic
psychrophobia
pterion
ptosis
puberty
pubescence
Pudenz'
    reservoir
    shunt
    tube
    valve
puerile
puerilism

pulvinar
puncture
    cisternal p.
    Corning's p.
    lumbar p.
    thecal p.
    ventricular p.
putamen
Puusepp's
    operation
    reflex
pyknic
pyknoepilepsy
pyknophrasia
pyramid
pyramidal
pyramidotomy
pyramis
pyrolagnia
pyromania
quadrantanopia
quadriplegia
Queckenstedt's sign
querulous
Quincke's meningitis
Quinquaud's sign
rachialbuminimetry
rachialgia
rachicentesis
rachidial
rachidian
rachigraph
rachilysis
rachiocampsis
rachiocentesis
rachiochysis
rachiodynia
rachiometer
rachiomyelitis
rachioscoliosis
rachiotomy
rachischisis

rachitis
rachitome
rachitomy
radicular
radiculectomy
radiculitis
radiculoganglionitis
radiculomedullary
radiculomeningomyelitis
radiculomyelopathy
radiculoneuritis
radiculoneuropathy
radiculopathy
radioactive brain scan
radioencephalogram
radioencephalography
radionuclide
Raeder's syndrome
rafe. See *raphe.*
rahpor. See *rapport.*
rake-. See words beginning
    rachi-.
rakeal-. See words beginning
    rachial-.
rakeo-. See words beginning
    rachio-.
rakiskisis. See *rachischisis.*
rakitis. See *rachitis.*
Ramirez' shunt
ramisection
ramitis
Ramsay-Hunt syndrome
ramus
Raney's
    clip
    curet
    drill
    forceps
raphe
rapport
Rathke's
    pouch

Rathke's (*continued*)
    tumor
rational
rationalization
Raymond's apoplexy
Ray's mania
reaction
    Cushing's r.
    r. formation
    Jolly's r.
reality testing
receptor
recess
recessus
    r. infundibuli
    r. lateralis fossae
      rhomboidei
    r. lateralis ventriculi
      quarti
    r. pinealis
    r. suprapinealis
    r. triangularis
recidivism
recidivist
Redlich-Fisher miliary plaques
red Robinson catheter
reflex
    Achilles tendon r.
    axon r.
    Babinski's r.
    Brain's r.
    Brissaud's r.
    carotid sinus r.
    cerebral cortex r.
    Chaddock's r.
    ciliospinal r.
    Hirschberg's r.
    H- r.
    Joffroy's r.
    Lust's r.
    McCarthy's r.
    Mendel-Bechterew r.

reflex (*continued*)
    palmomental r.
    proprioceptive r.
    Puusepp's r.
    quadrupedal extensor r.
    Remak's r.
    Riddoch's mass r.
    Rossolimo's r.
    Schaefer's r.
    Strümpell's r.
    tarsophalangeal r.
    Throckmorton's r.
    wrist clonus r.
regression
    atavistic r.
Reil
    island of R.
reinnervation
Reitan-Indiana aphasic screen-
    ing test
REM — rapid eye movement
Remak's reflex
Rendu-Osler-Weber disease
Rendu's tremor
repertoire
repression
reservoir
    Ommaya's r.
    Pecquet's r.
    Pudenz' r.
    Rickham's r.
    Rickham-Salmon r.
resistance
respiration
    Biot's r.
restibrachium
restiform
retardate
retardation
    psychomotor r.
rete
    r. canalis hypoglossi

retractor
 Adson's r.
 Barrett-Adson r.
 Beckman-Adson r.
 Beckman-Eaton r.
 Beckman's r.
 Bucy's r.
 Chandler's r.
 Cherry's r.
 Cloward-Hoen r.
 Cone's r.
 Contour's r.
 Cushing's r.
 Davidoff's r.
 Davidson's r.
 Davis' r.
 D'Errico-Adson r.
 D'Errico's r.
 Frazier's r.
 French s-shaped r.
 Gelpi's r.
 Gifford's r.
 Hamby's r.
 Jansen's r.
 Klemme's r.
 Love's r.
 Meyerding's r.
 Oldberg's r.
 Sachs' r.
 Scoville's r.
 Senn's r.
 Sheldon's r.
 Snitman's r.
 Taylor's r.
 Tower's r.
 Tuffier-Raney r.
 Tuffier's r.
 Ullrich's r.
 Weitlaner's r.
 Yasargil's r.
retrobulbar
retrogasserian

retropulsion
rhinencephalon
rhinorrhea
 cerebrospinal r.
rhizotomy
rhombencephalon
rhombocoele
rhomboid
rhythm
 alpha r.
 Berger r.
 beta r.
 gamma r.
Rickham-Salmon reservoir
Rickham's reservoir
Riddoch's mass reflex
rigidity
 cerebellar r.
 hemiplegic r.
 lead-pipe r.
 nuchal r.
rigor
 r. nervorum
 r. tremens
Rimbaud-Passouant-Vallat
 syndrome
rimula
rinensefalon. See
 rhinencephalon.
rinorea. See *rhinorrhea.*
risus
 r. caninus
 r. sardonicus
rizotomee. See *rhizotomy.*
RNA — ribonucleic acid
Rochester's
 connector
 elevator
Rolandi
 substantia r.
Rolando
 fasciculus of R.

Rolando (*continued*)
    tubercule of R.
rolandometer
rombensefalon. See
    rhombencephalon.
rombergism
Romberg's
    disease
    sign
rombosel. See *rhombocoele.*
rongeur
    DeVilbiss' r.
    gooseneck r.
    Kerrison's r.
    Leksell's r.
    Love-Gruenwald r.
    Schlesinger's r.
    Spurling's r.
    Stille-Luer r.
Rorschach test
Roser-Braun sign
Rossolimo's reflex
rostrum
    r. corporis callosi
Roth-Bernhardt disease
Roth's disease
Roussy-Cornil syndrome
rubrospinal
rule
    Jackson's r.
    M'Naghten r.
rumination
    obsessive r.
Rumpf's sign
Ruskin's forceps
Sachs'
    cannula
    guard
    needle
    retractor
    spatula
    suction tube

sacroiliac
sacrospinal
sacrovertebral
sadism
sadist
sadistic
sadomasochistic
Saenger's sign
sagittal
sal-. See words beginning *psal-.*
Salibi's clamp
saltation
saltereum. See *psalterium.*
Sanger-Brown's ataxia
Sarbó's sign
sarcoma
    reticulum cell s. of brain
satellitosis
satyriasis
satyromania
saw
    Gigli's s.
    Stille-Gigli s.
scan
    brain s.
    CAT s.
    CT s.
    EMI s.
scanner
scanning
    radioisotope s.
scanography
scaphocephalia
Schaefer's reflex
Schilder's disease
schizocephalia
schizogyria
schizoid
schizoidism
schizophasia
schizophrenia
    ambulatory s.

schizophrenia (*continued*)
    catatonic s.
    hebephrenic s.
    latent s.
    paranoid s.
    pseudoneurotic s.
    reactive s.
    schizoaffective s.
schizophreniac
schizophrenic
schizophreniform
schizophrenosis
Schlesinger's
    forceps
    rongeur
Schmorl's
    body
    disease
    nodule
Schrötter's chorea
Schutz's
    clip
    forceps
Schwalbe
    olivary peduncle of S.
schwannoma
Schwann's
    sheath
    white substance
Schwartz' clip
sciatica
scintiscanner
scissors
    Adson's s.
    Craig's s.
    craniotomy s.
    Dandy's s.
    Smellie's s.
    Stevenson's s.
    Strully's s.
    Taylor's s.
scleromeninx

sclerosis
    Alzheimer's s.
    amyotrophic lateral s.
    annular s.
    anterolateral s.
    arterial s.
    arteriolar s.
    arteriopapillary s.
    benign s.
    bone s.
    bulbar s.
    cerebellar s.
    cerebral s.
    cerebrospinal s.
    cervical s.
    s. circumscripta
      pericardii
    disseminated s.
    Erb's s.
    familial centrolobar s.
    hyperplastic s.
    insular s.
    Krabbe's s.
    Marie's s.
    miliary s.
    Mönckeberg's s.
    multiple s.
    nodular s.
    posterolateral s.
    presenile s.
    s. redux
    renal arteriolar s.
    s. tuberosa
    tuberous s.
    unicellular s.
    vascular s.
    venous s.
    ventrolateral s.
scoliosis
scotoma
scotomization
scotophobia

Scott's cannula
Scoville-Lewis clip
Scoville's
    clip
    forceps
    retractor
sedative
sefal-. See words beginning
   cephal-.
Seguin's signal symptom
seizure
    audiogenic s.
    cerebral s.
    photogenic s.
    psychic s.
    psychomotor s.
sejunction
selenoplegia
selenoplexia
Seletz's cannula
self-suspension
sella
    s. turcica
semicoma
semicomatose
semicretinism
seminarcosis
Senn's retractor
sensorial
sensorineural
sensorium
sensory
separator
    Horsley's s.
septum
    s. pellucidum
    s. pontis
serotonin
Setchenow's centers
Sewall's forceps
sexual
    s. masochism

sexual (*continued*)
    s. sadism
sfeno-. See words beginning
   spheno-.
sfenoid. See *sphenoid*.
sheath
    myelin s.
    Schwann's s.
Sheldon-Pudenz' dissector
Sheldon's retractor
shingles
shunt
    Holter's s.
    Javid's s.
    Pudenz' s.
    Ramirez' s.
    Silastic ventricular-
      peritoneal s.
    ventricular atrial s.
shwonnoma. See *schwannoma*.
Shy-Drager syndrome
siatika. See *sciatica*.
sibling
Siegert's sign
sifilis. See *syphilis*.
sifilo-. See words beginning
   syphilo-.
sign
    André-Thomas s.
    Babinski's s.
    Ballet's s.
    Barré's pyramidal s.
    Bragard's s.
    Brudzinski's s.
    Chaddock's s.
    Chvostek's s.
    Claude's hyperkinesis s.
    Dejerine's s.
    de la Camp's s.
    Fajersztajn's s.
    Gowers' s.
    Hoffmann's s.

sign (*continued*)
Holmes' s.
Kernig's s.
Lafora's s.
Lasègue's s.
Leichtenstern's s.
Leri's s.
Lhermitte's s.
Lichtheim's s.
Morquio's s.
Myerson's s.
Nothnagel's s.
Oppenheim's s.
Parrot's s.
Perez's s.
Piotrowski's s.
Queckenstedt's s.
Quinquaud's s.
Romberg's s.
Roser-Braun s.
Rumpf's s.
Saenger's s.
Sarbo's s.
Siegert's s.
Signorelli's s.
Soto-Hall s.
Stewart-Holmes s.
Strümpell's s.
Thomas' s.
Tinel's s.
Trousseau's s.
Turyn's s.
Vanzetti's s.
Wartenberg's s.
Weber's s.
Westphal's s.
Signorelli's sign
sika-. See words beginning
psycha-.
sikal-. See words beginning
psychal-.

sikan-. See words beginning
psychan-.
sikas-. See words beginning
psychas-.
sike-. See words beginning
psyche-.
siki-. See words beginning
psychi-.
siko-. See words beginning
psycho-.
Silastic ventricular-peritoneal
shunt
siliqua
s. olivae
Simmonds' disease
sin-. See also words beginning
cin- and *syn-*.
sinciput
sinerea. See *cinerea*.
singulum. See *cingulum*.
singulumotome. See
cingulumotomy.
sinistrocerebral
sinistrosis
sinus
carotid s.
cavernous s.
cerebral s.
s. durae matris
s. pericranii
sagittal s.
s. sagittalis inferior
s. sagittalis superior
subarachnoidal s.
siringo-. See words beginning
syringo-.
Sjögren-Larssen syndrome
skafosefalea. See
scaphocephalia.
skizo-. See words beginning
schizo-.

sklero-. See words beginning
   sclero-.
skull
SLR — straight leg raising
Smellie's scissors
Smith's clip
Smithwick's
    forceps
    operation
Snitman's retractor
SOA-MCA — superficial occipital artery to middle
   cerebral artery
sociology
sociopath
sodomy
soma
somatic
somatization
somatophrenia
somatopsychic
somatopsychosis
somnambulism
somniloquism
somnipathy
somnolence
somnolentia
somnolism
somopsychosis
Sonneberg's operation
Soto-Hall sign
space
    Broca's s.
    Magendie's s's
    subarachnoid s.
    subdural s.
spasm
spastic
spatula
    Cushing's s.
    Davis' s.
    Sachs' s.

spatula (*continued*)
    Woodson's s.
Spence-Adson forceps
Spence's forceps
sphenoethmoid
sphenofrontal
sphenoid
sphenoidal
sphenoidostomy
sphenoidotomy
sphenotemporal
Spielmeyer-Sjögren syndrome
Spielmeyer-Vogt disease
spina
    s. bifida
    s. bifida occulta
spinal cord
spine
spinobulbar
spinocerebellar
spinogalvanization
spinogram
spinous
splanchnicectomy
splanchnicotomy
splanknekotome. See
   splanchnicotomy.
splanknesektome. See
   splanchnicectomy.
splenium
    s. corporis callosi
spondylitis
spondylodesis
spondylolisthesis
spondylolysis
spondylomalacia
spondylopathy
spondylopyosis
spondyloschisis
spondylosis
    s. chronica ankylopoi-
      etica

spondylosis (*continued*)
    rhizomelic s.
spondylosyndesis
spondylotomy
spongioblast
spongioblastoma
spongiocyte
spoon
    Cushing's s.
spot
    Trousseau's s.
spreader
    Turek's s.
    Wiltberger's s.
Spurling's
    forceps
    rongeur
stability
STA-MCA — superficial
    temporal artery to middle
    cerebral artery
stammering
Stanford-Binet test
stasiphobia
status
    s. choreicus
    s. convulsivus
    s. cribalis
    s. cribrosus
    s. dysgraphicus
    s. dysmyelinatus
    s. dysmyelinisatus
    s. dysraphicus
    s. epilepticus
    s. hemicranicus
    s. lacunaris
    s. lacunosus
    s. marmoratus
    petit mal s.
    s. spongiosus
    s. verrucosus
    s. vertiginosus

Stearn's alcoholic amentia
stefaneon. See *stephanion*.
Steiner's disease
stellate
stellectomy
stenion
stephanion
stereoencephalotomy
stereognosis
stereotactic
stereotaxis
stereotypy
Stevenson's
    forceps
    scissors
Stewart-Holmes sign
Stille-Gigli saw
Stille-Liston forceps
Stille-Luer
    forceps
    rongeur
Stille's
    drill
    osteotome
stimulate
stimuli
stimulus
stratum
    s. album profundum
      corporis quadrigemini
    s. gangliosum cerebelli
    s. gelatinosum
    s. granulosum cerebelli
    s. griseum centrale
      cerebri
    s. griseum colliculi
      superioris
    s. interolivare lemnisci
    s. moleculare cerebelli
    s. nucleare medullae
      oblongatae
    s. olfactorium

stratum (*continued*)
    s. opticum
    s. pyramidale
    s. reticulatum
    s. zonale corporis
       quadrigemini
    s. zonale thalami
strephosymbolia
stria
    s. fornicis
    habenular s.
    s. lancisii
    s. medullaris thalami
    meningitic s.
    olfactory s.
    s. pinealis
    s. terminalis
striae
    Francke's s.
    s. medullares acusticae
    s. medullares fossae
       rhomboideae
    s. medullares ventriculi
       quarti
strikninomanea. See
    strychninomania.
stroke
Stromeyer's cephalhematocele
strontium
    radioactive s.
Strully's scissors
Strümpell's
    reflex
    sign
strychninomania
Stryker's frame
stupor
    anergic s.
    delusion s.
    epileptic s.
    lethargic s.
    postconvulsive s.

stuporous
Sturge's disease
Sturge-Weber-Dimitri disease
Sturge-Weber syndrome
stuttering
    labiochoreic s.
St. Vitus' dance
subarachnoid
subarachnoiditis
subconscious
subconsciousness
subcortical
subdural
subgaleal
subjective
sublimate
sublimation
subpial
subpontine
substance
    white s. of Schwann
substantia
    s. alba
    s. cinerea
    s. corticalis cerebelli
    s. gelatinosa
    s. grisea
    s. innominata
    s. nigra
    s. perforata
    s. reticularis alba gyri
       fornicati
    s. reticularis alba
       medullae oblongatae
    s. reticularis grisea
       medullae oblongatae
    s. Rolandi
substitution
subthalamus
suction tube
    Adson's s.t.
    Frazier's s.t.

suction tube (*continued*)
    Sachs' s.t.
sudo-. See words beginning
    pseudo-.
Sugar's clip
suicidal
suicide
sulci
sulcus
    anterolateral s.
    s. basilaris pontis
    calcarine s.
    callosal s.
    cingulate s.
    s. circularis
    s. collateralis
    s. corporis callosi
    s. hippocampi
    s. hypothalamicus
    lateral s.
    s. limitans
    s. lunatus
    medial frontal s.
    median s.
    oculomotor s.
    paramedial s.
superdural
superego
supination
suppression
surgical procedures. See
    operation.
surrogate
suture. See *General Surgical*
    Terms.
Sweet's forceps
Sydenham's chorea
sylvian
Sylvii
    cisterna S.
    cisterna fossae S.

Sylvius
    aqueduct of S.
    cistern of fossa of S.
    cistern of S.
    fissure of S.
    ventricle of S.
symbiosis
symbol
    phallic s.
symbolism
symbolization
symbolophobia
sympathectomy
    chemical s.
    lumbar s.
    periarterial s.
sympathetic
sympatheticomimetic
sympatheticoparalytic
sympatheticotonia
sympatheticotonic
sympathicoblastoma
sympathicodiaphtheresis
sympathicogonioma
sympathicopathy
sympathicotherapy
sympathicotripsy
sympathicus
sympathin
sympatholytic
sympathomimetic
sympathy
symptom
    Bonhoeffer's s.
    Ganser's s.
    Haenel's s.
    Oehler's s.
    Seguin's signal s.
    Trendelenburg's s.
synapse
    axodendritic s.

synapse (*continued*)
    axodendrosomatic s.
    axosomatic s.
synclonus
syncopal
syncope
syndrome
    acute organic brain s.
    Adie's s.
    alcohol withdrawal s.
    Alzheimer's s.
    Apert's s.
    Arnold-Chiari s.
    Baastrup's s.
    Babinski-Nageotte s.
    Babinski's s.
    Balint's s.
    Bárány's s.
    Barré-Liéou s.
    Bärtschi-Rochain's s.
    Beard's s.
    Beck's s.
    Blackfan-Diamond s.
    Bonnet's s.
    Briquet's s.
    Brissaud-Sicard s.
    Bristowe's s.
    Brown-Séquard s.
    Bruns' s.
    callosal s.
    Capgras's s.
    capsular thrombosis s.
    capsulothalamic s.
    Céstan-Chenais s.
    Claude's s.
    Cotard's s.
    Cushing's s.
    Dandy-Walker s.
    Dejerine-Roussy s.
    Dejerine's s.
    Dennie-Marfan s.
    De Sanctis-Cacchione s.

syndrome (*continued*)
    Devic's s.
    Down's s.
    Erb's s.
    Foix-Alajouanine s.
    Foville's s.
    Friderichsen-Waterhouse s.
    Friedmann's vasomotor s.
    Fröhlich's s.
    Froin's s.
    Ganser's s.
    Garcin's s.
    Gélineau's s.
    Gerstmann's s.
    Gilles de la Tourette's s.
    Gowers' s.
    Gradenigo's s.
    Guillain-Barré s.
    Hallervorden-Spatz s.
    Homén's s.
    Horton's s.
    Hunt's striatal s.
    Hurler's s.
    Jackson's s.
    Jakob-Cruetzfeldt s.
    Kanner's s.
    Kiloh-Nevin s.
    Klippel-Feil s.
    Klippel-Feldstein s.
    Klüver-Bucy s.
    Korsakoff's s.
    Lennox's s.
    Marchiafava-Bignami s.
    Ménière's s.
    Millard-Gubler s.
    Möbius' s.
    Munchausen's s.
    Naffziger's s.
    Nothnagel's s.
    organic brain s.
    Parinaud's s.

syndrome (*continued*)
    Parkinson's s.
    Parry-Romberg s.
    Raeder's s.
    Ramsay-Hunt s.
    Rimbaud-Passouant-
      Vallat s.
    Roussy-Cornil s.
    scalenus anticus s.
    Shy-Drager s.
    Sjögren-Larssen s.
    Spielmeyer-Sjögren s.
    Sturge-Weber s.
    subclavian steal s.
    trisomy D s.
    trisomy E s.
    trisomy 13-15 s.
    trisomy 16-18 s.
    trisomy 18 s.
    trisomy 21 s.
    Vogt-Koyanagi-Harada's
      s.
    Vogt's s.
    Wallenberg's s.
    Waterhouse-Friderichsen
      s.
    Wernicke-Korsakoff s.
synesthesia
synesthesialgia
synkinesis
synreflexia
syntactic
syntaxis
synthesis
syntonic
syphilis
syphilophobia
syphilopsychosis
syringobulbia
syringocele
syringocoele

syringoencephalia
syringoencephalomyelia
syringomeningocele
syringomyelia
    s. atrophica
syringomyelitis
syringomyelocele
syringomyelus
syringopontia
system
    autonomic nervous s.
    central nervous s.
    Conolly's s.
    peripheral nervous s.
    Pinel's s.
tabes
    cerebral t.
    diabetic t.
    t. dorsalis
    t. ergotica
    Friedreich's t.
    t. spinalis
    vessel t.
tabetic
taboparesis
tache
    t. cerebrale
    t. meningeale
    t. spinale
tachyphrasia
tachyphrenia
taedium
    t. vitae
taenia
    t. chorioidea
    t. cinerea
    t. fimbriae
    t. fornicis
    t. hippocampi
    t. medullaris thalami
      optici

taenia (*continued*)
- t. pontis
- t. semicircularis corporis striati
- t. tectae
- t. thalami
- t. violacea

taeniae
- t. acusticae
- t. telarum

tahsh. See *tache.*

tantalum sheet

tapeinocephaly

tapetum
- t. corporis callosi
- t. ventriculi

tasikinesia

TAT — thematic apperception test

Taylor's
- retractor
- scissors

Tay-Sachs disease

tectospinal

tedeum. See *taedium.*

tegmental

tegmentum
- hypothalamic t.
- t. of pons
- t. rhombencephali
- subthalamic t.

tela
- t. choroidea

telencephalon

telepathy

temp. dext. — to the right temple

tempora

temporal

temporalis

temporoauricular

temporofacial

temporofrontal

temporohyoid

temporomalar

temporomandibular

temporomaxillary

temporo-occipital

temporoparietal

temporopontile

temporosphenoid

temporozygomatic

temp. sinist. — to the left temple

tenia
- t. choroidea
- t. telae

teniola

tentorium
- t. cerebelli
- t. of hypophysis

tephromalacia

tephromyelitis

tereon. See *pterion.*

test
- Bárány's pointing t.
- Bender-Gestalt t.
- Ebbinghaus' t.
- edrophonium t.
- finger-nose t.
- finger-to-finger t.
- Halstead-Reitan t.
- heel-knee t.
- Janet's t.
- Minnesota Multiphasic Personality Inventory t.
- Pandy's t.
- Patrick's t.
- projective human figure drawing t.
- Reitan-Indiana aphasic screening t.
- Rorschach t.
- Stanford-Binet t.

test (*continued*)
    thematic apperception t.
    Tobey-Ayer t.
    Wada's t.
    Walter's bromide t.
    Wechsler's Adult Intelligence Scale t.
    Wechsler's Intelligence Scale for Children t.
    Wittenborn Psychiatric Rating Scale t.
    Yerkes-Bridges t.
    Ziehen's t.
tetraplegia
thalamencephalic
thalamencephalon
thalami
thalamic
thalamocele
thalamocortical
thalamolenticular
thalamotegmental
thalamotomy
thalamus
theory
    Adler's t.
    Freud's t.
    Gestalt t.
    Meyer's t.
therapy
    beam t.
    behavior t.
    carbon dioxide t.
    convulsive shock t.
    drug t.
    electric convulsive t.
    electroshock t.
    family t.
    group t.
    Indoklon t.
    lithium t.
    milieu t.

therapy (*continued*)
    play t.
    sex t.
    shock t.
Thomas' sign
Thomsen's disease
Throckmorton's reflex
thromboangiitis
    t. obliterans
thrombosis
thrombus
thymergastic
thymopathy
TIA — transient ischemic attack
tic
    t. de pensée
    t. de sommeil
    t. douloureux
    t. nondouloureux
Tinel's sign
titubation
    lingual t.
tizeo-. See words beginning *phthisio-*.
Tobey-Ayer test
Todd's paralysis
tolerance
tomography
    computed t.
tongs
    Barton-Cone t.
    Cherry's t.
    Crutchfield-Raney t.
    Crutchfield's t.
tonsil
    t. of cerebellum
tonsilla
    t. cerebelli
    t. of cerebellum
tonus
    neurogenic t.

topagnosis
topectomy
Torkildsen's operation
torticollis
tosis. See *ptosis.*
Tourette's disease
Tower's retractor
toxiphrenia
trabecula
    t. cerebri
    t. cinerea
    t. cranii
trabs
    t. cerebri
trachelism
trachelismus
tract
    Burdach's t.
    cerebellorubral t.
    cerebellorubrospinal t.
    cerebellospinal t.
    extrapyramidal t.
    Foville's t.
    Goll's t.
    Gowers' t.
    Helweg's t.
    Lissauer's t.
    Meynert's t.
    spinocerebellar t.
    tectospinal t.
tractotomy
    mesencephalic t.
trait
trance
tranquilizer
transference
transorbital
transsexual
transsexualism
transvestism
trauma
    psychic t.

traumasthenia
treatment
    Weir Mitchell t.
tremor
    epileptoid t.
    flapping t.
    Hunt's t.
    intention t.
    intermittent t.
    kinetic t.
    t. linguae
    motofacient t.
    t. potatorum
    Rendu's t.
    striocerebellar t.
    volitional t.
tremulous
Trendelenburg's symptom
trephination
trephine
    DeVilbiss' t.
    Galt's t.
trichologia
trichotillomania
tricyclic
trigone
trigonocephaly
trigonum
    t. acustici
    t. cerebrale
    t. collaterale
    t. habenulae
    t. lemnisci
    t. nervi hypoglossi
    t. olfactorium
triplegia
trismus
trisomy D, E, 13-15, 16-18, 18, 21
Trousseau's
    phenomenon
    sign

Trousseau's (*continued*)
    spot
    twitching
truncal
truncus
    t. corporis callosi
    t. lumbosacralis
    t. sympathicus
trypanosomiasis
tube
    Pudenz' t.
tuber
    t. annulare
    t. anterius hypothalami
    t. cinereum
    t. vermis
tubercle
    Babès' t.
    t. of Rolando
tuberculoma
    t. en plaque
tuberculum
Tuffier-Raney retractor
Tuffier's retractor
tumor
    Cushing's t.
    Rathke's t.
Turek's spreader
Turyn's sign
twitch
twitching
    fascicular t.
    fibrillar t.
    Trousseau's t.
type
    Kretschmer t's
ufor-. See words beginning
   euphor-.
ulegyria
Ullrich's retractor
ululation
uncinate

unconscious
uncus
underhorn
unoia. See *eunoia*.
Unverricht's disease
urolagnia
urophobia
vadum
vagabondage
vagal
vagotomy
vagotonia
vallecula
    v. cerebelli
    v. sylvii
Valsalva's maneuver
valve
    Pudenz' v.
Vanzetti's sign
varix
    aneurysmoid v.
varolian
velamenta cerebri
velum
    medullary v.
ventral
ventricle
    v. of Arantius
    v's of the brain
    v. of cerebrum
    v. of cord
    Duncan's v.
    Krause's v.
    v. of myelon
    v. of Sylvius
    terminal v. of spinal cord
    Verga's v.
    Vieussen's v.
ventricornu
ventricornual
ventricose
ventricular

ventriculitis
ventriculoatriostomy
ventriculocisternostomy
ventriculogram
ventriculography
ventriculometry
ventriculoperitoneal
ventriculopuncture
ventriculoscope
ventriculoscopy
ventriculostium
ventriculostomy
ventriculosubarachnoid
ventriculus
    v. dexter cerebri
    v. lateralis cerebri
    v. quartus cerebri
    v. sinister cerebri
    v. terminalis medullae
      spinalis
    v. tertius cerebri
Veraguth's fold
verbigeration
verbomania
Verga's ventricle
vermis
    v. cerebelli
Verneuil's neuroma
vertebra
    basilar v.
    v. dentata
    v. magnum
    odontoid v.
    v. plana
    prominent v.
    sternal v.
vertebrae
    cervical v.
    coccygeal v.
    lumbar v.
    sacral v.
    thoracic v.

vertebral
vertex
    v. cranii
    v. cranii ossei
vertiginous
vertigo
    central v.
    encephalic v.
    epileptic v.
    hysterical v.
    neurasthenic v.
    paralyzing v.
    vestibular v.
vesania
vibratory
vicious
Vieussen's
    ansa
    ventricle
visuopsychic
vitselzookt. See *witzelsucht.*
Vogt-Koyanagi-Harada's
    syndrome
Vogt's
    disease
    syndrome
volatile
volition
volitional
Volkman's curet
von Hippel-Lindau disease
von Recklinghausen's disease
voyeurism
vulnerability
vulnerable
Vulpian's atrophy
Wada's test
WAIS — Wechsler's Adult
          Intelligence Scale
Wallenberg's syndrome
wallerian
    degeneration

wallerian (*continued*)
    law
Walter's bromide test
Ward-French needle
Wartenberg's sign
Waterhouse-Friderichsen
    syndrome
wave
    alpha w's
    beta w's
    brain w's
    delta w's
    random w's
    theta w's
Weber's
    disease
    sign
Wechsler's Adult Intelligence
    Scale test
Wechsler's Intelligence Scale
    for Children test
Weck's clip
WEE — western equine
    encephalomyelitis
Weir Mitchell treatment
Weitlaner's retractor
Werdnig-Hoffmann
    atrophy
    paralysis
Wernicke-Korsakoff syndrome
Wernicke's
    area
    disease
    encephalopathy
Wertheim's clamp
Westphal's sign
Wilde's forceps
Willis' circle
Wiltberger's spreader
wing
    sphenoid w.
Winkelman's disease

WISC — Wechsler's Intelligence
    Scale for Children
withdrawal
Wittenborn Psychiatric Rating
    Scale test
witzelsucht
Woodson's
    elevator
    spatula
WPRS — Wittenborn Psychi-
    atric Rating Scale
xanthochromia
xanthochromic
xanthocyanopsia
xanthogranulomatosis
xenophobia
Yasargil's
    clip
    retractor
Yerkes-Bridges test
zan-. See words beginning *xan-*.
zelotypia
zenophobia. See *xenophobia*.
Ziehen-Oppenheim disease
Ziehen's test
zona
    z. reticularis
    z. rolandica
    z. spongiosa
zoophobia
Zuckerkandl's convolution
zygion
zygoma
zygomatic
zygomaticofacial
zygomaticofrontal
zygomaticomaxillary
zygomatico-orbital
zygomaticosphenoid
zygomaticotemporal
zygomaxillary

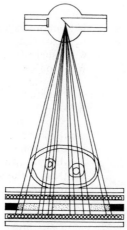

CASSETTE
FRONT FLUORESCING SCREEN
FILM WITH LATENT IMAGE
BACK FLUORESCING SCREEN
CASSETTE

Cassette Front		Bakelite
Intensifying Screen		Cardboard Backing / Calcium Tungstate
X-ray Film		Silver Bromide Crystals / Cellulose Acetate Base / Silver Bromide Crystals
Intensifying Screen		Calcium Tungstate / Cardboard Backing
Backing		Felt Cushion Back
Cassette Back		Steel Back

SPRING STEEL

(Courtesy of Meschan, I.: Radiographic Positioning and Related Anatomy, 2nd ed. Fig. 2-9, p. 26. Philadelphia, W. B. Saunders Company, 1978.)

RADIOLOGY AND
NUCLEAR MEDICINE

abduction
aberrant
aberration
    chromatid-type a.
    chromosome a.
    commatic a.
abnormalities
abscopal
absorbance
absorbed fraction
absorber
absorptiometer
absorption
    a. coefficient
Acacia
acanthus
accelerated
accelerator
    linear a.
acetabular rim
acetabulum
acetic anhydride
acetrizoate sodium
acetylated
acetylation
acinar-like
actinium

actinogen
actinogenesis
actinogram
actinograph
actinography
actinokymography
actinon
actinopraxis
actinoscopy
activation
adduction
AEC — Atomic Energy Com-
    mission
afterglow
agent
    contrast a.
aggregated
air
    a. bronchogram
    a. insufflation
    a. monitor
air-space disease
Albers-Schönberg position
albumin
    iodinated I 125 serum a.
    iodinated I 131 serum a.
    macroaggregated a.

771

aldosterone
algebraic reconstruction technique
alignment
allowed beta transition
alpha
    a. chamber
    a. decay
    a. particle
    a. radiation
    a. ray
    a. threshold
alumina
aluminum
alveolar
alveoli
americium
Amipaque contrast medium
amniography
A-mode — amplitude modulation
    A-m. ultrasonography
ampere
amphoteric
amplification
    gas a.
amplifier
    buffer a.
    linear a.
    nuclear pulse a.
    pulse a.
    voltage a.
ampulla
    a. of Vater
a.m.u. — atomic mass unit
analog
    a. computations
    a. photo
    a. rate meter
analog-to-digital converter
analysis
    activation a.

analysis (*continued*)
    chemical a.
    correlation a.
    least-squares a.
    regression a.
    saturation a.
analyzers
    multichannel a.
ancillary
Anger camera
angiocardiogram
angiocardiography
    intravenous a.
    radionuclide a.
    selective a.
    venous a.
Angioconray contrast medium
angiogram
angiography
    biliary a.
    carotid a.
    cerebral a.
    peripheral a.
    renal a.
    vertebral a.
    visceral a.
angiology
angioscintigraphy
angle
    a. board
    cardiophrenic a.
    subcarinal a.
Angstrom unit
anion
annihilation radiation
anode
    rotating a.
    stationary a.
anomalous
anteflexion
antegrade
anteroposterior view

anteversion
antibody
anticoincidence circuit
antigenic
antimony
antineutrino
antiparticle
antiproton
antrum
aortic
    a. arch
    a. knob
aortogram
aortography
    abdominal a.
    catheter a.
    lumbar a.
    retrograde a.
    selective visceral a.
    thoracic a.
    translumbar a.
    venous a.
    visceral a.
AP — anteroposterior
apical
appearance
    "coiled-spring" a.
    double-bubble a.
    "inverse comma" a.
    "pruned-tree" a.
applecore-like
areae gastricae
argon
ARRT — American Registry of Radiologic Technologists
arsenic
arteriogram
    coronary a.
    "pruned-tree" a.
    wedge a.

arteriography
    brachiocephalic a.
    carotid a.
    celiac a.
    cerebral a.
    coronary a.
    femoral a.
    mesenteric a.
    peripheral a.
    pulmonary a.
    renal a.
    selective a.
    vertebral a.
    visceral a.
arterioles
arthrogram
    double-contrast a.
arthrography
    air a.
    double-contrast a.
    opaque a.
articulation
artifact
ASRT — American Society of Radiologic Technologists
assay
    erythropoietin a.
astatine
asymmetry
atelectasis
atlas (C-1) (vertebra)
atom
    Na a's
    a. smasher
    tagged a.
atomic
    a. energy
    a. mass unit
    a. number
    a. spectrum

atomic (*continued*)
    a. weight
atrophy
attenuation
    a. coefficient
attenuator
Auger
    effect
    electron
autocorrelation function
autofluoroscope
    digital a.
autoradiograph
autoradiography
    contact a.
    dip-coating a.
    film-stripping a.
    thick-layer a.
    two-emulsion a.
autotomography
autotransformer formula
avalanche
    Townsend's a.
average life
Avogadro's number
axial
axis (C-2) (vertebra)
axis
    vertical a.
azygography
azygos vein
B — Bucky (film in cassette in
    Potter-Bucky diaphragm)
    tomogram with oscillating
    Bucky
BA — barium
background
    b. activity
    b. count
    b. erase

background (*continued*)
    b. radiation
backscatter
    b. peak
Ball's method
balsa wood block
barium
    b. enema
    b. meal
    b. sulfate
    b. swallow
barn
"barrel chest"
barreling distortion
basilar
basket cells
Bayes' theorem
BBB — blood-brain barrier
BE — barium enema
beam
    useful b.
Béclére's position
BEI — butanol-extractable
    iodine
Benassi's position
berkelium
beryllium
beta
    b. decay
    b. emitter
    b. particle
    b. radiation
    b.-ray
    b. transition
betatron
BEV — billion electron volts
bevatron
bezoar
biliary
Bilopaque contrast medium

bimolecular
binding energy
bioassay
    erythropoietin b.
biological half life
biopsy
biosynthesis
bisacodyl tannex
bismuth
Blackett-Healy position
block
    alveolar-capillary b.
    balsa wood b.
blood flow study
    cerebral b.f.s.
    pulmonary b.f.s.
blood pool
    b.p. imaging
    b.p. scan
blood volume measurements
blurring
B-mode − brightness modula-
        tion
BOBA − beta-oxybutyric acids
Bohr
    B. equation
    B. radius
bolus
bombardment
bone
    b. marrow scanning
    b. scan
    b. seeker
boron
brachytherapy
Bragg
    curve
    peak
brain scan
"braking" radiation
branch

branching
    b. decay
    b. fraction
    b. ratio
breeder reactor
bregma
bremsstrahlung
broad-beam scattering
Broden's position
bromine
bronchogram
bronchography
    Cope-method b.
    percutaneous trans-
        tracheal b.
bronchopulmonary
bronchoradiography
bronchoscopy
    fiberoptic b.
    nonfiberoptic b.
bronchus
    lower lobe b.
    main stem b.
    middle lobe b.
    upper lobe b.
BSP − Bromsulphalein
bubble-like
Bucky grid
bunamiodyl
c. − curie
cadmium
calcific
    c. shadows
calcification
calcium (with scandium 47)
calculogram
calculography
calculus
    ureteral c.
Caldwell-Moloy method
Caldwell's position

calibration
  E-dial c.
calibrator
  digital isotope c.
  radioisotope c.
calices
caliectasis
californium
calorie
camera
  Anger c.
  gamma c.
  Medx c.
  positron scintillation c.
  radioisotope c.
  scintillation c.
  video display c.
Camp-Coventry position
Camp-Gianturco method
Cannon's ring
Cantor's tube
capacitance
capture
  cross section
  gamma rays
carbon
  c. dioxide
cardiac
  c. output
  c. shunt detection
cardioangiography
  retrograde c.
Cardiografin contrast medium
cardiophrenic
cardiopulmonary
cardioscan
carina
carrier
  c.-free radioisotope
cartilaginous
cassette
  camp grid c.

CAT — chlormerodrin accumulation test
  computed axial tomography
catabolism
cataphoresis
catenary system
catheterization
  cardiac c.
cathode
caudad
caudal
cavography
cb — cardboard or plastic film holder without intensifying screens
CBG — corticosteroid-binding globulin
CCK — cholecystokinin
cecum
cell
  polygonal c.
  reticuloendothelial c.
cephalad
cephalic
cephalometry
  ultrasonic c.
Cerenkov radiation production
cerium
ceruloplasmin
cesium (with barium 137m)
chamber
  ionization c.
  multiwire proportional c.
  spark c.
  Wilson c.
charcoal
Chassard-Lapiné projection
Chausse's view
chemotherapeutic
chemotherapy
Cherenkov counter

chlorine
chlormerodrin
    c.-cysteine
    c. Hg 197
    c. Hg 203
cholangiogram
    endoscopic retrograde c.
    intraoperative c.
    intravenous c.
    operative c.
    percutaneous trans-
       hepatic c.
    retrograde c.
    transhepatic c.
    T-tube c.
cholangiography
    delayed operative c.
    direct percutaneous
       transhepatic c.
    intraoperative c.
    intravenous c.
    operative c.
    percutaneous hepato-
       biliary c.
    percutaneous trans-
       hepatic c.
    postoperative c.
    transabdominal c.
    transhepatic c.
    T-tube c.
cholangiopancreatography
    endoscopic retrograde c.
cholangiotomogram
Cholebrine contrast medium
cholecystocholangiography
cholecystogram
cholecystography
    intravenous c.
    oral c.
cholecystokinin
choledochogram
choledochograph

choledochography
cholegraphy
cholescintigram
Cholografin contrast medium
    C. methylglucamine
chromatid-type aberration
chromatoelectrophoretic
chromatography
chromic phosphate P 32
chromium
    c. Cr 51 serum albumin
chromosome
    c.-type aberration
Ci — curie
cineangiocardiography
cineangiograph
cineangiography
cinedensigraphy
cinefluorography
cinefluoroscopy
cinematography
cinematoradiography
cinephlebography
cineradiography
cineroentgenofluorography
cineroentgenography
circle of confusion
circuit
    anticoincidence c.
    coincidence c.
    magnetic c.
    phototube output c.
circuitry
cisternal puncture
cisternography
    radionuclide c.
cisternomyelography
clavicle
Cleaves' position
clinoids
cloud chamber
Clysodrast contrast medium

coarsening
cobalt
Cobb's method
coded-aperture imaging
Codman's triangle
coefficient
    linear absorption c.
    mass absorption c.
    partition c.
coeur en sabot
coffin
coincidence
    c. circuit
    c. counting
    c. loss
    c. sum peak
coinlike
Colcher-Sussman method
cold
    c. lesion
    c. spot
collecting system
collimate
collimation
collimator
    automatic c.
    converging c.
    diverging c.
    focusing c.
    multihole c.
    parallel-hole c.
    pin-hole c.
    single-hole c.
    thick-septa c.
    thin-septa c.
colloid
colloidal gold
colon
    ascending c.
    descending c.
    transverse c.
colorimetric

colorimetrically
combined transmission-emission scintiphoto
compartmental analysis
complex
    chlormerodrin-cysteine c.
compression
Compton
    C. edge
    C. effect
    C. electron
    C. photon
    C. scattering
    C. wavelength
computed tomography
computer
computerized
concept
    "ring of bone" c.
condenser
conductivity
    thermal c.
conductor
cone
coned-down view
confluent
conical
Conray contrast medium
constant
    permeability c.
    Planck's c.
constriction
contamination
contour
contrast media
    acetrizoate sodium
    Amipaque
    Angioconray
    barium sulfate
    Bilopaque
    bunamiodyl
    Cardiografin

coprecipitation
coprolith
Corbin technique
coronal
corresponding ray
cortex
corticosteroids
cosmotron
costophrenic
costotransverse
costovertebral
cotton-wool appearance
coulomb force
count density
counter
    boron c.
    Cherenkov c.
    Geiger-Müller c.
    proportional c.
    radiation c.
    scintillation c.
    whole-body c.
counting rate meter
craniad
crater
    ulcer c.
^{51}Cr-heated RBC's
critical mass
cross-fire treatment
cryptoscope
    Satvioni's c.
cryptoscopy
CT — computed tomography
CT body scanner
curie
curium
current
    alternating c.
    direct c.
    eddy c.
    pulsating c.
    saturation c.

current (*continued*)
    single-phase c.
    three-phase c.
    unidirectional c.
curve
    Bragg c.
cut
    tomographic c.
Cutie Pie
CXR — chest x-ray
cyanocobalamin Co 57, Co 58, Co 60
cycle
    Krebs c.
    pentose c.
cyclotron
cysteine
Cystografin contrast medium
cystogram
    triple-voiding c.
cystography
    radionuclide c.
    retrograde c.
    triple-voiding c.
Cystokon contrast medium
cystoscopy
cystoureterography
cystourethrogram
    micturition c.
    retrograde c.
    voiding c.
cystourethrography
    expression c.
    radionuclide voiding c.
    retrograde c.
    voiding c.
D — mean dose
dacryocystography
data
    ferrokinetic d.
datacamera
daughter nuclide

DDC — direct display console
de Broglie wavelength
decade scaler
decay
     alpha d.
     beta d.
     d. constant
     exponential d.
     isomeric d.
     d. mode
     positron d.
     d. product
     radioactive d.
     d. scheme
decontamination
decubitus
dee
de-excitation
defecography
defect
     filling d.
     napkin-ring d.
deflation
deflection
deformity
     cloverleaf d.
     valgus d.
     varus d.
delimitation
delineation
delta ray
demarcation
     no line of d.
     "shell-like" d.
denatured
densitometer
densitometry
density
     background d.
     calcific d.
     inherent d.
     ionization d.

densography
6-deoxy-1-galactose
deoxyribonucleic acid
descending
detection
     beta d.
detector
     dielectric track d.
     semiconductor d.
     tissue-equivalent d.
deuterium
deuteron
dextrogram
DI — diagnostic imaging
diaphragm
     Potter-Bucky d.
diaphragmatic
diapositive
diatrizoate meglumine
diatrizoate sodium
diethyltriamine-penta-acetic
     acid
diffusion
digital
diisofluorophosphate
dimerization
Diodrast contrast medium
Dionosil contrast medium
dioxide
diphenyloxazole
diphosphonate
diploë
dipolar
dipole
diprotrizoate
discography
discoid
discriminator
disintegration
diskogram
diskography
distal

distended
distortion
    pin-cushion d.
distribution
    depth dose d.
    gaussian d.
    maxwellian d.
    Poisson d.
    spatial dose d.
DNA — deoxyribonucleic acid
Doerner-Hoskins distribution
    law
dominance
Dooley, Caldwell and Glass
    method
Doppler
    D. effect
    D. ultrasound
dorsal
dose
    absorbed d.
    cumulative d.
    depth d.
    doubling d.
    erythema d.
    d. estimate
    exit d.
    genetically significant d.
    integral d.
    lethal d.
    maximum permissible d.
    mean d.
    nominal single d.
    organ tolerance d.
    d. reciprocity theorem
    threshold erythema d.
    tissue tolerance d.
    tumor lethal d.
dosimeter
    pencil d.
    pocket d.
    thermoluminescent d.

dosimeter (*continued*)
    ultraviolet fluorescent d.
    Victoreen d.
dosimetric
dosimetry
    pion d.
dot scan
"double-bubble"
double-contrast
"doughnut" sign
DPTA — diethylenetriamine
        penta-acetic acid
drugs. See *Drugs and
    Chemistry* section.
DTPA — diethyltriamine penta-
        acetic acid
duct
    common bile d.
    cystic d.
    hepatic d.
    pancreatic d.
ductography
    peroral retrograde pan-
        creaticobiliary d.
duodenal
    d. bulb
    d. loop
    d. papilla
duodenogram
duodenography
    hypotonic d.
duodenum
Duografin contrast medium
D-xylose
dye
    halogenated phenol-
        phthalein d.
    rose bengal d.
Dynapix
Dyne
dynode
dysphagia

dysprosium
echocardiography
echoencephalography
echogram
echolaminography
edge
> Compton e.
> e. packing

E-dial calibration
EDR — effective direct radiation
>> electrodermal response

EEG — electroencephalogram
effect
> Auger e.
> Compton e.
> Doppler e.
> isotope e.

effective
> e. half-life
> e. renal plasma flow

einsteinium
ejection fraction
elastic collision
electrokymogram
electrokymograph
electrokymography
electrolyte
electromagnetic
> e. induction
> e. radiation

electrometer
> dynamic-condenser e.
> vibrating-reed e.

electron
> Auger e.
> bound e.
> e. capture
> Compton e.
> e. multiplier tube
> secondary e.

electron (*continued*)
> e. volt

electronneutrino
electrophoretically
electrophoresis
electroscope
electrostatic
element
> daughter e.
> parent e.

ellipsoid
elliptical
Elon
elutriation
Embden-Meyerhof glycolytic pathway
EMI — Electric and Musical Industries (scanner)
emission
> photoelectric e.
> thermonic e.

emitter
emulsion
> nuclear e.

encephalogram
encephalography
encephalometry
endoergic reaction
endoscopy
enema
> barium e.
> cleansing e.
> opaque e.

energy
> binding e.
> e. frequency
> kinetic e.
> photon e.
> potential e.
> radiant e.
> e. resolution

energy (*continued*)
    thermal e.
    e. wavelength
enteropathy
    exudative e.
enzyme
epididymography
epididymovesiculography
epigastrium
equation
    Bohr e.
equilibrium
    radioactive e.
    secular e.
    transient e.
equivalence
    mass energy e.
erbium
ERCP — endoscopic retrograde
       cholangiopancre-
       atography
Erlenmeyer flask–like
ERPF — effective renal plasma
       flow
erythropoietin
esofa-. See words beginning
    esopha-.
esophagogram
esophagography
esophagram
Ethiodane contrast medium
ethiodized oil
Ethiodol contrast medium
Euler's number
europium
eV — electron volt
eversion
examination
    double-contrast e.
expiration
exponential
extension

extrapolate
E-zero offset
faceted
faceting
factor
    intrinsic f.
    geometry f.
fasciagram
fasciagraphy
fatty meal
feather analysis
Feist-Mankin position
femoral
    f. head
    f. neck
    f. shaft
Ferguson's method
fermium
ferrokinetics
ferrous citrate Fe 59
fetography
FEV — forced expiratory
      volume
fibrosis
Fick's
    law
    position
    principle
filling defect
film
    f. badge
    comparison f.
    f. density calibration
    lateral decubitus f.
    plain f.
    prone f.
    rapid processing f.
    sequential f.
    serial f.
filter
    inherent f.
    Thoreau's f.

filtration
fission
fistulogram
fistulography
fixer
fixing time
flail chest
"flank stripe"
flask-like
    Erlenmeyer f.-l.
fleb-. See words beginning
    phleb-.
Fleischner's position
flexion
flexure
flocculent
flood source
floppy disk
fluorescence
fluorescent scan
fluorine F 18
fluoroscope
fluoroscopic
fluoroscopy
    digital f.
    image-amplified f.
flurescence. See *fluorescence*.
fluroskope. See *fluoroscope*.
fluroskopic. See *fluoroscopic*.
fluoroskopy. See *fluoroscopy*.
flux
fluxes
focal
    f. spot
    f. zone
foramen
    f. lacerum
    f. magnum
    obturator f.
    f. ovale
    f. spinosum
foreign body

formatter
formula
    autotransformer f.
    projection f.
fossa
fraction
    penetration f.
    scatter f.
fractional
fractionation
francium
free peritoneal air
Fresnel zone plate
Friedman's position
fucose
full-width at half-maximum
fundus
fusion
FWHM — full width at half
          maximum
FZ — focal zone
Ga — gallium
gadolinium
    g.-159 hydroxycitrate
galactose
gallium
    g. citrate Ga 67
    g. scanning
    radioactive g. Ga 67
galvanometer
gamma-aminobutyrate
gamma camera
gammaphoto
gamma-ray
    g.-r. spectra
gamma well counter
gantry
Gastrografin contrast medium
gastrointestinal
gaussian distribution
Gaynor-Hart position
Geiger-Müller counter

generator
    electrostatic g.
    polyphase g.
    resonance g.
    supervoltage g.
    three-phase g.
    Van de Graaff g.
genetic
geographic
geometrical efficiency
geometry factor
germanium
GFR — glomerular filtration
    rate
GI — gastrointestinal
Girout's method
glabella
glow modular tube
glucagon
gluconeogenesis
glucose
glutamate
gold Au 198
gonion
graininess
granuloma
Grashey's position
grid
    Bucky g.
    g. cassette (or oscillating
      g.)
    focused g.
    Potter-Bucky g.
ground state
GSD — genetically significant
    dose
gynecography
gynogram
Haas position
hafnium
"hair-on-end"
"hairpin" loop

half-life
    biological h.
    effective h.
    physical h.
half-thickness
half-time of exchange
half-value layer
"Hampton's hump"
haustra
heavy particle therapy
helium
hematocrit
    mean circulatory h.
"hemi-diaphragms"
hemithorax
hepatic flexure
hepatography
hepatosplenography
Heublein's method
Hg meralluride
Hickey's position
hilum
Hippuran contrast medium
histogram mode
historadiography
holmium
holography
homogeneous
homogeneously
honeycomb
    h. lung
hot lesion
Hounsfield unit
hourglass chest
HSA — human serum albumin
HVL — half-value layer
hybrid
hydrogen
    h. atom
hydronephrosis
hydroquinone
hydrothorax

hydroxycitrate
Hypaque contrast media
    H.-Cysto
    H. M.
    H. Meglumine
    H. Sodium
hyperlucency
hypertrophy
hypoaeration
hysterosalpingogram
hysterosalpingography
I — iodine
ilium
ill-defined
image
    i. converter
    x-ray i.
imaging
    diagnostic i.
    electrostatic i.
    gray-scale i.
immobilization device
    Pigg-O-Stat i.d.
immunoadsorbent
immunoassay
immunoelectrophoresis
immunofiltration
immunofluorescence
immunogenetics
immunoglobulin
IMPH — 1-iodomercuri-2-
    hydroxypropane
I_n chelate
indium
induction
industrial monitoring
inferior ramus
inflation
inherent
inhibition
inion

injection
    perinephric air i.
    transduodenal fiberscopic
      duct i.
insoluble
inspiration
insufflation
    perirenal i.
    retroperitoneal gas i.
insulinase
insulin-iodine
intensification factor
intensity
interaction
intercartilaginous rim
internal conversion
interspace
interstitial disease
interstitium
intertrochanteric
^{113m}In-transferrin
intraperitoneal
intrinsic
Intropaque contrast medium
intubation
intussusception
inverse square law
inversion
in vitro
in vivo
iodinated
    i. contrast media
    i. I 125 fibrinogen
    i. I 125 serum albumin
    i. I 131 aggregated
      albumin (human)
    i. I 131 serum albumin
      (human)
iodination
iodine
    i. PVP bond

iodine (*continued*)
    radioactive i.
iodipamide
iodoalphionic acid
iodohippurate sodium
iodomethamate
iodophthalein sodium
iodopyracet
ion
    amphoteric dipolar i.
ionization
ionizing
iopanoic acid
iophendylate
iophenoxic acid
iopydol
iopydone
iothalamate
ipodate calcium
IRA-400 resin
iridium
iron
    i. hydroxide
    radioactive i.
irradiated
irradiation
ischium
Isherwood's position
isobar
isobaric transition
isoelectric
isomer
isomeric transition
Isopaque contrast medium
isotone
isotope
    radioactive i.
IVC — intravenous cholangio-
       gram
IVP — intravenous pyelogram
jejunum

Johnson's position
joint mice
junction
    myoneural j.
    rectosigmoid j.
K-capture
Kerley's
    A line
    B line
ker-on-sa-bo. See *coeur en
    sabot.*
ketone bodies
kev. — kilo electron volts
kidney washout
kilocalorie
kilocurie
kilomegacycle
kilovolt
kilovoltage
kineradiography
kinescope
kinetic energy
kinetics
Kinevac contrast medium
kol. See words beginning *chol-.*
kolangi-. See words beginning
    cholangi-.
kole-. See words beginning
    chole-.
kolo-. See words beginning
    cholo-.
Krebs cycle
krypton
K-shell
KUB — plain view of abdomen
      (kidneys, ureters,
      bladder)
Kurzbauer's position
kymograph
kymography
    roentgen k.

lacelike
lambda
lambdoidal suture
laminagram
laminagraph
laminagraphy
laminated
lamination
laminogram
laminography
lamp
    Wood's l.
lanthanum
LAO — left anterior oblique
Laquerrière-Pierquin position
Larkin's position
laryngogram
laryngography
    contrast l.
laryngopharyngography
laser beam
laterality
latitude
Lauenstein and Hickey projection
law
    Doerner-Hoskins distribution l.
    Fick's l.
    l. of inertia
    inverse-square l.
    Ohm's l.
    l. of reciprocity
    l. of thermodynamics
Lawrence's position
lawrencium
Law's position
LD_{50} — median lethal dose
lead
lens
    Thorpe plastic l.

Leonard-George position
lepton
lesion
    annular l.
    sessile l.
LET — linear energy transfer
levogram
Lewis' position
licorice powder
ligament of Treitz
Lilienfeld's position
Lindblom's position
line
    acanthomeatal l.
    auricular l.
    canthomeatal l.
    glabelloalveolar l.
    glabellomeatal l.
    infraorbital l.
    infraorbitomeatal l.
    interorbital l.
    interpupillary l.
    Kerley's A l.
    Kerley's B l.
    McGregor's l.
    pubococcygeal l.
    Reid's base l.
linear
    l. accelerator
    l. attenuation
    l. compartmental system
    l. energy transfer
    l. focus
Lipiodol contrast medium
lipogenesis
lipping
Liquipake contrast medium
lithium
localization
loopogram
loose bodies

lopamidol
lordotic
>anteroposterior l. projection
>apical l. projection
Lorenz' position
Löw-Beer position
LPO – left posterior oblique
lucent
lumen
lung
>l. markings
>l. root
lutetium
lymphangiogram
lymphangiography
lymphography
MAA – macroaggregated albumin
macroaggregated
>m. albumin
macromolecules
magenblase
magic numbers
magnesium
magnet
>beam-bending m.
magnetic circuit
magnification
malum coxae senilis
mamillary system
mammogram
mammography
mandible
manganese
Mannitol
maplike
mass
>atomic m.
>intraluminal m.
>relativistic m.
Massiot polytome

mastogram
mastography
maxicamera
maxwellian distribution
Mayer's
>position
>view
mc., mCi – millicurie
μc., μCi – microcurie
McGregor's line
mean
>m. free path
>m. life
media
>contrast m.
medial
mediastinal
mediastinum
medium
>contrast m.
Medx
>M. camera
>M. scanner
Meese's position
megavoltage
meglumine
>m. diatrizoate
>m. iodipamide
>m. iothalamate
mendelevium
Mercuhydrin
mercurihydroxypropane
mercury
meson
metallic
metastable state
method
>Ball's m.
>Caldwell-Moloy m.
>Camp-Gianturco m.
>Cobb's m.
>Colcher-Sussman m.

method (*continued*)
    Dooley, Caldwell, and
      Glass m.
    Ferguson's m.
    Girout's m.
    Heublein's m.
    Monte Carlo m.
    Ottonello's m.
    parallax m.
    Parama's m.
    Pfeiffer-Comberg m.
    Sommer-Foegella m.
    Sweet's m.
    Thoms' m.
    Wolf's m.
    Zimmer's m.
methylcellulose gel
metoclopramide
metric
    m. system
metrizamide
metrizoate sodium
Mev. — million electron volts
MHP — 1-mercuri-2-hydroxy-
     propane
microangiogram
microcurie
microdosimetry
micron
microradiogram
microradiography
microsphere
microtron
Miller-Abbott tube
Miller's position
milliamperage
milliampere-minute
milliampere-second
millicurie
    m.-hour
milliequivalent
milligamma

milliliter
millimicrocurie
millimicrogram
milliroentgen
millisecond
milliunit
millivolt
minometer
MLD — median lethal dose
MMFR — maximum midexpira-
     tory flow rate
M-mode scanning
modulation
    image m.
    object m.
molar volume
molecular
    m. vibrations
molecule
molybdenum
monitor
    beam m.
    radiation m.
monitoring
Monte Carlo method
mosaic
Mossbauer spectrometer
mottled
MPD — maximum permissible
     dose
MTF — modulation transfer
     function
mucosa
multilanigraph
multiple-nuclide
multiscaler
mutation
myelogram
myelography
    opaque m.
Na atoms
nanocurie

narrow-beam half-thickness
nasion
nasopharyngography
nc., nCi — nanocurie
negatron
    n. emission
neodymium
Neo-Iopax contrast medium
neon
neostigmine
nephrogram
nephrography
nephrosonography
nephrostogram
nephrotomography
    infusion n.
nephrourography
neptunium
neuroradiology
neutrino
neutron
    epithermal n.
    fast n.
    intermediate n.
    n. number
    slow n.
    thermal n.
niche
nickel
niobium
nitrogen
nitrous oxide
nobelium
node
    lymph n's
    mesenteric n.
nodular
Nölke's position
nomogram
nonhomogeneous
nonlinearity
normalized plateau slope

Novopaque contrast medium
NSD — nominal single dose
nuclear
    n. emulsion
    n. energy
    n. fission
    n. medicine
    n. reactor
nuclease
nuclei
nucleide
nucleiform
nucleography
nucleoid
nucleoliform
nucleon
    n. number
nucleonics
nucleoprotein
nucleoreticulum
nucleoside
nucleotherapy
nucleotide
nucleus
nuclide
number
    Avogadro's n.
    Euler's n.
numo-. See words beginning
    pneumo-.
oblique
obliquity
obturator foramen
OCG — oral cholecystogram
odontoid
Ohm's law
OIH — orthoiodohippurate
oleic acid I 125
oncology
    radiation o.
opacification
opacified

opaque
operating voltage
Orabilex contrast medium
oragrafin calcium
oragrafin sodium
orbit
orbitography
orthodiagram
orthodiagraph
orthodiagraphy
orthodiascope
orthodiascopy
orthoiodohippurate
orthopantomography
orthoroentgenography
orthoskiagraph
orthovoltage
oscilloscope
osmium
osteoporosis
OTD — organ tolerance dose
Ottonello's method
overexposure
"overlap shadow"
overvoltage
oxidation
oxygen
^{32}P — radioactive phosphorus
PA — posteroanterior
packing fraction
PAH — para-aminohippurate
pair production
palatograph
palatography
palatomyograph
palladium
palliative
palmitate
palmitic acid
pancreatography
pangynecography
panography

Panorex
pantomographic
pantomography
        concentric p.
        eccentric p.
Pantopaque contrast medium
para-aminohippuric acid
parallax method
Parama's method
parameter
parenchyma
parent nuclide
parietography
particle
        viral p.
pathway
        Embden-Meyerhof gly-
        colytic p.
Pauli's exclusion principle
Pawlow's position
PC — pentose cycle
pc., pCi — picocurie
peak
        Bragg p.
Pearson's position
pectus excavatum
pedicle
PEG — pneumoencephalog-
        raphy
peizoelectric
pelves
pelvicephalography
pelvicephalometry
pelvimetry
pelviography
pelvioradiography
pelvioscopy
pelviradiography
pelviroentgenography
pelvis
penetrology
penetrometer

pentose cycle
penumbra
percussion
percutaneous
perinephric
peripheral
periphery
peristalsis
peristaltic
peritoneal fluid
peritoneography
permeability constant
perpendicular
pertechnetate
petrous tips
PETT — positron emission
      transverse tomog-
      raphy
Pfeiffer-Comberg method
pharmacoradiology
pharyngography
phenolphthalein
phenolsulfonphthalein
phenoltetrachlorophthalein
phenomenon
    interference p.
    vacuum p.
phentetiothalein
phenylalanine
phenyldiphenyloxadiazole
phenyloxazolyl
phlebogram
phlebography
phlebolith
phonation
phosphate
phosphor
phosphorated
phosphorescence
phosphorus

phosphorus-32 diisofluoro-
      phosphate
Phospho-soda
photocathode
photodisintegration
photodisplay unit
photoelectric
      p. absorption
      p. effect
      p. interaction
photoelectron
photoflow
photofluorographic
photomicrograph
photomultiplier tube
photon
      Compton p.
      degraded p.
photoneutron
photonuclear
      p. effect
      p. reaction
photorecording
photosensitivity
photosensitization
phototimer
phototube output circuit
picocurie
picture-frame–like
pig
Pigg-O-Stat immobilization
      device
pile
pion beam
Pirie transoral projection
PIT — plasma iron turnover
pitchblende
Pitressin
pixel — picture element
placentography

Planck's
    constant
    quantum theory
plane
    coronal p.
    cross-sectional p.
    median-sagittal p.
planigram
planigraphy
plasma
plasmapheresis
plateau
platelets
platelike
platinum
pleura
pleural
    p. effusion
pleurography
plutonium
pneumarthrogram
pneumarthrography
pneumatogram
pneumatograph
pneumencephalography
pneumoalveolography
pneumoangiogram
pneumoangiography
pneumoarthrogram
pneumoarthrography
pneumocardiograph
pneumocardiography
pneumocystography
pneumocystotomography
pneumoencephalogram
pneumoencephalography
    cerebral p.
pneumoencephalomyelogram
pneumoencephalomyelography
pneumofasciogram
pneumogastrography

pneumogram
pneumography
    cerebral p.
    retroperitoneal p.
pneumogynogram
pneumomediastinogram
pneumomediastinography
pneumomyelography
pneumonograph
pneumonography
pneumoperitoneum
    diagnostic p.
pneumopyelogram
pneumopyelography
pneumoradiography
    retroperitoneal p.
pneumoretroperitoneum
pneumoroentgenogram
pneumoroentgenography
pneumothorax
    diagnostic p.
pneumotomography
pneumoventriculography
pocket chamber
Poisson distribution
"poker" spine
polarity
polonium
polymer
polyp
polytome
    Massiot p.
polytomography
polyvinylpyrrolidone
popcorn-like
POPOP — 1,4-bis-2-(5-phenyl-
            oxazolyl)-benzene
pork insulin
porous
portacamera
portosplenography

portwine marks
position
    abduction p.
    adduction p.
    Albers-Schönberg p.
    AP (anteroposterior) p.
    Béclères p.
    Benassi's p.
    Blackett-Healy p.
    Broden's p.
    brow-down p.
    brow-up p.
    Caldwell's p.
    Camp-Coventry p.
    Cleaves' p.
    cross-table lateral p.
    decubitus p.
    erect p.
    eversion p.
    extension p.
    Feist-Mankin p.
    Fick's p.
    Fleischner's p.
    flexion p.
    Friedman's p.
    frog-leg p.
    Gaynor-Hart p.
    Grashey's p.
    Haas p.
    Hickey's p.
    inlet p.
    inversion p.
    Isherwood's p.
    Johnson's p.
    Kurzbauer's p.
    Laquerrière-Pierquin p.
    Larkin's p.
    lateral p.
    Lawrence's p.
    Law's p.
    Leonard-George p.
    Lewis' p.

position (*continued*)
    Lilienfeld's p.
    Lindblom's p.
    Lorenz' p.
    Löw-Beer p.
    Mayer's p.
    Meese's p.
    Miller's p.
    Nölke's p.
    oblique p.
    PA (posteroanterior) p.
    Pawlow's p.
    Pearson's p.
    prone p.
    recumbent p.
    Schüller's p.
    semierect p.
    semirecumbent p.
    Settegast's p.
    Staunig's p.
    Stecher's p.
    Stenver's p.
    supine p.
    Tarrant's p.
    Taylor's p.
    Titterington's p.
    Towne's p.
    Trendelenburg p.
    Twining's p.
    Wigby-Taylor p.
    Zanelli's p.
positrocephalogram
positron
    p.-coincidence
    p. decay
positronium
posteroanterior view
postirradiation
potassium
    p. perchlorate
potential
    p. difference

potential (*continued*)
    p. gradient
Potter-Bucky
    diaphragm
    grid
PPD — phenyldiphenyloxadia-
    zole
PPO-(2,5-diphenyloxazole)
praseodymium
preamplifier
predetector
principle
    Fick's p.
    Pauli's exclusion p.
Priodax contrast medium
Pro-Banthine
probe
    fiberoptic p.
    scintillation p.
process
    bremsstrahlung p.
    neutron absorption p.
    spinous p.
    superior articulating p.
    transverse p.
projection
    anteroposterior lordotic
      p.
    apical lordotic p.
    axial p.
    axillary p.
    ball-catcher's p.
    basilar p.
    basovertical p.
    biplane p.
    blowout view p.
    Chassard-Lapiné p.
    cone-down p.
    craniocaudad p.
    cross-sectional transverse
      p.
    dorsoplantar p.

projection (*continued*)
    erect fluoro spot p.
    flexion, extension p.
    p. formula
    frontal p.
    half-axial p.
    inferior-superior p.
    inferior-superior tangen-
      tial p.
    inferosuperior axial p.
    intraoral p.
    L-5, S-1 p.
    lateral oblique axial p.
    lateral transcranial p.
    lateral transfacial p.
    lateromedial oblique p.
    Lauenstein and Hickey p.
    lumbosacral p.
    medial oblique axial p.
    mediolateral p.
    navicular p.
    nuchofrontal p.
    oblique lateral p.
    parieto-orbital p.
    pillar p.
    Pirie transoral p.
    plantodorsal p.
    posteroanterior lordotic
      p.
    recumbent lateral p.
    Runström p.
    scaphoid p.
    semiaxial p.
    semiaxial anteroposterior
      p.
    semiaxial transcranial p.
    skyline p.
    stereo right lateral p.
    submentovertical axial p.
    "sunrise" p.
    superoinferior p.
    tangential p.

projection (*continued*)
    Templeton and Zim
      carpal tunnel p.
    transtabular AP (PA) p.
    transthoracic p.
    tunnel p.
    verticosubmental p.
    Waters' p.
promethium
pronate
pronation
prone
propagation
propantheline bromide
proportional counter
propyliodone
prostatography
Prostigmin
protactinium
protein
proton
protuberance
    external occipital p.
proximal
"pruned hilum"
psoas
PSP — phenolsulfonphthalein
ptosis
pubic rami
pubis
pulmonary pedicle
pulse-height spectrum
punctate
PVP — polyvinylpyrrolidone
pyelofluoroscopy
pyelogram
    hydrated p.
    retrograde p.
pyelography
    drip infusion p.
    intravenous p.

pyelography (*continued*)
    percutaneous antegrade
      p.
    retrograde p.
    washout p.
pyloric stenosis
pylorus
pyrogen
pyrogenic
quanta
quantification
quantitative
quantum
    q. theory
quenching
R — roentgen
rabbit
racemose
rachitic
rad — radiation adsorbed dose
radiation
    annihilation r.
    electromagnetic r.
    monochromatic r.
    scattered r.
radiation production
    Cerenkov r.p.
radioactive
    r. decay
    r. fallout
    r. nuclides
radioactivity
radioactor
radioanaphylaxis
radioassay
radioautograph
radiobe
radiobioassay
radiobiological
radiobiologist
radiobiology

radiocalcium
radiocarbon
radiocardiogram
radiocardiography
radiochemical purity
radiochemistry
radiochemotherapy
radiochemy
radiocholecystography
radiochroism
radiochromatography
radiocinematograph
radiocolloid
radiocurable
radiode
radiodensity
radiodiagnosis
radiodiagnostics
radiodiaphane
radioelectrocardiogram
radioelectrocardiograph
radioelectrocardiography
radioelement
radioencephalogram
radioencephalography
radiofluorine
radiogallium
radiogenic
radiogold
radiogram
radiograph
radiographic
    r. density
    r. effect
radiography
    biomedical r.
    body section r.
    pan-oral r.
    stereoscopic r.
radiohepatographic
radioimmunity
radioimmunoassay

radioimmunodiffusion
radioimmunoelectrophoresis
radioimmunoprecipitation
radioinduction
radioiodine
radioiron
radioisotope
radiokymography
radiolead
radiologic
radiological
radiologist
radiology
radiolucencies
radiolucency
radiolucent
radiometer
    pastille r.
    photographic r.
radiometric
    r. analysis
radiomicrometer
radiomimetic
radion
radionitrogen
radionuclide
    r. imaging
    r. kinetics
    r. purity
    r. scanning
radionuclides. See *Drugs and Chemistry* section.
radiopacity
radiopaque
radioparency
radioparent
radiopathology
radiopelvimetry
radiopharmaceutical
radiophosphorus
radiophotography
radiophylaxis

radiopotassium
radiopotentiation
radiopulmonography
radioreceptor
radioresistant
radioscope
radioscopy
radiosensitive
radiosensitivity
radiosodium
radiospirometry
radiostereoscopy
radiostrontium
radiosulfur
radiotellurium
radiotherapeutics
radiotherapy
radiothorium
radiotransparency
radiotransparent
radium
radius
    Bohr r.
radon
range
RAO — right anterior oblique
rate meter
ratio
    target-to-nontarget r.
ray
    alpha r.
    beta r.
    cathode r.
    central r.
    cosmic r.
    fluorescent r.
    gamma r.
    grenz r.
    parallel r.
    secondary r.
    vertical r.
Rayopak

RBC's — red blood cells
RBL — Reid's base line
rd. — rutherford
reaction
    biomolecular r.
    thermonuclear r.
reactor
    nuclear r.
recanalization
recovery time
recumbency
recumbent
redundancy
redundant
refractory
Reid's base line
relativistic mass
REM — roentgen equivalent–man
REMP — roentgen equivalent–man period
renocystogram
Renografin contrast medium
renogram
renography
Reno-M-30 contrast medium
Reno-M-60 contrast medium
Reno-M-dip contrast medium
Renovist contrast medium
rentgen. See *roentgen.*
rentgenogram. See *roentgenogram.*
rentgenologe. See *roentgenology.*
rentgenologic. See *roentgenologic.*
REP — roentgen equivalent–physical
resin
resolution
    spatial r.
resonance capture

reticular
reticulation
retrococcygeal
retrograde
retroperitoneal
rhenium
rhodium
ribose
ribosome
ribosyl
ribothymidine
ribulose
ring
    Cannon's r.
    "r. of bone"
ripple voltage
R-meter
RNA — ribonucleic acid
roentgen
roentgenogram
roentgenologic
roentgenologist
roentgenology
RP — retrograde pyelogram
RPM — rapid processing mode;
    par speed screens
RPO — right posterior oblique
rubidium
ruga
rugae
rugal pattern
Runström projection
RUQ — right upper quadrant
ruthenium
rutherford
s — screen containing cassette
sacrum
sagittal
saline solution
Salpix contrast medium
Salyrgan
samarium

sarcoidosis
saturation current
Satvioni's cryptoscope
SBFT — small bowel follow-
    through
scaler
scalloped
scan
    isotope bone s.
scandium
scanner
    CT body s.
    Medx s.
    neurodiagnostic s.
    nuclear s.
    radioisotope s.
    rectilinear s.
    supercam scintillation s.
    tomographic multiplane
    s.
    whole body s.
scanning
    A-mode (amplitude
    modulation) s.
    B-mode (brightness
    modulation) s.
    bone s.
    brain s.
    compound s.
    M-mode (motion) s.
    radioisotope s.
    renal s.
scanography
    slit s.
    spot s.
scattering
    Compton s.
Schüller's position
scintiangiography
scintigram
scintigraphic
scintigraphy

scintillation
scintiphotograph
scintiphotosplenoportography
scintiscan
scintiscanner
scintiview
scoliosis
Seidlitz powder test
selenium
selenomethionine Se 75
self
    s.-absorption
    s.-quenched counter tube
    s.-scattering
sella turcica
senograph
senography
sensitivity
    plane s.
    point s.
sensitometer
    electroluminescent s.
sensitometry
Sephadex
sequestration
series
    gastrointestinal s.
    small bowel s.
serpiginous
Settegast's position
shadow
    psoas s.
shadowgram
shadowgraph
shadowgraphy
shaggy
shape
    "baseball bat" s.
    "cricket bat" s.
shield
    lead gonad s.
shielding

sialadenitis
sialogram
sialography
sign
    air bronchogram s.
    air dome s.
    doughnut s.
    fat pad s.
    meniscus s.
    rim s.
    silhouette s.
    string s.
    Westmark's s.
silhouette
silicon
silver
    s. iodide
Sinografin contrast medium
sinogram
sinography
sinti-. See words beginning
    scinti-.
sinus
    costophrenic s.
    frontal s.
    sphenoid s.
sinusography
    cerebral s.
skeletal
skiagram
skiagraph
skiagraphy
Skiodan contrast medium
    S. Acacia
"skip areas"
slug
sodium
    s. bromide
    s. chromate Cr 51
    s. diatrizoate
    s. iodide I 123, I 125,
      I 131

sodium (*continued*)
    s. iodipamide
    s. iodohippurate I 131
    s. iodomethamate
    s. iothalamate I 125
    s. ipodate
    s. methiodal
    s. pertechnetate Tc 99m
    s. phosphate P 32
    s. radioiodide
    s. rose bengal I 131
    s. thorium tartrate
    s. tyropanoate
solarization
solid-state
    s.-s. physics
solubilize
soluble
solution
    hundredth-normal s.
    hypertonic s.
    molal s.
Sommer-Foegella method
sonarography
sonofluoroscope
sonogram
sonography
space
    retroperitoneal s.
    subarachnoid s.
spadelike
spallation
spatial
specific activity
speckled
spectrometer
    beta-ray s.
    gamma-ray s.
    mass s.
    Mossbauer s.
    scintillation s.
spectrometry
    pulse height s.

spectrophotofluorometer
spectrophotometer
    absorption s.
spectrophotometry
spectroscope
spectroscopic
spectroscopy
spectrum
    chromatic s.
    electromagnetic s.
    thermal s.
    x-ray s.
sphere
spherical
spiculated
spindling
spine
    lumbar s.
    sacral s.
spinogram
spinthariscope
spintherometer
spintometer
splenic flexure
splenoportogram
splenoportography
spot film
    s. f. device
    s. f. radiography
    s. f. study
Staunig's position
Stecher's position
Stenver's
    position
    view
stereocinefluorography
stereofluoroscopy
stereogram
stereoradiogram
stereoradiography
stereoroentgenography
stereoroentgenometry
stereosalpingography

stereoscope
stereoscopic
stereoscopy
stereoskiagraphy
straggling
stress films
stridor
strontium (with yttrium 90)
    s. nitrate Sr 85
    s. Sr 87m
study
    air contrast s.
    barium meal s.
    blood flow s.
    cine s.
    double-contrast s.
    dual-contrast s.
    horizontal beam s.
    iodized oil s.
    lumbar, flexion, and
      extension s.
    motility s.
    perfusion s.
    perirenal air s.
    phonation s.
    quantitative regional lung
      function s.
    retrococcygeal air s.
    retroperitoneal air s.
    single-contrast s.
    spot film s.
    tracer s.
    ventilation s.
    videotape s.
    washout s.
subluxation
subpleural
succinic semialdehyde
sulcus
    s. for optic chiasm

sulcus (*continued*)
    sigmoid s.
sulfur
superimposed
superimposition
superior
    s. ramus
supernumerary
supinate
supination
supine
swallow
    barium s.
Sweet's method
symmetrical
symphysis
    s. pubis
synchrotron
synthesis
system
    catenary s.
    linear s.
    mamillary s.
    metric s.
    three-compartment s.
    three-phase s.
    two-compartment s.
T_3 — triiodothyronine
tagged atom
tagging
tannic acid
tantalum
target
Tarrant's position
Taylor's position
Tc — technetium
    Tc 99m aggregated
      albumin kit
    Tc 99m albumin micro-
      spheres kit

Tc — technetium (*continued*)
    Tc 99m etidronate
      sodium kit
    Tc 99m generator
    Tc 99m medronate
      sodium kit
    Tc 99m pentetate sodium
      kit
    Tc 99m serum albumin
      kit
    Tc 99m stannous pyro-
      phosphate/polyphos-
      phate kit
    Tc 99m sulfur colloid
technetium
technique
    autoradiographic t.
    chromatographic-fluoro-
      metric t.
    Corbin t.
    drip infusion t.
    supervoltage t.
    Welin's t.
TED — threshold erythema
      dose
telecobolt
telemetry
teleoroentgenogram
teleoroentgenography
Telepaque contrast medium
teleradiography
teleroentgenogram
teleroentgenography
teleroentgentherapy
teletherapy
tellurium
Templeton and Zim carpal
    tunnel projection
terbium
test
    chlormerodrin accumula-
      tion t.

test (*continued*)
    fat absorption t.
    gastrointestinal blood
      loss t.
    gastrointestinal protein
      loss t.
    positive washout t.
    radioimmunoprecipita-
      tion t.
    radioiodine t.
    Seidlitz powder t.
    string t.
    triiodothyronine red cell
      uptake t.
    triiodothyronine resin t.
    washout t.
testosterone
thallium
thallous chloride Tl 201
theorem
    Bayes' t.
therapy
    beam t.
    deep roentgen ray t.
    megavolt t.
theory
    Planck's quantum t.
thermal neutrons
thermogram
thermographic
thermography
thermonuclear
thiosemicarbazide
thiosemicarbazone
Thixokon contrast medium
Thoms' method
Thoreau's filter
thorium
    t. dioxide
Thorotrast contrast medium
Thorpe plastic lens
three-phase system

thulium
thumb-printing
thymidine
thyratron
thyroxine
Thyrx timer
Ti – titanium
timer
    Thyrx t.
tin (with indium-113m)
titanium
Titterington's position
tl – thallium
TLD – thermoluminescent
      dosimeter
    tumor lethal dose
TM – time motion
tomogram
tomograph
tomography
    axial computed t.
    axial transverse t.
    computed t.
    focal plane t.
    panoramic t.
    plesiosectional t.
    polycycloidal t.
    positron emission trans-
      verse t. (PETT)
    transversal t.
tomolaryngography
tomoscopy
tortuous
tourniquet
Towne's
    position
    view
Townsend's avalanche
tracer
trachea
tracheobronchoscopy
transducer

transferrin
transformer
    filament t.
    high-voltage t.
    ratio t.
    step-down t.
    step-up t.
transillumination
transmutation
transverse
    t. colon
tree
    tracheobronchial t.
Treitz
    ligament of T.
Trendelenburg position
triangle
    Codman's t.
triangular
triangulation
trichloroacetic acid
triiodothyronine
triolein (glyceral trioleate)
    I 131
tritium
triton
trochanter
    greater t.
    lesser t.
TSC – technetium sulfur
      colloid
TTD – tissue tolerance dose
T-tube
    T-t. cholangiogram
    T-t. cholangiography
tube
    Cantor's t.
    Miller-Abbott t.
    photomultiplier t.
tungsten
Twining's position
tympanography

UGI — upper gastrointestinal
UIBC — unsaturated iron-
      binding capacity
ulceration
ultrasonogram
ultrasonograph
ultrasonographic
ultrasonography
    A-mode u.
ultrasound
    Doppler u.
    real-time u.
ultraviolet
undulating
unit
    Angstrom u.
    Hounsfield u.
unsaturated
    u. compounds
upper GI series
uptake
uranium
ureterogram
ureterography
urethrocystography
urethrogram
    excretory u.
urethrography
urogram
    drip-infusion u.
urography
    excretory u.
    intravenous u.
    percutaneous antegrade
    u.
    retrograde u.
urokymography
Uroselectan
uterosalpingogram
uterosalpingography
vaginogram
vaginography

vanadium
Van de Graeff generator
vascular
    v. groove
Vasopressin
Vater
    ampulla of V.
VCUG — voiding cystourethro-
    gram
velocity
Velpeau axillary view
venogram
venography
    limb v.
    peripheral v.
    selective v.
    splenoportal v.
ventriculogram
ventriculography
    cardiac v.
    cerebral v.
    contrast v.
vermiform
vermography
vertebra
vesiculogram
    seminal v.
vesiculography
Victoreen dosimeter
view
    anteroposterior v.
    Chausse's v.
    comparison v.
    coned-down v.
    dorsal v.
    frog-leg v.
    lateral v.
    lordotic v.
    Mayers' v.
    normal AP v.
    oblique v.
    panoramic v.

view (*continued*)
    pantomographic v.
    plantar v.
    posterior v.
    posteroanterior v.
    "scottie dog" v.
    skyline v.
    Stenver's v.
    Towne's v.
    tunnel v.
    Velpeau axillary v.
    Waters' v.
viscus
visualization
    double-contrast v.
voltage
volume
    atomic v.
    molar v.
volvulus
voxel — volume element
Waters'
    projection
    view
wave
    electromagnetic w.
wavelength
    Compton w.
    de Broglie w.
weight
    atomic w.
    w.-bearing
Welin's technique
Westmark's sign

whole-body counting
Wigby-Taylor position
Wilson chamber
wolfram
Wolf's method
Wood's lamp
Xe — xenon
xenon
    x. Xe 133
xeromammography
xeroradiograph
xeroradiographic
xeroradiography
x-ray
Xu — X-unit
xylose
Y — yttrium
Yb — ytterbium
ytterbium
    y. Yb pentetate sodium
yttrium
Zanelli's position
zero. See words beginning
    xero-.
Zimmer's method
zinc
zirconium (with niobium-95)
zone plate
    Fresnel z.p.
zonogram
zonography
    stereoscopic z.
zwitterion

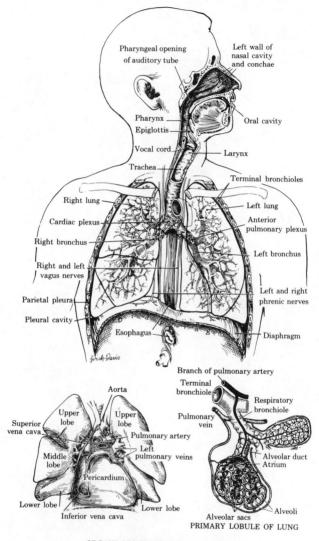

ORGANS OF RESPIRATORY SYSTEM

RESPIRATORY SYSTEM

aasmus
Abelson's cannula
Abraham's
    cannula
    sign
Abrams' needle
abscess
ACMI bronchoscope
Actinomyces
    A. bovis
actinomycosis
    pulmonary a.
Adair's forceps
adenocarcinoma
adenoma
    bronchial a.
    chondromatous a.
adenomatosis
    pulmonary a.
adenopathy
    hilar a.
adenovirus
adhesions
    a. of pleura
Adson's test
aeration
aerodermectasia
aeroemphysema
aeroionotherapy
aeroporotomy

aerosol
AFB — acid-fast bacillus
agenesis
airway
    a. resistance
Albert's bronchoscope
Allen's test
Allis' forceps
alveobronchiolitis
alveolar
alveoli
    a. pulmonis
alveolitis
    diffuse sclerosing a.
alveolus
Ambu bag
amebiasis
    pulmonary a.
amyloidosis
anapnoic
anapnotherapy
Andrews-Pynchon tube
Andrews' retractor
anesthesia. See *General*
    Surgical Terms.
aneurysm
    mycotic a.
angiogram
angiography
    pulmonary a.

anomaly
> Freund's a.

anthracosilicosis
anthracosis
anthropotoxin
aorta
> retroesophageal a.

A&P — auscultation and percussion
apex
apical
apices
apicolysis
apnea
> deglutition a.
> traumatic a.

apneic
apneumatosis
apneumia
apneusis
apparatus
> Fell-O'Dwyer a.

applicator
> Plummer-Vinson radium a.

arch
> aortic a.

arcus
> a. costarum

ARD — acute respiratory disease
area
> Krönig's a.

Argyle chest tube
Arloing-Courmont test
Arneth's syndrome
artery
> pulmonary a.
> subclavian a.

arytenoid
asbestosis

aspergillosis
> pulmonary a.

Aspergillus
asphyxia
aspiration
aspirator
> Broyles' a.

Assmann's
> focus
> infiltrate

asthma
> allergic a.
> alveolar a.
> bronchial a.
> cotton dust a.
> emphysematous a.
> essential a.
> grinders' a.
> intrinsic a.
> millers' a.
> miners' a.
> potters' a.
> steam-fitters' a.
> stone-strippers' a.

asthmatic
atelectasis
> absorption a.
> compression a.
> lobar a.
> lobular a.
> obstructive a.
> relaxation a.
> resorption a.
> secondary a.
> segmental a.

atelectatic
Atkins-Cannard tube
Atlee's clamp
atmograph
atmotherapy
atresia

atrium
  pulmonary a.
atrophy
  senile a. of lung
auscultation
Ayerza's
  disease
  syndrome
azygography
azygos
Babcock's forceps
Baccelli's sign
bacilli
bacillus
  Friedländer's b.
  rhinoscleroma b.
Bacillus pneumoniae
Bacteroides
bag
  Ambu b.
bagassosis
Bailey's catheter
Balme's cough
Bard's syndrome
baritosis
Bársony-Polgár syndrome
Beatty-Bright friction sound
Belsey's repair
Benedict-Roth spirometer
Benedict's gastroscope
Bernay's retractor
berylliosis
Bethea's sign
Bethune's tourniquet
Biermer's change
bifurcatio
  b. tracheae
bifurcation
bilharziasis
biopsy
  scalene lymph node b.

Biot's
  breathing
  respiration
bistoury
  Jackson's b.
Blakemore's tube
Blalock-Taussig operation
blastomycosis
bleb
  subpleural b.
blennothorax
Blumenau's test
Boies' forceps
bolus
Bornholm's disease
Boros' esophagoscope
bougie
  Hurst's b.
  Jackson's b.
  Trousseau's b.
BP — bronchopleural
Bragg-Paul pulsator
breathing
  Biot's b.
  bronchial b.
  frog b.
  glossopharyngeal b.
  intermittent positive-
    pressure b.
Brewster's retractor
Brock's syndrome
bronchadenitis
bronchi
  hyparterial b.
  lobar b.
  b. lobares
  segmental b.
  b. segmentales
bronchia
bronchial
  b. brushing

bronchiectasis
    capillary b.
    cylindrical b.
    cystic b.
    follicular b.
    pseudocylindrical b.
    saccular b.
bronchiectatic
bronchiloquy
bronchiocele
bronchiocrisis
bronchiole
    alveolar b's
    lobular b.
    respiratory b's
    terminal b's
bronchiolectasis
bronchioli respiratorii
bronchiolitis
    acute obliterating b.
    b. exudativa
    b. fibrosa obliterans
    vesicular b.
bronchiolus
bronchiospasm
bronchitic
bronchitis
    arachidic b.
    Castellani's b.
    catarrhal b.
    cheesy b.
    chronic b.
    croupous b.
    epidemic capillary b.
    ether b.
    exudative b.
    fibrinous b.
    hemorrhagic b.
    infectious asthmatic b.
    mechanic b.
    membranous b.
    b. obliterans

bronchitis (*continued*)
    phthinoid b.
    plastic b.
    polypoid b.
    productive b.
    pseudomembranous b.
    putrid b.
    secondary b.
    staphylococcus b.
    streptococcus b.
    suffocative b.
    verminous b.
    vesicular b.
bronchium
bronchoadenitis
bronchoalveolar
bronchoalveolitis
bronchoaspergillosis
bronchobiliary
bronchoblastomycosis
bronchoblennorrhea
bronchocandidiasis
bronchocavernous
bronchocele
bronchocephalitis
bronchoclysis
bronchoconstrictor
bronchodilatation
bronchodilation
bronchodilator
bronchoesophageal
bronchoesophagology
bronchoesophagoscopy
bronchogenic
bronchogram
bronchography
broncholith
broncholithiasis
bronchologic
bronchology
bronchomalacia
bronchomotor

bronchomycosis
bronchonocardiosis
broncho-oidiosis
bronchopathy
bronchophony
    pectoriloquous b.
    sniffling b.
    whispered b.
bronchoplasty
bronchoplegia
bronchopleural
bronchopleuropneumonia
bronchopneumonia
bronchopneumonitis
bronchopneumopathy
bronchopulmonary
bronchoradiography
bronchorrhagia
bronchorrhaphy
bronchorrhea
bronchoscope
    ACMI b.
    Albert's b.
    Broyles' b.
    Bruening's b.
    Chevalier Jackson b.
    coagulation b.
    costophrenic b.
    Davis' b.
    double-channel irrigating
      b.
    Emerson's b.
    fiberoptic b.
    Foregger's b.
    Haslinger's b.
    Holinger-Jackson b.
    Holinger's b.
    hook-on b.
    Jackson's b.
    Jesberg's b.
    Kernan-Jackson b.
    Michelson's b.

bronchoscope (*continued*)
    Moersch's b.
    Negus' b.
    Overholt-Jackson b.
    Pilling's b.
    Riecker's b.
    Safar's b.
    Staple's b.
    Storz' b.
    telescope b.
    Tucker's b.
    ventilation b.
    Waterman's b.
    Yankauer's b.
bronchoscopic
bronchoscopy
bronchosinusitis
bronchospasm
bronchospirochetosis
bronchospirography
bronchospirometer
bronchospirometry
bronchostaxis
bronchostenosis
bronchostomy
bronchotetany
bronchotome
bronchotomy
bronchotracheal
bronchotyphoid
bronchotyphus
bronchovesicular
bronchus
    apical b.
    cardiac b.
    eparterial b.
    lingular b.
    lobar b.
    main stem b.
    b. principalis dexter
    b. principalis sinister
    stem b.

bronchus (*continued*)
    tracheal b.
brong-. See words beginning
    bronch-.
Broyles'
    aspirator
    bronchoscope
    dilator
    esophagoscope
    forceps
    telescope
    tube
Bruening's
    bronchoscope
    esophagoscope
    forceps
bruit
    b. d'airain (brwe da ra)
    b. de bois (brwe duh
        bwah)
    b. de craquement (brwe
        duh krak maw)
    b. de cuir neuf (brwe
        duh kwer nuf)
    b. de frolement (brwe
        duh frol maw)
    b. de grelot (brwe duh
        gruh lo)
    b. de pot fêlé (brwe duh
        po fe la)
brwe. See *bruit*.
Buhl's desquamative
    pneumonia
bulla
    emphysematous b.
bullae
Burghart's symptom
button
    Moore's tracheostomy b's
byssinosis
calcicosilicosis
calcicosis

calcification
cancrocirrhosis
Candida
    C. albicans
candidiasis
cannula
    Abelson's c.
    Abraham's c.
    Pritchard's c.
    Rockey's c.
cannulation
capillary
Caplan's syndrome
Carabelli's tube
carcinoma
    alveolar cell c.
    anaplastic c.
    bronchiolar c.
    bronchogenic c.
    epidermoid c.
    squamous cell c.
cardia
    incompetent c.
cardiopulmonary
carina
    c. of trachea
Carlens'
    catheter
    mediastinoscope
Carswell's grapes
cartilage
    cricoid c.
caseation
Casoni's test
Castellani's bronchitis
catheter
    Bailey's c.
    Carlens' c.
    Lloyd's c.
    Metras' c.
    Thompson's c.
    Zavod's c.

caval
cavernoscopy
cavernostomy
cavernous
cavitary
cavitation
cavum
Cegka's sign
Celestin's tube
cell
    Langhans' c's
chalicosis
change
    Biermer's c.
    Gerhardt's c. of sound
Chaussier's tube
chemotherapy
Chevalier Jackson
    bronchoscope
    esophagoscope
    tube
Cheyne-Stokes respiration
cholesterohydrothorax
chondroadenoma
chondroma
chylomediastinum
chylopleura
chylopneumothorax
chylorrhea
chylothorax
cinebronchogram
cineradiography
circumscribed
clamp
    Atlee's c.
    Davidson's c.
    Hudson's c.
    Kantrowicz's c.
    Kapp-Beck c.
    Kinsella-Buie c.
    Lees' c.
    Mueller's c.

clamp (*continued*)
    Price-Thomas c.
    Ralks' c.
    Rockey's c.
    Rubin's c.
    Sarot's c.
    Thomson's c.
clavicle
clavicular
clavipectoral
coalescence
coarctation
Coccidioides
    C. immitis
coccidioidomycosis
coin lesion
collapse
    c. of the lung
collapsotherapy
Collins' respirometer-
    spirometer
congestion
    pleuropulmonary c.
coniosporosis
coniotoxicosis
COPD — chronic obstructive
        pulmonary disease
Cope's needle
cor
    c. pulmonale
Cordes' forceps
Corrigan's
    pneumonia
    respiration
Corynebacterium
costa
costal
costectomy
costophrenic
costopleural
costopneumopexy
costovertebral

cough
    Balme's c.
    barking c.
    compression c.
    extrapulmonary c.
    mechanical c.
    minute gun c.
    Morton's c.
    productive c.
    reflex c.
    Sydenham's c.
    tea taster's c.
    trigeminal c.
    whooping c.
    winter c.
Coxsackie virus
CPR — cardiopulmonary
    resuscitation
Crafoord's
    forceps
    scissors
Craig's test
crepitant
cricoid
cricopharyngeus
cricotracheotomy
croup
croupette
croupy
crura
crus
cryptococcosis
Cryptococcus
    C. neoformans
cupula
    c. of pleura
curse
    Ondine's c.
CVA — costovertebral angle
cyanosis
    pulmonary c.

cyst
    bronchogenic c.
    dermoid c.
    enteric c.
    neurenteric c.
    pericardial c.
    thymic c.
D'Amato's sign
Daniel's operation
Darling's disease
Davidson's clamp
Davis' bronchoscope
Debove's membrane
decannulation
decarbonization
décollement
decortication
    d. of lung
deficiency
    alpha-1-antitrypsin d.
degeneration
    trabecular d.
Delmege's sign
Delorme's operation
density
    conglomerate d.
Depaul's tube
Desnos'
    disease
    pneumonia
desquamative
DeVilbiss nebulizer
dextrocardia
diaphragm
diaphragmatic
dilator
    Broyles' d.
    Einhorn's d.
    Jackson's d.
    Jackson-Trousseau d.
    Laborde's d.

dilator (*continued*)
- Patton's d.
- Plummer's d.
- Plummer-Vinson d.
- Sippy's d.
- Steele's d.
- Trousseau-Jackson d.
- Trousseau's d.

diminution

DIP — desquamative interstitial pneumonitis

diphtheria

Diplococcus
- *D. pneumoniae*

discission
- d. of pleura

disease
- Ayerza's d.
- black lung d.
- Bornholm's d.
- brown lung d.
- Darling's d.
- Desnos' d.
- farmer's lung d.
- grinder's d.
- Hamman's d.
- Hodgkin's d.
- hyaline membrane d.
- Kartagener's d.
- Löffler's d.
- Lucas-Championnière's d.
- pigeon breeder's d.
- Shaver's d.
- silo filler's d.
- Woillez' d.

dissector
- Lynch's d.

diverticulum
- pharyngoesophageal d.
- Rokitansky's d.
- supradiaphragmatic d.

diverticulum (*continued*)
- Zenker's d.

Douglas' bag spirometer

drainage systems
- closed water seal d.s.
- continuous suction d.s.
- Glover's d.s.
- Monaldi's d.s.
- postural d.s.
- redivac d.s.
- Snyder's surgivac d.s.
- sump d.s.
- surgivac suction d.s.
- three-bottle d.s.
- tidal d.s.
- two-bottle d.s.
- underwater seal d.s.
- vacuum d.s.
- waterseal d.s.

Drinker respirator

drugs. See *Drugs and Chemistry* section.

Duguet's siphon

Durham's tube

Duval-Crile forceps

dysphagia

dyspnea
- expiratory d.
- inspiratory d.
- nocturnal d.
- nonexpansional d.
- orthostatic d.
- Traube's d.

dyspneic

Eaton agent pneumonia

ECHO virus

edema
- pulmonary e.
- vernal e.

Eder-Hufford esophagoscope

effusion
- pleural e.

EGL — eosinophilic granuloma
      of the lung
egophony
Einhorn's dilator
electrocardiogram
elevator
      Jackson's e.
Ellis' sign
Eloesser's
      flap
      operation
embolism
      pulmonary e.
Emerson's bronchoscope
emphysema
      alveolar e.
      atrophic e.
      bullous e.
      centrilobular e.
      compensatory e.
      cystic e.
      diffuse e.
      false e.
      focal-dust e.
      gangrenous e.
      generalized e.
      glass blower's e.
      hypertrophic e.
      hypoplastic e.
      idiopathic unilobar e.
      interlobular e.
      interstitial e.
      Jenner's e.
      lobar e.
      loculated e.
      mediastinal e.
      obstructive e.
      panacinar e.
      panlobular e.
      paracicatricial e.
      paraseptal e.
      pulmonary e.

emphysema (*continued*)
      senile e.
      small-lunged e.
      subcutaneous e.
      subfascial e.
      surgical e.
      traumatic e.
      unilateral e.
      vesicular e.
emphysematous
empyema
      e. benignum
      interlobar e.
      metapneumonic e.
      pneumococcal e.
      putrid e.
      sacculated e.
      streptococcal e.
      synpneumonic e.
      thoracic e.
      tuberculous e.
empyemic
endobronchial
endobronchitis
endoscopic
endoscopy
endotracheal
endotracheitis
eparterial
epicardia
epidermoid
epiglottis
Equen's magnet
Erich's forceps
Escherichia
      E. coli
Escherich's test
esofa-. See words beginning
      esopha-.
esophagalgia
esophageal
esophagectasia

esophagectomy
esophagism
    hiatal e.
esophagitis
    reflux e.
esophagocele
esophagocologastrostomy
esophagoduodenostomy
esophagodynia
esophagoenterostomy
esophagofundopexy
esophagogastrectomy
esophagogastroanastomosis
esophagogastroplasty
esophagogastroscopy
esophagogastrostomy
esophagogram
esophagography
esophagojejunogastrostomosis
esophagojejunostomy
esophagolaryngectomy
esophagomalacia
esophagometer
esophagomycosis
esophagomyotomy
esophagopharynx
esophagoplasty
esophagoplication
esophagoptosis
esophagosalivation
esophagoscope
    Boros' e.
    Broyles' e.
    Bruening's e.
    Chevalier Jackson e.
    Eder-Hufford e.
    Haslinger's tracheo-
      broncho- e.
    Holinger's e.
    Jackson's e.
    Jesberg's e.
    Lell's e.

esophagoscope (*continued*)
    Moersch's e.
    Mosher's e.
    Moure's e.
    Roberts' e.
    Schindler's e.
    Tucker's e.
    Yankauer's e.
esophagoscopy
esophagospasm
esophagostenosis
esophagostoma
esophagostomy
esophagotome
esophagotomy
esophagus
Estlander's operation
eupnea
evagination
eventration
    diaphragmatic e.
Ewart's sign
expansion
expectorant
expectoration
expiration
expiratory
exsufflation
exsufflator
extratracheal
faringo-. See words beginning
    pharyngo-.
farinjeal. See *pharyngeal.*
farinks. See *pharynx.*
Fauvel's granules
FEF — forced expiratory flow
Fell-O'Dwyer apparatus
fever
    Q f. (Q for query)
fiberscope
    Hirschowitz's gastro-
      duodenal f.

fibrogastroscopy
fibroma
    f. of lung
fibrosis
    cystic f.
    diffuse interstitial pul-
      monary f.
    idiopathic f.
    interstitial f.
    mediastinal f.
    pulmonary f.
fibrothorax
fibrotic
fibrous
field
    Krönig's f.
FIF — forced inspiratory flow
Finochietto's forceps
Fischer's needle
fissure
    f. of lung
fistula
    bronchocutaneous f.
    bronchopleural f.
    esophagobronchial f.
    pulmonary arteriovenous
      f.
    tracheal f.
    tracheoesophageal f.
flap
    Eloesser's f.
flem. See *phlegm.*
Floyd's needle
fluoroscopy
flutter
    mediastinal f.
focus
    Assmann's f.
foramen
    f. ovale basis cranii
    f. ovale ossis sphenoidalis

forceps
    Adair's f.
    Allis' f.
    Babcock's f.
    Boies' f.
    Broyles' f.
    Bruening's f.
    Cordes' f.
    Crafoord's f.
    Duval-Crile f.
    Erich's f.
    Finochietto's f.
    Fraenkel's f.
    Harrington-Mayo f.
    Holinger's f.
    Jackson's f.
    Johnson's f.
    Julian's f.
    Kahler's f.
    Killian's f.
    Kocher's f.
    Kolb's f.
    Krause's f.
    Leyro-Diaz f.
    Lovelace's f.
    Lynch's f.
    Mayo-Russian f.
    Moersch's f.
    Myerson's f.
    Nelson's f.
    New's f.
    Patterson's f.
    Pennington's f.
    Price-Thomas f.
    Roberts' f.
    Rockey's f.
    Russian f.
    Sam Roberts f.
    Sarot's f.
    Scheinmann's f.
    Seiffert's f.

forceps (*continued*)
    Tobold-Fauvel f.
    Tuttle's f.
    Yankauer-Little f.
Foregger's bronchoscope
Forlanini's treatment
fossa
    supraclavicular f.
Fowler's operation
Fraenkel's forceps
Frederick's needle
fremitus
    bronchial f.
    pleural f.
    rhonchal f.
    tactile f.
    tussive f.
fren-. See words beginning
    phren-.
Freund's anomaly
Friedländer's
    bacillus pneumonia
    pneumobacillus
    pneumonia
Friedreich's sign
Friedrich's operation
furrow
    Schmorl's f.
Gabriel Tucker tube
gangrene
    g. of lung
gastrocamera
    Olympus model GTF-A g.
gastroscope
    Benedict's g.
geotrichosis
Gerhardt's change of sound
Ghon tubercle
Gibson's rule
glanders
    g. of lung
Glenn's operation

Glover's drainage system
Goldstein's hemoptysis
Goodpasture's syndrome
granule
    Fauvel's g's
granuloma
    eosinophilic g.
granulomatosis
    pulmonary g.
    Wegener's g.
granulomatous
grape
    Carswell's g's
Guisez's tube
Haight's retractor
hamartoma
    intrapulmonary h.
    h. of lung
Hamburger's test
Hamman-Rich syndrome
Hamman's
    disease
    sign
Harrington-Mayo forceps
Haslinger's
    bronchoscope
    tracheo-broncho-
      esophagoscope
Heaf test
heaves
Hecht's pneumonia
Heimlich's maneuver
hemangioendothelioma
hemangioma
hemidiaphragm
hemithorax
Hemophilus
    H. influenzae
    H. pertussis
hemopneumothorax
hemoptysis
    endemic h.

hemoptysis (*continued*)
    Goldstein's h.
    Manson's h.
    parasitic h.
hemosiderosis
    idiopathic pulmonary h.
hemothorax
hernia
    diaphragmatic h.
    hiatal h.
    hiatus h.
    h. of lung
hernial
hiatus
    esophageal h.
hibernoma
hiccup
hilar
hilum
hilus
    h. pulmonis
Himmelstein's valvulotome
Hirschowitz's gastroduodenal
    fiberscope
Hirtz's rale
histiocytosis
    h. X.
Histoplasma
    H. capsulatum
histoplasmosis
Hitzenberg's test
Hodgkin's disease
Holinger-Jackson
    bronchoscope
Holinger's
    bronchoscope
    esophagoscope
    forceps
    laryngoscope
    telescope
    tube

hook
    New's h.
Hopp's laryngoscope
Horner's syndrome
Hudson's clamp
Hurst's bougie
Hurwitz's trocar
hyalinization
hydropneumothorax
hydrops
    h. of pleura
hydrothorax
    chylous h.
hygroma
hyparterial
hypercapnia
hyperinflation
hyperlucency
hyperlucent
hyperplasia
hyperresonance
hypertrophy
hyperventilation
hypoxemia
hypoxia
IC – inspiratory capacity
I/E – inspiratory-expiratory
    ratio
impaction
    mucoid i.
impressio
    i. cardiaca pulmonis
incarcerated
incision. See *General Surgical
    Terms.*
infarction
    pulmonary i.
infiltrate
    Assmann's i.
infiltration
inflammation

inflation
influenza
infrapulmonic
INH — isoniazid
inhalant
    antifoaming i.
inhalation
inhaler
inspiration
inspiratory
inspissated
insufficiency
    pulmonary i.
insufflation
    endotracheal i.
interlobar
intermedius
interstitial
intrabronchial
intracavitary
intractable
intrapleural
intrathoracic
intratracheal
intubation
    endotracheal i.
IPPB — intermittent positive
        pressure breathing
IPPO — intermittent positive
        pressure inflation
        with oxygen
isotope
    radioactive i.
isthmus
    Krönig's i.
IT — inhalation test
    inhalation therapy
    intratracheal tube
Jackson's
    bistoury
    bougie
    bronchoscope

Jackson's (*continued*)
    dilator
    elevator
    esophagoscope
    forceps
    laryngoscope
    retractor
    scalpel
    scissors
    tenaculum
    tube
Jackson-Trousseau dilator
Jacobaeus operation
Jenner's emphysema
Jesberg's
    bronchoscope
    esophagoscope
Johnson's forceps
jugular
Julian's forceps
Jürgensen's sign
Kahler's forceps
Kantrowicz's clamp
Kaplan's needle
Kapp-Beck clamp
Kartagener's
    disease
    syndrome
    triad
Kaufman's pneumonia
kemotherapy. See *chemo-*
        therapy.
Kernan-Jackson bronchoscope
Killian's
    forceps
    tubes
kilo-. See words beginning
        chylo-.
Kinsella-Buie clamp
Kistner's tube
Klebsiella
    K. pneumoniae

knife
    Lynch's k.
Kocher's forceps
Kolb's forceps
kondro-. See words beginning
    chondro-.
Krause's forceps
krico-. See words beginning
    crico-.
Krogh's apparatus spirometer
Krönig's
    area
    field
    isthmus
    percussion
Kussmaul-Kien respiration
Kussmaul's
    respiration
    sign
Kveim test
Laborde's dilator
Laennec's
    pearls
    sign
Langhans' cells
Lanz' tube
laparothoracoscopy
laringo-. See words beginning
    laryngo-.
larinjeal. See *laryngeal*.
larinks. See *larynx*.
laryngeal
laryngitis
laryngopharyngitis
laryngopharynx
laryngoscope
    Holinger's l.
    Hopp's l.
    Jackson's l.
    Lewy's l.
    Welch-Allyn l.
laryngoscopy

laryngospasm
laryngotomy
laryngotracheal
laryngotracheitis
laryngotracheobronchitis
laryngotracheobronchoscopy
laryngotracheoscopy
laryngotracheotomy
larynx
Lautier's test
lavage
Lees' clamp
Legroux's remission
leiomyoma
Leitner's syndrome
Lell's esophagoscope
Lennarson's tube
Lepley-Ernst tube
leptospirosis
Leredde's syndrome
lesion
    coin l.
Lewis' tube
Lewy-Rubin needle
Lewy's laryngoscope
Leyro-Diaz forceps
Lignières' test
Linguatula
lingula
    l. pulmonis sinistri
lingulectomy
Linton's tube
lipoma
LL — left lung
    lower lobe
LLL — left lower lobe
Lloyd's catheter
lobar
lobectomy
lobitis
lobostomy
loculated

Löffler's
    disease
    pneumonia
    syndrome
Lore-Lawrence tube
Louisiana pneumonia
Lovelace's forceps
Lowenstein's medium
LTB — laryngotracheobron-
      chitis
Lucas-Championnière's
    disease
Luer's tube
Lukens' retractor
LUL — left upper lobe
lung
    arc-welder l.
    artificial l.
    bird-breeder's l.
    black l.
    brown l.
    cardiac l.
    coalminer's l.
    drowned l.
    eosinophilic l.
    farmer's l.
    fibroid l.
    harvester's l.
    honeycomb l.
    hyperlucent l.
    iron l.
    masons' l.
    miners' l.
    pigeon-breeder's l.
    polycystic l.
    silo filler's l.
    thresher's l.
    trench l.
    vanishing l.
    wet l.
    white l.
lungmotor

lungworm
lymphadenitis
lymphadenopathy
    subcarinal l.
lymphangiectasis
    congenital pulmonary l.
lymphoblastoma
lymphoma
lymphosarcoma
Lynch's
    dissector
    forceps
    knife
    scissors
magnet
    Equen's m.
malformation
Malm-Himmelstein valvulo-
    tome
maneuver
    Heimlich's m.
    Müller's m.
    Valsalva's m.
Manson's hemoptysis
Mantoux test
manubrium
Martin's tube
Maugeri's syndrome
Mayo-Russian forceps
Mayo's scissors
mediastinal
mediastinitis
mediastinography
mediastinopericarditis
mediastinoscope
    Carlens' m.
mediastinoscopy
mediastinotomy
mediastinum
medications. See *Drugs and*
    Chemistry section.
medicolegal

medicothorax
medium
    Lowenstein's m.
Meigs' syndrome
melioidosis
    pulmonary m.
membrane
    Debove's m.
Mendelson's syndrome
mesothelioma
metastases
    hematogenous m.
    lymphangitic m.
    mediastinal m.
    miliary m.
    nodular m.
    pleural m.
metastasis
metastatic
Metras' catheter
Metzenbaum's scissors
Michelson's bronchoscope
microlithiasis
    pulmonary alveolar m.
midthorax
mist
    ultrasonic m.
Moersch's
    bronchoscope
    esophagoscope
    forceps
Monaldi's
    drainage system
    operation
Monilia
    M. albicans
Moore's tracheostomy
    buttons
Morch's tube
Morton's cough
Mosher's
    esophagoscope

Mosher's (*continued*)
    tube
Mounier-Kuhn syndrome
Moure's esophagoscope
mucoid
mucopurulent
Mucor
mucormycosis
mucoviscidosis
mucus
Mueller's clamp
Müller's
    maneuver
    test
murmur
    cardiopulmonary m.
    cardiorespiratory m.
    respiratory m.
muscle
    scalenus m.
    serratus m.
    strap m.
Mycobacterium
    M. tuberculosis
Mycoplasma
    M. pneumoniae
Myerson's
    forceps
    saw
Nachlas' tube
Naffziger's syndrome
Nathan's test
nebulizer
    DeVilbiss n.
needle
    Abrams' n.
    Cope's n.
    Fischer's n.
    Floyd's n.
    Frederick's n.
    Kaplan's n.
    Lewy-Rubin n.

Negus' bronchoscope
Nelson's
    forceps
    scissors
neurofibroma
New's
    forceps
    hook
    tube
Nocardia
    N. asteroides
nocardial
nocardiosis
node
    bronchopulmonary
        lymph n.
    mediastinal lymph n.
    pulmonary lymph n.
    tracheobronchial lymph
        n.
nodular
nodularity
numektome. See
    pneumectomy.
numo-. See words beginning
    pneumo-.
obturator
Octomyces
    O. etiennei
oleothorax
Olympus model GTF-A
    gastrocamera
Ondine's curse
operation
    Blalock-Taussig o.
    Daniel's o.
    Delorme's o.
    Eloesser's o.
    Estlander's o.
    Fowler's o.
    Friedrich's o.
    Glenn's o.

operation (*continued*)
    Jacobaeus o.
    Monaldi's o.
    Overholt's o.
    Potts-Smith-Gibson o.
    Ransohoff's o.
    Schede's o.
    Semb's o.
    Tuffier's o.
    Wilms' o.
ornithosis
orthopnea
orthopneic
Overholt-Jackson
    bronchoscope
Overholt's operation
oxyetherotherapy
P & A — percussion and
        auscultation
Pancoast's
    syndrome
    tumor
PAP — positive airway pressure
        primary atypical pneu-
        monia
papilloma
paracentesis
    p. pulmonis
    p. thoracis
paragonimiasis
Paragonimus
    P. westermani
para-influenzal
parenchyma
paries
    p. membranaceus
        bronchi
    p. membranaceus
        tracheae
parietal
paroksizm. See *paroxysm.*
paroksizmal. See *paroxysmal.*

paroxysm
paroxysmal
pars
    p. thoracalis esophagi
Patterson's
    forceps
    trocar
Patton's dilator
patulous
pCO_2 — carbon dioxide pressure
PE — pharyngoesophageal
    pleural effusion
    pulmonary edema
    pulmonary embolism
pearl
    Laennec's p's
pectoral
pectoralis
pectoriloquy
pectorophony
pectus
    p. carinatum
    p. excavatum
    p. gallinatum
    p. recurvatum
pedunculated
PEEP — positive end-expiratory pressure
penicilliosis
Penicillium
Pennington's forceps
percussion
    Krönig's p.
    respiratory p.
Perez' sign
peribronchial
peribronchiolar
peribronchiolitis
peribronchitis

pericarditis
    tuberculous p.
periesophageal
periesophagitis
perihilar
peripneumonia
    p. notha
pertussis
Peyrot's thorax
PFT — pulmonary function test
Pfuhl-Jaffe sign
Pfuhl's sign
pharyngeal
pharyngitis
pharyngoesophageal
pharyngospasm
pharyngostenosis
pharyngotomy
pharynx
phlegm
phonation
photofluorogram
photofluorography
phrenic nerve
phrenicectomy
phreniclasia
phrenicoexeresis
phrenicotomy
phrenicotripsy
phrenitis
phthisis
    bacillary p.
    colliers' p.
    diabetic p.
    fibroid p.
    flax dressers' p.
    grinders' p.
    miner's p.
    nodosa p.

phthisis (*continued*)
    potters' p.
    pulmonary p.
    stone cutters' p.
PI – pulmonary incompetence
    pulmonary infarction
PIE – pulmonary infiltration
        and eosinophilia
    pulmonary interstitial
        emphysema
Pilling's
    bronchoscope
    tube
piriform
planigram
plaque
plasmacytoma
platysma
plethysmograph
    body p.
plethysmography
pleura
    cervical p.
    costal p.
    diaphragmatic p.
    mediastinal p.
    parietal p.
    pericardial p.
    pulmonary p.
    visceral p.
pleuracentesis
pleuracotomy
pleural
    p. cavity
    p. shock
pleuralgia
pleurectomy
pleurisy
    adhesive p.
    blocked p.
    circumscribed p.

pleurisy (*continued*)
    costal p.
    diaphragmatic p.
    diffuse p.
    encysted p.
    exudative p.
    fibrinous p.
    hemorrhagic p.
    ichorous p.
    indurative p.
    interlobular p.
    mediastinal p.
    metapneumonic p.
    plastic p.
    pulmonary p.
    pulsating p.
    purulent p.
    sacculated p.
    serofibrinous p.
    serous p.
    suppurative p.
    visceral p.
    wet p.
pleuritic
pleuritis
pleurobronchitis
pleurocele
pleurocentesis
pleuroclysis
pleurodynia
    epidemic p.
pleurogenous
pleurography
pleurohepatitis
pleurolith
pleurolysis
pleuroparietopexy
pleuropericardial
pleuropericarditis
pleuroperitoneal
pleuroperitoneum

pleuropneumonia
pleuropneumonia-like
pleuropneumonolysis
pleuropulmonary
pleurorrhea
pleuroscopy
pleurothoracopleurectomy
pleurotome
pleurotomy
pleurotyphoid
pleurovisceral
plexus
    p. aorticus thoracicus
    brachial p.
    esophageal p.
    mediastinal p.
    p. pulmonalis
    subpleural mediastinal p.
plication
    fundal p.
plombage
    extraperiosteal p.
Plummer's dilator
Plummer-Vinson
    dilator
    radium applicator
PND — paroxysmal nocturnal
    dyspnea
pneogram
pneograph
pneometer
pneoscope
pneumal
pneumatic
pneumatocele
pneumatodyspnea
pneumatometer
pneumatometry
pneumatophore
pneumatosis
    p. pulmonum

pneumectomy
pneumoalveolography
pneumoangiography
pneumobacillus
    Friedländer's p.
pneumobronchotomy
pneumobulbar
pneumocardial
pneumocentesis
pneumochirurgia
pneumocholecystitis
pneumochysis
pneumococcal
pneumococcic
pneumococcus
pneumoconiosis
    bauxite p.
    coal workers' p.
    collagenous p.
    mica p.
    noncollagenous p.
    rheumatoid p.
    p. siderotica
    talc p.
pneumocystic
Pneumocystis
    P. carinii
pneumoenteritis
pneumoerysipelas
pneumogastric
pneumogram
pneumography
pneumohemothorax
pneumohydrothorax
pneumolithiasis
pneumomalacia
pneumomediastinography
pneumomediastinum
pneumomelanosis
pneumomycosis
pneumonectasis

pneumonectomy
pneumonedema
pneumonemia
pneumonere
pneumonia
    abortive p.
    acute p.
    p. alba
    amebic p.
    anthrax p.
    p. apostematosa
    aspiration p.
    atypical p.
    bacterial p.
    bilious p.
    bronchial p.
    Buhl's desquamative p.
    caseous p.
    catarrhal p.
    cheesy p.
    cold agglutinin p.
    Corrigan's p.
    croupous p.
    deglutition p.
    Desnos' p.
    desquamative p.
    desquamative interstitial
      p.
    p. dissecans
    double p.
    Eaton agent p.
    embolic p.
    ephemeral p.
    fibrinous p.
    Friedländer's bacillus p.
    Friedländer's p.
    gangrenous p.
    giant cell p.
    Hecht's p.
    hypostatic p.
    indurative p.

pneumonia (*continued*)
    influenzal p.
    p. interlobularis puru-
      lenta
    interstitial plasma cell p.
    Kaufman's p.
    Klebsiella p.
    lingular p.
    lipoid p.
    lobar p.
    lobular p.
    Löffler's p.
    Louisiana p.
    metastatic p.
    migratory p.
    mycoplasmal p.
    obstructive p.
    parenchymatous p.
    pleurogenetic p.
    pneumococcal p.
    Pneumocystis carinii p.
    purulent p.
    rheumatic p.
    Riesman's p.
    septic p.
    staphylococcal p.
    Stoll's p.
    streptococcal p.
    suppurative p.
    toxemic p.
    transplantation p.
    tuberculous p.
    tularemic p.
    typhoid p.
    unresolved p.
    vagus p.
    varicella p.
    viral p.
    wandering p.
    woolsorter's p.
pneumonic

pneumonitis
    aspiration p.
    cholesterol p.
    desquamative interstitial
      p.
    eosinophilic p.
    granulomatous p.
    malarial p.
    pneumocystis p.
    uremic p.
pneumonocentesis
pneumonochirurgia
pneumonocirrhosis
pneumonocyte
    granular p.
    membranous p.
pneumonograph
pneumonography
pneumonolipoidosis
pneumonolysis
pneumonomelanosis
pneumonomoniliasis
pneumonopathy
    eosinophilic p.
pneumonopexy
pneumonophthisis
pneumonoresection
pneumonorrhaphy
pneumonosis
pneumonotherapy
pneumonotomy
pneumoparesis
pneumopericardium
pneumoperitoneum
pneumopexy
pneumopleuritis
pneumopleuroparietopexy
pneumopyothorax
pneumoresection
pneumorrhagia
pneumosepticemia
pneumoserothorax

pneumosilicosis
pneumotachograph
pneumotachometer
pneumotachygraph
pneumotherapy
pneumothorax
    artificial p.
    clicking p.
    closed p.
    diagnostic p.
    extrapleural p.
    spontaneous p.
    tension p.
    valvular p.
pneumotoxin
pneumotropic
pneumotropism
pneumotyphoid
pneumotyphus
PO_2 — oxygen pressure
Polisar-Lyons tube
polycythemia
position. See *General Surgical Terms.*
postpneumonic
post-tussis
Pottenger's sign
Potts-Smith-Gibson operation
poudrage
    pleural p.
PP — pink puffers (emphysema)
PPB — positive pressure breathing
PPD — purified protein derivative
PPLO — pleuropneumonia-like organism
pretracheal
Price-Thomas
    clamp
    forceps

Pritchard's cannula
profundoplasty
proteinosis
    pulmonary alveolar p.
Proteus
pseudobronchiectasis
pseudocoarctation
Pseudomonas
    P. aeruginosa
psittacosis
pulmogram
pulmolith
pulmometer
pulmometry
pulmonary
    p. abscess
    p. edema
    p. embolism
pulmonic
pulmonitis
pulmonohepatic
pulmonology
pulmonoperitoneal
pulmotor
pulsator
    Bragg-Paul p.
purulent
PX – pneumothorax
pyopneumothorax
pyothorax
Q fever (Q for query)
radiogram
radiography
radioisotope
radiolucent
radiopaque
rale
    amphoric r.
    atelectatic r.
    bronchial r.
    bubbling r.
    cavernous r.

rale (*continued*)
    cellophane r.
    clicking r.
    collapse r.
    consonating r.
    crackling r.
    crepitant r.
    r. de retour
    extrathoracic r.
    gurgling r.
    guttural r.
    Hirtz's r.
    r. indux
    moist r.
    r. muqueux
    pleural r.
    r. redux
    sibilant r.
    Skoda's r.
    sonorous r.
    subcrepitant r.
    tracheal r.
    vesicular r.
    whistling r.
Ralks' clamp
Ramond's sign
Ransohoff's operation
RDS – respiratory distress
    syndrome
reflux
regurgitation
    esophageal r.
remission
    Legroux's r's
rentgenograhfe. See *roentgen-
    ography.*
repair
    Belsey's r.
resonance
    bandbox r.
    bell-metal r.
    cracked-pot r.

resonance (*continued*)
   shoulder-strap r.
   skodaic r.
resonant
respiration
   amphoric r.
   anaerobic r.
   asthmoid r.
   Biot's r.
   bronchial r.
   bronchocavernous r.
   bronchovesicular r.
   cavernous r.
   Cheyne-Stokes r.
   cogwheel r.
   Corrigan's r.
   external r.
   internal r.
   Kussmaul-Kien r.
   Kussmaul's r.
   paradoxical r.
   puerile r.
   Seitz's metamorphosing
      r.
   stertorous r.
   tubular r.
   vesicular r.
   vesiculocavernous r.
   vicarious r.
respirator
   cabinet r.
   cuirass r.
   Drinker r.
respiratory
respirometer
retractor
   Andrews' r.
   Bernay's r.
   Brewster's r.
   flexible shaft r.
   Haight's r.
   Jackson's r.

retractor (*continued*)
   Lukens' r.
   Robinson's r.
   Shurly's r.
retrosternal
rhonchal
rhonchial
rhonchus
RI — respiratory illness
rib spreader
   Tuffier's r.s.
rickettsial
Riecker's bronchoscope
Riesman's pneumonia
ring
   Schatzki's r.
Riviere's sign
RL — right lung
RLC — residual lung capacity
RLL — right lower lobe
RM — respiratory movement
RML — right middle lobe
Roberts'
   esophagoscope
   forceps
Robinson's retractor
Rockey's
   cannula
   clamp
   forceps
   scope
roentgenography
Rokitansky's diverticulum
rong-. See words beginning
   rhonc-.
Roussel's sign
RS — respiratory syncytial
RTF — respiratory tract fluid
Rubin's clamp
RUL — right upper lobe
rule
   Gibson's r.

Russian forceps
RV — respiratory volume
Safar's bronchoscope
Salvatore-Maloney tracheo-
    tome
Sam Roberts forceps
sarcoid
sarcoidosis
sarcoma
Sarot's
        clamp
        forceps
saw
        Myerson's s.
scalene
scalenectomy
scalenotomy
scalpel
        Jackson's s.
Schatzki's ring
Schede's operation
Scheinmann's forceps
Schindler's esophagoscope
schistosomiasis
        pulmonary s.
Schmorl's furrow
scissors
        Crafoord's s.
        Jackson's s.
        Lynch's s.
        Mayo's s.
        Metzenbaum's s.
        Nelson's s.
        Sweet's s.
scleroderma
        pulmonary s.
scope
        Rockey's s.
segment
        bronchopulmonary s.
segmenta
        s. bronchopulmonalia

segmental
Seiffert's forceps
Seitz's metamorphosing
    respiration
Semb's operation
Sengstaken-Blakemore tube
septum
        s. bronchiale
        s. mediastinale
sequestration
        pulmonary s.
sequoiosis
serosanguineous
serpiginous
Shaver's disease
Shenstone's tourniquet
Shibley's sign
shunt
        portacaval s.
Shurly's retractor
siderosilicosis
siderosis
Sierra-Sheldon tracheotome
sign
        Abraham's s.
        Baccelli's s.
        Bethea's s.
        Cegka's s.
        D'Amato's s.
        Delmege's s.
        Ellis' s.
        Ewart's s.
        Friedreich's s.
        Hamman's s.
        Jürgensen's s.
        Kussmaul's s.
        Laennec's s.
        Perez' s.
        Pfuhl-Jaffe s.
        Pfuhl's s.
        Pottenger's s.
        Ramond's s.

sign (*continued*)
    Riviere's s.
    Roussel's s.
    Shibley's s.
    Skoda's s.
    Sternberg's s.
    Westermark's s.
    Williams' s.
    Williamson's s.
silicatosis
silicosiderosis
silicosis
    infective s.
silicotuberculosis
singultus
sinobronchitis
sinus
    s. trunci pulmonalis
siphon
    Duguet's s.
Sippy's dilator
sitakosis. See psittacosis.
situs
    s. inversus viscerum
Skoda's
    rale
    sign
    tympany
Snyder's surgivac drainage
   system
solitary nodule
sonorous
sound
    Beatty-Bright friction s.
    cracked-pot s.
    esophageal s.
    hippocratic s.
    respiratory s.
    to-and-fro s.
Souttar's tube
space
    Traube's s.

Spinhaler
spirochetosis
    bronchopulmonary s.
spirogram
spirograph
spirography
spirometer
    Benedict-Roth s.
    Collins' respirometer-s.
    Douglas' bag s.
    Krogh's apparatus s.
    Tissot's s.
    Venturi's meter s.
    Wright's respirometer-s.
spirometry
    bronchoscopic s.
spirophore
splenization
    hypostatic s.
splenopneumonia
sputum
    s. aeroginosum
    albuminoid s.
    s. coctum
    s. crudum
    s. cruentum
    egg yolk s.
    globular s.
    green s.
    icteric s.
    moss-agate s.
    nummular s.
    prune juice s.
    rusty s.
squama
    s. alveolaris
stannosis
Staphylococcus
    S. aureus
Staple's bronchoscope
status
    s. asthmaticus

Steele's dilator
stenosis
stereoscopy
sternal
Sternberg's sign
sternoclavicular
sternocostal
sternotomy
sternotracheal
sternum
stethoscope
Stoll's pneumonia
Storz' bronchoscope
stricture
stridor
    s. serraticus
study
    cytological s.
    enzyme s.
subpleural
substernal
succussion
    hippocratic s.
suctioning
    endotracheal-bronchial s.
sudo-. See words beginning
    pseudo-.
suffocation
sulcate
sulcus
    s. pulmonalis thoracis
    subclavian s. of lung
    s. subclavius pulmonis
surgical procedures. See
    operation.
suture. See *General Surgical*
    Terms.
Sweet's scissors
Sydenham's cough
symptom
    Burghart's s.

syndrome
    Arneth's s.
    Ayerza's s.
    Bard's s.
    Bársony-Polgár s.
    Brock's s.
    Caplan's s.
    Goodpasture's s.
    Hamman-Rich s.
    Horner's s.
    hyperlucent lung s.
    Kartagener's s.
    Leitner's s.
    Leredde's s.
    Löffler's s.
    Maugeri's s.
    Meigs' s.
    Mendelson's s.
    middle lobe s.
    Mounier-Kuhn s.
    Naffziger's s.
    Pancoast's s.
    Wilson-Mikity s.
system
    respiratory s.
talcosis
TB — tuberculosis
telescope
    Broyles' t.
    Holinger's t.
    right-angle t.
tenaculum
    Jackson's t.
teratodermoid
teratoma
test
    Adson's t.
    Allen's t.
    Arloing-Courmont t.
    Blumenau's t.
    Casoni's t.

test (*continued*)
    coccidioidin t.
    Craig's t.
    Escherich's t.
    Hamburger's t.
    Heaf t.
    histoplasmin skin t.
    Hitzenberg's t.
    Kveim t.
    Lautier's t.
    Lignières' t.
    Mantoux t.
    Müller's t.
    Nathan's t.
    patch t.
    pulmonary function t.
    tine tuberculin t.
    tuberculin t.
    Valsalva's t.
    Vollmer's t.
    Weinberg's t.
    Youman-Parlett t.
Thompson's catheter
Thomson's clamp
thoracentesis
thoracic
thoracicoabdominal
thoracobronchotomy
thoracocautery
thoracocentesis
thoracocyllosis
thoracocyrtosis
thoracodynia
thoracogastroschisis
thoracograph
thoracolaparotomy
thoracolysis
    t. praecordiaca
thoracometer
thoracometry
thoracoplasty
    costoversion t.

thoracopneumograph
thoracopneumoplasty
thoracoschisis
thoracoscope
thoracoscopy
thoracostenosis
thoracostomy
thoracotomy
thorax
    barrel-shaped t.
    cholesterol t.
    Peyrot's t.
    pyriform t.
thrombosis
thymectomy
thymoma
thymus
thymusectomy
tine test
tisis. See *phthisis.*
Tissot's spirometer
TLC — total lung capacity
    total lung compliance
Tobold-Fauvel forceps
tomography
torulosis
tourniquet
    Bethune's t.
    Shenstone's t.
toxoplasmosis
trachea
tracheaectasy
tracheal
trachealgia
tracheitis
tracheobronchial
tracheobronchitis
tracheobronchomegaly
tracheobronchoscopy
tracheocele
tracheoesophageal
tracheofissure

tracheofistulization
tracheogenic
tracheomalacia
tracheopathia
    t. osteoplastica
tracheophony
tracheoplasty
tracheopyosis
tracheorrhagia
tracheorrhaphy
tracheoschisis
tracheoscopy
tracheostenosis
tracheostoma
tracheostomy
tracheotome
    Salvatore-Maloney t.
    Sierra-Sheldon t.
tracheotomize
tracheotomy
transillumination
transthoracic
transthoracotomy
transtracheal
Traube's
    dyspnea
    space
treatment
    Forlanini's t.
tree
    bronchial t.
    tracheobronchial t.
triad
    Kartagener's t.
Trichomonas
    T. pulmonalis
trocar
    Hurwitz's t.
    Patterson's t.
Trousseau-Jackson dilator
Trousseau's
    bougie

Trousseau's (*continued*)
    dilator
truncus
    t. bronchomediastinalis
     dexter
    t. pulmonalis
tube
    Andrews-Pynchon t.
    Argyle chest t.
    Atkins-Cannard t.
    Blakemore's t.
    Broyles' t.
    Carabelli's t.
    Celestin's t.
    Chaussier's t.
    Chevalier Jackson t.
    Depaul's t.
    Durham's t.
    fiberoptic t.
    Gabriel Tucker t.
    Guisez's t.
    Holinger's t.
    intubation t.
    Jackson's t.
    Killian's t's
    Kistner's t.
    Lanz' t.
    Lennarson's t.
    Lepley-Ernst t.
    Lewis' t.
    Linton's t.
    Lore-Lawrence t.
    Luer's t.
    Martin's t.
    Morch's t.
    Mosher's t.
    Nachlas' t.
    New's t.
    Pilling's t.
    Polisar-Lyons t.
    Sengstaken-Blakemore t.
    Souttar's t.

tube (*continued*)
    thoracostomy t.
    tracheostomy t.
    Tucker's t.
tubercle
    Ghon t.
    scalene t.
tubercular
tuberculin
tuberculoid
tuberculoma
tuberculomyces
tuberculosilicosis
tuberculosis
    acute miliary t.
    anthracotic t.
    cestodic t.
    exudative t.
    hilus t.
    miliary t.
    pulmonary t.
    tracheobronchial t.
tuberculous
Tucker's
    bronchoscope
    esophagoscope
    tube
Tuffier's
    operation
    rib spreader
tumor
    alveolar cell t.
    amyloid t.
    epidermoid t.
    oat cell t.
    Pancoast's t.
    sulcus t.
    teratoid t.
    thymic t.
tunica
    t. adventitia esophagi
    t. mucosa bronchiorum

tunica (*continued*)
    t. mucosa esophagi
    t. mucosa laryngis
    t. mucosa tracheae
    t. muscularis esophagi
    t. muscularis tracheae
Tuttle's forceps
tympanic
tympany
    bell t.
    skodaic t.
    Skoda's t.
ulceration
underwater seal drainage
URI — upper respiratory
    infection
Valsalva's
    maneuver
    test
valvulotome
    Himmelstein's v.
    Malm-Himmelstein v.
varices
varix
vein
    azygos v.
    brachial v.
    cephalic v.
    innominate v.
    thymic v.
vena
    v. cava
venesection
venogram
Venti-mask
Venturi's meter spirometer
virus
    v. bronchopneumonia
    Coxsackie v.
    ECHO (enteric cyto-
    pathogenic human
    orphan v.

virus (*continued*)
    parainfluenza v.
    respiratory syncytial v.
visceropleural
visualization
    laryngoscopic v.
Vollmer's test
Waterman's bronchoscope
Wegener's granulomatosis
Weinberg's test
Welch-Allyn laryngoscope
Westermark's sign
wheeze
whooping cough
Williams' sign
Williamson's sign
Wilms' operation

Wilson-Mikity syndrome
windpipe
Woillez' disease
Wright's respirometer-
    spirometer
X histiocytosis
xiphocostal
xiphoid
Yankauer-Little forceps
Yankauer's
    bronchoscope
    esophagoscope
Youman-Parlett test
Zavod's catheter
Zenker's diverticulum
zifo-. See words beginning
    xipho-.

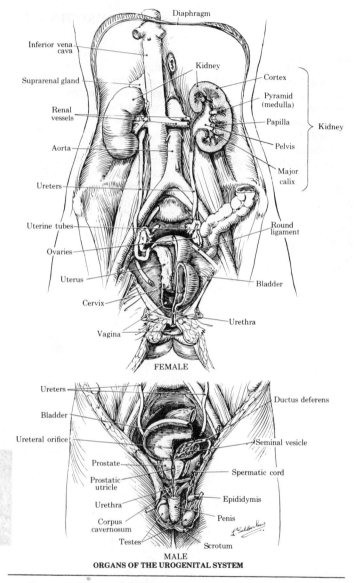

FEMALE

- Diaphragm
- Inferior vena cava
- Suprarenal gland
- Kidney
- Cortex
- Pyramid (medulla)
- Renal vessels
- Papilla
- Aorta
- Pelvis
- Ureters
- Major calix
- Kidney
- Uterine tubes
- Round ligament
- Ovaries
- Uterus
- Bladder
- Cervix
- Urethra
- Vagina

MALE

- Ureters
- Ductus deferens
- Bladder
- Ureteral orifice
- Seminal vesicle
- Prostate
- Spermatic cord
- Prostatic utricle
- Urethra
- Epididymis
- Corpus cavernosum
- Penis
- Testes
- Scrotum

ORGANS OF THE UROGENITAL SYSTEM

(Courtesy of Dorland's Illustrated Medical Dictionary, 26th ed. Plate L. Philadelphia, W. B. Saunders Company, 1981.)

UROLOGY

aberrant
abscess
acetone
acetonuria
achromaturia
acidosis
    renal tubular a.
Acmistat catheter
Acmi-Valentine tube
aconuresis
acraturesis
actinomycosis
acuminata
    condylomata a.
    verruca a.
adapter
    Ralks' a.
Addison's disease
Addis's method
adenitis
adenoacanthoma
adenocarcinoma
adenoma
    cortical a's
adenomyosarcoma
adenosarcoma
    embryonal a.
ADH — antidiuretic hormone
adiposis
    a. orchalis

adiposis (*continued*)
    a. orchica
adrenal
    Marchand's a's
adrenalectomy
adrenalinuria
adrenalism
adrenalitis
adrenalopathy
adrenic
adrenin
adrenitis
adrenocortical
adrenogenous
adrenokinetic
adrenomedullotropic
adrenomegaly
adrenopathy
adrenopause
adrenoprival
adrenostatic
adrenotoxin
adrenotropic
adrenotropin
adrenotropism
adventitia
aerocystography
aerocystoscope
aerocystoscopy
afferent

agenesis
agenitalism
agenosomia
aglomerular
aidoiitis
Albarran's
    gland
    test
    tubules
albiduria
albuginea
    a. penis
albugineotomy
albumin
albuminaturia
albuminuria
    adventitious a.
    globular a.
    nephrogenous a.
    postrenal a.
    renal a.
    residual a.
albuminuric
Alcock-Hendrickson's lithotrite
Alcock's
    catheter
    lithotrite
Alcock-Timberlake obturator
alcoholuria
alginuresis
alkaline
Allemann's syndrome
Allis' forceps
allograft
Alyea's clamp
amebiasis
    a. of bladder
ampulla
    a. ductus deferentis
    Henle's a.
    a. of vas deferens
amyloidosis

anastomosis
    pyeloileocutaneous a.
    transuretero-ureteral a.
Andrews' operation
androgen
anesthesia. See *General
    Surgical Terms.*
aneurysm
aneurysmal
aneurysmatic
angiogram
    renal a.
angiography
angle
    costovertebral a.
angulation
anischuria
ankylurethria
annulus
    a. urethralis
anorchia
anorchid
anorchidic
anorchidism
anorchis
anorchism
anovesical
anuresis
anuretic
anuria
    angioneurotic a.
    calculous a.
    obstructive a.
    postrenal a.
    prerenal a.
    renal a.
    suppressive a.
anuric
aorta
aorticorenal
apex
    a. of bladder

apex (*continued*)
    a. prostatae
    a. vesicae urinariae
aponeurosis
    Denonvilliers' a.
arcuate
ardor
    a. urinae
areolar
Arnold and Gunning's method
arteriole
    glomerular a.
    glomerular a., afferent
    glomerular a., efferent
    Isaacs-Ludwig a.
    postglomerular a.
    preglomerular a.
    renal a.
arteriorenal
arteriosclerotic
arteriovenous
artery
    arcuate a.
    cremasteric a.
    dorsal a.
    gluteal a.
    helcine a.
    hypogastric a.
    iliac a.
    interlobar a.
    interlobular a.
    perineal a.
    pudendal a.
    renal a.
    spermatic a.
    vesical a.
ascites
aspermatism
aspermatogenesis
aspermia
asthenospermia

atonic
atony
atresia
atrophic
atrophy
azoospermatism
azoospermia
azotemia
    extrarenal a.
    prerenal a.
azotemic
    a. osteodystrophy
azoturia
azoturic
Babcock's clamp
backflow
    pyelovenous b.
bacteriuria
bah-fon. See *bas-fond.*
balanic
balanitis
    b. circinata
    b. diabetica
    Follmann's b.
    b. gangraenosa
    gangrenous b.
    b. xerotica obliterans
balanoblennorrhea
balanocele
balanoplasty
balanoposthitis
balanoposthomycosis
balanopreputial
balanorrhagia
balanus
Balkan nephritis
bar
    Mercier's b.
Bardex's catheter
Bard's catheter
Bartter's syndrome

bas-fond
basket
    Browne's b.
    Councill's b.
    Dormia's b.
    Ferguson's b.
    Howard's b.
    Johnson's b.
    Mitchell's b.
Bates' operation
Baumrucker's resectoscope
Belfield's operation
Bellini's
    ducts
    tubules
Bell's muscle
Bence-Jones
    cylinders
    protein method
    proteinuria
    urine
Benedict and Franke's method
Benedict and Osterberg's
    method
Bengt-Johanson repair
benign
Bennett's operation
Bergenhem's operation
Bertin's column
Bertrand's method
Bethune's rib cutter
Bevan-Rochet operation
Bevan's operation
bifid
bifurcation
Bigelow's
    lithotrite
    operation
bilabe
bilirubin
bilirubinuria

biopsy
    renal b.
Bittorf's reaction
bladder
    atonic b.
    autonomic b.
    dome of b.
    fasciculated b.
    ileocecal b.
    irritable b.
    nervous b.
    neurogenic b.
    sacculated b.
    stammering b.
    urinary b.
Blake's forceps
Blasucci's catheter
blennorrhagia
blennorrhea
blennuria
Boari's operation
body
    b. of Highmore
    wolffian b.
boggy
boo-zhe. See *bougie.*
Bottini's operation
bougie
    b. à boule
    acorn-tipped b.
    b. coudé
    LeFort's b.
    olive tip b.
    Otis' b.
    Philips' b.
    Ruschelit's b.
boutonnière
Bowman's capsule
Bozeman's forceps
BPH — benign prostatic hyper-
    trophy

Braasch's
    catheter
    cystoscope
    forceps
Brewer's infarcts
Bricker's operation
brightism
Bright's disease
Brodny's clamp
Brödel's line
Brown-Buerger cystoscope
Browne's basket
bubo
    chancroidal b.
    gonorrheal b.
    venereal b.
bubonulus
Buck's fascia
Buerger-McCarthy forceps
Bugbee's electrode
bulbitis
bulbocavernosus
bulbourethral
bulbous
bulbus
    b. penis
    b. urethrae
bullous
Bumpus'
    forceps
    resectoscope
BUN — blood urea nitrogen
Bunim's forceps
Buschke-Loewenstein tumor
Butterfield's cystoscope
Bywaters' syndrome
Cacchi-Ricci syndrome
cachexia
    urinary c.
calcification
calculi

calculus
    alternating c.
    coral c.
    cystine c.
    decubitus c.
    dendritic c.
    encysted c.
    fibrin c.
    gonecystic c.
    hemp seed c.
    indigo c.
    matrix c.
    mulberry c.
    nephritic c.
    oxalate c.
    prostatic c.
    renal c.
    spermatic c.
    stag-horn c.
    struvite c.
    ureteral c.
    urethral c.
    uric acid c.
    urinary c.
    urostealith c.
    vesical c.
    vesicoprostatic c.
    xanthic c.
caliber
calibrated
calibration
calibrator
caliceal
calicectasis
calicectomy
calices
calices renales
    c.r. majores
    c.r. minores
calicine
caliectasis

caliectomy
calix
calyceal
calycectasis
calycectomy
calyces
calyces renales
    c.r. majores
    c.r. minores
calyx
Campbell's
    catheter
    forceps
    retractor
    sound
    trocar
cannulation
capillaries
capistration
capsula
    c. adiposa renis
    c. fibrosa renis
    c. glomeruli
capsulae renis
capsular
capsule
    adipose c.
    Bowman's c.
    fibrous c. of corpora
      cavernosa penis
    Gerota's c.
    glomerular c.
    c. of glomerulus
    müllerian c.
    pelvioprostatic c.
    perinephric c.
    suprarenal c.
capsulectomy
capsuloma
capsuloplasty
capsulorrhaphy
capsulotomy

caput
    c. gallinaginis
carcinoma
    epibulbar c.
    c. scroti
    squamous cell c.
    transitional cell c.
Carson's catheter
caruncle
    morgagnian c.
castrate
castration
cast
    blood c.
    epithelial c.
    fat c.
    wax c.
Cathelin's segregator
catheter
    Acmistat c.
    acorn tip c.
    Alcock's c.
    Bard's c.
    Bardex's c.
    Blasucci's c.
    Braasch's c.
    Campbell's c.
    Carson's c.
    cathematic c.
    c. coudé
    Councill's c.
    Coxeter's c.
    de Pezzer c.
    Emmett-Foley c.
    filiform c.
    Foley c.
    Foley-Alcock c.
    French-Robinson c.
    Furniss' c.
    indwelling c.
    latex c.
    LeFort's c.

catheter (*continued*)
    Malecot's c.
    McIver's c.
    Nélaton's c.
    olive tip c.
    Owens' c.
    Pezzer's c.
    Philips' c.
    polyethylene c.
    red Robinson c.
    retention c.
    return flow hemostatic c.
    Silastic mushroom c.
    spiral tip c.
    Tiemann's c.
    ureteral c.
    whistle tip c.
    Winer's c.
    Wishard's c.
catheterization
    retrourethral c.
catheterize
cauda
    e. epididymidis
cavernous
cavum
    c. retzii
C-clamp
Cecil's
    operation
    repair
cell
    Leydig's c's
    Sertoli's c.
cellule
cervix
chancre
    Nisbet's c.
chancroid
chemolysis
chorda
    c. gubernaculum

chorda (*continued*)
    c. spermatica
chordae
chordee
chorditis
choriocarcinoma
chorioepithelioma
chylocele
    parasitic c.
chyloderma
chyluria
cinefluorography
cineurography
circumcise
circumcision
circumferential
Civiale's operation
Cl – chloride
clamp
    Alyea's c.
    Babcock's c.
    Brodny's c.
    C-c.
    Cunningham's c.
    Goldblatt's c.
    Gomco's c.
    Guyon-Pean c.
    Guyon's c.
    Halsted's c.
    Herrick's c.
    Hyams' c.
    Kantor's c.
    Mayo's c.
    Ockerblad's c.
    pedicle c.
    penile c.
    rubber-shod c.
    Stille's c.
    Stockman's c.
    Tatum's c.
    Walther-Crenshaw c.
    Walther's c.

clamp (*continued*)
    Wertheim-Cullen c.
    Wertheim-Reverdin c.
    Wertheim's c.
    Young's c.
    Zipser's c.
Clark's operation
cloaca
    congenital c.
    persistent c.
CMV — cytomegalovirus
Cock's operation
colic
    renal c.
collecting system
Colles' fascia
colliculectomy
colliculi
colliculitis
colliculus
    bulbar c.
    seminal c.
    c. seminalis
Collings' electrode
colloid
collum
    c. glandis penis
colony count
column
    Bertin's c.
    c. of Sertoli
concentric
concrement
concretion
condyloma
    c. acuminatum
    c. latum
continence
continent
contracture
convoluted

Cooke-Apert-Gallais
    syndrome
cooler
    Eissner's prostatic c.
Cooper's irritable testis
Coppridge's forceps
copulation
copulatory
Corbus' disease
cord
    genital c.
    gubernacular c.
    nephrogenic c.
    spermatic c.
corditis
corona
    c. glandis penis
    c. of glans penis
coronal
corpora
corpus
    c. cavernosum penis
    c. cavernosum urethrae
      virilis
    c. epididymidis
    c. glandulae bulbo-
      urethralis
    c. glandulare prostatae
    c. Highmori
    c. highmorianum
    c. penis
    c. spongiosum penis
    c. vesicae urinariae
    c. vesiculae seminalis
    c. Wolffi
cortex
    adrenal c.
    c. glandulae suprarenalis
    renal c.
    c. renis
cortiadrenal

cortical
costovertebral angle
coudé
    bougie c.
    catheter c.
Councill's
    basket
    catheter
    stone dislodger
Cowper's gland
Coxeter's catheter
creatinine
Creevy's evacuator
cremaster
    internal c. of Henle
cremasteric
Crenshaw's forceps
CRF – chronic renal failure
crisis
    Dietl's c.
crista
    c. urethralis masculinae
    c. urethralis virilis
crura
crus
    c. penis
cryogenic
cryptorchid
cryptorchidectomy
cryptorchidism
cryptorchidopexy
cryptorchidy
cryptorchism
crystalloid
crystalluria
crystalluridrosis
C & S – culture and sensitivity
Culp's ureteropelvioplasty
cuneiform
Cunningham's clamp
CVA – costovertebral angle

cylinders
    Bence Jones c's
cylindruria
cyst
    medullary c.
    pyelogenic c.
    renal c.
    wolffian c.
cystalgia
cystathioninuria
cystatrophia
cystauchenitis
cystauchenotomy
cystauxe
cystectasia
cystectasy
cystectomy
cysteine
cystelcosis
cystendesis
cysterethism
cysthypersarcosis
cystic
cystidolaparotomy
cystidotrachelotomy
cystine
cystinosis
cystinuria
cystistaxis
cystitis
    allergic c.
    amicrobic c.
    bacterial c.
    catarrhal c.
    chemical c.
    c. colli
    croupous c.
    cystic c.
    c. cystica
    diphtheritic c.
    c. emphysematosa

cystitis (*continued*)
    eosinophilic c.
    exfoliative c.
    c. follicularis
    gangrenous c.
    c. glandularis
    hemorrhagic c.
    incrusted c.
    interstitial c.
    mechanical c.
    panmural c.
    c. papillomatosa
    c. senilis feminarum
    subacute c.
    submucous c.
cysto — cystoscopic examination
cystocele
cystochrome
cystochromoscopy
cystocolostomy
cystodynia
cystoenterocele
cystoepiplocele
cystogram
    air c.
    excretory c.
    gravity c.
    postvoiding c.
    voiding c.
cystography
cystolith
cystolithectomy
cystolithiasis
cystolithic
cystolithotomy
cystometer
    Lewis' c.
cystometric
cystometrogram
cystometrography
cystometry

cystonephrosis
cystoneuralgia
cystoparalysis
cystopexy
cystophotography
cystophthisis
cystoplasty
    cecal c.
cystoplegia
cystoproctostomy
cystoptosis
cystopyelitis
cystopyelogram
cystopyelography
cystopyelonephritis
cystoradiography
cystorectostomy
cystorrhagia
cystorrhaphy
cystorrhea
cystoschisis
cystoscirrhus
cystoscope
    Braasch's c.
    Brown-Buerger c.
    Butterfield's c.
    fiberoptic c.
    Kelly's c.
    Lowsley-Peterson c.
    McCarthy-Campbell c.
    McCarthy-Peterson c.
    McCarthy's c.
    National c.
    Nesbit's c.
    Ravich's c.
    Storz' c.
    Wappler's c.
cystoscopic
cystoscopy
cystospasm
cystospermitis
cystostaxis

cystostomy
cystotome
cystotomy
    suprapubic c.
cystotrachelotomy
cystoureteritis
cystoureterogram
cystoureteropyelitis
cystoureteropyelonephritis
cystourethritis
cystourethrocele
cystourethrogram
cystourethropexy
cystourethroscope
cystous
dartoic
dartoid
dartos
dartrous
Davat's operation
Davis'
    sound
    stone dislodger
Deaver's retractor
decapsulation
decortication
    renal d.
Dees' needle
Defer's method
Del Castillo's syndrome
demasculinization
Deming's operation
Demme's method
Dennis-Brown technique
Denonvilliers'
    aponeurosis
    fascia
    operation
de Pezzer catheter
descending
descensus
    d. testis

Desjardin's forceps
detrusor
    d. urinae
diabetes
    d. insipidus
    d. mellitus
dialysance
dialysate
dialysis
    peritoneal d.
    renal d.
dialyzer
diaphragm
    urogenital d.
Dietl's crisis
diffusion
dilatation
dilator
    French's d. Nos. 8 to 36
    Guyon's d.
    Kollmann's d.
    Leader-Kollmann d.
    Van Buren's d.
    Walther's d.
disease
    Addison's d.
    Bright's d.
    Corbus' d.
    Ducrey's d.
    Durand-Nicholas-Favre d.
    Ebstein's d.
    Fournier's d.
    Klebs' d.
    Lindau's d.
    medullary cystic d.
    Peyronie's d.
    polycystic d.
    Reiter's d.
    Stühmer's d.
Dittel's
    operation
    sound

diureses
diuresis
tubular d.
diuretic
hydragogue d.
refrigerant d.
diuria
diverticula
d. ampullae ductus
deferentis
diverticulectomy
diverticuleve
diverticulitis
diverticulum
calyceal d.
vesical d.
Doppler's operation
Dorian's rib stripper
Dormia's
basket
stone dislodger
Douglas' pouch
Doyen's operation
drain
Malecot's d.
Penrose d.
Pezzer's d.
sump d.
dressing. See *General Surgical Terms.*
dribbling
drugs. See *Drugs and Chemistry* section.
Ducrey's disease
duct
Bellini's d's
ejaculatory d.
Leydig's d.
mesonephric d.
d. of Wolff
wolffian d.

ductuli
d. aberrantes
d. prostatica
ductulus
d. aberrans superior
ductus
d. aberrans
d. deferens
d. ejaculatorius
d. epididymidis
d. excretorius glandulae bulbourethrales
d. excretorius vesiculae seminalis
d. glandulae bulbourethralis
d. mesonephricus
d. Muelleri
d. paraurethrales
d. prostatica
d. spermaticus
d. wolffi
Duplay's operation
Dupuytren's hydrocele
Durand-Nicholas-Favre disease
dynamoscope
dynamoscopy
dysgenesis
gonadal d.
dysgenitalism
dysgerminoma
dysgonesis
dysuresia
dysuria
psychic d.
spastic d.
dysuriac
dysuric
dyszoospermia
Ebstein's disease
echinococcosis

ectasia
ectopia
    e. testis
    e. vesicae
Edebohls' operation
edema
efferent
efflux
Eissner's prostatic cooler
ejaculate
ejaculatio
    e. deficiens
    e. praecox
    e. retardata
ejaculation
ejaculatory
ejaculum
electrocystography
electrode
    ball tip e.
    bayonet tip e.
    Bugbee's e.
    Collings' e.
    conical tip e.
    Hamm's e.
    McCarthy's e.
    Neil-Moore e.
    ureteral meatotomy e.
electrolyte
electromyography
    ureteral e.
electrotome
    Stern-McCarthy e.
elephantiasis
    e. scroti
Ellik's evacuator
embolism
embryonal
emission
Emmett-Foley catheter

endometriosis
    e. vesicae
endoscope
    Kelly's e.
endoscopic
endoscopy
endourethral
enorchia
enucleation
enucleator
    Young's e.
enuresis
    diurnal e.
    nocturnal e.
enuretic
epicystitis
epicystotomy
epidermoid
epididymal
epididymectomy
epididymis
epididymitis
    spermatogenic e.
epididymodeferentectomy
epididymodeferential
epididymo-orchitis
epididymotomy
epididymovasectomy
epididymovasostomy
epinephrectomy
epinephritis
epinephroma
epinephros
epispadia
epispadiac
epispadial
epispadias
    balanitic e.
    penile e.
    penopubic e.

epistaxis
    Gull's renal e.
epithelial
Epstein's
    nephrosis
    syndrome
erectile
erection
erythroplasia
    e. of Queyrat
    Zoon's e.
Esbach's method
evacuator
    Creevy's e.
    Ellik's e.
    McCarthy's e.
    Toomey's e.
Everett-TeLinde operation
excretion
excretory
    e. cystogram
    e. urogram
exophytic
exsanguinate
exstrophy
    e. of the bladder
extravasation
exudate
exudative
fal-. See words beginning *phal-.*
Fanconi's syndrome
Farr's retractor
fascia
    Buck's f.
    Colles' f.
    cremasteric f.
    f. cremasterica
    dartos f. of scrotum
    Denonvilliers' f.
    Gerota's f.
    inferior f.
    f. penis profunda

fascia (*continued*)
    f. penis superficialis
    f. propria cooperi
    f. of prostate
    rectovesical f.
    renal f.
    f. renalis
    Scarpa's f.
    spermatic f., external
    spermatic f., internal
    f. spermatica externa
    f. spermatica interna
    subserous f.
    transversalis f.
    f. of urogenital trigone
Feleki's instrument
feminization
    testicular f.
feo-. See words beginning
    pheo-.
Ferguson's basket
fi-. See words beginning *phi-.*
fibrosis
    retroperitoneal f.
filariasis
filiform
filtration
Fishberg's method
fistula
flagellum
flebo-. See words beginning
    phlebo-.
fluid
    straw-colored f.
fluoresceinuria
Foley
    catheter
    forceps
    Y-type ureteropelvio-
        plasty
Foley-Alcock catheter
Folin and Bell's method

Folin and Berglund's method
Folin and Denis' method
Folin and Farmer's method
Folin and Flander's method
Folin and Hart's method
Folin and Macallum's method
Folin and Wright's method
Folin and Youngburg's method
Folin, Benedict and Myers'
    method
Folin, McEllroy and Peck's
    method
Folin's
    gravimetric method
    method
Follmann's balanitis
follower
forceps
    Allis' f.
    Blake's f.
    Bozeman's f.
    Braasch's f.
    Buerger-McCarthy f.
    Bumpus' f.
    Bunim's f.
    Campbell's f.
    Coppridge's f.
    Crenshaw's f.
    Desjardin's f.
    Foley f.
    Harris' f.
    Kelly's f.
    Lewis' f.
    Lewkowitz's f.
    Lowsley's f.
    Mathieu's f.
    McCarthy-Alcock f.
    McCarthy's f.
    McNealy-Glassman-
      Babcock f.
    Millin's f.
    Pitha's f.

forceps (*continued*)
    Poutasse's f.
    Randall's f.
    Ratliff-Blake f.
    Ray's f.
    Rochester-Pean f.
    Skillern's f.
    White-Oslay f.
    Young's f.
foreskin
    redundant f.
Formad's kidney
foroblique
fossa
    f. of Morgagni
    navicular f. of male
      urethra
    f. navicularis urethrae
    f. ovalis
    paravesical f.
Fournier's disease
Fowler's sound
Franco's operation
Franklin-Silverman needle
French-McCarthy panendo-
    scope
French-Robinson catheter
French's dilator
frenulum
    f. of prepuce of penis
    f. preputii penis
frenum
frequency
Freyer's operation
friable
FTA-ABS — fluorescent trepo-
      nemal antibody-
      absorption test

fulguration
Fuller's operation
fundic

fundiform
fundus
    f. of bladder
    f. of urinary bladder
    f. vesicae urinariae
funiculitis
funiculopexy
funiculus
    f. spermaticus
Furniss' catheter
galactosuria
galacturia
GC – gonococcus
Gelpi's retractor
genital
genitalia
genitocrural
genitofemoral
genitoinfectious
genitoplasty
genitourinary
germinoma
Gerota's
    capsule
    fascia
Gibbon's hydrocele
Gilbert-Dreyfus syndrome
Gilbert's
    sign
    syndrome
Giraldes' organ
gland
    adrenal g.
    Albarran's g.
    bulbourethral g.
    Cowper's g.
    Littre's g's
    paraurethral g.
    preputial g.
    prostate g.
    Skene's g.
    suprarenal g.

glans
    g. penis
gleet
Glenn's technique
glischruria
globulinuria
globus
    g. major epididymidis
    g. minor epididymidis
glomerular
glomeruli
    g. renis
    Ruysch's g.
glomerulitis
glomerulonephritis
glomerulopathy
glomerulosclerosis
glomerulose
glomerulus
glycosuria
Goldblatt's
    clamp
    hypertension
    kidney
Gomco's clamp
gonad
gonadal
gonadectomize
gonadectomy
gonadial
gonadopathy
gonadotherapy
gonadotropin
    chorionic g.
gonadotropism
gonaduct
gonangiectomy
gonecyst
gonecystis
gonecystitis
gonecystolith
gonecystopyosis

gonocele
gonococcal
gonococci
gonococcus
gonophore
gonorrhea
gonorrheal
Goodpasture's syndrome
gorget
    Teale's g.
graft
    Thiersch's g.
granuloma
    g. inguinale
gravity
    specific g.
Grawitz's tumor
groin
GU – genitourinary
gubernaculum
    chorda g.
    Hunter's g.
    g. testis
Gull's renal epistaxis
gumma
Guyon-Pean clamp
Guyon's
    clamp
    dilator
    sound
Hacker's operation
Hagner's operation
Halsted's clamp
Hamm's electrode
Harrington's retractor
Harris'
    forceps
    segregator
HCO_3 – bicarbonate
Heintz's method
Heitz-Boyer procedure
Heller-Nelson syndrome

hemangioma
hemangiosarcoma
hematocele
    scrotal h.
hematoma
hematoscheocele
hematospermatocele
hematospermia
hematuria
    angioneurotic h.
    endemic h.
    essential h.
    microscopic h.
    renal h.
    urethral h.
    vesical h.
hemaurochrome
heminephrectomy
heminephroureterectomy
hemodialysis
hemospermia
hemostatic bag
    Pilcher's h.b.
Hendrickson's lithotrite
Henle's
    ampulla
    internal cremaster
    loop
    sphincter
    tubules
hermaphrodism
hermaphrodite
hermaphroditism
herpes
    genital h.
    h. praeputialis
    h. progenitalis
    h. simplex
    h. zoster
Herrick's clamp
Hesselbach's triangle
Hess' operation

Heyd's syndrome
Highmore
    corpus of H.
    H.'s body
hilar
hili
hilum
hilus
    h. glandulae suprarenalis
    h. of kidney
    h. renalis
    h. of suprarenal gland
hind-kidney
Hinman's reflux
Hippel-Lindau syndrome
homotransplant
hook
    Kimball's h.
Howard's basket
Huggins' operation
Hunner's stricture
Hunter's gubernaculum
Hurwitz's trocar
Hutchins' needle
hyaline
Hyams' clamp
hydatid
    h. of Morgagni
    sessile h.
hydatidocele
hydatiduria
hydration
hydrocele
    chylous h.
    h. colli
    communicating h.
    Dupuytren's h.
    encysted h.
    funicular h.
    Gibbon's h.
    Maunoir's h.
    noncommunicating h.

hydrocele (*continued*)
    scrotal h.
hydrocelectomy
hydronephrosis
hydronephrotic
hydroperinephrosis
hydropyonephrosis
hydrosarcocele
hydroscheocele
hydroureter
hydroureterosis
hydrouria
hyperbilirubinemia
hyperemia
hypernephritis
hypernephroid
hypernephroma
hyperorchidism
hyperoxaluria
hyperparathyroidism
hyperplasia
hypertension
    adrenal h.
    essential h.
    Goldblatt's h.
    renal h.
    secondary h.
hypertonic
hypertrophy
    prostatic h.
hypogastric
hypogonadism
hypoplasia
hypoproteinemia
hypospadiac
hypospadias
hypotonia
hypotonic
Hyrtl's sphincter
Iglesias' resectoscope
ileocystoplasty
ileocystostomy

iliac
iliocostal
iliohypogastric
ilioinguinal
Immergut's tube
immune
immunosuppressive
implant
    Silastic i.
impotence
impotentia
    i. coeundi
    i. erigendi
incision. See *General Surgical Terms.*
incontinence
    paradoxical i.
    paralytic i.
    stress i.
    urinary i.
    i. of urine
incontinent
incontinentia
    i. urinae
indoluria
indoxyl
indoxyluria
induration
    penile i.
indwelling
infarct
    bilirubin i's
    Brewer's i's
    uric acid i.
infarction
    renal i.
inferior vena cava
inflammatory
infundibula
    i. of kidney
infundibular

infundibuliform
infundibulopelvic
infundibulum
    i. of urinary bladder
inguinal
inguinocrural
inguinoscrotal
insertion
    cystoradium i.
insipidus
instrument
    Feleki's i.
insufficiency
    renal i.
integument
intercostal
intercourse
interlobar
interlobular
interstitial
interureteral
interureteric
intrarenal
intratesticular
intraureteral
intraurethral
intravenous
intravesical
intussusception
irradiation
Isaacs-Ludwig arteriole
ischemia
ischiopubic
ischiorectal
Israel's operation
isthmus
    i. prostatae
    i. urethrae
isuria
IVP — intravenous pyelogram
Jacobson's retractor

Jewett's sound
Johnson's
    basket
    needle holder
    stone dislodger
Judd-Masson retractor
Judd's retractor
junction
    ureteropelvic j.
    ureterovesical j.
K — potassium
Kantor's clamp
Keitzer's urethrotome
Kelly-Deming operation
Kelly's
    cystoscope
    endoscope
    forceps
    operation
Kelly-Stoeckel operation
ketone body
ketonuria
ketosis
Keyes' lithotrite
kidney
    amyloid k.
    arteriosclerotic k.
    artificial k.
    atrophic k.
    cake k.
    cicatricial k.
    cirrhotic k.
    clump k.
    congested k.
    contracted k.
    crush k.
    cyanotic k.
    cystic k.
    disk k.
    doughnut k.
    ectopic k.
    fatty k.

kidney (*continued*)
    flea-bitten k.
    floating k.
    Formad's k.
    fused k.
    Goldblatt's k.
    granular k.
    hind k.
    horseshoe k.
    hypermobile k.
    hypoplastic k.
    lardaceous k.
    large red k.
    lump k.
    medullary sponge k.
    mortar k.
    mural k.
    myelin k.
    pelvic k.
    polycystic k.
    primordial k.
    putty k.
    Rokitansky's k.
    Rose-Bradford k.
    sacciform k.
    sclerotic k.
    sigmoid k.
    soapy k.
    sponge k.
    supernumerary k.
    wandering k.
    waxy k.
kilo-. See words beginning
    chylo-.
Kimball's hook
Kimmelstiel-Wilson syndrome
Klebs' disease
Klinefelter's syndrome
Kocher's retractor
Kollmann's dilator
kor-. See words beginning
    chor-.

Korean hemorrhagic nephrosonephritis
kraurosis
  k. penis
KUB — kidney, ureter and
  bladder
Labbé's syndrome
lactosuria
lacuna
  great l. of urethra
  l. magna
lacunae
  l. of Morgagni
  l. Morgagnii urethrae
    muliebris
  l. of urethra
  l. urethrales
lamella
lamina
  l. visceralis tunicae
    vaginalis propriae testis
  l. visceralis tunicae vagi-
    nalis testis
Lancereaux's nephritis
laparonephrectomy
Lapides' needle holder
Lashmet and Newburgh
  method
Leader-Kollmann dilator
LeFort's
  bougie
  catheter
  sound
Legueu's retractor
leiomyoma
leiomyosarcoma
Leriche's syndrome
leukoplakia
  l. penis
Levant's stone dislodger
Lewis'
  cystometer

Lewis' (*continued*)
  forceps
Lewkowitz's forceps
leydigarche
Leydig's
  cells
  duct
libidogen
lichen
  l. planus
lienorenal
ligament
  lateral false l.
  lateral puboprostatic l.
  medial puboprostatic l.
  middle umbilical l.
  pubovesical l.
  round l.
Lightwood's syndrome
Lindau's disease
line
  Brödel's l.
linea
  l. alba
lipoma
liposarcoma
liquor
  l. prostaticus
  l. seminis
lithangiuria
lithectasy
lithiasis
lithocenosis
lithoclysmia
lithocystotomy
lithodialysis
lithokonion
litholabe
litholapaxy
litholysis
litholyte
lithometer

lithomyl
lithonephria
lithonephritis
lithonephrotomy
lithophone
lithoscope
lithotripsy
lithotriptic
lithotriptor
lithotriptoscope
lithotriptoscopy
lithotrite
    Alcock's l.
    Alcock-Hendrickson's l.
    Bigelow's l.
    Hendrickson's l.
    Keyes' l.
    Lowenstein's l.
    Lowsley's l.
    Reliquet's l.
    Thompson's l.
lithotrity
lithous
lithoxiduria
lithuresis
lithureteria
lithuria
Littre's glands
Lloyd's sign
lobulation
lobule
    cortical l's of kidney
    l's of testis
lobuli
    l. corticales renis
    l. epididymidis
    l. testis
lobulus
Löhlein's nephritis
Longuet's operation
loop
    Henle's l.

Lowenstein's lithotrite
Lowsley-Peterson cystoscope
Lowsley's
    forceps
    lithotrite
    operation
    tractor
Luder-Sheldon syndrome
lumbosacral
lumen
luxation
Luy's segregator
lymphangiogram
lymphangioma
lymphangiosarcoma
lymphogranuloma
    l. inguinale
    venereal l.
    l. venereum
lymphopathia
    l. venereum
Maisonneuve's urethrotome
Makka's operation
malacoplakia
    m. vesicae
Malecot's
    catheter
    drain
malrotation
Marañon's syndrome
Marchand's adrenals
Marian's operation
Marshall-Marchetti-Birch
    operation
Marshall-Marchetti-Krantz
    operation
Marshall-Marchetti operation
Marshall's
    surgical sucker
    test
Martin's operation
Martius-Harris operation

Martius' operation
Masson-Judd retractor
Mathieu's forceps
Maunoir's hydrocele
Mayo's clamp
Mays' operation
McCarthy-Alcock forceps
McCarthy-Campbell cystoscope
McCarthy-Peterson cystoscope
McCarthy's
      cystoscope
      electrode
      evacuator
      forceps
      foroblique panendoscope
      resectoscope
      telescope
McCrea's sound
McGill's operation
McIver's catheter
McNealy-Glassman-Babcock
      forceps
meatal
meatome
meatometer
meatorrhaphy
meatoscope
meatoscopy
meatotome
meatotomy
meatus
      m. urinarius
median-bar
mediastinum
      m. testis
medications. See *Drugs and
      Chemistry* section.
medorrhea
medulla
      adrenal m.
      m. glandulae suprarenalis
      m. of kidney

medulla (*continued*)
      m. nephrica
      m. renis
      m. of suprarenal gland
      suprarenal m.
medullae
medullary
medullectomy
medulliadrenal
medulloadrenal
medulloid
medullosuprarenoma
megabladder
megalopenis
megaloureter
melanoma
melasma
      m. addisonii
      m. suprarenale
mellitus
Mercier's
      bar
      operation
mesangium
mesenchymal
mesonephric
mesonephroma
mesonephron
mesonephros
mesothelioma
metanephrine
metanephroi
metanephros
method
      acid hematin m.
      Addis's m.
      Arnold and Gunning's m.
      Bence Jones protein m.
      Benedict and Franke's m.
      Benedict and Osterberg's
          m.
      Bertrand's m.

method (*continued*)

Defer's m.
Demme's m.
Esbach's m.
Fishberg's m.
Folin and Bell's m.
Folin and Berglund's m.
Folin and Denis' m.
Folin and Farmer's m.
Folin and Flander's m.
Folin and Hart's m.
Folin and Macallum's m.
Folin and Wright's m.
Folin and Youngburg's m.
Folin, Benedict, and Myers' m.
Folin, McEllroy, and Peck's m.
Folin's gravimetric m.
Folin's m.
Heintz's m.
Lashmet and Newburgh m.
Naunyn-Minkowski m.
Osborne and Folin's m.
permutit m.
Power and Wilder's m.
Shohl and Pedley's m.
Sjöqvist's m.
Sumner's m.
Volhard and Fahr m.
Metzenbaum's scissors
microrchidia
miction
micturate
micturition
Miller's syndrome
Millin-Bacon
retractor
spreader

Millin's
forceps
tube
Mitchell's basket
mononephrous
morcellement
Morgagni
fossa of M.
hydatid of M.
lacunae of M.
mosaicism
Mosher's speculum
Moynihan's
probe
scoop
Muelleri
ductus M.
muscle
Bell's m.
bulbocavernous m.
cremaster m.
detrusor urinae m.
external oblique m.
internal oblique m.
ischiocavernous m.
latissimus dorsi m.
levator ani m.
psoas m.
pubovesicalis m.
rectourethralis m.
rectovesicalis m.
transversalis m.
transverse perinei m.
musculus
m. levator prostate
m. obturatorius externus
m. obturatorius internus
m. pubovaginalis
m. pubovesicalis
m. quadratus lumborum
m. rectourethralis

musculus (*continued*)
    m. rectovesicalis
    m. spyincter urethrae
    m. sphincter vesicae
       urinariae
    m. transversus abdominis
    m. transversus perinei
       superficialis
myoma
myxocystitis
myxoma
myxosarcoma
Na — sodium
Narath's operation
National cystoscope
Naunyn-Minkowski method
necrosis
    renal papillary n.
needle
    Dees' n.
    Franklin-Silverman n.
    Hutchins' n.
    Travenol n.
    Turkel's n.
    Veenema-Gusberg n.
    Vim-Silverman n.
needle holder
    Johnson's n.h.
    Lapides' n.h.
    Stratte's n.h.
    Young-Millin n.h.
    Young's n.h.
Neil-Moore electrode
Nélaton's
    catheter
    sphincter
neoplastic
nephradenoma
nephralgia
    idiopathic n.
nephralgic
nephrapostasis

nephrasthenia
nephratonia
nephratony
nephrauxe
nephrectasia
nephrectasis
nephrectasy
nephrectomize
nephrectomy
    abdominal n.
    lumbar n.
    paraperitoneal n.
    posterior n.
nephredema
nephrelcosis
nephremia
nephremphraxis
nephria
nephric
nephridium
nephrism
nephritic
nephritides
nephritis
    albuminous n.
    arteriosclerotic n.
    azotemic n.
    bacterial n.
    Balkan n.
    capsular n.
    n. caseosa
    catarrhal n.
    cheesy n.
    chloroazotemic n.
    clostridial n.
    congenital n.
    croupous n.
    degenerative n.
    desquamative n.
    diffuse n.
    n. dolorosa
    dropsical n.

nephritis (*continued*)
    exudative n.
    fibrolipomatous n.
    fibrous n.
    focal n.
    glomerular n.
    glomerulocapsular n.
    n. gravidarum
    hemorrhagic n.
    hydremic n.
    hydropigenous n.
    hypogenetic n.
    idiopathic n.
    indurative n.
    interstitial n.
    Lancereaux's n.
    lipomatous n.
    Löhlein's n.
    n. mitis
    parenchymatous n.
    phenacetin n.
    pneumococcus n.
    potassium-losing n.
    n. of pregnancy
    productive n.
    radiation n.
    n. repens
    salt-losing n.
    saturnine n.
    scarlatinal n.
    subacute n.
    suppurative n.
    syphilitic n.
    tartrate n.
    transfusion n.
    trench n.
    tubal n.
    tuberculous n.
    vascular n.
    Volhard's n.
    war n.
nephritogenic

nephroabdominal
nephroangiosclerosis
nephroblastoma
nephrocalcinosis
nephrocapsectomy
nephrocardiac
nephrocele
nephrocirrhosis
nephrocolic
nephrocolopexy
nephrocoloptosis
nephrocystanastomosis
nephrocystitis
nephrocystosis
nephroerysipelas
nephrogastric
nephrogenic
nephrogenous
nephrogram
nephrography
nephrohemia
nephrohydrosis
nephrohypertrophy
nephroid
nephrolith
nephrolithiasis
nephrolithotomy
nephrologist
nephrology
nephrolysis
nephroma
    embryonal n.
nephromalacia
nephromegaly
nephron
nephroncus
nephro-omentopexy
nephroparalysis
nephropathic
nephropathy
    analgesic n.
    dropsical n.

nephropathy (*continued*)
    gouty n.
    hypazoturic n.
    hypercalcemic n.
    hypochloruric n.
    toxic n.
nephropexy
nephrophagiasis
nephropoietic
nephropoietin
nephroptosia
nephroptosis
nephropyelitis
nephropyelolithotomy
nephropyeloplasty
nephropyosis
nephrorosein
nephrorrhagia
nephrorrhaphy
nephroscleria
nephrosclerosis
    arteriolar n.
    benign n.
    hyaline arteriolar n.
    hyperplastic arteriolar n.
    intercapillary n.
    malignant n.
    senile n.
nephroses
nephrosis
    amyloid n.
    cholemic n.
    Epstein's n.
    glycogen n.
    hydropic n.
    hypokalemic n.
    larval n.
    lipid n.
    lipoid n.
    lower nephron n.
    necrotizing n.
    osmotic n.

nephrosis (*continued*)
    toxic n.
    vacuolar n.
nephrosonephritis
    hemorrhagic n.
    Korean hemorrhagic n.
nephrosonography
nephrospasis
nephrosplenopexy
nephrostomy
nephrotic
nephrotome
nephrotomogram
nephrotomography
nephrotomy
    abdominal n.
    lumbar n.
nephrotoxic
nephrotoxicity
nephrotoxin
nephrotresis
nephrotropic
nephrotuberculosis
nephrotyphoid
nephrotyphus
nephroureterectomy
nephroureterocystectomy
nephrozymase
nephrozymosis
Nesbit's
    cystoscope
    resectoscope
neurofibroma
Nisbet's chancre
nocturia
Nonnenbruch's syndrome
nonopaque
Nourse's syringe
NSU — nonspecific urethritis
obstruction
obstructive
    o. uropathy

obturator
 Alcock-Timberlake o.
 Timberlake's o.
Ochsner's
 probe
 trocar
Ockerblad's clamp
O'Conor's operation
oligohydruria
oligonecrospermia
oligophosphaturia
oligospermatism
oligospermia
oliguria
Ombrédanne's operation
opacity
opaque
operation
 Andrews' o.
 Bates' o.
 Belfield's o.
 Bennett's o.
 Bergenhem's o.
 Bevan-Rochet o.
 Bevan's o.
 Bigelow's o.
 Boari's o.
 Bottini's o.
 Bricker's o.
 Cecil's o.
 Civiale's o.
 Clark's o.
 Cock's o.
 Davat's o.
 Deming's o.
 Denonvilliers' o.
 Dittel's o.
 Doppler's o.
 Doyen's o.
 Duplay's o.
 Edebohls' o.
 Everett-TeLinde o.

operation (*continued*)
 Franco's o.
 Freyer's o.
 Fuller's o.
 Hacker's o.
 Hagner's o.
 Hess' o.
 Huggins' o.
 interposition o.
 Israel's o.
 Kelly-Deming o.
 Kelly's o.
 Kelly-Stoeckel o.
 Longuet's o.
 Lowsley's o.
 Makka's o.
 Marian's o.
 Marshall-Marchetti-Birch o.
 Marshall-Marchetti-Krantz o.
 Marshall-Marchetti o.
 Martin's o.
 Martius-Harris o.
 Martius' o.
 Mays' o.
 McGill's o.
 Mercier's o.
 mika o.
 morcellement o.
 Narath's o.
 O'Conor's o.
 Ombrédanne's o.
 Petersen's o.
 Poncet's o.
 Rigaud's o.
 sling o.
 Spivack's o.
 Stanischeff's o.
 Steinach's o.
 Torek's o.
 Tuffier's o.

operation (*continued*)
    van Hook's o.
    Vidal's o.
    Vogel's o.
    Volkmann's o.
    von Bergmann's o.
    von Hacker's o.
    Voronoff's o.
    Wheelhouse's o.
    White's o.
    Wood's o.
    Young's o.
orchialgia
orchichorea
orchidalgia
orchidectomy
orchidic
orchiditis
orchidocelioplasty
orchidoepididymectomy
orchidoncus
orchidopathy
orchidopexy
orchidoplasty
orchidoptosis
orchidorrhaphy
orchidotherapy
orchidotomy
orchiectomy
orchiencephaloma
orchiepididymitis
orchilytic
orchiocatabasis
orchiocele
orchiococcus
orchiodynia
orchiomyeloma
orchioncus
orchioneuralgia
orchiopathy
orchiopexy
orchioplasty

orchiorrhaphy
orchioscheocele
orchioscirrhus
orchiotomy
orchis
orchitic
orchitis
    metastatic o.
    o. parotidea
    o. variolosa
orchitolytic
orchotomy
organ
    o. of Giraldes
orgasm
orifice
    o. of male urethra
    o. of ureter
    ureteral o.
    o. of urethra
    vesicourethral o.
os
    o. penis
    o. pubis
Osborne and Folin's method
osteoma
Otis'
    bougie
    sound
    urethrotome
ovaries
ovary
Owens' catheter
pampiniform
panendoscope
    French-McCarthy p.
    McCarthy's foroblique p.
panendoscopy
papilla
papillary
papilloma
    squamous cell p.

paradidymal
paradidymis
paragenitalis
paraglobulinuria
paranephric
paranephritis
    lipomatous p.
paranephroma
paranephros
paraphimosis
pararenal
paraurethra
paraurethral
paraurethritis
paravesical
parenchyma
    p. of kidney
    p. testis
    p. of testis
parenchymal
parietal
pars
    p. abdominalis ureteris
    p. cavernosa urethrae
        virilis
    p. convoluta lobuli
        corticalis renis
    p. membranacea
        urethrae masculinae
    p. membranacea
        urethrae virilis
    p. pelvina ureteris
    p. prostatica urethrae
        masculinae
    p. prostatica urethrae
        virilis
    p. radiata lobuli
        corticalis renis
    p. spongiosa urethrae
        masculinae

partes
    p. genitales externae
        viriles
    p. genitales masculinae
        externae
pedicle
pelves
pelvilithotomy
pelvioileoneocystostomy
pelviolithotomy
pelvioneostomy
pelvioperitonitis
pelvioplasty
pelvioradiography
pelvioscopy
pelviostomy
pelviotomy
pelviradiography
pelvirectal
pelviroentgenography
pelvis
    renal p.
penial
penile
penis
    clubbed p.
    ligamentum fundiforme
        p.
    p. plastica
penischisis
penitis
penoscrotal
Penrose drain
periarteritis
    p. gummosa
    p. nodosa
pericystitis
perineal
perineoscrotal
perineostomy

perinephric
perinephritic
perinephritis
perinephrium
perineum
periorchitis
    p. adhaesiva
    p. purulenta
periorchium
peripenial
periprostatic
periprostatis
perirenal
perispermatitis
    p. serosa
peritoneal
peritoneum
periureteric
periureteritis
periurethral
periurethritis
perivesical
perivesicular
perivesiculitis
permutit method
Petersen's operation
Peyronie's disease
Pezzer's
    catheter
    drain
pH — hydrogen ion concentration
phallalgia
phallanastrophe
phallaneurysm
phallectomy
phallic
phallitis
phallocampsis
phallocrypsis
phallodynia

phalloncus
phalloplasty
phallorrhagia
phallorrhea
phallotomy
phallus
Pheifer-Young retractor
phenolsulfonphthalein
phenylketonuria
pheochromocytoma
Philips'
    bougie
    catheter
phimosiectomy
phimosis
phimotic
phlebolith
photoscan
pielo-. See words beginning
    pyelo-.
Pilcher's hemostatic bag
pio-. See words beginning *pyo-*.
Pitha's forceps
Pitres' sign
PKU — phenylketonuria
plaque
    Randall's p's
plexus
    p. cavernosus penis
    cavernous p. of penis
    hypogastric p.
    pampiniform p.
    p. pampiniformis
    prostatic p.
    prostaticovesical p.
    p. prostaticus
    renal p.
    p. renalis
    sacral p.
    Santorini's p.
    spermatic p.

plexus (*continued*)
    p. spermaticus
    suprarenal p.
    p. suprarenalis
    testicular p.
    p. testicularis
    ureteric p.
    p. uretericus
    p. venosus prostaticus
    vesical p.
    p. vesicale
    p. vesicalis
    vesicoprostatic p.
plica
    p. pubovesicalis
    p. vesicalis transversa
pneumaturia
polycystic
polydipsia
polyorchidism
polyorchis
polyspermia
polyspermism
polyspermy
polyuria
Poncet's operation
porphyria
porphyrinuria
porphyruria
position. See *General Surgical Terms.*
posthetomy
posthioplasty
posthitis
postholith
Potain's trocar
pouch
    p. of Douglas
Poutasse's forceps
Power and Wilder's method
Pratt's sound
Prehn's sign

preperitoneal
prepuce
    p. of penis
preputial
preputiotomy
preputium
    p. penis
preurethritis
prevesical
priapism
priapitis
priapus
probe
    Moynihan's p.
    Ochsner's p.
procedure
    Heitz-Boyer p.
progenital
pronephros
properitoneal
prostata
prostatalgia
prostatauxe
prostate
prostatectomy
    perineal p.
    retropubic prevesical p.
    suprapubic transvesical p.
    transurethral p.
prostatelcosis
prostateria
prostatic
prostaticovesical
prostaticovesiculectomy
prostatism
    vesical p.
prostatisme
    p. sans prostate
prostatitic
prostatitis
    granulomatous p.
    tuberculous p.

prostatocystitis
prostatocystotomy
prostatodynia
prostatography
prostatolith
prostatolithotomy
prostatomegaly
prostatometer
prostatomy
prostatomyomectomy
prostatorrhea
prostatotomy
prostatotoxin
prostatovesiculectomy
prostatovesiculitis
prosthesis
    Silastic testicular p.
proteinuria
    adventitious p.
    Bence-Jones p.
    cardiac p.
    colliquative p.
    cyclic p.
    emulsion p.
    enterogenic p.
    febrile p.
    globular p.
    gouty p.
    hematogenous p.
    intrinsic p.
    nephrogenous p.
    palpatory p.
    postrenal p.
    residual p.
proteinuric
pseudohermaphrodism
pseudohermaphrodite
pseudohermaphroditism
psoas muscle
PSP — phenolsulfonphthalein
ptosis
    p. of kidney

ptosis (*continued*)
    renal p.
pubes
pubetrotomy
pubic
pubioplasty
pubiotomy
pubis
    symphysis p.
puboprostatic
pubovesical
pudendal
punch
    Turkel's p.
purulent
pustule
PVC — postvoiding cystogram
pyelectasia
pyelectasis
pyelic
pyelitic
pyelitis
    calculous p.
    p. cystica
    defloration p.
    encrusted p.
    p. glandularis
    p. granulosa
    p. gravidarum
    hematogenous p.
    hemorrhagic p.
    suppurative p.
    urogenous p.
pyelocaliectasis
pyelocystanastomosis
pyelocystitis
pyelocystostomosis
pyelofluoroscopy
pyelogram
    dragon p.
    infusion p.
    intravenous p.

pyelograph
pyelography
    air p.
    ascending p.
    drip p.
    excretion p.
    infusion p.
    intravenous p.
    respiration p.
    retrograde p.
    washout p.
pyeloileocutaneous
pyelointerstitial
pyelolithotomy
pyelometer
pyelometry
pyelonephritis
    acute p.
    chronic p.
    xanthogranulomatous p.
pyelonephrosis
pyelopathy
pyelophlebitis
pyeloplasty
pyeloplication
pyeloscopy
pyelostomy
pyelotomy
pyelotubular
pyeloureterectasis
pyeloureteritis cystica
pyeloureterogram
pyeloureterography
pyeloureterolysis
pyeloureteroplasty
pyelovenous
pyocalix
pyocele
pyogenic
pyonephritis
pyonephrolithiasis
pyonephrosis

pyonephrotic
pyospermia
pyoureter
pyovesiculosis
pyramid
    p's of kidney
    renal p's
pyuria
Queyrat's erythroplasia
rabdo-. See words beginning
    rhabdo-.
radioactive gold
radiolucent
radiopaque
rafe. See *raphe*.
Ralks' adapter
Randall's
    forceps
    plaque
Rankin's retractor
raphe
    r. penis
    r. of perineum
    r. scroti
    r. of scrotum
Ratliff-Blake forceps
Ravich's cystoscope
Ray's forceps
reabsorption
reaction
    Bittorf's r.
recessus
    r. hepatorenalis
rectourethral
rectovesical
rectovestibular
red Robinson catheter
reflux
    Hinman's r.
    urethrovesiculodifferen-
      tial r.
Reifenstein's syndrome

Reiter's disease
rejection
Reliquet's lithotrite
ren
    r. mobilis
    r. unguliformis
renal
    r. artery
    r. cortex
    r. cortical necrosis
    r. cyst
    r. ectopia
    r. failure
    r. fascia
    r. hyperplasia
    r. insufficiency
    r. lithiasis
    r. osteodystrophy
    r. papillae
    r. pedicle
    r. pelvis
    r. plexus
    r. pouch
    r. rickets
    r. sinus
    r. tubular acidosis
    r. tubule
    r. vein
    r. venogram
renculi
renes
renicapsule
renicardiac
reniculi
reniculus
renin
renipelvic
reniportal
renipuncture
renocortical
renocutaneous
renogastric

renogram
renography
renointestinal
renoprival
renopulmonary
renotrophic
renotropic
repair
    Bengt-Johanson r.
    Cecil's r.
resection
resectoscope
    Baumrucker's r.
    Bumpus' r.
    cold punch r.
    Iglesias' r.
    McCarthy's r.
    Nesbit's r.
    Stern-McCarthy r.
    Thompson's r.
residual
rete
    r. testis
retention
retractor
    Campbell's r.
    Deaver's r.
    Farr's r.
    Gelpi's r.
    Harrington's r.
    Jacobson's r.
    Judd-Masson r.
    Judd's r.
    Kocher's r.
    Legueu's r.
    Masson-Judd r.
    Millin-Bacon r.
    Pheifer-Young r.
    Rankin's r.
    self-retaining r.
    Tuffier-Raney r.
    Tuffier's r.

retractor (*continued*)
    Veenema's r.
    Young's r.
retrograde
    r. pyelography
    r. urography
retroperitoneal
Retzius' space
rhabdomyoma
rhabdosarcoma
    renal r.
rib cutter
    Bethune's r.c.
rib stripper
    Dorian's r.s.
ridge
    interureteric r.
Rigaud's operation
Robinson's stone dislodger
Roche's sign
Rochester-Pean forceps
Rokitansky's kidney
Rose-Bradford kidney
Rosenthal's speculum
RP – retrograde pyelogram
ruga
rugae
Ruschelit's bougie
Ruysch's glomeruli
sacculation
sacculus
sacral
Santorini's plexus
sarcocele
sarcoma
scapus
    s. penis
Scardino's ureteropelvioplasty
Scarpa's fascia
schistosomiasis
    urinary s.
    vesical s.

Schmidt's syndrome
scissors
    Metzenbaum's s.
sclerosis
    renal arteriolar s.
scoop
    Moynihan's s.
scrotal
scrotectomy
scrotitis
scrotocele
scrotoplasty
scrotum
    s. lapillosum
    lymph s.
    watering-can s.
secretion
segregator
    Cathelin's s.
    Harris' s.
    Luy's s.
semen
semenuria
seminal
semination
seminiferous
seminologist
seminology
seminoma
seminuria
septa of testis
septum
    s. bulbi urethrae
    s. glandis penis
    s. of glans penis
    s. pectiniforme
    s. penis
    rectovesical s.
    s. rectovesicale
    s. renis
    s. scroti
    s. of scrotum

serosa
Sertoli's
 cell
 column
shangker. See *chancre.*
Shiley's tube
Shohl and Pedley's method
sign
 Gilbert's s.
 Lloyd's s.
 Pitres' s.
 Prehn's s.
 Roche's s.
 Thornton's s.
Silastic
 S. implant
 S. mushroom catheter
 S. testicular prosthesis
sinus
 s. epididymidis
 s. of epididymis
 prostatic s.
 s. prostaticus
 renal s.
 s. renalis
Sjöqvist's method
Skene's gland
Skillern's forceps
skis-. See words beginning
 schis-.
smegma
 s. praeputii
sois. See *psoas.*
sound
 Campbell's s.
 Davis' s.
 Dittel's s.
 Fowler's s.
 Guyon's s.
 Jewett's s.
 LeFort's s.
 McCrea's s.

sound (*continued*)
 Otis' s.
 Pratt's s.
 Van Buren's s.
 Walther's s.
space
 intravesical s.
 preperitoneal s.
 prevesical s.
 Retzius' s.
specific gravity
speculum
 Mosher's s.
 Rosenthal's s.
sperm
 muzzled s.
spermacrasia
spermagglutination
spermalist
spermatemphraxis
spermatic
spermaticide
spermatid
spermatin
spermatism
spermatitis
spermatoblast
spermatocele
spermatocelectomy
spermatocidal
spermatocyst
spermatocystectomy
spermatocystitis
spermatocystotomy
spermatocytal
spermatocyte
spermatocytogenesis
spermatogenesis
spermatogenic
spermatogenous
spermatogeny
spermatogone

spermatogonium
spermatoid
spermatology
spermatolysin
spermatolysis
spermatolytic
spermatomere
spermatomerite
spermatopathia
spermatopoietic
spermatorrhea
spermatoschesis
spermatovum
spermatozoa
spermatozoal
spermatozoon
spermaturia
spermectomy
spermia
spermiation
spermicidal
spermicide
spermiduct
spermiocyte
spermiogenesis
spermioteleosis
spermioteleotic
spermium
spermoblast
spermoculture
spermolith
spermoloropexy
spermolytic
spermoneuralgia
spermophlebectasia
spermoplasm
spermosphere
spermotoxic
spermotoxin
sphincter
    Henle's s.
    Hyrtl's s.

sphincter (*continued*)
    inguinal s.
    Nélaton's s.
    s. urethrae
    s. vesicae
Spivack's operation
spreader
    Millin-Bacon s.
stain
    Ziehl-Neelsen s.
Stanischeff's operation
stasis
    urinary s.
Steinach's operation
stellate
stenosis
    meatal s.
stenotic
sterile
sterility
sterilization
Stern-McCarthy
    electrotome
    resectoscope
Stille's clamp
Stockman's clamp
stone
    bladder s.
    cystine s.
    kidney s.
    s. searcher
stone dislodger
    Councill's s.d.
    Davis' s.d.
    Dormia's s.d.
    Johnson's s.d.
    Levant's s.d.
    Robinson's s.d.
    woven loop s.d.
Storz' cystoscope
strangulation
    s. of bladder

stranguria
strangury
Stratte's needle holder
stricture
    Hunner's s.
stroma
Stühmer's disease
stuttering
    urinary s.
stylet
sucker
    Marshall's surgical s.
sulcus
Sulkowitch's test
summit
    s. of bladder
Sumner's method
suprapubic
suprarenal
suprarenalectomy
suprarenalism
suprarenalopathy
suprarene
suprarenoma
surgical procedures. See
    operation.
suspensory
suture. See *General Surgical*
    Terms.
symphysis
    s. pubica
    s. pubis
syndrome
    adrenogenital s.
    Allemann's s.
    Bartter's s.
    Bywaters' s.
    Cacchi-Ricci s.
    Cooke-Apert-Gallais s.
    Del Castillo's s.
    Epstein's s.
    Fanconi's s.

syndrome (*continued*)
    Gilbert-Dreyfus s.
    Gilbert's s.
    Goodpasture's s.
    Heller-Nelson s.
    Heyd's s.
    Hippel-Lindau s.
    Kimmelstiel-Wilson s.
    Klinefelter's s.
    Labbé's s.
    Leriche's s.
    Lightwood's s.
    Luder-Sheldon s.
    Marañon's s.
    Miller's s.
    nephrotic s.
    Nonnenbruch's s.
    Reifenstein's s.
    Schmidt's s.
    suprarenogenic s.
    Thorn's s.
    Turner's s.
    Waterhouse-Friderichsen
      s.
synorchidism
synorchism
synoscheos
syphilis
syphilitic
syringe
    Nourse's s.
    Toomey's s.
Tatum's clamp
Teale's gorget
technique
    Dennis-Brown t.
    Glenn's t.
telescope
    McCarthy's t.
    Vest's t.
tenesmus
    vesical t.

teratocarcinoma
teratoma
test
    Albarran's t.
    blood urea nitrogen
      (BUN) t.
    creatinine clearance t.
    FTA-ABS t.
    glucose t.
    ketone body t.
    Marshall's t.
    nitrogen retention t.
    pH t.
    proteinuria t.
    radioisotope renogram t.
    semen analysis t.
    serum creatinine t.
    specific gravity t.
    Sulkowitch's t.
    urine chloride t.
    urine concentration t.
    VDRL test
    Watson-Schwartz t.
testes
testicle
testicular
testiculoma
testiculus
testis
    Cooper's irritable t.
    ectopic t.
    inverted t.
    obstructed t.
    pulpy t.
    t. redux
    retained t.
    undescended t.
testitis
testitoxicosis
testoid
testopathy
testosterone

Thiersch's graft
Thompson's
    lithotrite
    resectoscope
Thorn's syndrome
Thornton's sign
thrombosis
    renal vein t.
Tiemann's catheter
Timberlake's obturator
Toomey's
    evacuator
    syringe
Torek's operation
torsion
torus
    t. uretericus
tosis. See *ptosis.*
tour
    t. de maitre
trabecula
trabeculae
trabeculae corporis spongiosi
    penis
trabeculae corporum caverno-
    sorum penis
trabecular
trabeculation
tractor
    Lowsley's t.
    Young's t.
transillumination
transitional
transplant
transplantation
    renal t.
transureteroureterostomy
transurethral
transversalis
transverse
transversourethralis
transversus

transvesical
transvestism
transvestite
Travenol needle
triangle
    Hesselbach's t.
trichiasis
Trichomonas
    T. urethritis
trichomoniasis
trigone
    urogenital t.
trigonectomy
trigonitis
trigonotome
trigonum
    t. urogenitale
    t. vesicae
triplication
trocar
    Campbell's t.
    Hurwitz's t.
    Ochsner's t.
    Potain's t.
tube
    Acmi-Valentine t.
    Immergut's t.
    Millin's t.
    rectal t.
    Shiley's t.
    U-t.
    Valentine's t.
tuberculosis
    adrenal t.
    t. of kidney and bladder
tubule
    Albarran's t's
    Bellini's t's
    Henle's t's
    mesonephric t's
    metanephric t's
    renal t's

tubule (*continued*)
    seminiferous t's
    urine-collecting t.
    uriniferous t's
    uriniparous t's
Tuffier-Raney retractor
Tuffier's
    operation
    retractor
tuft
    malpighian t.
    renal t.
tumor
    Buschke-Loewenstein t.
    Grawitz's t.
    Wilms' t.
tunica
    t. adnata testis
    t. adventitia
    t. adventitia ductus
      deferentis
    t. adventitia ureteris
    t. adventitia vesiculae
      seminalis
    t. albuginea
    t. albuginea corporis
      spongiosi
    t. albuginea corporum
      cavernosorum
    t. albuginea testis
    t. dartos
    t. mucosa ductus
      deferentis
    t. mucosa ureteris
    t. mucosa vesicae
      urinariae
    t. mucosa vesiculae
      seminalis
    t. muscularis ductus
      deferentis
    t. muscularis renis
    t. muscularis ureteris

tunica (*continued*)
    t. muscularis vesicae
      urinariae
    t. muscularis vesiculae
      seminalis
    t. propria tubuli testis
    t. serosa testis
    t. serosa vesicae urinariae
    t. vaginalis communis
      testis et funiculi
      spermatica
    t. vaginalis propria testis
    t. vaginalis testis
    t. vasculosa
tunicae
    t. funiculi spermatici
    t. funiculi spermatici et
      testis
TUR — transurethral resection
turbid
Turkel's
    needle
    punch
Turner's syndrome
TURP — transurethral resec-
      tion of prostate
U/A — urine analysis
ulceration
ulcus
    u. syphiliticum
ultrasonogram
    renal u.
ultrasonography
undescended testis
UPJ — ureteropelvic junction
urachal
urachovesical
urachus
uracrasia
uracratia
uragogue
uraturia

urea
uremia
    azotemic u.
    extrarenal u.
    prerenal u.
    retention u.
uremic
ureter
    ectopic u.
    postcaval u.
    retrocaval u.
    retroiliac u.
ureteral
ureteralgia
ureterectasia
ureterectasis
ureterectomy
ureteric
    u. ridge
ureteritis
    u. cystica
    u. glandularis
ureterocele
ureterocelectomy
ureterocervical
ureterocolostomy
ureterocutaneostomy
ureterocutaneous
ureterocystanastomosis
ureterocystoneostomy
ureterocystoscope
ureterocystostomy
ureterodialysis
ureteroduodenal
ureteroenteric
ureteroenteroanastomosis
ureteroenterostomy
ureterogram
ureterography
ureteroheminephrectomy
ureteroileostomy
ureterointestinal

ureterolith
ureterolithiasis
ureterolithotomy
ureterolysis
ureteromeatotomy
ureteroneocystostomy
ureteroneopyelostomy
ureteronephrectomy
ureteropathy
ureteropelvic
ureteropelvioneostomy
ureteropelvioplasty
    Culp's u.
    Foley Y-type u.
    Scardino's u.
ureterophlegma
ureteroplasty
ureteroproctostomy
ureteropyelitis
ureteropyelography
ureteropyeloneostomy
ureteropyelonephritis
ureteropyelonephrostomy
ureteropyeloplasty
ureteropyelostomy
ureteropyosis
ureterorectal
ureterorectoneostomy
ureterorectostomy
ureterorrhagia
ureterorrhaphy
ureterosigmoid
ureterosigmoidostomy
ureterostegnosis
ureterostenoma
ureterostenosis
ureterostoma
ureterostomosis
ureterostomy
    cutaneous u.
ureterotomy
ureterotrigonoenterostomy

ureterotrigonosigmoidostomy
ureteroureteral
ureteroureterostomy
ureterouterine
ureterovaginal
ureterovesical
ureterovesicoplasty
ureterovesicostomy
urethra
    u. masculina
    u. virilis
urethral
urethralgia
urethratresia
urethrectomy
urethremphraxis
urethreurynter
urethrism
urethritis
    u. cystica
    u. glandularis
    gonorrheal u.
    gouty u.
    u. granulosa
    nonspecific u.
    u. orificii externi
    u. petrificans
    polypoid u.
    prophylactic u.
    specific u.
    u. venerea
urethroblennorrhea
urethrobulbar
urethrocele
urethrocystitis
urethrocystogram
urethrocystography
urethrocystopexy
urethrodynia
urethrogram
urethrograph
urethrography

urethrometer
urethrometry
urethropenile
urethroperineal
urethroperineoscrotal
urethropexy
urethrophraxis
urethrophyma
urethroplasty
urethroprostatic
urethrorectal
urethrorrhagia
urethrorrhaphy
urethrorrhea
urethroscope
urethroscopic
urethroscopy
urethroscrotal
urethrospasm
urethrostaxis
urethrostenosis
urethrostomy
urethrotome
 Keitzer's u.
 Maisonneuve's u.
 Otis' u.
urethrotomy
urethrovaginal
urethrovesical
uretic
urhidrosis
uric acid
uricaciduria
uricometer
uricosuria
urina
 u. chyli
 u. cibi
 u. cruenta
 u. galactodes
 u. jumentosa
 u. potus

urina (*continued*)
 u. sanguinus
 u. spastica
urinable
urinacidometer
urinal
urinalysis
urinary
 u. bladder
 u. frequency
 u. meatus
 u. retention
 u. sphincter
 u. tract
urinate
urination
 precipitant u.
 stuttering u.
urine
 anemic u.
 Bence-Jones u.
 black u.
 chylous u.
 clean catch u.
 crude u.
 diabetic u.
 dyspeptic u.
 febrile u.
 gouty u.
 milky u.
 nebulous u.
 nervous u.
 residual u.
 straw-colored u.
 voided u.
urinemia
urine-mucoid
uriniferous
uriniparous
urinocryoscopy
urinogenital
urinogenous

urinoglucosometer
urinologist
urinology
urinoma
urinometer
urinometry
urinosexual
urinous
urobilinogenuria
urobilinuria
urocele
urochezia
urochrome
urochromogen
uroclepsia
urocrisia
urocrisis
urocriterion
urocyanogen
urocyst
urocystic
urocystis
urocystitis
urodeum
urodialysis
urodochium
urodynia
uroedema
uroerythrin
uroflavin
uroflometer
urofuscin
urofuscohematin
urogenital
    u. trigone
urogenous
uroglaucin
urogram
    excretory u.
    intravenous u.
urography
    ascending u.

urography (*continued*)
    cystoscopic u.
    descending u.
    excretion u.
    excretory u.
    intravenous u.
    oral u.
    retrograde u.
urohematin
urohematonephrosis
urohematoporphyrin
urohypertensin
urokinase
urokinetic
urokymography
urolith
urolithiasis
urolithic
urolithology
urologic
urological
urologist
urology
urolutein
uromancy
uromantia
uromelanin
urometer
uromucoid
uroncus
uronephrosis
uronology
urononcometry
uronophile
uronoscopy
uropathogen
uropathy
    obstructive u.
uropenia
uropepsin
uropepsinogen
urophanic

urophein
urophobia
urophosphometer
uroplania
uropoiesis
uropoietic
uroporphyrin
uropsammus
uropterin
uropyonephrosis
uropyoureter
uroreaction
urorhythmography
urorrhagia
urorrhea
urorrhodin
urorrhodinogen
urorubin
urorubinogen
urorubrohematin
urosaccharometry
uroscheocele
uroschesis
uroscopic
uroscopy
urosemiology
urosepsin
urosepsis
uroseptic
urosis
urospectrin
urostalagmometry
urostealith
urotherapy
urotoxia
urotoxic
urotoxicity
urotoxin
uroureter
uroxanthin
uterine
uterus

UTI — urinary tract infection
utricle
    prostatic u.
    urethral u.
utricular
utriculi
utriculitis
utriculosaccular
utriculus
    u. masculinus
    u. prostaticus
    u. vestibuli
U-tube
UVJ — ureterovesical junction
uvula
    u. of bladder
    u. vesicae
vagina
Valentine's tube
Van Buren's
    dilator
    sound
van Hook's operation
varicocele
varicocelectomy
varix
vas
    v. aberrans
    v. afferens glomeruli
    v. deferens
    v. efferens glomeruli
    v. epididymidis
vasectomized
vasectomy
vasitis
vasoepididymostomy
vasoligation
vaso-orthidostomy
vasopuncture
vasoresection
vasorrhaphy
vasosection

vasostomy
vasotomy
vasovasotomy
vasovesiculectomy
vasovesiculitis
VCU — voiding cystourethro-
    gram
VDRL — Venereal Disease Re-
    search Laboratory
Veenema-Gusberg needle
Veenema's retractor
vein
    arcuate v.
    interlobar v.
venae cavernosae penis
venereal
venogram
    renal v.
ventral
venulae
    v. rectae renis
    v. stellatae renis
venule
    stellate v's of kidney
    straight v's of kidney
verruca
    v. acuminata
vertex
    v. of urinary bladder
    v. vesicae urinariae
verumontanitis
verumontanum
Ves. (vesica) — bladder
vesica
    v. prostatica
    v. urinaria
vesicae
vesical
vesicle
    prostatic v.
    seminal v.
    spermatic v.

vesicoabdominal
vesicocele
vesicocervical
vesicoclysis
vesicocolonic
vesicoenteric
vesicofixation
vesicointestinal
vesicoperineal
vesicoprostatic
vesicopubic
vesicopustule
vesicorectal
vesicorenal
vesicosigmoid
vesicosigmoidostomy
vesicospinal
vesicotomy
vesicoumbilical
vesicourachal
vesicoureteral
vesicourethral
vesicouterine
vesicouterovaginal
vesicovaginal
vesicovaginorectal
vesicula
    v. prostatica
    v. seminalis
vesiculase
vesiculectomy
vesiculitis
vesiculogram
vesiculography
vesiculotomy
vessel
    internal spermatic v.
Vest's telescope
Vidal's operation
Vim-Silverman needle
visceral
viscus

Vogel's operation
void
voiding
Volhard and Fahr method
Volhard's nephritis
Volkmann's operation
von Bergmann's operation
von Hacker's operation
Voronoff's operation
Walther-Crenshaw clamp
Walther's
      clamp
      dilator
      sound
Wappler's cystoscope
waste
      nitrogenous w.
Waterhouse-Friderichsen
  syndrome
Watson-Schwartz test
Wertheim-Cullen clamp
Wertheim-Reverdin clamp
Wertheim's clamp
Wheelhouse's operation
White-Oslay forceps
White's operation

Wilms' tumor
Winer's catheter
Wishard's catheter
Wolff
      corpus of W.
      duct of W.
wolffian
      body
      cyst
      duct
Wood's operation
XC — excretory cystogram
XU — excretory urogram
Young-Millin needle holder
Young's
      clamp
      enucleator
      forceps
      needle holder
      operation
      retractor
      tractor
Ziehl-Neelsen stain
Zipser's clamp
Zoon's erythroplasia
zoospermia

III

GUIDES TO TERMINOLOGY

ABBREVIATIONS AND SYMBOLS*

ABBREVIATIONS

A absolute temperature
    absorbance
    accommodation
    acetum
    age
    allergy
    ampere
    Angström unit
    anode
    anterior
    artery
    atropine
    axial
    before (*ante*)
    mass number
    start of anesthesia
    total acidity
    water (*aqua*)
A. *Actinomyces*
    Anopheles
a or A ampere
    anode
A_2 aortic second sound
AA acetic acid
    achievement age
    alveolar-arterial
    aminoacetone
    ascending aorta
    of each (*ana*)

aa arteries
A & A aid and attendance
AAA abdominal aortic aneurysm
    amalgam
    androgenic anabolic agent
AAL anterior axillary line
AAR antigen-antiglobulin reaction
AAS aortic arch syndrome
AAT alpha-antitrypsin
AB abnormal
    abortion
    alcian blue
    asbestos body
    asthmatic bronchitis
    axiobuccal
A/B acid-base ratio
ABA antibacterial activity
ABC absolute basophil count
    axiobuccocervical
ABD,
Abd or
abd abdomen
    abdominal
ABDOM,
Abdom or
abdom abdomen
    abdominal
ABE acute bacterial endocarditis
ABG axiobuccogingival

*Symbols start on page 971.

ABL   abetalipoproteinemia
     axiobuccolingual
ABLB   alternate binaural loudness
     balance
ABN,
Abn or
abn   abnormal
ABO   blood groups (named for
     agglutinogens)
ABP   arterial blood pressure
abs feb   while the fever is absent
     (*absente febre*)
AC   acromioclavicular
     adrenal cortex
     air conduction
     alternating current
     anodal closure
     anterior chamber
     anticoagulant
     anticomplementary
     anti-inflammatory corticoid
     aortic closure
     atriocarotid
     auriculocarotid
     axiocervical
     before meals (*ante cibum*)
ac   acute
     before meals (*ante cibum*)
ACA   adenocarcinoma
ACAD   academy
ACC   adenoid cystic carcinoma
     anodal closure contraction
Acc   accommodation
ACCL   anodal closure clonus
accom   accommodation
ACD   absolute cardiac dullness
     acid, citrate, dextrose
     anterior chest diameter
ACE   adrenocortical extract
ACG   apexcardiogram
AcG   accelerator globulin
ACH   adrenal cortical hormone
ACh   acetylcholine
ACHE   acetylcholinesterase
ACl   aspiryl chloride
ACM   albumin-calcium-magnesium

ACO   anodal-closing odor
ACP   acid phosphatase
     acyl-carrier protein
     anodal-closing picture
     aspirin, caffeine, phenacetin
ACS   anodal-closing sound
     antireticular cytotoxic serum
ACSV   aortocoronary saphenous
     vein
ACT   activated coagulation time
     anticoagulant therapy
ACTe   anodal-closure tetanus
ACTH   adrenocorticotropic
     hormone
ACTP   adrenocorticotropic
     polypeptide
ACVD   acute cardiovascular
     disease
AD   admitting diagnosis
     Aleutian disease
     anodal duration
     average deviation
     axiodistal
     axis deviation
     right ear (*auris dextra*)
A & D   ascending and descending
ad   add (*adde*)
     let there be added (*addetur*)
Ad lib   as desired (*ad libitum*)
ADA   adenosine deaminase
     anterior descending artery
ADA#   American Diabetes Asso-
     ciation diet number
ADC   anodal-duration contraction
     average daily census
     axiodistocervical
ADEM   acute disseminated
     encephalomyelitis
ADG   atrial diastolic gallop
     axiodistogingival
ADH   alcohol dehydrogenase
     antidiuretic hormone
adhib   to be administered
     (*adhibendus*)
ADI   axiodistoincisal
ADL   activities of daily living

ADM administrative medicine
administrator
adm or
admit admission
admov let there be added
(*admove*)
ADO axiodisto-occlusal
ADP adenosine diphosphate
automatic data processing
ADPL average daily patient load
ADS antibody deficiency
syndrome
antidiuretic substance
ADT adenosine triphosphate
anything desired (*placebo*)
adv against (*adversum*)
ad 2 vic for two doses (*ad duas
vices*)
AE antitoxineinheit (antitoxin
unit)
AEC Atomic Energy Commission
AEG air encephalogram
aeg the patient (*aeger*)
AEP average evoked potential
AEq age equivalent
AER aldosterone excretion rate
auditory evoked response
average evoked response
AET absorption-equivalent thickness
aet age (*aetas*)
aetat aged, of age (*aetatis*)
AF acid-fast
aldehyde fuchsin
amniotic fluid
antibody-forming
aortic flow
atrial fibrillation
atrial flutter
AFB acid-fast bacilli
AFC antibody-forming cells
AFI amaurotic familial idiocy
AFIB atrial fibrillation
AFL atrial flutter
AFP anterior faucial pillar
AG antiglobulin

AG (*continued*)
atrial gallop
axiogingival
A/G albumin-globulin ratio
AGA appropriate for gestational
age
AGG agammaglobulinemia
agg aggravated
agit shake (*agita*)
AGL acute granulocytic leukemia
aminoglutethimide
AGMK African green monkey
kidney
AGN acute glomerulonephritis
AGS adrenogenital syndrome
AGT antiglobulin test
AGTT abnormal glucose tolerance
test
AGV aniline gentian violet
AH abdominal hysterectomy
acetohexamide
amenorrhea and hirsutism
aminohippurate
antihyaluronidase
arterial hypertension
hypermetropic astigmatism
AHA acquired hemolytic anemia
autoimmune hemolytic
anemia
AHD arteriosclerotic heart disease
atherosclerotic heart disease
AHF antihemophilic factor
AHG antihemophilic globulin
antihuman globulin
AHH alpha-hydrazine analogue of
histidine
arylhydrocarbon hydroxy-
lase
AHLE acute hemorrhagic leukoencephalitis
AHLS antihuman lymphocyte
serum
AHP air at high pressure
AHT augmented histamine test
AI accidentally incurred
aortic incompetence

AI (*continued*)
    aortic insufficiency
    apical impulse
    axioincisal
AIBA aminoisobutyric acid
AIC aminoimidazole carboxamide
AID acute infectious disease
    artificial insemination donor
AIEP amount of insulin extract-
    able from the pancreas
AIH artificial insemination, homol-
    ogous
AIHA autoimmune hemolytic
    anemia
AIP acute intermittent porphyria
    average intravascular pressure
AITT arginine insulin tolerance
    test
AIU absolute iodine uptake
AJ ankle jerk
AK above knee
AKA above-knee amputation
AL albumin
    axiolingual
ALA aminolevulinic acid
    axiolabial
ALAD abnormal left axis devia-
    tion
    aminolevulinic acid dehy-
    drase
ALAG axiolabiogingival
ALAL axiolabiolingual
alb albumin
    white
ALC approximate lethal concen-
    tration
    axiolinguocervical
ALD aldolase
ALG antilymphocyte globulin
    axiolinguogingival
ALH anterior lobe hormone
    anterior lobe of the hy-
    pophysis
alk alkaline
alk phos alkaline phosphatase
ALL acute lymphoblastic leu-
    kemia

ALL (*continued*)
    acute lymphocytic leukemia
all allergies
ALME acetyl-lysine methyl ester
ALMI anterior lateral myocardial
    infarct
ALN anterior lymph node
ALO axiolinguo-occlusal
ALP alkaline phosphatase
    antilymphocyte plasma
ALS amyotrophic lateral sclerosis
    antilymphatic serum
    antilymphocyte serum
ALTEE acetyl-L-tyrosine ethyl
    ester
ALW arch-loop-whorl
AM alveolar macrophage
    ametropia
    amperemeter
    anovular menstruation
    arithmetic mean
    aviation medicine
    axiomesial
    morning
    myopic astigmatism
am meter-angle
AMA against medical advice
    American Medical Associa-
    tion
AMB ambulatory
AMC axiomesiocervical
AMD alpha-methyldopa
    axiomesiodistal
AMG antimacrophage globulin
    axiomesiogingival
AMH automated medical history
Amh mixed astigmatism with
    myopia predominating
AMI acute myocardial infarction
    amitriptyline
    axiomesioincisal
AML acute monocytic leukemia
    acute myelocytic leukemia
AMLS antimouse lymphocyte
    serum
AMM agnogenic myeloid meta-
    plasia

AMM (*continued*)
    ammonia
AMML acute myelomonocytic
      leukemia
AMO axiomesio-occlusal
A-mode amplitude modulation
AMOL acute monocytic leukemia
AMP acid mucopolysaccharide
    adenosine monophosphate
    ampicillin
    amputation
    average mean pressure
amp ampere
AMPS abnormal mucopolysac-
      chariduria
    acid mucopolysaccharides
AMS aggravated in military service
    antimacrophage serum
    automated multiphasic
      screening
AMT alpha-methyltyrosine
    amethopterin
amt amount
amu atomic mass unit
AMY amylase
An anisometropia
    anodal
    anode
ANA acetylneuraminic acid
    antinuclear antibodies
    aspartyl naphthylamide
anal analysis
    analyst
anat anatomical
    anatomy
AnCC anodal-closure contraction
AnDTe anodal-duration tetanus
anes anesthesia
    anesthesiology
ANF alpha-naphthoflavone
    antinuclear factor
ang angiogram
ank ankle
ANLL acute nonlymphocytic
      leukemia
AnOC anodal-opening contraction
ANOV analysis of variance

ANS antineutrophilic serum
    arteriolonephrosclerosis
    autonomic nervous system
ant anterior
ante before
ANTR apparent net transfer rate
ANTU alpha-naphthylthiourea
AO anodal opening
    anterior oblique
    aorta
    aortic opening
    axio-occlusal
    opening of the atrioventricular
      valves
AOB alcohol on breath
AOC anodal-opening contraction
AOCl anodal-opening clonus
AOD arterial occlusive disease
AOO anodal-opening odor
AOP anodal-opening picture
AOS anodal-opening sound
AOTe anodal-opening tetanus
AP acid phosphatase
    action potential
    acute proliferative
    alkaline phosphatase
    aminopeptidase
    angina pectoris
    antepartum
    anterior pituitary
    anteroposterior
    appendix
    arterial pressure
    association period
    axiopulpal
A & P anterior and posterior
    auscultation and percussion
APA aldosterone-producing
      adenoma
    aminopenicillanic acid
    antipernicious anemia factor
APB atrial premature beat
    auricular premature beat
APC acetylsalicylic acid, phenace-
      tin, caffeine
    adenoidal-pharyngeal-
      conjunctival

APC (*continued*)
    aspirin, phenacetin, caffeine
    atrial premature contraction
APC-C aspirin, phenacetin, caffeine; with codeine
APD action-potential duration
APE aminophylline, phenobarbital, ephedrine
    anterior pituitary extract
APF animal protein factor
APGL alkaline phosphatase activity of the granular leukocytes
APH antepartum hemorrhage
APHP anti-*Pseudomonas* human plasma
APL accelerated painless labor
    acute promyelocytic leukemia
    anterior pituitary-like
APN average peak noise
APP alum-precipitated pyridine
app appendix
appy appendectomy
APR amebic prevalence rate
APT alum-precipitated toxoid
APTT activated partial thromboplastin time
AQ achievement quotient
aq water (*aqua*)
AQS additional qualifying symptoms
AR alarm reaction
    aortic regurgitation
    Argyll Robertson (pupil)
    artificial respiration
    at risk
ara-C cytosine arabinoside
ARC anomalous retinal correspondence
ARD acute respiratory disease
    anorectal dressing
ARDS adult respiratory distress syndrome
ARF acute respiratory failure
arg silver (*argentum*)
ARL average remaining lifetime

ARM artificial rupture of the membranes
ARP at risk period
ARRT American Registry of Radiologic Technologists
ARS antirabies serum
art artery
AS acetylstrophanthidin
    Adams-Stokes (disease)
    androsterone sulfate
    antistreptolysin
    aortic stenosis
    arteriosclerosis
    astigmatism
    left ear (*auris sinistra*)
ASA acetylsalicylic acid
    Adams-Stokes attack
    argininosuccinic acid
    arylsulfatase-A
ASCVD arteriosclerotic cardiovascular disease
    atherosclerotic cardiovascular disease
ASD aldosterone secretion defect
    atrial septal defect
ASF aniline, sulfur, formaldehyde
ASH asymmetrical septal hypertrophy
AsH hypermetropic astigmatism
ASHD arteriosclerotic heart disease
ASIS anterior superior iliac spine
ASK antistreptokinase
ASL antistreptolysin
ASLO antistreptolysin-O
AsM myopic astigmatism
ASMI anteroseptal myocardial infarct
ASN alkali-soluble nitrogen
ASO antistreptolysin-O
    arteriosclerosis obliterans
ASP area systolic pressure
ASR aldosterone secretion rate
    aldosterone secretory rate
ASRT American Society of Radiologic Technologists
ASS anterior superior spine

asst   assistant
AST   aspartate aminotransferase
Ast   astigmatism
Asth   asthenopia
ASTO   antistreptolysin-O
ASV   antisnake venom
AT   antitrypsin
      old tuberculin (alt tuberculin)
AT_{10} dihydrotachysterol
ATA   anti-*Toxoplasma* antibodies
      atmosphere absolute
      aurintricarboxylic acid
ATB   at the time of the bomb
      (A-bomb in Japan)
ATD   asphyxiating thoracic
      dystrophy
ATE   adipose tissue extract
ATEE   acetyltyrosine ethyl ester
ATG   antithyroglobulin
ATL   antitension line
ATN   acute tubular necrosis
ATP   adenosine triphosphate
ATPS   ambient temperature and
      pressure, saturated
ATR   Achilles tendon reflex
atr fib   atrial fibrillation
ATS   antitetanic serum
      antithymocyte serum
      anxiety tension state
      arteriosclerosis
ATT   aspirin tolerance time
att   attending
at wt   atomic weight
AU   Angström unit
      antitoxin unit
      arbitrary units
      azauridine
Au   Australia (antigen)
au   both ears (*aures unitas*)
      each ear (*auris uterque*)
AUL   acute undifferentiated
      leukemia
aur fib   auricular fibrillation
ausc   auscultation
AV   arteriovenous
      atrioventricular

av   average
AV/AF   anteverted, anteflexed
AVCS   atrioventricular conduction
      system
avdp   avoirdupois
AVF   arteriovenous fistula
AVH   acute viral hepatitis
AVI   air velocity index
AVN   atrioventricular node
AVR   aortic valve replacement
AVRP   atrioventricular refractory
      period
AVT   Allen vision test
AW   anterior wall
A & W   alive and well
AWI   anterior wall infarction
AWMI   anterior wall myocardial
      infarction
ax   axis
Az   azote (French for nitrogen)
azg   azaguanine
AZO   (indicates presence of the
      group) −N:N−
AZT   Aschheim-Zondek test
AZ test   Aschheim-Zondek test
AZUR   azauridine
B   bacillus
      base
      bath (*balneum*)
      Baume's scale
      behavior
      Benoist's scale
      bicuspid
      boron
      buccal
      Bucky (film in cassette in
      Potter-Bucky diaphragm)
      symbol for gauss
      tomogram with oscillating
      Bucky
B4   before
B. Brucella
b   born
BA   bacterial agglutination
      betamethasone acetate
      blocking antibody

BA (*continued*)
    bone age
    bovine albumin
    branchial artery
    bronchial asthma
    buccoaxial
    sand bath (*balneum arenae*)
Ba barium
BAC blood alcohol concentration
    buccoaxiocervical
bact bacterium
BaE barium enema
BAEE benzoyl arginine ethyl ester
    benzylarginine ethyl ester
BAG buccoaxiogingival
BAIB beta-aminoisobutyric acid
BAL British anti-lewisite
bal bath (*balneum*)
bals balsam
BAME benzoylarginine methyl
    ester
BAO basal acid output
BAP blood agar plate
BASH body acceleration given
    synchronously with the
    heartbeat
baso basophile
BB blood bank
    blood buffer base
    blue bloaters (emphysema)
    both bones
    breakthrough bleeding
    breast biopsy
    buffer base
BBA born before arrival
BBB blood-brain barrier
    bundle branch block
BBT basal body temperature
BC bactericidal concentration
    battle casualty
    bone conduction
    buccocervical
BCB brilliant cresyl blue
BCE basal cell epithelioma
BCG bacille Calmette Guérin
    (vaccine)

BCG (*continued*)
    ballistocardiogram
    bicolor guaiac (test)
BCNU bischloroethylnitrosourea
    bischloronitrosourea
BCW biological and chemical war-
    fare
BD base deficit
    base of prism down
    bile duct
    buccodistal
    twice a day (*bis die*)
BDE bile duct exploration
BE Bacillen Emulsion (tuberculin)
    bacterial endocarditis
    barium enema
    base excess
    bovine enteritis
BEI butanol-extractable iodine
BEV billion electron volts
BF blood flow
bf bouillon filtrate (tuberculin)
B/F bound-free ratio
BFC benign febrile convulsion
BFP biologic false-positive
BFR biologic false-positive reactor
    blood flow rate
    bone formation rate
BFT bentonite flocculation test
BG blood glucose
    bone graft
    buccogingival
BGH bovine growth hormone
BGP beta-glycerophosphatase
BGSA blood granulocyte-specific
    activity
BGTT borderline glucose
    tolerance test
BH benzalkonium and heparin
BHA butylated hydroxyanisole
BHC benzene hexachloride
BHI brain-heart infusion
BHS beta-hemolytic streptococcus
BHT butylated hydroxytoluene
BH/VH body hematocrit-venous
    hematocrit ratio

BI bacteriological index
base of prism in
burn index
bib drink (*bibe*)
BID or
bid twice a day (*bis in die*)
BIDLB block in the posteroinferior division of the left
branch
BIH benign intracranial hypertension
BIL bilirubin
bil bilateral
bilat bilateral
BIN or
bin twice a night (*bis in nocte*)
BIP bismuth iodoform paraffin
bis twice
BJ Bence Jones
BJP Bence Jones protein
BK below knee
BKA below-knee amputation
bkfst breakfast
BL baseline
Bessey-Lowry (units)
bleeding
blood loss
buccolingual
Burkitt's lymphoma
bl cult blood culture
bl pr blood pressure
BLB Boothby, Lovelace, Bul-
bulian (mask)
BLG beta-lactoglobulin
BLN bronchial lymph nodes
BLT blood-clot lysis time
BLU Bessey-Lowry units
BM basement membrane
body mass
bone marrow
bowel movement
buccomesial
bm sea-water bath (*balneum
maris*)
bmk birthmark
B-mode brightness modulation

BMR basal metabolic rate
BN branchial neuritis
BNO bladder neck obstruction
BNPA binasal pharyngeal airway
BO base (of prism) out
bowel obstruction
bucco-occlusal
B & O belladonna and opium
BOBA beta-oxybutyric acids
BOEA ethyl biscoumacetate
bol pill (*bolus*)
BOM bilateral otitis media
BP back pressure
bathroom privileges
behavior pattern
benzpyrene
birthplace
blood pressure
boiling point
bronchopleural
buccopulpal
bypass
BPH benign prostatic hypertrophy
BPL beta-propiolactone
BPO benzylpenicilloyl
BPRS brief psychiatric rating scale
brief psychiatric reacting
scale
BR bathroom
bed rest
bilirubin
Br. *Brucella*
BRBC bovine red blood cells
brkf or
brkt breakfast
BRM biuret reactive material
BRP bathroom privileges
bilirubin production
brth breath
BS blood sugar
bowel sounds
breaking strength
breath sounds
BSA bismuth-sulphite agar
body surface area
bovine serum albumin

BSAP   brief short-action potential
BSB   body surface burned
BSDLB   block in the antero-
        superior division of the
        left branch
BSE   bilateral symmetrical and
        equal
BSF   back scatter factor
BSI   bound serum iron
BSO   bilateral salpingo-oophorec-
        tomy
BSP   Bromsulphalein
BSR   basal skin resistance
BSS   balanced salt solution
        black silk suture
        buffered saline solution
BT   bladder tumor
        brain tumor
BTB   breakthrough bleeding
BTPS   body temperature, ambient
        pressure, saturated
BTR   Bezold-type reflex
BTU   British thermal unit
BU   base (of prism) up
        Bodansky units
        burn unit
BUDR   bromodeoxyuracil
        bromodeoxyuridine
bull   let it boil (*bulliat*)
BUN   blood urea nitrogen
BUS   Bartholin's, urethral, Skene's
        (glands)
but   butter (*butyrum*)
BV   biologic value
        blood vessel
        blood volume
        bronchovesicular
bv   vapor bath (*balneum vaporis*)
BVH   biventricular hypertrophy
BVI   blood vessel invasion
BVV   bovine vaginitis virus
BW   biological warfare
        birth weight
        body water
        body weight
BX   biopsy

C   calculus
        calorie (large)
        canine
        carbohydrate
        cathode
        Caucasian
        Celsius
        centigrade
        certified
        cervical
        chest
        clearance rate
        clonus
        closure
        color sense
        compound
        contracture
        correct
        curie
        cylinder
        gallon (*congius*)
        hundred
        velocity of light
C.   *Clostridium*
        Cryptococcus
C'   complement
c   calorie (small)
        cup
        curie
        with (*cum*)
C_{alb} albumin clearance
C_{am} amylase clearance
C_{cr} creatinine clearance
C_{in} insulin clearance
C_{pah} para-aminohippurate clear-
        ance
C_u urea clearance
CA   cancer
        carcinoma
        cardiac arrest
        cathode
        cervicoaxial
        chronological age
        cold agglutinin
        common antigen
        coronary artery

CA (*continued*)
    corpora amylacea
    croup-associated (virus)
Ca calcium
ca about (*circa*)
CAB coronary artery bypass
CABG coronary artery bypass
    graft
CACC cathodal closure contraction
CAD computerized assisted design
    coronary artery disease
CADTe cathodal-duration tetanus
CAG chronic atrophic gastritis
CAH chronic active hepatitis
    congenital adrenal hyperplasia
CAHD coronary atherosclerotic heart disease
CAI computer-assisted instruction
CAL computer-assisted learning
Cal large calorie
cal small calorie
calef warmed (*calefactus*)
CAM chorioallantoic membrane
    contralateral axillary metastasis
CAMP computer-assisted menu planning
    cyclic adenosine monophosphate
CAO chronic airway obstruction
CAP capsule
    cellulose acetate phthalate
    chloramphenicol
    cystine aminopeptidase
cap let him take (*capiat*)
card cardiology
CAT children's apperception test
    chlormerodrin accumulation test
    computed axial tomography
    computer of average transients
    computerized axial tomography

cath cathartic
    catheter
    catheterize
CAV congenital absence of vagina
    congenital adrenal virilism
CB chronic bronchitis
cb cardboard or plastic film holder without intensifying screens
CBA chronic bronchitis with asthma
CBC complete blood count
CBD common bile duct
CBF cerebral blood flow
    coronary blood flow
CBG corticosteroid-binding globulin
    cortisol-binding globulin
CBOC completion bed occupancy care
CBS chronic brain syndrome
CBV central blood volume
    circulating blood volume
    corrected blood volume
CBW chemical and biological warfare
CC cardiac cycle
    chief complaint
    clinical course
    commission certified
    compound cathartic
    cord compression
    costochondral
    creatinine clearance
cc cubic centimeter
CCA chick-cell agglutination
    chimpanzee coryza agent
    common carotid artery
CCAT conglutinating complement absorption test
CCC cathodal-closing contraction
    chronic calculous cholecystitis
    consecutive case conference
CCCl cathodal-closure clonus
CCF cephalin-cholesterol flocculation

CCF (*continued*)
    compound comminuted fracture
    congestive cardiac failure
CCK cholecystokinin
CCK-PZ cholecystokinin-pancreozymin
CCN coronary care nursing
CCP ciliocytophthoria
CCS casualty clearing station
CCT composite cyclic therapy
CCTe cathodal-closure tetanus
CCU cardiac care unit
    Cherry-Crandall units
    community care unit
    coronary care unit
CCW counterclockwise
CD cadaver donor
    cardiac disease
    cardiac dullness
    cardiovascular disease
    caudal
    common duct
    conjugata diagonalis
    consanguineous donor
    curative dose
    cystic duct
C/D cigarettes per day
C & D cystoscopy and dilatation
CD_{50} median curative dose
CDC calculated date of confinement
    Center for Disease Control
    chenodeoxycholate
    Communicable Disease Center
CDD certificate of disability for discharge
CDE canine distemper encephalitis
    chlordiazepoxide
    common duct exploration
CDH ceramide dihexoside
    congenital dislocation of the hip
CDL chlorodeoxylincomycin
CDP coronary drug project

CDSS clinical decision support system
CE California encephalitis
    cardiac enlargement
    chick embryo
    cholesterol esters
    contractile element
CEA carcinoembryonic antigen
    crystalline egg albumin
CEEV Central European encephalitis virus
CEF chick embryo fibroblast
Cel Celsius
Cent Centigrade
cent centimeter
Cert certified
CES central excitatory state
CF carbolfuchsin
    cardiac failure
    carrier-free
    chemotactic factor
    chest and left leg
    Chiari-Frommel syndrome
    Christmas factor
    citrovorum factor
    complement fixation
    complement-fixing
    contractile force
    count fingers
    counting finger
    cystic fibrosis
cf compare (*confer*)
CFA complement-fixing antibody
    complete Freund adjuvant
CFF critical flicker fusion test
    critical fusion frequency
CFP chronic false-positive
    cystic fibrosis of the pancreas
CFT clinical full-time
    complement-fixation test
CFU colony-forming units
    color-forming units
CFWM cancer-free white mouse
CG cardiogreen
    chorionic gonadotropin
    chronic glomerulonephritis

CG (*continued*)
    colloidal gold
    phosgene (choking gas)
Cg or
cg centigram
CGD chronic granulomatous
    disease
CGI clinical global impression
CGL chronic granulocytic
    leukemia
c gl correction with glasses
cgm centigram
CGN chronic glomerulonephritis
CG/OQ cerebral glucose oxygen
    quotient
CGP choline glycerophosphatide
    chorionic growth hormone
    prolactin
    circulating granulocyte pool
CGS or
cgs centimeter-gram-second
CGT chorionic gonadotropin
CGTT cortisone glucose tolerance
    test
CH cholesterol
    crown-heel (length of fetus)
    wheelchair
CHA congenital hypoplastic
    anemia
    cyclohexylamine
Chart paper (*charta*)
CHB complete heart block
CHD congestive heart disease
CHE cholinesterase
Chem chemotherapy
CHF congestive heart failure
CHH cartilage-hair hypoplasia
CHL chloramphenicol
CHO carbohydrate
Chol cholesterol
Chol est cholesterol esters
CHP child psychiatry
    comprehensive health plan-
    ning
Chr. *Chromobacterium*
chr chronic

CHS Chediak-Higashi syndrome
CI cardiac index
    cardiac insufficiency
    cerebral infarction
    chemotherapeutic index
    clinical investigator
    colloidal iron
    color index
    coronary insufficiency
    crystalline insulin
Ci curie
cib food (*cibus*)
CICU cardiology intensive care
    unit
    coronary intensive care unit
CID cytomegalic inclusion disease
CIDS cellular immunity deficiency
    syndrome
CIN cervical intra-epithelial neo-
    plasia
circ circulation
CIS carcinoma in situ
    central inhibitory state
CIXA constant infusion excretory
    urogram
CK creatine kinase
ck check
CL chest and left arm
Cl. *Clostridium*
Cl chlorine
cl centiliter
CLAS congenital localized absence
    of skin
CLBBB complete left bundle
    branch block
CLD chronic liver disease
    chronic lung disease
cldy cloudy
clin clinic
    clinical
CLL chronic lymphatic leukemia
    chronic lymphocytic leu-
    kemia
CLO cod liver oil
CLSL chronic lymphosarcoma
    (cell) leukemia

CLT   clot-lysis time
CM   capreomycin
      chloroquine-mepacrine
      cochlear microphonic
      complications
      costal margin
      cow's milk
cm   centimeter
      tomorrow morning (*cras mane*)
cm³   cubic centimeter
CMB   carbolic methylene blue
CMC   carboxymethyl cellulose
      critical micellar concentration
CMF   chondromyxoid fibroma
      Cytoxan, methotrexate, 5-fluorouracil
CMGN   chronic membranous glomerulonephritis
CMI   carbohydrate metabolism index
      cellular-mediated immune (response)
CMID   cytomegalic inclusion disease
c/min   cycles per minute
CML   chronic myelocytic leukemia
      chronic myelogenous leukemia
CMM   cutaneous malignant melanoma
cmm   cubic millimeter
CMN   cystic medial necrosis
CMN-AA   cystic medial necrosis of the ascending aorta
CMO   cardiac minute output
      card made out
CMP   cytidine monophosphate
CMR   cerebral metabolic rate
      crude mortality ratio
CMRG   cerebral metabolic rate of glucose
CMRO   cerebral metabolic rate of oxygen
CMS   Clyde Mood Scale

cms   to be taken tomorrow morning (*cras mane sumendus*)
CMU   chlorophenyldimethylurea
CMV   cytomegalovirus
CN   clinical nursing
      cyanogen
cn   tomorrow night (*cras nocte*)
CNE   chronic nervous exhaustion
CNH   community nursing home
CNHD   congenital nonspherocytic hemolytic disease
CNL   cardiolipin natural lecithin
CNS   central nervous system
cns   to be taken tomorrow night (*cras nocte sumendus*)
CNV   conative negative variation
      contingent negative variation
CO   carbon monoxide
      cardiac output
      castor oil
      cervicoaxial
      coenzyme
      corneal opacity
      compound
C/O   complains of
CO₂   carbon dioxide
CoA   coenzyme A
coag   coagulation
COC   cathodal-opening clonus
      coccygeal
      combination-type oral contraceptive
cochl   spoonful (*cochleare*)
COCL   cathodal-opening clonus
coct   boiling (*coctio*)
COD   cause of death
COGTT   cortisone-primed oral glucose tolerance test
COHB   carboxyhemoglobin
col   strain (*cola*)
colat   strained (*colatus*)
COLD   chronic obstructive lung disease
coll   eyewash (*collyrium*)
collut   mouthwash (*collutorium*)
collyr   eyewash (*collyrium*)

COMP   complaint
       complication
       compound
COMT   catechol-O-methyl trans-
       ferase
ConA   concanavalin A
conc   concentration
concis   cut (*concisus*)
cong   gallon (*congius*)
cont   continue
       continuously
conv   convalescent
COP   colloid osmotic pressure
       Cytoxan, Oncovin, pred-
       nisone
COPD   chronic obstructive pul-
       monary disease
coq   boil (*coque*)
coq sa   boil properly (*coque secun-
       dum artem*)
CORA   conditioned orientation
       reflex audiometry
cort   bark (*cortex*)
       cortex
COT   critical off-time
CP   candle power
       cerebral palsy
       chemically pure
       chloropurine
       chloroquine and primaquine
       chronic pyelonephritis
       closing pressure
       cochlear potential
       combination product
       combining power
       coproporphyrin
       creatine phosphate
C/P   cholesterol-phospholipid ratio
C & P   compensation and pension
CPA   cerebellar pontine angle
       chlorophenylalanine
CPAP   continuous positive airway
       pressure
CPB   cardiopulmonary bypass
CPC   cetylpyridinium chloride

CPC (*continued*)
       chronic passive congestion
       clinicopathologic conference
CPD   cephalopelvic disproportion
       citrate-phosphate-dextrose
cpd   compound
CPE   chronic pulmonary emphy-
       sema
       compensation, pension, and
       education
       cytopathic effect
CPI   constitutional psychopathic
       inferiority
       coronary prognostic index
CPIB   chlorophenoxyisobutyrate
CPK   creatine phosphokinase
cpm   counts per minute
CPN   chronic pyelonephritis
CPP   cyclopentenophenanthrene
CPPB   continuous positive-pressure
       breathing
CPPD   calcium pyrophosphate
       dihydrate
CPR   cardiopulmonary resuscita-
       tion
       cerebral-cortex perfusion
       rate
       cortisol production rate
CPS   clinical performance score
       cumulative probability of
       success
cps   cycles per second
CPT   chest physiotherapy
CPZ   chlorpromazine
CQ   chloroquine-quinine
       circadian quotient
CR   calculus removed
       chest and right arm
       clinical research
       colon resection
       complete remission
       conditioned reflex
       crown-rump (length of fetus)
Cr   chromium
CRA   central retinal artery

cran   cranial
CRBBB   complete right bundle
    branch block
CRD   chronic renal disease
    complete reaction of degen-
    eration
creat   creatinine
CRF   chronic renal failure
    corticotropin-releasing factor
CRI   concentrated rust-inhibitor
CRM   cross-reacting material
CROS   contralateral routing of
    signal
CRP   C-reactive protein
CRS   Chinese restaurant syndrome
    colon-rectal surgery
CRST   calcinosis cutis, Raynaud's
    phenomenon, sclero-
    dactyly, and telangiec-
    tasia
CRT   cathode ray tube
CRU   clinical research unit
CRV   central retinal vein
crys   crystal
CS   Central Service
    Central Supply
    cesarean section
    chondroitin sulfate
    conditioned stimulus
    conscious
    coronary sinus
    corticosteroid
    current strength
    cycloserine
C & S   conjunctiva and sclera
    culture and sensitivity
CSA   canavaninosuccinic acid
    chondroitin sulfate A
CSF   cerebrospinal fluid
    colony-stimulating factor
CSH   chronic subdural hematoma
    cortical stromal hyperplasia
CSL   cardiolipin synthetic lecithin
CSM   cerebrospinal meningitis
    corn-soy milk
CSN   carotid sinus nerve

CSR   Cheyne-Stokes respiration
    corrected sedimentation rate
    cortisol secretion rate
CSS   carotid sinus stimulation
CST   convulsive shock therapy
CT   cardiothoracic (ratio)
    carotid tracing
    carpal tunnel
    cerebral thrombosis
    chlorothiazide
    circulation time
    classic technique
    clotting time
    coagulation time
    collecting tubule
    computed tomography
    connective tissue
    contraction time
    Coombs' test
    coronary thrombosis
    corrected transposition
    corrective therapy
    crest time
    cytotechnologist
CTAB   cetyltrimethylammonium
    bromide
CTC   chlortetracycline
CTD   carpal tunnel decompression
    congenital thymic dysplasia
CTFE   chlorotrifluoroethylene
CTH   ceramide trihexoside
CTR   cardiothoracic ratio
CTZ   chlorothiazide
CU   color unit
    convalescent unit
CUC   chronic ulcerative colitis
cu cm   cubic centimeter
CUG   cystourethrogram
cuj   of which (*cujus*)
cuj lib   of any you desire (*cujus
    libet*)
cu mm   cubic millimeter
CV   cardiovascular
    cell volume
    central venous
    cerebrovascular

CV (*continued*)
    coefficient of variation
    color vision
    conjugate diameter of pelvic
      inlet
    conversational voice
    corpuscular volume
    cresyl violet
cv tomorrow evening (*cras vespere*)
CVA cardiovascular accident
    cerebrovascular accident
    costovertebral angle
CVD cardiovascular disease
    color vision deviant
    color vision deviate
cvd curved
CVH combined ventricular hyper-
      trophy
    common variable hypogam-
      maglobulinemia
CVO conjugate diameter of pelvic
      inlet
CVOD cerebrovascular obstructive
      disease
CVP cell volume profile
    central venous pressure
    Cytoxan, vincristine,
      prednisone
CVR cardiovascular-renal
    cerebrovascular resistance
CVRD cardiovascular renal disease
CVS cardiovascular surgery
    cardiovascular system
    clean-voided specimen
CW cardiac work
    casework
    chemical warfare
    chest wall
    children's ward
    continuous wave
cw clockwise
CWDF cell wall–deficient bacterial
      forms
CWI cardiac work index
CWP childbirth without pain

cwt hundredweight
CX cervix
Cx or
cx convex
CXR chest x-ray film
Cy cyanogen
cy copy
Cyclo cyclophosphamide
    cyclopropane
cyl cylinder
    cylindrical lens
cysto cystoscopic examination
D daughter
    day
    dead
    deciduous
    density
    dermatology
    deuterium
    deuteron
    dextro
    died
    diopter
    diplomate
    distal
    divorced
    dorsal
    duration
    mean dose
    vitamin D unit
d dose (*dosis*)
    give (*da*)
    right (*dexter*)
D_{CO} diffusing capacity for
      carbon monoxide
D_L diffusing capacity of lung
DA degenerative arthritis
    dental assistant
    direct agglutination
    disaggregated
    dopamine
    ductus arteriosus
DAB dimethylaminoazobenzene
DAH disordered action of the
      heart
DALA delta-aminolevulinic acid

DAM degraded amyloid
    diacetyl monoxime
DAO diamine oxidase
DAP dihydroxyacetone phosphate
    direct agglutination preg-
    nancy (test)
DAPT direct agglutination preg-
    nancy test
Dapt Daptazole
DAT differential agglutination
    titer
    diphtheria antitoxin
DB date of birth
    dextran blue
    disability
    distobuccal
db decibel
DBA dibenzanthracene
DBC dye-binding capacity
DBCL dilute blood clot lysis
    (method)
DBI development-at-birth index
DBM dibromomannitol
DBO distobucco-occlusal
DBP diastolic blood pressure
    distobuccopulpal
DC daily census
    deoxycholate
    diagnostic code
    diphenylarsine cyanide
    direct current
    discontinue
    distocervical
D & C dilatation and curettage
    dilation and curettage
DCA deoxycholate-citrate agar
    desoxycorticosterone acetate
DCC double concave
DCF direct centrifugal flotation
DCG disodium cromoglycate
DCHFB dichlorohexafluorobutane
DCI dichloroisoproterenol
DCT direct Coombs' test
DCTMA desoxycorticosterone
    trimethylacetate

DCTPA desoxycorticosterone
    triphenylacetate
DCx double convex
DD died of the disease
    differential diagnosis
    disk diameter
dd let it be given to (*detur ad*)
DDC diethyldithiocarbamic acid
    direct display console
DDD dichlorodiphenyldichloro-
    ethane
DDS diaminodiphenylsulfone
    dystrophy-dystocia syn-
    drome
DDT dichlorodiphenyltrichloro-
    ethane
DE dream elements
    duration of ejection
D & E dilation and evacuation
DEA dehydroepiandrosterone
DEAE diethylaminoethanol
    diethylaminoethyl
DEAE-D diethylaminoethyl
    dextran
DEBA diethylbarbituric acid
dec deceased
    deciduous
    decrease
dec pour off (*decanta*)
decoct decoction
decr decrease
decub lying down (*decubitus*)
def deficiency
deg degeneration
    degree
deglut let it be swallowed
    (*deglutiatur*)
del delivery
Dem Demerol (meperidine)
dep dependents
DeR reaction of degeneration
derm dermatology
DES diethylstilbestrol
dest distilled (*destilla*)
DET diethyltryptamine

det give (*detur*)
DEV duck embryo vaccine
DF decapacitation factor
    deficiency factor
    degree of freedom
    desferrioxamine
    diabetic father
    discriminant function
    disseminated foci
DFDT difluorodiphenyltrichloro-
    ethane
DFO deferoxamine
DFP diisopropylfluorophosphate
DFU dead fetus in utero
    dideoxyfluorouridine
DG deoxyglucose
    diagnosis
    diastolic gallop
    diglyceride
    distogingival
dg or
dgm decigram
DH delayed hypersensitivity
DHA dehydroepiandrosterone
    dihydroxyacetone
DHAP dihydroxyacetone phos-
    phate
DHAS dehydroepiandrosterone
    sulfate
DHE dihydroergotamine
DHEA dehydroepiandrosterone
DHEAS dehydroepiandrosterone
    sulfate
DHFR dihydrofolate reductase
DHIA dehydroisoandrosterone
DHL diffuse histiocytic lymphoma
DHT dihydrotachysterol
DI diabetes insipidus
    diagnostic imaging
diag diagnosis
DIC diffuse intravascular coagula-
    tion
    disseminated intravascular
    coagulation
DID dead of intercurrent disease
DIE died in Emergency Room

diff differential
dig let it be digested (*digeratur*)
dil dilute (*dilue*)
DILD diffuse infiltrative lung
    disease
diluc at daybreak (*diluculo*)
dilut dilute (*dilutus*)
DIM divalent ion metabolism
dim one half (*dimidius*)
DIP desquamative interstitial
    pneumonia
    diisopropyl phosphate
    distal interphalangeal
DIPJ distal interphalangeal joint
dis disease
disc discontinue
disch discharge
disp dispensatory
    dispense
dist distill
DIT diiodotyrosine
div divide
DJD degenerative joint disease
DK decay
    diseased kidney
    dog kidney
DL danger list
    difference limen
    diffusing capacity of lung
    distolingual
    Donath-Landsteiner (test)
dl deciliter
DLA distolabial
DLAI distolabioincisal
DLCO diffusing capacity of lung
    for carbon monoxide
DLE discoid lupus erythematosus
    disseminated lupus
    erythematosus
DLI distolinguoincisal
DLO distolinguo-occlusal
DLP distolinguopulpal
DM diabetes mellitus
    diabetic mother
    diastolic murmur
    dopamine

DMA   dimethyladenosine
DMAB   dimethylaminobenzalde-
       hyde
DMBA   dimethylbenzanthracene
DMCT   demethylchlortetracycline
DMD   Duchenne's muscular
       dystrophy
DME   dimethyl ether (of
       D-tubocurarine)
DMF   decayed, missing or filled
       (teeth)
DMM   dimethylmyleran
DMN   dimethylnitrosamine
DMO   dimethyloxazolidinedione
DMPA   depomedroxyprogesterone
       acetate
DMPE or
DMPEA   dimethoxyphenylethyla-
       mine
DMPP   dimethylphenylpiperazin-
       ium
DMS   dimethylsulfoxide
DMSO   dimethylsulfoxide
DMT   dimethyltryptamine
DN   dextrose-nitrogen (ratio)
DNA   deoxyribonucleic acid
DNase   deoxyribonuclease
DNB   dinitrobenzene
DNC   dinitrocarbanilide
DNCB   dinitrochlorobenzene
DND   died a natural death
DNFB   dinitrofluorobenzene
DNP   deoxyribonucleoprotein
       dinitrophenol
DNPH   dinitrophenylhydrazine
DNPM   dinitrophenylmorphine
DNT   did not test
DO   diamine oxidase
       disto-occlusal
DOA   dead on arrival
DOB   date of birth
DOC   deoxycholate
       deoxycorticosterone
       died of other causes
DOCA   deoxycorticosterone
       acetate
DOCS   deoxycorticoids

DOD   date of death
       dead of disease
DOE   dyspnea on exercise
       dyspnea on exertion
DOM   deaminated-O-methyl
       metabolite
       dimethoxymethyl ampheta-
       mine
DOMA   dihydroxymandelic acid
DON   diazo-oxonorleucine
DOPA   dihydroxyphenylalanine
DOPAC   dihydroxyphenylacetic
       acid
DP   dementia praecox
       diastolic pressure
       directional preponderance
       disability pension
       distopulpal
dp   with proper direction (*direc-
       tione propria*)
DPA   dipropylacetate
DPC   delayed primary closure
DPD   diffuse pulmonary disease
DPDL   diffuse poorly differenti-
       ated lymphoma
DPG   diphosphoglycerate
       displacement placentogram
DPGM   diphosphoglyceromutase
DPGP   diphosphoglycerate phos-
       phatase
DPH   diphenylhydantoin
DPI   disposable personal income
DPL   distopulpolingual
dpm   disintegrations per minute
DPN   diphosphopyridine nucleo-
       tide
DPO   dimethoxyphenyl penicillin
DPS   dimethylpolysiloxane
DPT   diphtheria, pertussis, and
       tetanus
       dipropyltryptamine
DPTA   diethylenetriamine penta-
       acetic acid
DQ   developmental quotient
DR   diabetic retinopathy
       doctor
       reaction of degeneration

Dr doctor
dr drachm
    dram
DRF dose-reduction factor
DRI Discharge Readiness Inventory
DS dead space
    dehydroepiandrosterone sulfate
    dextrose-saline
    Down's syndrome
    dry swallow
D & S dermatology and syphilology
DSAP disseminated superficial actinic porokeratosis
DSC or
DSCG disodium cromoglycate
DSM dextrose solution mixture
DST dexamethasone suppression test
DT delirium tremens
    distance test
    duration tetany
    dye test
DTBC D-tubocurarine
DTBN di-t-butyl nitroxide
DTC D-tubocurarine
dtd let such a dose be given (*datur talis dosis*)
D time dream time
DTM dermatophyte test medium
DTMP deoxythymidine monophosphate
DTN diphtheria toxin normal
DTNB dithiobisnitrobenzoic acid
DTP diphtheria, tetanus, and pertussis
    distal tingling on percussion
DTPA diethylenetriaminepentacetic acid
DTR deep tendon reflex
DTZ diatrizoate
DU deoxyuridine
    diagnosis undetermined
    dog unit
    duodenal ulcer

DUMP deoxyuridine monophosphate
duod duodenum
DV double vibration
DVA distance visual acuity
DW distilled water
    dry weight
D/W dextrose in water
D5W,
D5 & W or
D_5W 5 per cent dextrose in water
DX dextran
Dx diagnosis
DXD discontinued
DXM dexamethasone
DXT deep x-ray therapy
DZ dizygous
E cortisone (compound E)
    electric charge
    electromotive force
    electron
    emmetropia
    energy
    epinephrine
    experimenter
    eye
E. Entamoeba
    Escherichia
EA ethacrynic acid
ea each
EAC Ehrlich ascites carcinoma
    external auditory canal
EACA epsilon aminocaproic acid
ead the same (*eadem*)
EAE experimental allergic encephalomyelitis
EAHF eczema, asthma, hay fever
EAHLG equine antihuman lymphoblast globulin
EAHLS equine antihuman lymphoblast serum
EAM external auditory meatus
EAP epiallopregnanolone
EB elementary body
    epidermolysis bullosa
    Epstein-Barr (virus)
    estradiol benzoate

EBI   emetine bismuth iodide
EBL   estimated blood loss
EBV   Epstein-Barr virus
EC   electron capture
    enteric-coated
    entrance complaint
    Escherichia coli
    excitation-contraction
    experimental control
    extracellular
    eyes closed
ECA   ethacrynic acid
ECBO   enteric cytopathogenic bovine orphan (virus)
ECBV   effective circulating blood volume
ECC   extracorporeal circulation
ECDO   enteric cytopathogenic dog orphan (virus)
ECF   effective capillary flow
    extended care facility
    extracellular fluid
ECFA   eosinophil chemotactic factor of anaphylaxis
ECFV   extracellular fluid volume
ECG   electrocardiogram
ECHO   enteric cytopathogenic human orphan (virus)
ECI or
ECIB   extracorporeal irradiation of blood
ECIL   extracorporeal irradiation of lymph
eclec   eclectic
ECLT   euglobulin clot lysis time
ECM   extracellular material
ECMO   enteric cytopathogenic monkey orphan (virus)
E. coli   *Escherichia coli*
ECS   electroconvulsive shock
ECSO   enteric cytopathogenic swine orphan (virus)
ECT   electroconvulsive therapy
ECV   extracellular volume
ECW   extracellular water
ED   effective dose

ED (*continued*)
    Ehlers-Danlos syndrome
    epileptiform discharge
    erythema dose
ED_{50} median effective dose
EDC   estimated date of confinement
    expected date of confinement
EDD   effective drug duration
    expected date of delivery
EDP   electronic data processing
    end-diastolic pressure
EDR   effective direct radiation
    electrodermal response
EDS   Ehlers-Danlos syndrome
EDTA   edetic acid
    ethylenediaminotetra-acetate
EDV   end-diastolic volume
EE   end-to-end
    eye and ear
EEA   electroencephalic audiometry
EEC   enteropathogenic *Escherichia coli*
EEE   Eastern equine encephalitis
EEG   electroencephalogram
EEME   ethinylestradiol methyl ether
EENT   eyes, ears, nose and throat
EER   electroencephalic response
EF   ectopic focus
    ejection fraction
    encephalitogenic factor
EFA   essential fatty acids
    extrafamily adoptees
EFC   endogenous fecal calcium
EFE   endocardial fibroelastosis
EFV   extracellular fluid volume
EFVC   expiratory flow-volume curve
EG   esophagogastrectomy
EGG   electrogastrogram
EGL   eosinophilic granuloma of the lung

EGM   electrogram
EGOT   erythrocyte glutamic
            oxaloacetic transaminase
EH   essential hypertension
EHBF   estimated hepatic blood
            flow
            exercise hyperemia blood
            flow
EHC   enterohepatic circulation
            essential hypercholesterol-
            emia
EHDP   ethane hydroxydiphos-
            phate
EHF   exophthalmos-hyperthyroid
            factor
EHL   endogenous hyperlipidemia
EHO   extrahepatic obstruction
EHP   excessive heat production
EI   enzyme inhibitor
E/I   expiration-inspiration ratio
EID   egg-infective dose
            electroimmunodiffusion
EIP   extensor indicis proprius
EK   erythrokinase
EKC   epidemic keratoconjunctiv-
            itis
EKG   electrocardiogram
EKY   electrokymogram
el   elixir
elb   elbow
ELISA   enzyme-linked immuno-
            sorbent assay
elix   elixir
ELT   euglobulin lysis time
EM   ejection murmur
            electron microscopy
            erythrocyte mass
Em   emmetropia
EMB   embryology
            eosin methylene blue
            ethambutol
            ethambutol-myambutol
EMC   electron microscopy
            encephalomyocarditis
EMF   electromagnetic flowmeter
            electromotive force
            endomyocardial fibrosis

EMF (*continued*)
            erythrocyte maturation
            factor
EMG   electromyogram
            exophthalmos, macroglossia,
            gigantism
EMI   Electric and Musical Indus-
            tries
emp   a plaster (*emplastrum*)
            as directed
emul   emulsion
EN   enema
            erythema nodosum
ENA   extractable nuclear antigen
enem   enema
ENG   electronystagmograph
ENL   erythema nodosum leproti-
            cum
ENT   ear, nose, and throat
EO   eosinophils
            ethylene oxide
            eyes open
EOD   entry on duty
eod   every other day
EOG   electro-oculogram
EOM   extraocular movement
eos   eosinophils
EOT   effective oxygen transport
EP   ectopic pregnancy
            erythrocyte protoporphyrin
EPC   epilepsia partialis continua
EPEC   enteropathogenic *Esche-
            richia coli*
EPF   exophthalmos-producing
            factor
Epi   epinephrine
epith   epithelium
EPP   erythropoietic protoporphy-
            ria
EPR   electron paramagnetic
            resonance
            electrophrenic respiration
            estradiol production rate
EPS   exophthalmos-producing
            substance
EPTE   existed prior to enlistment
EPTS   existed prior to service

eq   equivalent
ER   ejection rate
     emergency room
     endoplasmic reticulum
     estrogen receptors
     external resistance
     evoked response
ERA   evoked response audiometry
ERBF   effective renal blood flow
ERCP   endoscopic retrograde chol-
     angiopancreatography
ERG   electroretinogram
ERP   effective refractory period
     equine rhinopneumonitis
ERPF   effective renal plasma flow
ERV   expiratory reserve volume
ES   end-to-side
     Expectation Score
ESB   electrical stimulation to brain
ESC   electromechanical slope com-
     puter
Esch.   *Escherichia*
ESD   electronic summation device
ESF   erythropoietic-stimulating
     factor
ESL   end-systolic length
ESM   ejection systolic murmur
eso   esophagoscopy
     esophagus
ESP   end-systolic pressure
     extrasensory perception
ESR   erythrocyte sedimentation
     rate
ESS   erythrocyte-sensitizing sub-
     stance
ess   essential
ess neg   essentially negative
EST   electroshock therapy
est   estimated
ESU   electrostatic unit
ESV   end-systolic volume
ET   effective temperature
     ejection time
     endotracheal
     etiology
     eustachian tube

Et   ethyl
et al   and others (*et alii*)
ETA   ethionamide
ETF   eustachian tube function
ETH   elixir terpin hydrate
ETH/C   elixir terpin hydrate with
     codeine
etiol   etiology
ETKM   every test known to man
ETM   erythromycin
ETOH   ethyl alcohol
ETOX   ethylene oxide
ETP   entire treatment period
     eustachian tube pressure
ETT   extrathyroidal thyroxine
ETV   educational television
EU   Ehrlich units
     enzyme units
EUA   examination under anes-
     thesia
EV   extravascular
ev   electron volt
eval   evaluation
EW   Emergency Ward
ew   elsewhere
EWB   estrogen withdrawal bleed-
     ing
EWL   egg-white lysozyme
ex   excision
     exophthalmos
exam   examination
EXBF   exercise hyperemia blood
     flow
exc   excision
exhib   let it be given (*exhibeatur*)
exp or
expir   expired
     expiration
     expiratory
ext   exterior
     external
     extract
     spread (*extende*)
F   Fahrenheit
     fat
     father

F (*continued*)
  fellow
  female
  field of vision
  foramen
  formula
  French (catheter size)
  gilbert (unit of magnetomotive force)
  hydrocortisone (compound F)
F. Filaria
  Fusiformis
f make (*fiat*)
F_1 first filial generation
F_2 second filial generation
FA far advanced
  fatty acid
  femoral artery
  field ambulance
  first aid
  fluorescent antibody
  forearm
  free acid
FAD flavin adenine dinucleotide
FADF fluorescent antibody dark-field
Fahr Fahrenheit
fam doc family doctor
FAN fuchsin, amido black, and naphthol yellow
FANA fluorescent antinuclear antibody
FAT fluorescent antibody test
FAV feline ataxia virus
FB fingerbreadth
  foreign body
FBE full blood examination
FBP femoral blood pressure
  fibrinogen breakdown products
FBS fasting blood sugar
  fetal bovine serum
FC finger clubbing
  finger counting
fc foot candles

FCA ferritin-conjugated antibodies
FD fatal dose
  focal distance
  foot drape
  forceps delivery
  freeze-dried
FD_{50} median fatal dose
FDA frontodextra anterior
FDE final drug evaluation
FDP fibrin degradation product
  flexor digitorum profundus
  frontodextra posterior
  fructose 1,6-diphosphate
FDS flexor digitorum superficialis
FDT frontodextra transversa
feb dur while the fever lasts (*febre durante*)
FEC free erythrocyte coproporphyrin
FECG fetal electrocardiogram
FECP free erythrocyte coproporphyria
FECVC functional extracellular fluid volume
FEF forced expiratory flow
FEKG fetal electrocardiogram
fem female
FEP or
FEPP free erythrocyte protoporphyrin
FES forced expiratory spirogram
FET forced expiratory time
FETS forced expiratory time, in seconds
FEV forced expiratory volume
FF fat free
  father factor
  fecal frequency
  filtration fraction
  finger-to-finger
  flat feet
  force fluids
  forearm flow
  foster father

FFA   free fatty acids
FFDW   fat-free dry weight
FFM   fat-free mass
FFP   fresh frozen plasma
FFT   flicker fusion threshold
FFWW   fat-free wet weight
FG   fibrinogen
FGD   fatal granulomatous disease
FGF   father's grandfather
    fresh gas flow
FGM   father's grandmother
FH   family history
    fetal head
    fetal heart
fh   let a draft be made (*fiat
    haustus*)
FHR   fetal heart rate
FHS   fetal heart sound
FHT   fetal heart
    fetal heart tones
FI   fever caused by infection
    fibrinogen
    forced inspiration
fib   fibrillation
    fibrinogen
FID   flame ionization detector
FIF   forced inspiratory flow
fig   figure
FIGLU   formiminoglutamic acid
filt   filter
fist   fistula
FJN   familial juvenile nephro-
    phthisis
fl   fluid
fl dr   fluid dram
fl oz   fluid ounce
Fl up   flare-up
FLA   left frontoanterior (*fronto-
    laevo anterior*)
fla   according to rule (*fiat lege
    artis*)
fld   fluid
flor   flowers
FLP   left frontoposterior (*fronto-
    laevo posterior*)
FLSA   follicular lymphosarcoma

FLT   left frontotransverse (*fronto-
    laeva transversa*)
FM   flowmeter
fm   make a mixture (*fiat mistura*)
FME   full-mouth extraction
FMF   familial Mediterranean fever
FMG   foreign medical graduate
FMN   flavin mononucleotide
FMS   fat-mobilizing substance
    full-mouth series
FN   false-negative
    finger-to-nose
FO   foramen ovale
    fronto-occipital
FOAVF   failure of all vital forces
FOD   free of disease
fol   leaves (*folia*)
FP   false-positive
    family practice
    freezing point
    frontoparietal
    frozen plasma
fp   let a potion be made (*fiat
    potio*)
FPA   fluorophenylalanine
FPC   fish protein concentrate
f pil   let pills be made (*fiant
    pilulae*)
FPM   filter paper microscopic
    (test)
fps   frames per second
FR   Fisher-Race (notation)
    flocculation reaction
    flow rate
Fr   French (catheter gauge)
Fr BB   fracture of both bones
F & R   force and rhythm
fract   fracture
frag   fragility
FRC   frozen red cells
    functional reserve capacity
    functional residual capacity
frict   friction
FROM   full range of motion
FRP   functional refractory period
FRS   furosemide

FS   full scale (IQ)
      function study
fsa   let it be made skillfully (*fiat
      secundum artem*)
FSD   focal skin distance
FSF   fibrin-stabilizing factor
FSH   follicle-stimulating hormone
FSP   fibrinogen split products
      fibrinolytic split products
FSR   fusiform skin revision
FSW   field service worker
FT   false transmitter
      family therapy
      fibrous tissue
      free thyroxine
      full term
ft   foot
      make (*fiat*)
ft pulv   make a powder (*fiat pulvis*)
FTA   fluorescent treponemal anti-
      body
FTA-AB or
FTA-ABS   fluorescent treponemal
          antibody absorption
          test
FTI   free thyroxine index
FTLB full term living birth
FTND full term normal delivery
FTT   failure to thrive
FU   fecal urobilinogen
      fluorouracil
      follow-up
FUDR fluorodeoxyuridine
FUO   fever of undetermined origin
      fever of unknown origin
FUR   fluorouracil riboside
FV   fluid volume
FVC   forced vital capacity
FVL   femoral vein ligation
f vs let the patient be bled (*fiat
      venaesectio*)
FW   Felix-Weil (reaction)
      Folin and Wu's (method)
      fragment wound
FWHM full width at half-
      maximum

FWR   Felix-Weil reaction
fx   fracture
FY   fiscal year
FYI   for your information
FZ   focal zone
G   an immunoglobulin
      gauge
      gingival
      glucose
      gonidial (colony)
      good
      gravida
      Greek
g   force (the pull of gravity)
      gram
GA   Gamblers Anonymous
      gastric analysis
      general anesthesia
      gestational age
      gingivoaxial
      glucuronic acid
      gut-associated
Ga   gallium
GABA gamma-aminobutyric acid
gal   gallon
GALT gut-associated lymphoid
      tissue
galv galvanic
GAPD or
GAPDH glyceraldehyde phosphate
      dehydrogenase
garg gargle
GB   gallbladder
      Guillain-Barré syndrome
GBA   ganglionic-blocking agent
      gingivobuccoaxial
GBH   graphite-benzalkonium-
      heparin
GBM   glomerular basement mem-
      brane
GBS   gallbladder series
GC   ganglion cells
      gas chromatography
      glucocorticoid
      gonococcus
      gonorrhea

GC (*continued*)
    granular casts
    guanine cytosine
g-cal gram-calorie
g-cm gram-centimeter
GCS general clinical service
GDA germine diacetate
GDH glycerophosphate dehydro-
    genase
GDS Gradual Dosage Schedule
GE gastroemotional
    gastroenterology
    gastroenterostomy
G/E granulocyte-erythroid ratio
GEMS good emergency mother
    substitute
gen general
ger geriatrics
GET gastric emptying time
GET½ gastric emptying half-time
GF germ-free
    gluten-free
    grandfather
GFD gluten-free diet
GFR glomerular filtration rate
GG gamma globulin
GG or S glands, goiter, or stiff-
    ness (the neck)
GGA general gonadotropic
    activity
GGG gamboge
GGT gamma glutamyl transferase
GGTP gamma-glutamyl trans-
    peptidase
GH growth hormone
GHD growth hormone deficiency
GHRF growth hormone–releasing
    factor
GI gastrointestinal
    globin insulin
GIK glucose, insulin, and potas-
    sium
GIM gonadotropin-inhibitory
    material
GIS gas in stomach
    gastrointestinal system

GIT gastrointestinal tract
GITT glucose-insulin tolerance
    test
GK glycerol kinase
GL greatest length
Gl gill
    gland
GLA gingivolinguoaxial
GLC gas-liquid chromatography
glob globulin
GLP group-living program
glu or
gluc glucose
GM gastric mucosa
    general medical
    geometric mean
    grandmother
    grand multiparity
gm gram
GMA glyceryl methacrylate
GMC general medical council
GMK green monkey kidney
g-m gram-meter
GM & S general medical and
    surgical
GMT geometric mean titer
GMW gram-molecular weight
GN glomerulonephritis
    glucose nitrogen (ratio)
    gram-negative
GNID gram-negative intracellular
    diplococci
GOE gas, oxygen and ether
GOK God only knows
GOT glutamic oxaloacetic trans-
    aminase
GP general paresis
    general practice
    general practitioner
    glycoprotein
    guinea pig
    gutta-percha
gp group (muscle)
GPA grade-point averages
GPAIS guinea pig anti-insulin
    serum

GPD or
GPDH   glucose phosphate dehy-
           drogenase
G6PD or
G6PDH   glucose-6-phosphate de-
            hydrogenase
GPI   general paralysis of the insane
        glucose phosphate isomerase
GPIPID   guinea pig intraperitoneal
             infectious dose
GPK   guinea pig kidney (antigen)
GPKA   guinea pig kidney absorp-
             tion (test)
GPS   guinea pig serum
GPT   glutamic pyruvic trans-
         aminase
GPUT   galactose phosphate uridyl
            transferase
GR   gastric resection
       glutathione reductase
gr   grain
GRA   gonadotropin-releasing agent
grad   gradually, by degrees
GRAS   generally recognized as safe
grav I   pregnancy one
             primigravida
GRF   gonadotropin-releasing
          factor
GS   general surgery
G/S   glucose and saline
GSA   Gross virus antigen
          guanidinosuccinic acid
GSC   gas-solid chromatography
          gravity-settling culture
GSD   genetically significant dose
          glycogen storage disease
GSE   gluten-sensitive enteropathy
GSH   glomerular-stimulating
          hormone
          (reduced) glutathione
GSR   galvanic skin response
          generalized Shwartzman
          reaction
GSSG   (oxidized) glutathione
GSSR   generalized Sanarelli-
            Shwartzman reaction

GSW   gunshot wound
GT   gingiva, treatment of
       glucose tolerance
       glutamyl transpeptidase
G & T   gowns and towels
gt   drop
GTH   gonadotropic hormone
GTN   glyceryl trinitrate
GTP   glutamyl transpeptidase
         guanosine triphosphate
GTT   glucose tolerance test
gtt   drops
GU   gastric ulcer
       genitourinary
       gonococcal urethritis
GUS   genitourinary system
GV   gentian violet
GVH   graft versus host
GVHR   graft-versus-host reaction
GW   group work
GXT   graded exercise test
gyn   gynecology
GZ   Guilford-Zimmerman
        personality test
H   a draft (*haustus*)
      height
      henry
      high
      Holzknecht unit
      horizontal
      hormone
      hour
      hypermetropia
      hypo
H   Hauch (motile microorganism)
H.   *Hemophilus*
H+   hydrogen ion
HA   headache
       height age
       hemagglutinating antibody
       hemagglutination
       hemolytic anemia
       high anxiety
       hospital admission
       Hounsfield unit
       hydroxyapatite

HAA   hepatitis-associated antigen
HABA   hydroxybenzeneazoben-
      zoic acid
HAD   hemadsorption
HAHTG   horse antihuman thymus
      globulin
HAI   hemagglutination inhibition
     hemagglutinin inhibition
hal   halothane
HAP   heredopathia atactica poly-
      neuritiformis
     histamine phosphate acid
HAPA   hemagglutinating anti-
      penicillin antibody
HASHD   hypertensive arterio-
      sclerotic heart disease
haust   a draft (*haustus*)
HB   heart block
   housebound
Hb   hemoglobin
HBABA   hydroxybenzeneazoben-
      zoic acid
HBB   hydroxybenzyl benzimida-
     zole
HBD or
HBDH   hydroxybutyrate dehydro-
      genase
HBF   hepatic blood flow
HBI   high serum-bound iron
HBO   hyperbaric oxygen
HBP   high blood pressure
HBW   high birth weight
HC   hair cell
   head compression
   hepatic catalase
   house call
   Huntington's chorea
   hyaline casts
   hydroxycorticoid
HCC   hydroxycholecalciferol
hCG   human chorionic gonado-
     tropin
HCH   hexachlorocyclohexane
HCO_3 – bicarbonate
HCP   hepatocatalase peroxidase
   hereditary coproporphyria

hCS or
hCSM   human chorionic somato-
      mammotropin
HCT   hematocrit
   homocytotrophic
   hydrochlorothiazide
HCU   homocystinuria
HCVD   hypertensive cardiovascular
      disease
HD   hearing distance
   heart disease
   high dosage
   Hodgkin's disease
   hydatid disease
hd   at bedtime (*hora decubitus*)
HDBH   hydroxybutyric dehydro-
      genase
HDC   histidine decarboxylase
HDH   heart disease history
HDL or
HDLP   high-density lipoprotein
HDLW   distance at which a watch
      is heard by the left ear
HDN   hemolytic disease of the
     newborn
HDP   hydroxydimethylpyrimidine
HDRW   distance at which a watch
      is heard by the right ear
HDS   herniated disk syndrome
HE   human enteric
H & E   hematoxylin and eosin
HEAT   human erythrocyte agglu-
     tination test
hebdom   a week (*hebdomada*)
HEC   hydroxyergocalciferol
HED   unit of roentgen-ray dosage
     (*Haut-Einheits-Dosis*)
HEENT   head, eyes, ears, nose and
     throat
HEK   human embryo kidney
   human embryonic kidney
hematol   hematology
HEPA   high-efficiency particulate
     air (filter)
HES   hydroxyethyl starch
HET   helium equilibration time

HETP hexaethyltetraphosphate
HF Hageman factor
    hay fever
    heart failure
    hemorrhagic fever
    high flow
    high frequency
HFI hereditary fructose intoler-
    ance
HFP hexafluoropropylene
hG or
hGB hemoglobin
HGF hyperglycemic-glycogen-
    olytic factor
HGG human gamma globulin
hGH human growth hormone
HGPRT hypoxanthine guanine
    phosphoribosyl trans-
    ferase
HH hydroxyhexamide
HHA hereditary hemolytic anemia
HHb un-ionized hemoglobin
HHD hypertensive heart disease
H & Hm compound hyperme-
    tropic astigmatism
HHT hereditary hemorrhagic
    telangiectasia
HI hemagglutination inhibition
    high impulsiveness
    hydroxyindole
HIA hemagglutination-inhibition
    antibody
HIAA hydroxyindoleacetic acid
HIHA high impulsiveness, high
    anxiety
HILA high impulsiveness, low
    anxiety
HIOMT hydroxyindole-O-methyl
    transferase
HIT hemagglutination-inhibition
    test
    hypertrophic infiltrative
    tendinitis
HJ Howell-Jolly (bodies)
HK heat-killed
    heel-to-knee

HK (*continued*)
    hexokinase
HKLM heat-killed *Listeria mono-*
    cytogenes
HL hearing level
    hearing loss
    histocompatibility locus
    hypermetropia, latent
H & L heart and lungs
HLA histocompatibility complex
HLDH heat-stable lactic dehydro-
    genase
hLH human luteinizing hormone
H-L-K heart, liver, kidney
HLR heart-lung resuscitator
HLT human lymphocyte trans-
    formation
hlth health
HLV herpes-like virus
HM hand movement(s)
    human milk
    hydatidiform mole
Hm manifest hyperopia
HMD hyaline membrane disease
HME heat and moisture exchanger
HMF hydroxymethylfurfural
HMG human menopausal gonado-
    tropin
    hydroxymethylglutaryl
HML human milk lysozyme
HMM hexamethylolmelamine
HMP hexose monophosphate
    hexose monophosphate
    pathway
    hot moist packs
HMPG hydroxymethoxyphenyl-
    glycol
HMPS hexose monophosphate
    shunt
HMSAS hypertrophic muscular
    subaortic stenosis
HN hereditary nephritis
    hilar node
hn tonight (*hac nocte*)
HN_2 nitrogen mustard, mechlor-
    ethamine

HNP   herniated nucleus pulposus
HNSHA   hereditary nonsphero-
　　　　cytic hemolytic anemia
HO   high oxygen
　　　hyperbaric oxygen
H/O   history of
H₂O   water
HOC   hydroxycorticoid
HOCM   hypertrophic obstructive
　　　　cardiomyopathy
HOOD   hereditary osteo-onycho
　　　　dysplasia
HOP   high oxygen pressure
hosp   hospital
HP   high protein
　　　human pituitary
H & P   history and physical
hp   haptoglobin
HPA   hypothalamic-pituitary-
　　　adrenal
HPAA   hydroxyphenylacetic acid
HPE   history and physical exam-
　　　　ination
HPF   heparin-precipitable fraction
　　　high-power field
hPFSH   human pituitary follicle-
　　　　stimulating hormone
hPG   human pituitary gonado-
　　　　tropin
HPI   history of present illness
hPL   human placental lactogen
HPLA   hydroxyphenyllactic acid
HPO   high pressure oxygen
HPP   hydroxypyrazolopyrimidine
HPPA   hydroxyphenylpyruvic acid
HPPH   hydroxyphenyl-phenylhy-
　　　　dantoin
HPS   hematoxylin-phloxine-saffron
　　　hypertrophic pyloric stenosis
HPT   hyperparathyroidism
HPV   *Hemophilus pertussis* vaccine
HPVD   hypertensive pulmonary
　　　　vascular disease
HPVG   hepatic portal venous gas
HR   heart rate
　　　hospital record
　　　hospital report

Hr   blood type factor
hr   hour
H & R   hysterectomy and radiation
HRBC   horse red blood cells
HRIG   human rabies immune
　　　　globulin
HRS   Hamilton Rating Scale
HRT   heart rate
HS   heat stable
　　　heme synthetase
　　　hereditary spherocytosis
　　　herpes simplex
　　　horse serum
　　　Hurler's syndrome
hs   on retiring (*hora somni*)
HSA   human serum albumin
HSG   hysterosalpingogram
HSV   herpes simplex virus
HT   hemagglutination titer
　　　histologic technician
　　　hydroxytryptamine
　　　hypermetropia, total
　　　hypertension
　　　hypodermic tablet
Ht   total hyperopia
ht   heart
　　　height
HTA   hydroxytryptamine
HTHD   hypertensive heart disease
HTOH   hydroxytryptophol
HTP   hydroxytryptophan
HTV   herpes-type virus
HU   hemagglutinating unit
　　　hydroxyurea
　　　hyperemia unit
HUS   hemolytic-uremic syndrome
　　　hyaluronidase unit for semen
HUTHAS   human thymus anti-
　　　　serum
HV   hepatic vein
　　　herpes virus
　　　hospital visit
H & V   hemigastrectomy and
　　　　vagotomy
HVA   homovanillic acid
HVD   hypertensive vascular disease
HVE   high-voltage electrophoresis

HVH   herpes virus hominis
HVL   half-value layer
HVM   high-velocity missile
HVSD hydrogen-detected ventric-
      ular septal defect
Hx   history
Hy   hypermetropia
hy   hysteria
hypo injection
      under
hys   hysteria
Hz   Hertz
I   intensity of magnetism
      permanent incisor
^{131}I   radioactive iodine
i   deciduous incisor
      optically inactive
IA   impedance angle
      internal auditory
      intra-aortic
      intra-arterial
IABP intra-aortic balloon pump
IAC   internal auditory canal
IADH inappropriate antidiuretic
      hormone
IADHS inappropriate antidiuretic
      hormone syndrome
IAM   internal auditory meatus
IAS   interatrial septum
      intra-amniotic saline infusion
IASD interatrial septal defect
IAT   invasive activity test
      iodine-azide test
IB   inclusion body
IBB   intestinal brush border
IBC   iron-binding capacity
IBR   infectious bovine rhino-
      tracheitis
IBU   international benzoate unit
IC   inspiratory capacity
      intensive care
      intercostal
      intermediate care
      intermittent claudication
      intracavitary
      intracellular

IC (*continued*)
      intracerebral
      intracranial
      intracutaneous
      irritable colon
      isovolumic contraction
ICA   internal carotid artery
      intracranial aneurysm
ICAO internal carotid artery
      occlusion
ICC   immunocompetent cells
      Indian childhood cirrhosis
      intensive coronary care
ICCU intensive coronary care unit
ICD or
ICDH isocitric dehydrogenase
ICF   intensive care facility
      intracellular fluid
ICG   indocyanine green
ICM   intercostal margin
ICS   intercostal space
ICSH interstitial cell-stimulating
      hormone
ICT   indirect Coombs' test
      inflammation of connective
      tissue
      insulin coma therapy
      isovolumic contraction time
ict ind icterus index
ICU   intensive care unit
ICW   intracellular water
ID   identification
      infant deaths
      infective dose
      inside diameter
      internal diameter
      intradermal
id   the same (*idem*)
I & D incision and drainage
ID$_{50}$ median infective dose
IDA   image display and analysis
      iron deficiency anemia
IDI   induction-delivery interval
IDM   infant of diabetic mother
IDP   initial dose period
IDR   intradermal reaction

IDS immunity deficiency state
IDU idoxuridine
 iododeoxyuridine
IDVC indwelling venous catheter
IE immunizing unit (*immunitäts Einheit*)
I/E inspiratory-expiratory ratio
IEMG integrated electromyogram
IEOP immunoelectro-osmophoresis
IEP immunoelectrophoresis
IF immunofluorescence
 interstitial fluid
 intrinsic factor
IFA indirect fluorescent antibody
IFC intrinsic factor concentrate
IFR inspiratory flow rate
IFRA indirect fluorescent rabies antibody (test)
IFV intracellular fluid volume
IG immune globulin
 intragastric
Ig immunoglobulin
IgA gamma A immunoglobulin
IgD gamma D immunoglobulin
IgE gamma E immunoglobulin
IgG gamma G immunoglobulin
IgM gamma M immunoglobulin
IGDM infant of gestational diabetic mother
IGV intrathoracic gas volume
IH infectious hepatitis
 inner half
IHA indirect hemagglutination
IHBTD incompatible hemolytic blood transfusion disease
IHC idiopathic hypercalciuria
 inner hair cell
IHD ischemic heart disease
IHO idiopathic hypertrophic osteoarthropathy
IHR intrinsic heart rate
IHSA iodinated human serum albumin
IHSS idiopathic hypertrophic sub-aortic stenosis

IIF indirect immunofluorescent
IJP internal jugular pressure
ILA insulin-like activity
ILB or
ILBW infant, low birth weight
ILD ischemic leg disease
 ischemic limb disease
IM infectious mononucleosis
 internal medicine
 intramedullary
 intramuscularly
im- (indicates presence of) NH group
IMA internal mammary artery
IMAA iodinated macroaggregated albumin
IMB intermenstrual bleeding
IMBC indirect maximum breathing capacity
IMH idiopathic myocardial hypertrophy
IMHP 1-iodomercuri-2-hydroxypropane
IMI intramuscular injection
imp impression
 improved
IMR infant mortality rate
IMRAD introduction, methods, results, and discussion
IMS incurred in military service
IN intranasal
in inch
INAD infantile neuroaxonal dystrophy
INAH isonicotinic acid hydrazide
inc increase
 incurred
incr increase
ind independents
in d daily (*in die*)
INDM infant of nondiabetic mother
INE infantile necrotizing encephalomyelopathy
inf inferior
 infusion
 pour in (*infunde*)

info   information
INH   isoniazid
       isonicotinic acid hydrazide
inj   inject
inl   inlay
inoc   inoculate
INPV   intermittent negative-
       pressure assisted ventila-
       tion
INS   idiopathic nephrotic syn-
       drome
inspir   inspiration
int   intermediates
       intermittent
       internal
int med   internal medicine
IO   internal os
       intestinal obstruction
       intraocular
I & O   in and out
       intake and output
IOFB   intraocular foreign body
IOP   intraocular pressure
IOU   intensive therapy observation
       unit
IP   incisoproximal
       incubation period
       instantaneous pressure
       interphalangeal
       intraperitoneal
       isoelectric point
I-para   primipara
IPC   isopropyl chlorophenyl
IPD   inflammatory pelvic disease
IPG   impedance plethysmography
IPH   idiopathic pulmonary hemo-
       siderosis
IPL   intrapleural
IPP   intermittent positive pressure
IPPB   intermittent positive-
       pressure breathing
IPPI   interruption of pregnancy for
       psychiatric indication
IPPO   intermittent positive-
       pressure inflation with
       oxygen

IPPR   intermittent positive-
       pressure respiration
IPPV   intermittent positive-
       pressure ventilation
IPRT   interpersonal reaction test
IPS   initial prognostic score
IPU   inpatient unit
IPV   inactivated poliovaccine
IQ   intelligence quotient
IR   immunoreactive
       index of response
       internal resistance
IRBBB   incomplete right bundle
       branch block
IRDS   idiopathic respiratory dis-
       tress syndrome
IRG   immunoreactive glucagon
IRHCS   immunoradioassayable
       human chorionic so-
       matomammotropin
IRhGH   immunoreactive human
       growth hormone
IRI   immunoreactive insulin
irr   irradiation
IRS   infrared spectrophotometry
IRV   inspiratory reserve volume
IS   intercostal space
       interspace
is   in place (in situ)
ISC   irreversibly sickled cells
ISD or
ISDN   isosorbide dinitrate
ISF   interstitial fluid
ISG   immune serum globulin
ISH   icteric serum hepatitis
iso   isoproterenol
ISP   interspace
IST   insulin sensitivity test
       insulin shock therapy
ISW   interstitial water
IT   implantation test
       inhalation test
       inhalation therapy
       intradermal test
       intrathecal
       intratracheal

IT (*continued*)
  intratracheal tube
  intratumoral
  isomeric transition
ITC imidazolyl-thioguanine chemotherapy
ITLC instant thin-layer chromatography
ITP idiopathic thrombocytopenic purpura
ITPA Illinois Test of Psycholinguistic Abilities
ITT insulin tolerance test
ITU intensive therapy unit
IU immunizing unit
  international unit
  intrauterine
IUCD intrauterine contraceptive device
IUD intrauterine death
  intrauterine device
IUDR iododeoxyuridine
IUFB intrauterine foreign body
IUGR intrauterine growth rate
IUM intrauterine fetally malnourished
IUT intrauterine transfusion
IV interventricular
  intervertebral
  intravascular
  intravenous
  intraventricular
  invasive
IVAP in vivo adhesive platelet
IVC inferior vena cava
  intravenous cholangiogram
IVCC intravascular consumption coagulopathy
IVCD intraventricular conduction defect
IVCP inferior vena cava pressure
IVCV inferior venacavography
IVD intervertebral disk
IVF intravascular fluid
IVGTT intravenous glucose tolerance test

IVH intraventricular hemorrhage
IVM intravascular mass
IVP intravenous pyelogram
IVS interventricular septum
IVSD interventricular septal defect
IVT intravenous transfusion
IVTTT intravenous tolbutamide tolerance test
IVU intravenous urography
IWL insensible water loss
IWMI inferior wall myocardial infarction
J Joule's equivalent
  journal
JBE Japanese B encephalitis
jej jejunum
JG juxtaglomerular
JGC juxtaglomerular cell
JGI juxtaglomerular granulation index
JND just noticeable difference
JPS joint position sense
JRA juvenile rheumatoid arthritis
jt joint
JV jugular vein
  jugular venous
JVP jugular venous pulse
K absolute zero
  electrostatic capacity
  kathode (cathode)
  Kell blood system
  Kelvin
  potassium
KA kathode
  ketoacidosis
  King-Armstrong (units)
KAP knowledge, attitudes, and practice
KAU King-Armstrong units
KB ketone bodies
KC kathodal closing
kc kilocycle
kcal kilocalorie
KCC kathodal-closing contraction
KCG kinetocardiogram

KCl potassium chloride
kcps kilocycles per second
KCT kathodal-closing tetanus
KD kathodal duration
KDT kathodal-duration tetanus
KE kinetic energy
kev kilo electron volts
KFAB kidney-fixing antibody
KFS Klippel-Feil syndrome
kg kilogram
kg-cal kilogram-calorie
KGS ketogenic steroid
kHz kilohertz
KIA Kliger iron agar
KIU kallikrein-inhibiting unit
KJ knee jerk
KK knee kick
KLH keyhole-limpet hemocyanin
KLS kidney, liver, spleen
KM kanamycin
km kilometer
KMnO potassium permanganate
KMV killed measles virus vaccine
kn knee
KOC kathodal-opening contrac-
tion
KOH potassium hydroxide
KP keratitic precipitates
KPTT kaolin partial thrombo-
plastin time
KRB Krebs-Ringer bicarbonate
buffer
KRP Kolmer's test with Reiter
protein
Krebs-Ringer phosphate
KS ketosteroid
Klinefelter's syndrome
Kveim-Siltzbach (test)
KSC kathodal-closing contraction
KST kathodal-closing tetanus
KU Karmen units
KUB kidney, ureter, and bladder
KV killed vaccine
kv kilovolt
kvp kilovolt peak

KW Keith-Wagener
kw kilowatt
KWB Keith, Wagener, Barker
(classification)
kw-hr kilowatt-hour
L coefficient of induction
Latin
left
length
lethal (*letha*)
levo-
ligament
light sense
liter
low
lower
lumbar
pound (*libra*)
L. Lactobacillus
Leishmania
l liter
LA lactic acid
left arm
left atrial
left atrium
leucine aminopeptidase
linguoaxial
local anesthesia
low anxiety
L & A light and accommodation
LAA leukocyte ascorbic acid
lab laboratory
LAD left anterior descending
left axis deviation
LAE left atrial enlargement
LAF laminar air flow
LAG labiogingival
lymphangiogram
LAH lactalbumin hydrolysate
left atrial hypertrophy
LAI labioincisal
LAIT latex agglutination-inhibi-
tion test
LAO left anterior oblique
LAP left atrial pressure

LAP (*continued*)
    leucine aminopeptidase
    leukocyte alkaline phosphatase
    lyophilized anterior pituitary
LAR left arm recumbent
LAS linear alkylate sulfonate
LASER light amplification by stimulated emission of radiation
lat lateral
LATS long-acting thyroid stimulator
LB laboratory data
    lipid body
    live births
    loose body
lb pound (*libra*)
LBB left bundle branch
LBBB left bundle branch block
LBCD left border of cardiac dullness
LBF *Lactobacillus bulgaricus* factor
LBI low serum-bound iron
LBM lean body mass
LBNP lower-body negative pressure
LBW low birth weight
LBWI low birth weight infant
LBWR lung–body weight ratio
LC late clamped
    lethal concentration
    lipid cytosomes
    living children
LCA left coronary artery
LCD liquor carbonis detergens
LCFA long-chain fatty acid
LCL Levinthal-Coles-Lillie (bodies)
    lymphocytic lymphosarcoma
LCM left costal margin
    lymphatic choriomeningitis
    lymphocytic choriomeningitis
LCT long-chain triglyceride

LD labyrinthine defect
    lactic dehydrogenase
    left deltoid
    lethal dose
    light difference
    linguodistal
    living donor
    low dosage
    lymphocyte-defined
L-D Leishman-Donovan (bodies)
L/D light-dark ratio
LD$_{50}$ median lethal dose
LDA left dorsoanterior
    linear displacement analysis
LDD light-dark discrimination
LDDS local dentist
LDH lactic dehydrogenase
LDL loudness discomfort level
    low-density lipoprotein
LDLP low-density lipoprotein
LDP left dorsoposterior
LDV lactic dehydrogenase virus
LE left eye
    leukoerythrogenetic
    lower extremity
    lupus erythematosus
LED lupus erythematosus disseminatus
LES local excitatory state
LET linear energy transfer
LF laryngofissure
    limit flocculation
    low forceps
LFA left femoral artery
    left frontoanterior
LFD lactose-free diet
    least fatal dose
    low forceps delivery
LFN lactoferrin
LFP left frontoposterior
LFT latex flocculation test
    left frontotransverse
    liver function test
LG laryngectomy
    left gluteal
    linguogingival

lg   large
LGB   Landry-Guillain-Barré
    (syndrome)
LGN   lateral geniculate nucleus
LGV   lymphogranuloma venereum
LH   lower half
    luteinizing hormone
LHL   left hepatic lobe
LHRF   luteinizing hormone–
    releasing factor
LI   linguoincisal
    low impulsiveness
LIAFI   late infantile amaurotic
    familial idiocy
lib   pound (*libra*)
LIBC   latent iron-binding capacity
LIF   left iliac fossa
lig   ligament
LIHA   low impulsiveness, high
    anxiety
LILA   low impulsiveness, low
    anxiety
liq   liquid
    liquor
LIQ   lower inner quadrant
LIS   lobular in situ
LK   left kidney
LL   left leg
    left lower
    left lung
    lower lobe
    lysolecithin
LLC   lymphocytic leukemia
LLF   Laki-Lorand factor
LLL   left lower lobe
LLM   localized leukocyte mobili-
    zation
LLQ   left lower quadrant
LM   light microscopy
    linguomesial
LMA   left mentoanterior
LMD   local medical doctor
    low molecular weight dex-
    tran
LMDX   low molecular weight dex-
    tran

LMP   last menstrual period
    left mentoposterior
LMT   left mentotransverse
LMW   low molecular weight
LMWD   low molecular weight dex-
    tran
LN   lipoid nephrosis
    lupus nephritis
    lymph node
L/N   letter-numerical (system)
LNMP   last normal menstrual
    period
LNPF   lymph node permeability
    factor
LO   linguo-occlusal
    low
LOA   leave of absence
    left occipitoanterior
loc dol   to the painful spot (*loco
    dolenti*)
LOD   line of duty
LOM   limitation of motion
    loss of motion
LOP   left occipitoposterior
LOQ   lower outer quadrant
LOT   left occipitotransverse
LOWBI   low birth weight infant
LP   latency period
    leukocyte-poor
    light perception
    linguopulpal
    lipoprotein
    low protein
    lumbar puncture
    lymphoid plasma
L/P   lactate-pyruvate ratio
LPA   left pulmonary artery
LPC   late positive component
LPE   lipoprotein electrophoresis
LPF   leukocytosis-promoting
    factor
    localized plaque formation
    low-power field
    lymphocytosis-promoting
    factor
LPL   lipoprotein lipase

lpm   liters per minute
LPO   left posterior oblique
     light perception only
LPS   lipopolysaccharide
LPV   left pulmonary veins
LR   laboratory references
     lactated Ringer's solution
     light reaction
L/R   left to right ratio
L & R   left and right
L→R   left to right
LRF   luteinizing hormone–
     releasing factor
LRH   luteinizing hormone–
     releasing hormone
LRQ   lower right quadrant
LRS   lactated Ringer's solution
LRT   lower respiratory tract
LS   left side
     legally separated
     liver and spleen
     lumbosacral
     lymphosarcoma
LSA   left sacroanterior
     lymphosarcoma
LSA/RCS   lymphosarcoma-reticu-
     lum cell sarcoma
LSB   left sternal border
LScA   left scapuloanterior
LScP   left scapuloposterior
LSCS   lower segment cesarean
     section
LSD   lysergic acid diethylamide
LSM   late systolic murmur
LSP   left sacroposterior
LST   left sacrotransverse
LSV   left subclavian vein
LT   left thigh
     levothyroxine
     long-term
     lymphotoxin
lt   left
LTB   laryngotracheobronchitis
LTH   lactogenic hormone
     luteotropic hormone

lt lat   left lateral
LTPP   lipothiamide pyrophosphate
LU   left upper
L & U   lower and upper
LUL   left upper lobe
LUQ   left upper quadrant
LV   left ventricle
     leukemia virus
     live virus
LVDP   left ventricular diastolic
     pressure
LVE   left ventricular enlargement
LVEDP   left ventricular end-
     diastolic pressure
LVEDV   left ventricular end-
     diastolic volume
LVET   left ventricular ejection
     time
LVF   left ventricular failure
     low-voltage fast
     low-voltage foci
LVH   left ventricular hypertrophy
LVP   left ventricular pressure
     lysine-vasopressin
LVS   left ventricular strain
LVSP   left ventricular systolic
     pressure
LVSV   left ventricular stroke
     volume
LVSW   left ventricular stroke work
LVW   left ventricular work
LVWI   left ventricular work index
LW   lacerating wound
     Lee-White (method)
L & W or
L/W   living and well
LX   local irradiation
lymphs   lymphocytes
lzm   lysozyme
M   macerate (*macerare*)
     male
     married
     minim
     minute
     mix

M (*continued*)
  molar
  month
  mother
  multipara
  murmur
  muscle
  myopia
  permanent molar
  strength of pole
  thousand (*mil, milli*)

M. *Micrococcus*
  Microsporum
  Mycobacterium
  Mycoplasma

m handful (*manipulus*)

μ micron
  mu

m meter
  minim
  deciduous molar

M_1 mitral first sound

MA mandelic acid
  mean arterial (blood pressure)
  medical audit
  mental age
  Miller-Abbott (tube)
  moderately advanced

ma meter-angle
  milliampere

MAA macroaggregated albumin

MABP mean arterial blood pressure

mac macerate

MAC maximum allowable concentration
  minimum alveolar concentration

MAFH macroaggregated ferrous hydroxide

magn large (*magnus*)

MAM methylazomethanol

M+Am myopic astigmatism

mam milliampere-minute

man handful (*manipulus*)

man (*continued*)
  manipulate

manip manipulation

MANOVA multivariate analysis of variance

man pr early in the morning (*mane primo*)

MAO maximal acid output
  monoamine oxidase

MAOI monoamine oxidase inhibitor

MAP mean aortic pressure
  mean arterial pressure
  megaloblastic anemia of pregnancy
  methylacetoxyprogesterone
  methylaminopurine
  muscle-action potential

MAPF microatomized protein food

mas milliampere-second

MASER microwave amplification by stimulated emission of radiation
  molecular application by stimulated emission of radiation

matut in the morning (*matutinus*)

max maximum

MB mesiobuccal
  methylene blue

mb mix well (*misce bene*)

MBA methylbovine albumin

MBAS methylene blue active substance

MBC maximal breathing capacity
  minimal bactericidal concentration

MBD methylene blue dye
  minimal brain damage
  minimal brain dysfunction
  Morquio-Brailsford disease

MBF myocardial blood flow

MBFLB monaural bifrequency loudness balance

MBL   minimal bactericidal level
MBO   mesiobucco-occlusal
MBP   antigen prepared from
          melitensis
        mean blood pressure
        mesiobuccopulpal
MBSA methylated bovine serum
          albumin
MC   mast cell
        maximum concentration
        metacarpal
        mineralocorticoid
        myocarditis
        mytomycin-C
Mc   megacurie
        megacycle
mc,
mCi or
MCU   millicurie
MCA   methylcholanthrene
        middle cerebral artery
MCB   membranous cytoplasmic
          body
MCBR minimum concentration of
          bilirubin
MCC   mean corpuscular hemo-
          globin concentration
        minimum complete-killing
          concentration
MCCU mobile coronary care unit
MCD   mean cell diameter
        mean corpuscular diameter
        medullary cystic disease
MCFA medium-chain fatty acid
mcg or
μg   microgram
MCH   mean corpuscular hemo-
          globin
mch   millicurie-hour
MCHC mean corpuscular hemo-
          globin concentration
MCI   mean cardiac index
mCi   millicurie
MCL   midclavicular line
        midcostal line

MCL (*continued*)
        most comfortable loudness
          level
MCP   metacarpophalangeal
        mitotic-control protein
mc p s megacycles per second
MCQ   multiple choice question
MCR   message competition ratio
        metabolic clearance rate
MCT   mean circulation time
        mean corpuscular thickness
        medium-chain triglyceride
MCV   mean clinical value
        mean corpuscular volume
MD   malic dehydrogenase
        manic depressive
        Mantoux diameter
        Marek's disease
        maternal deprivation
        medium dosage
        movement disorder
        muscular dystrophy
        myocardial damage
        myocardial disease
MDA   mentodextra anterior
        methylenedioxyampheta-
          mine
        motor discriminative acuity
MDC   minimum detectable concen-
          tration
MDD   mean daily dose
MDF   mean dominant frequency
        myocardial depressant factor
MDH   malic dehydrogenase
MDHV Marek's disease herpesvirus
m dict as directed (*moro dicto*)
MDM   minor determinant mixture
MDP   mentodextra posterior
MDT   median detection threshold
        mentodextra transversa
MDTR mean diameter-thickness
          ratio
MDUO myocardial disease of un-
          known origin
MDY   month, date, year

ME   medical education
    mercaptoethanol
    middle ear
M/E   myeloid-erythroid ratio
Me   methyl
MEA   mercaptoethylamine
    multiple endocrine adeno-
      matosis
MED   minimal effective dose
    minimal erythema dose
med   median
    medical
    medicine
meds   medications
    medicines
MEF   maximal expiratory flow
MEFR   maximum expiratory flow
      rate
MEG   mercaptoethylguanidine
meg   megakaryocytes
MEM   minimum essential medium
mep   meperidine
MEPP   miniature end-plate poten-
      tial
mEq or
meq   milliequivalent
MER   mean ejection rate
    methanol-extruded residue
MER-29   triparanol
Mets   metastases
m et sig   mix and label (*misce et
      signa*)
mev   million electron volts
MF   medium frequency
    mycosis fungoides
    myelin figures
M/F   male-female ratio
M & F   mother and father
mf   microfilaria
MFB   metallic foreign body
MFD   midforceps delivery
    minimum fatal dose
μf or
μfd   microfarad
MFP   monofluorophosphate

MFR   mucus flow rate
m ft   make a mixture (*mistura
      fiat*)
MFW   multiple fragment wounds
MG   mesiogingival
    methyl glucoside
    muscle group
Mg   magnesium
mg   milligram
MGF   mother's grandfather
MGGH   methylglyoxal guanyl-
      hydrazone
MGH or
mgh   milligram-hour
MGM   mother's grandmother
mgm   milligram
MGN   membranous glomerulo-
      nephritis
MGP   marginal granulocyte pool
mg%   milligrams per 100 milliliters;
      milligrams per deciliter
MGR   modified gain ratio
mgtis   meningitis
MH   mammotropic hormone
    marital history
    medical history
    mental health
MHA   methemalbumin
    microangiopathic hemolytic
      anemia
    mixed hemadsorption
MHB   maximum hospital benefit
MHb   methemoglobin
MHD   mean hemolytic dose
    minimum hemolytic dose
mHg   millimeters of mercury
MHN   massive hepatic necrosis
MHP   1-mercuri-2-hydroxypropane
MHPG   methoxyhydroxyphenyl-
      glycol
MHR   maximal heart rate
MI   mercaptoimidazole
    mitral incompetence
    mitral insufficiency
    myocardial infarction

MIC   Maternity and Infant Care
     minimum inhibitory concentration
mic pan   bread crumb (*mica panis*)
MICU   mobile intensive care unit
MID   maximum inhibiting dilution
     mesioincisodistal
     minimum infective dose
midnoc   midnight
MIF   macrophage-inhibiting factor
     migration inhibition factor
     mixed immunofluorescence
MIFR   maximal inspiratory flow rate
min   minim
     minimal
     minute
MIO   minimum identifiable odor
MIP   maximum inspiratory pressure
MIRD   medical internal radiation dose
MIRU   myocardial infarction research unit
mist   mixture (*mistura*)
MIT   monoiodotyrosine
mit   send (*mitte*)
mixt   mixture
MK   monkey kidney
MKS   meter-kilogram-second
MKV   killed-measles vaccine
ML   mesiolingual
     middle lobe
     midline
M:L   monocyte-lymphocyte ratio
ml   milliliter
MLA   mentolaeva anterior
     mesiolabial
     monocytic leukemia, acute
MLAI   mesiolabioincisal
MLAP   mean left atrial pressure
MLC   minimum lethal concentration
     mixed leukocyte culture
     mixed lymphocyte culture
     multilamellar cytosome

MLC (*continued*)
     myelomonocytic leukemia, chronic
MLD   metachromatic leukodystrophy
     minimum lethal dose
MLI   mesiolinguoincisal
MLO   mesiolinguo-occlusal
MLP   left mentoposterior (*mentolaeva posterior*)
     mesiolinguopulpal
MLS   mean lifespan
     myelomonocytic leukemia, subacute
MLT   left mentotransverse (*mentolaeva transversa*)
MLV   Moloney's leukemogenic virus
     mouse leukemia virus
MM   malignant melanoma
     Marshall-Marchetti
     medial malleolus
     mucous membrane
     multiple myeloma
     muscularis mucosa
     myeloid metaplasia
M & M   milk and molasses
mM   millimolar
     millimole
mm   millimeter
     muscles
MMA   methylmalonic acid
MMC   minimum medullary concentration
MMD   minimum morbidostatic dose
MMEF   maximal midexpiratory flow
MMEFR   maximal midexpiratory flow rate
MMF   maximal midexpiratory flow
MMFR   maximal midexpiratory flow rate
     maximal midflow rate
mM/L or
mM/l   millimols per liter

MMM   myeloid metaplasia with myelofibrosis
myelosclerosis with myeloid metaplasia
MMPI   Minnesota Multiphasic Personality Inventory
mmpp   millimeters partial pressure
MMPR   methylmercaptopurine riboside
MMR   mass miniature radiography
mobile mass x-ray
myocardial metabolic rate
mμ   millimicron
mμc   millimicrocurie (nanocurie)
mμg   millimicrogram (nanogram)
μl   microliter
μmg   micromilligram
μmm   micromillimeter
μμ   micromicron
μμc   micromicrocurie (picocurie)
μμg   micromicrogram (picogram)
MN   midnight
multinodular
myoneural
M/N   or
mn   midnight
M & N   morning and night
Mn   manganese
mN   millinormal
MNA   maximum noise area
MNCV   motor nerve conduction velocity
MNU   methylnitrosourea
MO   mesio-occlusal
mineral oil
mo   month
MOD   mesio-occlusodistal
mod   moderate
mol wt   molecular weight
moll   soft (*mollis*)
MOM   milk of magnesia
MOMA   methoxyhydroxymandelic acid
Monos   monocytes
MOPP   nitrogen mustard, Oncovin, prednisone, procarbazine

MOPV   monovalent oral poliovirus vaccine
mor dict   in the manner directed (*more dicto*)
mor sol   in the usual way (*more solito*)
mOs   milliosmolal
mOsm   milliosmol, milliosmole
MP   mean pressure
melting point
menstrual period
mercaptopurine
mesiopulpal
metacarpophalangeal
monophosphate
mucopolysaccharide
multiparous
mp   as directed (*modo prescripto*)
MPA   main pulmonary artery
medroxyprogesterone acetate
methylprednisolone acetate
MPAP   mean pulmonary arterial pressure
MPC   marine protein concentrate
maximum permissible concentration
meperidine, promethazine, chlorpromazine
minimum mycoplasmacidal concentration
MPD   maximum permissible dose
MPEH   methylphenylethylhydantoin
MPJ   metacarpophalangeal joint
MPL   mesiopulpolingual
MPLA   mesiopulpolabial
MPN   most probable number
MPO   myeloperoxidase
MPP   mercaptopyrazidopyrimidine
MPS   mucopolysaccharide
MR   mental retardation
metabolic rate
methyl red
mitral reflux
mitral regurgitation

MR (*continued*)
    mortality rate
    mortality ratio
    muscle relaxant
mr   milliroentgen
MRAP   mean right atrial pressure
MRD   minimum reacting dose
MRF   mesencephalic reticular
      formation
    mitral regurgitant flow
mRNA   messenger RNA
MRT   median recognition thresh-
      old
    milk-ring test
MRVP   mean right ventricular
      pressure
MS   mental status
    mitral stenosis
    morphine sulfate
    mucosubstance
    multiple sclerosis
    musculoskeletal
ms   manuscript
msec   millisecond
MSER   mean systolic ejection rate
MSG   monosodium glutamate
MSH   medical self-help
    melanocyte-stimulating
      hormone
    melanophore-stimulating
      hormone
MSK   medullary sponge kidney
MSL   midsternal line
MSLA   mouse-specific lymphocyte
      antigen
MSN   mildly subnormal
MSRPP   multidimensional scale for
      rating psychiatric
      patients
MSS   mental status schedule
MSU   monosodium urate
MSUD   maple syrup urine disease
MSV   Moloney sarcoma virus
    murine sarcoma virus
MT   empty
    malignant teratoma

MT (*continued*)
    maximal therapy
    medical technologist
    membrana tympani
    metatarsal
    methyltyrosine
    more than
    music therapy
MTD   maximum tolerated dose
MTDT   modified tone decay test
MTF   maximum terminal flow
    modulation transfer function
MTHF   methyltetrahydrofolic acid
MTI   malignant teratoma inter-
      mediate
    minimum time interval
MTP   metatarsophalangeal
MTR   Meinicke turbidity reaction
MTT   malignant teratoma tropho-
      blastic
    mean transit time
    monotetrazolium
MTU   methylthiouracil
MTV   mammary tumor virus
MTX   methotrexate
MU   Mache unit
    Montevideo unit
mU   milliunit
mu   micron
    mouse unit
muc   mucilage
multip   pregnant woman who has
      borne two or more
      children
MUST   medical unit, self-
      contained, transportable
MUU   mouse uterine units
MV   minute volume
    mitral valve
    mixed venous
mv   millivolt
MVM   microvillose membrane
MVP   mitral valve prolapse
MVR   massive vitreous retraction
MVV   maximum voluntary ventila-
      tion

MW   molecular weight
mw   microwave
My   myopia
my   mayer (unit of heat capacity)
MyG   myasthenia gravis
MZ   monozygotic
N   nasal
     neurology
     normal
     size of sample
     unit of neutron dosage
N.   *Neisseria*
     Nocardia
n   index of refraction
     nerve
NA   neutralizing antibody
     Nomina Anatomica
     noradrenaline
     not admitted
     not applicable
     not available
     numerical aperture
Na   sodium
NAA   no apparent abnormalities
NAD   nicotinamide adenine di-
     nucleotide
     no appreciable disease
     normal axis deviation
NADH   nicotinamide adenine di-
     nucleotide (reduced
     form)
NADP   nicotinamide adenine di-
     nucleotide phosphate
NADPH   nicotinamide adenine di-
     nucleotide phosphate
     (reduced form)
NANA   *N*-acetylneuraminic acid
NAPA   *N*-acetyl-*p*-aminophenol
NB   newborn
     nitrous oxide–barbiturate
nb   note well (*nota bene*)
NBM   nothing by mouth
NBO   nonbed occupancy
NBS   normal blood serum
NBT   nitroblue tetrazolium

NBTE   nonbacterial thrombotic
     endocarditis
NBW   normal birth weight
NC   no casualty
     no change
     noise criterion
     noncontributory
     not cultured
N/C   no complaints
nc   nanocurie
NCA   neurocirculatory asthenia
NCD   not considered disabling
nCi   nanocurie
NCV   nerve conduction velocity
ND   neonatal death
     neurotic depression
     Newcastle disease
     New Drugs
     no data
     no disease
     nondisabling
     normal delivery
     not detectable
     not detected
     not determined
     not done
n_D refractive index
NDA   no data available
     no demonstrable antibodies
NDF   new dosage form
NDGA   nordihydroguaiaretic acid
NDI   nephrogenic diabetes in-
     sipidus
NDMA   nitrosodimethylaniline
NDP   net dietary protein
NDV   Newcastle disease virus
NE   nerve ending
     neurologic examination
     no effect
     nonelastic
     norepinephrine
     not evaluated
     not examined
NEC   not elsewhere classifiable
     not elsewhere classified

NED   no evidence of disease
NEFA   nonesterified fatty acid
NEG   negative
NEM   *N*-ethylmaleimide
NER   no evidence of recurrence
NERD   no evidence of recurrent
    disease
neur   neurology
neuro   neurologic
neurol   neurologic
NF   none found
    normal flow
    not found
NFTD   normal full-term delivery
NG   nasogastric
ng   nanogram
NGF   nerve growth factor
NGU   nongonococcal urethritis
NH   nonhuman
    nursing home
NHA   nonspecific hepatocellular
    abnormality
NHS   normal horse serum
    normal human serum
NI   no information
    not identified
    not isolated
NIA   no information available
NIH   National Institutes of Health
NK   not known
NKH   nonketotic hyperosmotic
Nl   normal
NLA   neuroleptanalgesia
NLP   no light perception
NLT   normal lymphocyte transfer
    test
NM   neuromuscular
    not measurable
    not measured
    not mentioned
    nuclear medicine
nm   nanometer
    nutmeg (*nux moschata*)
NMA   neurogenic muscular
    atrophy
NMP   normal menstrual period

N:N   (indicates presence of) the
    azo group
nn   nerves
NND   neonatal death
    New and Nonofficial Drugs
NNI   noise and number index
NNN   Nicolle-Novy-MacNeal
    (medium)
NO   none obtained
No   number
noc   night
noct   at night (*nocte*)
non-REM   nonrapid eye movement
non rep   do not repeat (*non
    repetatur*)
NOS   not otherwise specified
NP   nasopharyngeal
    nasopharynx
    neuropathology
    neuropsychiatric
    normal plasma
    not performed
    nucleoplasmic index
    nucleoprotein
    nursing procedure
NPB   nodal premature beat
NPC   near point of convergence
NPD   Niemann-Pick disease
NPDL   nodular, poorly differen-
    tiated lymphocytes
NPH   neutral protamine Hagedorn
    (insulin)
NPN   nonprotein nitrogen
NPO, npo   nothing by mouth
    (*nulla per os*)
NPO/HS   nothing by mouth at
    bedtime (*nulla per os
    hora somni*)
NPT   neoprecipitin test
NPU   net protein utilization
NR   do not repeat (*non repetatur*)
    no radiation
    no response
    nonreactive
    normal
    not readable

NR (*continued*)
    not recorded
    not resolved
nr do not repeat (*non repetatur*)
NRBC nucleated red blood cell
NRC National Research Council
    normal retinal correspon-
      dence
NRD nonrenal death
NREM nonrapid eye movement
NRS normal rabbit serum
    normal reference serum
NS nephrotic syndrome
    nervous system
    neurologic survey
    neurosurgery
    no sample
    no specimen
    nonspecific
    nonsymptomatic
    normal saline
    not significant
    not sufficient
N/S normal saline
NSA no serious abnormality
    no significant abnormality
NSC no significant change
    not service-connected
NSCD nonservice-connected dis-
      ability
NSD no significant defect
    no significant deviation
    no significant difference
    no significant disease
    nominal single dose
    normal spontaneous delivery
nsg nursing
NSM neurosecretory material
NSND nonsymptomatic, non-
      disabling
NSQ not sufficient quantity
NSR normal sinus rhythm
NSS normal saline solution
    not statistically significant
NSU nonspecific urethritis

NT nasotracheal
    neutralization test
    neutralizing
    nontypable
    not tested
NTAB nephrotoxic antibody
NTG nontoxic goiter
NTN nephrotoxic nephritis
NTP normal temperature and
      pressure
NUG necrotizing ulcerative gin-
      givitis
NV negative variation
N & V nausea and vomiting
Nv naked vision
NVA near visual acuity
NVD nausea, vomiting, and diar-
      rhea
    Newcastle virus disease
NWB no weight bearing
NYD not yet diagnosed
O eye (*oculus*)
    none
    obstetrics
    opening
    oral
    orderly
    oxygen
    respirations (anesthesia chart)
    suture size (zero)
O nonmotile organism
O_2 both eyes
    oxygen
o pint (*octarius*)
o- ortho-
OA occipital artery
    osteoarthritis
    oxalic acid
OAAD ovarian ascorbic acid
      depletion
OAD obstructive airway disease
OAP osteoarthropathy
OAR other administrative reasons
OAV oculoauriculovertebral dys-
      plasia

OB objective benefit
    obstetrics
O & B opium and belladonna
OBG or
OB-GYN obstetrics and gyne-
        cology
obl oblique
OBS obstetrical service
    organic brain syndrome
obs or
obst obstetrics
OC occlusocervical
    office call
    on call
    oral contraceptive
    original claim
O_2cap oxygen capacity
occ occasional
OCG oral cholecystogram
OCR optical character recognition
OCT ornithine carbamyl transfer-
      ase
OCV ordinary conversational
      voice
OD once a day
    optical density
    outside diameter
    overdose
    right eye (*oculus dexter*)
ODA occipitodextra anterior
ODD oculodentodigital dysplasia
ODM ophthalmodynamometry
ODP occipitodextra posterior
ODT occipitodextra transversa
O & E observation and examina-
      tion
OER oxygen enhancement ratio
OF Ovenstone factor
Off official
OFC occipitofrontal circumfer-
      ence
OFD oral-facial-digital
OG or
O & G obstetrics and gynecology
OGS oxogenic steroid
OGTT oral glucose tolerance test

OH hydroxycorticosteroids
    occupational history
OHC outer hair cell
OHCS hydroxycorticosteroid
OHP oxygen under high pressure
OIF oil immersion field
OIH orthoiodohippurate
OJ orange juice
OKN optokinetic nystagmus
OL left eye (*oculus laevus*)
ol oil
ol res oleoresin
OLA occipitolaeva anterior
OLH ovine lactogenic hormone
OLP occipitolaeva posterior
OL & T owners, landlords, and
      tenants
OM otitis media
om every morning (*omni mane*)
OMD ocular muscle dystrophy
OMI old myocardial infarction
omn bih every two hours (*omni
      bihora*)
omn hor every hour (*omni hora*)
OMPA octamethylpyrophosphora-
      mide
    otitis media, purulent,
      acute
ON,
On or
on every night (*omni nocte*)
OOB out of bed
OP opening pressure
    operation
    osmotic pressure
    outpatient
O & P ova and parasites
OPC outpatient clinic
OPD outpatient department
OPG oxypolygelatin
oph or
ophth ophthalmology
OPK optokinetic
OPS outpatient service
OPT outpatient
    outpatient treatment

OPV   oral poliovaccine
     oral poliovirus vaccine
OR   operating room
ORS   orthopedic surgery
orth or
ortho   orthopedics
OS   left eye (*oculus sinister*)
     opening snap
     oral surgery
os   mouth (*os*)
OSM   oxygen saturation meter
OST   object sorting test
OT   occlusion time
     occupational therapy
     old term
     old terminology
     old tuberculin
     orotracheal
     otolaryngology
OTC   ornithine transcarbamylase
     over-the-counter
     oxytetracycline
OTD   organ tolerance dose
oto   otolaryngology
     otology
otol   otology
otolar   otolaryngology
OTR   Ovarian Tumor Registry
OU   both eyes (*oculi unitas*)
     each eye (*oculus uterque*)
OURQ   outer upper right quadrant
OV   office visit
ov   egg (*ovum*)
OW   out of wedlock
O/W   oil in water
     oil-water ratio
ox   oxymel
oz   ounce
P   by weight (*pondere*)
     near (*proximum*)
     partial pressure
     pharmacopeia
     phosphorus
     position
     postpartum
     premolar

P (*continued*)
     presbyopia
     pressure
     primipara
     protein
     psychiatry
     pulse
     pupil
P.   *Pasteurella*
     Plasmodium
     Proteus
P_1 parental generation
P_2 pulmonic second sound
^{32}P radioactive phosphorus
p   after (*post*)
     handful (*pugillus*)
     probability
p-   para-
PA   paralysis agitans
     pathology
     pernicious anemia
     phakic-aphakic
     posteroanterior
     primary amenorrhea
     primary anemia
     pulmonary artery
     pulpoaxial
P & A   percussion & auscultation
pa   yearly (*per annum*)
PAB or
PABA   para-aminobenzoic acid
PAC   premature auricular contrac-
     tion
p ae   in equal parts (*partes
     aequales*)
PAF   pulmonary arteriovenous
     fistula
PAFIB   paroxysmal atrial fibrilla-
     tion
PAGMK   primary African green
     monkey kidney
PAH   para-aminohippurate
     polycyclic aromatic hydro-
     carbon
     pulmonary artery hyperten-
     sion

PAHA   para-aminohippuric acid
PAL   posterior axillary line
PAM   crystalline penicillin G in 2
 per cent aluminum mono-
 stearate
 phenylalanine mustard
 pralidoxime
 pulmonary alveolar macro-
 phage(s)
 pulmonary alveolar microlithiasis
 pyridine aldoxime methio-
 dide
PAN   periodic alternating nystagmus
 peroxyacetyl nitrate
PANS   puromycin aminonucleo-
 side
PAOD   peripheral arterial occlusive
 disease
 peripheral arteriosclerotic
 occlusive disease
PAP   Papanicolaou (stain, smear,
 test)
 positive airway pressure
 primary atypical pneumonia
 prostatic acid phosphatase
 pulmonary alveolar proteinosis
 pulmonary artery pressure
PAPP   para-aminopropiophenone
PAPS   phosphoadenosyl-phospho-
 sulfate
PAPVC   partial anomalous pulmonary venous connec-
 tion
PAR   postanesthesia room
 pulmonary arteriolar resistance
par aff   the part affected (*pars
 affecta*)
para   number of pregnancies
PAS   para-aminosalicylic acid
 periodic acid–Schiff (method,
 stain, technique, test)
 pulmonary artery stenosis

PASA   para-aminosalicylic acid
PAS-C   para-aminosalicylic acid
 crystallized with ascorbic
 acid
PASD   after diastase digestion
 periodic acid–Schiff tech-
 nique
PASM   periodic acid-silver methen-
 amine
Past.   *Pasteurella*
PAT   paroxysmal atrial tachycardia
path   pathology
PB   phenobarbital
 phonetically balanced
PBA   pulpobuccoaxial
PBC   prebed care
 primary biliary cirrhosis
PBF   pulmonary blood flow
PBG   porphobilinogen
PBI   protein-bound iodine
PBN   paralytic brachial neuritis
PBO   penicillin in beeswax
 placebo
PBS   phosphate-buffered saline
PBSP   prognostically bad signs
 during pregnancy
PBT_4 protein-bound thyroxine
PBV   predicted blood volume
 pulmonary blood volume
PBZ   pyribenzamine
PC   pentose cycle
 phosphate cycle
 phosphocreatine
 platelet concentrate
 platelet count
 portacaval
 pubococcygeus
 pulmonic closure
pc   after meals (*post cibum*)
 avoirdupois weight (*pondus
 civile*)
 picocurie
PCA   passive cutaneous anaphylaxis
PCB   paracervical block
PcB   near point of convergence

PCc   periscopic concave
PCD   phosphate-citrate-dextrose
          polycystic disease
          posterior corneal deposits
PCF   posterior cranial fossa
PCG   phonocardiogram
PCH   paroxysmal cold hemo-
          globinuria
pCi   picocurie
PCM   protein-calorie malnutrition
PCN   penicillin
PCO_2 or
pCO_2 carbon dioxide pressure
PCP   parachlorophenate
PCPA   parachlorophenylalanine
pcpt   perception
PCS   portacaval shunt
pcs   preconscious
PCT   plasmacrit
          porphyria cutanea tarda
          portacaval transposition
PCV   packed cell volume
          polycythemia vera
PCV-M   myeloid metaplasia with
              polycythemia vera
PCx   periscopic convex
PD   papilla diameter
        Parkinson's disease
        patent ductus
        pediatrics
        phosphate dehydrogenase
        plasma defect
        poorly differentiated
        potential difference
        pressor dose
        prism diopter
        progression of disease
        psychotic depression
        pulmonary disease
        pulpodistal
        pupillary distance
PDA   patent ductus arteriosus
          pediatric allergy
PDAB   para-dimethylamino-
              benzaldehyde
PDC   pediatric cardiology

PDD   pyridoxine-deficient diet
PDH   packaged disaster hospital
          phosphate dehydrogenase
pdl   pudendal
PDP   piperidino-pyrimidine
PE   pharyngoesophageal
        phenylephrine
        physical evaluation
        physical examination
        pleural effusion
        polyethylene
        probable error
        pulmonary edema
        pulmonary embolism
PEBG   phenethylbiguanide
ped or
peds   pediatrics
PEF   peak expiratory flow
PEFR   peak expiratory flow rate
PEG   pneumoencephalography
          polyethylene glycol
PEI   phosphate excretion index
        physical efficiency index
pen   penicillin
pent   pentothal
PEO   progressive external ophthal-
          moplegia
PEP   pre-ejection period
PEPP   positive expiratory pressure
            plateau
PER   protein efficiency ratio
PERLA   pupils equal, react to light
              and accommodation
perpad   perineal pad
PERRLA   pupils equal, round,
                regular, react to light
                and accommodation
PET   pre-eclamptic toxemia
PETN   pentaerythritol tetranitrate
PETT   positron emission transverse
            tomography
PF   personality factor
        picture-frustration (study)
        platelet factor
P/F   pass-fail system
PFC   plaque-forming cell

PFIB   perfluoroisobutylene
PFK   phosphofructokinase
PFO   patent foramen ovale
PFQ   personality factor question-
       naire
PFR   peak flow rate
PFT   posterior fossa tumor
       pulmonary function test
PFU   plaque-forming units
PG   plasma triglyceride
       postgraduate
       pregnant
       prostaglandin
       pyoderma gangrenosum
pg   picogram
PGA   pteroylglutamic acid
PGD   phosphogluconate dehydro-
       genase
       phosphoglyceraldehyde de-
       hydrogenase
PGDH   phosphogluconate dehy-
       drogenase
PGDR   plasma-glucose disappear-
       ance rate
PGH   pituitary growth hormone
PGI   phosphoglucoisomerase
       potassium, glucose, and
       insulin
PGK   phosphoglycerate kinase
PGM   phosphoglucomutase
PGP   postgamma proteinuria
PGTR   plasma glucose tolerance
       rate
PH   past history
       personal history
       pharmacopeia
       prostatic hypertrophy
       public health
       pulmonary hypertension
Ph   phenyl
pH   hydrogen ion concentration
PHA   phytohemagglutinin
phar or
pharm pharmacy
PHBB   propylhydroxybenzyl
       benzimidazole

PHC   posthospital care
PHI   phosphohexoisomerase
PHK   platelet phosphohexokinase
PHLA   postheparin lipolytic ac-
       tivity
PHP   primary hyperparathyroidism
       pseudohypoparathyroidism
phys   physiology
PI   pacing impulse
       performance intensity
       pre-induction (examination)
       present illness
       protamine insulin
       pulmonary incompetence
       pulmonary infarction
PIA   plasma insulin activity
PICA   posterior inferior cerebellar
       artery
PICU   pulmonary intensive care
       unit
PID   pelvic inflammatory disease
       plasma-iron disappearance
PIDT   plasma-iron disappearance
       time
PIE   pulmonary infiltration and
       eosinophilia
       pulmonary interstitial emphy-
       sema
PIF   peak inspiratory flow
       prolactin-inhibiting factor
PIFR   peak inspiratory flow rate
PII   plasma inorganic iodine
pil   pill
PIP   proximal interphalangeal
PIPJ   proximal interphalangeal
       joint
PIT   plasma iron turnover
PITR   plasma iron turnover rate
pixel picture element
PK   Prausnitz-Küstner (reaction)
       psychokinesis
       pyruvate kinase
PKU   phenylketonuria
PKV   killed poliomyelitis vaccine
PL   light perception
       phospholipid

PL (*continued*)
    placebo
    placental lactogen
    pulpolingual
PLA pulpolinguoaxial
    pulpolabial
PLD platelet defect
PLS prostaglandin-like substance
pls please
PLV live poliomyelitis vaccine
    panleukopenia virus
    phenylalanine-lysine-vaso-
      pressin
PM after noon
    night
    physical medicine
    polymorphs
    postmortem
    pulpomesial
PMA prevalence of gingivitis
    (papillary, marginal,
    attached)
    progressive muscular atrophy
PMB para-hydroxymercuribenzo-
    ate
    polymorphonuclear basophil
PMD primary myocardial disease
    progressive muscular dys-
    trophy
PME polymorphonuclear eosino-
    phil
PMH past medical history
PMI point of maximal impulse
    point of maximal intensity
PML progressive multifocal leuko-
    encephalopathy
PMN polymorphonuclear neutro-
    phil
PMP past menstrual period
    previous menstrual period
PMR perinatal mortality rate
    physical medicine and
      rehabilitation
    proportionate morbidity
      ratio

PMS phenazine methosulfate
    postmitochondrial super-
      natant
    pregnant mare serum
PMSG pregnant mare serum
      gonadotropin
PMT Porteus maze test
PN perceived noise
    percussion note
    periarteritis nodosa
    peripheral neuropathy
    pneumonia
    positional nystagmus
    pyelonephritis
P_{NA} plasma sodium
PND paroxysmal nocturnal
    dyspnea
    postnasal drainage
    postnasal drip
pnd pound
PNH paroxysmal nocturnal hemo-
    globinuria
PNP para-nitrophenol
PNPP para-nitrophenylphosphate
PNU protein nitrogen unit
PO by mouth (*per os*)
    parieto-occipital
    period of onset
    phone order
    posterior
    postoperative
po by mouth (*per os*)
PO_2 or
pO_2 oxygen partial pressure (ten-
    sion)
POA point of application
POB phenoxybenzamine
    place of birth
POC postoperative care
pocul cup (*poculum*)
POD place of death
    postoperative day
PODx preoperative diagnosis
pOH hydroxyl concentration
poik poikilocyte

polio poliomyelitis
poly polymorphonuclear leukocyte
POMP prednisone, Oncovin, methotrexate, 6-mercaptopurine
POP plasma oncotic pressure
POPOP 1,4-bis-a-(5-phenyloxazolyl)-benzene
pos positive
pos pr positive pressure
poss possible
post posterior
   postmortem
postop postoperative
pot potassa
   potion
PP near point (*punctum proximum*) of accommodation
   partial pressure
   pellagra preventive
   permanent partial
   pink puffers (emphysema)
   pinpoint
   postpartum
   postprandial
   private practice
   prothrombin-proconvertin
   protoporphyrin
   proximal phalanx
   pulse pressure
   pyrophosphate
PPA phenylpyruvic acid
PPA,
Ppa or
ppa first shake well (*phiala prius agitata*)
PPB platelet-poor blood
   positive-pressure breathing
ppb parts per billion
PPBS postprandial blood sugar
PPC progressive patient care
PPD paraphenylenediamine
   phenyldiphenyloxadiazole
   purified protein derivative

PPD-S purified protein derivative—standard
ppg picopicogram
PPH primary pulmonary hypertension
   protocollagen proline hydroxylase
   postpartum hemorrhage
PPHP pseudopseudohypoparathyroidism
PPLO pleuropneumonia-like organism
ppm parts per million
PPP pentose phosphate pathway
PPPI primary private practice income
PPR Price precipitation reaction
PPS postpump syndrome
PPT plant protease test
Ppt or
ppt precipitate
   prepared
PPV positive-pressure ventilation
PQ permeability quotient
   pyrimethamine-quinine
PR far point (*punctum remotum*)
   partial remission
   peer review
   peripheral resistance
   pregnancy rate
   production rate
   professional relations
   protein
   public relations
   pulse rate
Pr presbyopia
   prism
pr or
Pr far point (*punctum remotum*)
pr through the rectum (*per rectum*)
PRA plasma renin activity
PRBV placental residual blood volume
PRC packed red cells

PRCA   pure red cell agenesis
PRD   partial reaction of degeneration
    postradiation dysplasia
pre   preliminary
preg   pregnant
preop   preoperative
prep   prepare
PRFM   prolonged rupture of fetal membranes
PRI   phosphoribose isomerase
primip   woman bearing first child
PRL   prolactin
PRM   phosphoribomutase
    preventive medicine
prn   as the occasion arises (*pro re nata*)
pro   prothrombin
proct   proctology
prog   prognosis
PROM   premature rupture of membranes
    prolonged rupture of membranes
prot   protein
prox   proximal
PRP   pityriasis rubra pilaris
    platelet-rich plasma
    Psychotic Reaction Profile
PRPP   phosphoribosylpyrophosphate
PRRE   pupils round, regular, and equal
PRT   phosphoribosyltransferase
PRU   peripheral resistance unit
PS   performing scale (IQ)
    periodic syndrome
    physical status
    plastic surgery
    population sample
    Porter-Silber (chromogen)
    prescription
    psychiatric
    pulmonary stenosis
    pyloric stenosis
Ps.   *Pseudomonas*

P/S   polyunsaturated to saturated fatty acids ratio
ps   per second
PSA   apply to the affected region
    polyethylene sulfonic acid
PSC   Porter-Silber chromogen
    posterior subcapsular cataract
PSD   peptone-starch-dextrose
PSE   portal-systemic encephalopathy
PSG   peak systolic gradient
    presystolic gallop
PSGN   poststreptococcal glomerulonephritis
psi   pounds per square inch
PSP   periodic short pulse
    phenolsulfonphthalein
    positive spike pattern
    progressive supranuclear palsy
PSS   physiological saline solution
    progressive systemic sclerosis
PST   penicillin, streptomycin, and tetracycline
psy or
psych   psychiatry
    psychology
PT   parathyroid
    paroxysmal tachycardia
    permanent and total
    pharmacy and therapeutics
    physical therapy
    physical training
    pneumothorax
    prothrombin time
pt   patient
    pint
PTA   persistent truncus arteriosus
    phosphotungstic acid
    plasma thromboplastin antecedent
    post-traumatic amnesia
    prior to admission
    prior to arrival
PTAH   phosphotungstic acid hematoxylin
PTB   patellar tendon bearing

PTB (*continued*)
 prior to birth
PTC phenylthiocarbamide
 plasma thromboplastin component
PTD permanent and total disability
PTE parathyroid extract
 pulmonary thromboembolism
PTED pulmonary thromboembolic disease
PTH parathormone
 parathyroid hormone
 post-transfusion hepatitis
PTHS parathyroid hormone secretion (rate)
PTI persistent tolerant infection
PTM post-transfusion mononucleosis
PTMA phenyltrimethylammonium
PTP post-tetanic potentiation
 prior to program
PTR peripheral total resistance
PTS para-toluenesulfonic acid
PTT partial thromboplastin time
 particle transport time
PTU propylthiouracil
PTX parathyroidectomy
PU peptic ulcer
 pregnancy urine
PUD pulmonary disease
PUE pyrexia of unknown etiology
PUFA polyunsaturated fatty acid
pul pulmonary
pulm gruel (*pulmentum*)
 pulmonary
pulv powder (*pulvis*)
PUO pyrexia of unknown origin
PV peripheral vascular
 peripheral vein
 peripheral vessels
 plasma volume
 polycythemia vera
 portal vein
 postvoiding

PV (*continued*)
 through the vagina (*per vaginam*)
P & V pyloroplasty and vagotomy
PVA polyvinyl alcohol
PVC polyvinyl chloride
 postvoiding cystogram
 premature ventricular contraction
 pulmonary venous congestion
PVD peripheral vascular disease
PVF portal venous flow
PVM pneumonia virus of mice
PVP penicillin V potassium
 peripheral vein plasma
 polyvinylpyrrolidone
 portal venous pressure
PVR peripheral vascular resistance
 pulmonary vascular resistance
PVS premature ventricular systole
PVT paroxysmal ventricular tachycardia
 portal vein thrombosis
pvt private
PW posterior wall
PWB partial weight-bearing
PWC physical work capacity
PWI posterior wall infarct
Px physical examination
 pneumothorax
 prognosis
PXE pseudoxanthoma elasticum
PZ pancreozymin
PZA pyrazinamide
PZ-CCK pancreozymin-cholecystokinin
PZI protamine zinc insulin
Q coulomb (electric quantity)
q every (*quaque*)
 quart
qAM every morning
QC quinine-colchicine
qd every day (*quaque die*)
qh every hour (*quaque hora*)

q2h   every two hours
q3h   every three hours
q4h   every four hours
qhs   every hour of sleep
qid   four times a day (*quater in die*)
ql   as much as desired (*quantum libet*)
qm   every morning (*quaque mane*)
qn   every night (*quaque nocte*)
QNS   quantity not sufficient
qod   every other day
QO_2 or
qO_2 oxygen quotient
QP   quanti-Pirquet reaction
qP,
Qp or
QP   at will (*quantum placeat*)
qPM   every night
qq   each (*quaque*)
qqh   every four hours (*quaque quarta hora*)
qqhor   every hour (*quaque hora*)
QRZ   wheal reaction time
qs,
Qs or
QS   enough (*quantum satis*)
qsad   to a sufficient quantity
qsuff   as much as suffices (*quantum sufficit*)
qt   quiet
      quart
quant   quantity
quat   four (*quattuor*)
QUICHA   quantitative inhalation challenge apparatus
quint   fifth (*quintus*)
quotid   daily (*quotidie*)
qv   as much as you like (*quantum vis*)
      which see (*quod vide*)
R   Behnken's unit
    far point (*remotum*)
    organic radical
    radiology
    Rankine (scale)

R (*continued*)
    Réaumur (scale)
    rectal
    regression coefficient
    remote
    resistance
    respiration
    right
    Rinne test
    roentgen
    rough (colony)
    take (*recipe*)
R.   *Rickettsia*
RA   renal artery
     rheumatoid arthritis
     right arm
     right atrial
     right atrium
R_A airway resistance
RAD   right axis deviation
rad   radial
      radiation absorbed dose
      root (*radix*)
RADTS   rabbit antidog thymus serum
RAE   right atrial enlargement
RAF   rheumatoid arthritis factor
RAH   right atrial hypertrophy
RAI   radioactive iodine
RAIU   radioactive iodine uptake
RAMT   rabbit antimouse thymocyte
RAO   right anterior oblique
RAP   right atrial pressure
RAR   right arm recumbent
RARLS   rabbit antirat lymphocyte serum
RAS   renal artery stenosis
ras   scrapings (*rasurae*)
RAST   radioallergosorbent test
RATHAS   rat thymus antiserum
RATx   radiation therapy
RB   rating board
RBA   rose bengal antigen
RBB   right bundle branch
RBBB   right bundle branch block

RBC   red blood cell
       red blood count
RBCM   red blood cell mass
RBCV   red blood cell volume
RBE   relative biological effective-
       ness
RBF   renal blood flow
RBL   Reid's base line
RC   red cell
       red cell casts
       retrograde cystogram
RCA   right coronary artery
RCBV   regional cerebral blood
       volume
RCC   red cell count
RCD   relative cardiac dullness
RCF   red cell folate
       relative centrifugal force
RCM   red cell mass
       right costal margin
RCR   respiratory control ratio
RCS   reticulum cell sarcoma
RCU   respiratory care unit
RCV   red cell volume
RD   Raynaud's disease
       reaction of (to) degeneration
       resistance determinant
       respiratory disease
       right deltoid
rd   rutherford
RDA   recommended daily allow-
       ance
       recommended dietary allow-
       ance
       right dorsoanterior
RDDA   recommended daily di-
       etary allowance
RDE   receptor-destroying enzyme
RDI   rupture-delivery interval
RDP   right dorsoposterior
RDS   respiratory distress syndrome
RE   radium emanation
       regional enteritis
       resting energy
       reticuloendothelial
       right eye

R & E   research and education
rec   fresh (*recens*)
rect   rectified
REF   renal erythropoietic factor
REG   radioencephalogram
rehab   rehabilitation
REM   rapid eye movement
       roentgen-equivalent – man
rem   removal
REMP   roentgen-equivalent – man
       period
REP   roentgen equivalent – phys-
       ical
rep or
rept   let it be repeated (*repetatur*)
RER   rough endoplasmic reticulum
res   research
RES   reticuloendothelial system
resp   respectively
       respiratory
retic   reticulocyte
RF   Reitland-Franklin (unit)
       relative fluorescence
       releasing factor
       rheumatic fever
       rheumatoid factor
       root canal, filling of
RFA   right femoral artery
       right frontoanterior
RFB   retained foreign body
RFLA   rheumatoid factor–like
       activity
RFP   right frontoposterior
RFS   renal function study
RFT   right frontotransverse
       rod-and-frame test
RFW   rapid filling wave
RG   right gluteal
RH   reactive hyperemia
       relative humidity
Rh   Rhesus (factor)
rh   rheumatic
Rh neg   Rhesus factor negative
Rh pos   Rhesus factor positive
RHBF   reactive hyperemia blood
       flow

RHD   relative hepatic dullness
      rheumatic heart disease
rheum   rheumatic
RHL   right hepatic lobe
RHLN   right hilar lymph node
rhm   roentgen (per) hour (at one)
      meter
RI   refractive index
      regional ileitis
      respiratory illness
RIA   radioimmunoassay
RIF   right iliac fossa
RIFA   radioiodinated fatty acid
RIHSA   radioactive iodinated
      human serum albumin
RISA   radioactive iodinated serum
      albumin
RITC   rhodamine isothiocyanate
RIU   radioactive iodine uptake
RK   rabbit kidney
      right kidney
RKY   roentgen kymography
RL   right leg
      right lung
R-L, R→L   right-to-left
RLC   residual lung capacity
RLD   related living donor
RLF   retrolental fibroplasia
RLL   right lower lobe
RLN   recurrent laryngeal nerve
RLP   radiation-leukemia-protec-
      tion
RLQ   right lower quadrant
RLS   Ringer's lactate solution
RM   radical mastectomy
      respiratory movement
RMA   right mentoanterior
RMK   rhesus monkey kidney
RML   right middle lobe
RMP   rapidly miscible pool
      right mentoposterior
RMS   root-mean-square
RMSF   Rocky Mountain spotted
      fever
RMT   retromolar trigone
      right mentotransverse

RMV   respiratory minute volume
RNA   ribonucleic acid
RNase   ribonuclease
RND   radical neck dissection
RNP   ribonucleoprotein
RO   Ritter-Oleson (technique)
      rule out
ROA   right occipitoanterior
roent   roentgenology
ROH   rat ovarian hyperemia (test)
ROM   range of motion
      rupture of membranes
ROP   right occipitoposterior
ROS   review of systems
ROT   right occipitotransverse
rot   rotating
RP   reactive protein
      refractory period
      rest pain
      resting pressure
      retrograde pyelogram
R_P pulmonary resistance
RPA   right pulmonary artery
RPCF   Reiter protein comple-
      ment-fixation
RPCFT   Reiter protein comple-
      ment-fixation test
RPE   retinal pigment epithelium
RPF   renal plasma flow
RPG   retrograde pyelogram
RPGN   rapidly progressive glo-
      merulonephritis
RPM   rapid processing mode
rpm   revolutions per minute
RPO   right posterior oblique
RPR   rapid plasma reagin
RPS   renal pressor substance
RPV   right pulmonary veins
RQ   respiratory quotient
RR   radiation response
      recovery room
      renin release
      respiratory rate
      response rate
R & R   rest and recuperation
RR & E   round, regular, and equal

RR-HPO   rapid recompression–
         high pressure oxygen
RRP   relative refractory period
RRR   renin-release rate
RS   rating schedule
     respiratory syncytial
     right side
RSA   relative specific activity
      reticulum cell sarcoma
      right sacroanterior
RSB   right sternal border
RSC   rested-state contraction
RScA   right scapuloanterior
RScP   right scapuloposterior
RSP   right sacroposterior
RSR   regular sinus rhythm
RST   radiosensitivity test
      right sacrotransverse
RSTL   relaxed skin tension lines
RSV   respiratory syncytial virus
      right subclavian vein
      Rous sarcoma virus
RT   radiation therapy
     radiotherapy
     radium therapy
     reaction time
     reading test
     recreational therapy
     right thigh
     room temperature
rt   right
rt lat   right lateral
RTA   renal tubular acidosis
RTD   routine test dilution
rtd   retarded
RTF   replication and transfer
      resistance transfer factor
      respiratory tract fluid
rtn   return
RU   rat unit
     resistance unit
     retrograde urogram
     right upper
     roentgen unit
rub   red (*ruber*)

RUL   right upper lobe
RUQ   right upper quadrant
RUR   resin-uptake ratio
RURTI   recurrent upper respira-
        tory tract infection
RV   rat virus
     residual volume
     respiratory volume
     right ventricle
     rubella virus
RVB   red venous blood
RVD   relative vertebral density
RVE   right ventricular enlargement
RVEDP   right ventricular end-
        diastolic pressure
RVH   right ventricular hyper-
      trophy
RVI   relative value index
RVP   red veterinary petrolatum
RVR   renal vascular resistance
      resistance to venous return
RVRA   renal vein renin activity
       renal venous renin assay
RVRC   renal vein renin concentra-
       tion
RVS   Relative Value Schedule
      Relative Value Study
RVT   renal vein thrombosis
RW   ragweed
R_x prescription
     take (*recipe*)
     therapy
     treatment
S   half (*semis*)
    label (*signa*)
    left (*sinister*)
    sacral
    screen-containing cassette
    second
    single
    smooth (colony)
    soluble
    spherical lens
    subject
    supravergence

S (*continued*)
  surgery
  Svedberg unit of sedimentation
    coefficient
  write (*signa*)
S. *Salmonella*
  Schistosoma
  Spirillum
  Staphylococcus
  Streptococcus
s̄ without (*sine*)
SA salicylic acid
  sarcoma
  secondary amenorrhea
  secondary anemia
  serum albumin
  sinoatrial
  slightly active
  specific activity
  Stokes-Adams
  surface area
  sustained action
  sympathetic activity
sa according to art (*secundum artem*)
SAB significant asymptomatic bacteriuria
SACD subacute combined degeneration
SAD source to axis distance
SAG Swiss agammaglobulinemia
SAH subarachnoid hemorrhage
sal according to the rules of art (*secundum artis leges*)
  saline
SAM sulfated acid mucopolysaccharide
SAP serum alkaline phosphatase
  systemic arterial pressure
SAS supravalvular aortic stenosis
SAT Scholastic Aptitude Test
sat saturated
SB serum bilirubin
  single breath
  Stanford-Binet (test)

SB (*continued*)
  sternal border
  stillbirth
SBE subacute bacterial endocarditis
SBF splanchnic blood flow
SBFT small bowel follow-through
SBP systemic blood pressure
  systolic blood pressure
SBS social-breakdown syndrome
SBT single-breath test
SBTI soybean trypsin inhibitor
SC closure of the semilunar valves
  sacrococcygeal
  self-care
  semicircular
  semiclosed
  service-connected
  sick call
  sickle cell
  single chemical
  special care
  sternoclavicular
  subcutaneous
  succinylcholine
  sugar-coated
SCAT sheep cell agglutination test
scat a box (*scatula*)
SCC squamous cell carcinoma
SCD service-connected disability
ScDA scapulodextra anterior
ScDP scapulodextra posterior
SCG serum chemistry graft
SCH succinylcholine
sched schedule
schiz schizophrenia
SCI structured clinical interview
SCK serum creatine kinase
ScLA scapulolaeva anterior
ScLP scapulolaeva posterior
scop scopolamine
SCP single-celled protein
SCPK serum creatine phosphokinase
scr scruple

SCT   sex chromatin test
      staphylococcal clumping test
SCUBA self-contained underwater
        breathing apparatus
SD   septal defect
      serum defect
      skin dose
      spontaneous delivery
      standard deviation
      streptodornase
      sudden death
S/D   systolic to diastolic
SDA   sacrodextra anterior
      specific dynamic action
SDCL   symptom distress check list
SDH   serine dehydrase
      sorbitol dehydrogenase
      succinate dehydrogenase
SDM   standard deviation of the
      mean
SDO   sudden-dosage onset
SDP   sacrodextra posterior
SDS   Self-Rating Depression Scale
      sensory deprivation syn-
        drome
      sodium dodecyl sulfate
      sudden death syndrome
SDT   sacrodextra transversa
SE   himself, itself (*se*)
      standard error
      Starr-Edwards (prosthesis)
sec   second
SED   skin erythema dose
      spondyloepiphyseal dysplasia
sed   stool (*sedes*)
sed rate sedimentation rate
SEE   standard error of the estimate
SEG   sonoencephalogram
seg   segmented (leukocyte)
SEGS   segmented neutrophils
SEM   scanning electron micros-
        copy
      standard error of the mean
semi   half
semid half a drachm (dram)

semih half an hour
SEP   sensory evoked potential
      systolic ejection period
seq   sequela
      sequestrum
SER   smooth endoplasmic reticu-
        lum
      systolic ejection rate
serv   keep, preserve (*serva*)
SES   socioeconomic status
SET   systolic ejection time
sev   severe
      severed
SF   scarlet fever
      shell fragment
      shrapnel fragment
      spinal fluid
Sf   Svedberg flotation units
SFP   screen filtration pressure
      spinal fluid pressure
SFS   split function study
SFT   skinfold thickness
SFW   shell fragment wound
      shrapnel fragment wound
SG   serum globulin
      signs
      skin graft
      specific gravity
      surgeon general
S-G   Sachs-Georgi (test)
SGA   small for gestational age
s gl   without correction
SGOT   serum glutamic-oxaloacetic
        transaminase
SGP   serine glycerophosphatide
SGPT   serum glutamic-pyruvic
        transaminase
SGV   salivary gland virus
SH   serum hepatitis
      sex hormone
      sinus histiocytosis
      social history
      sulfhydryl
      surgical history
sh   shoulder

SHB   sulfhemoglobin
SHBD   serum hydroxybutyrate
      dehydrogenase
SHG   synthetic human gastrin
SHO   secondary hypertrophic
      osteoarthropathy
SI   sacroiliac
    saturation index
    self-inflicted
    seriously ill
    serum iron
    soluble insulin
    stroke index
SIADH   syndrome of inappropriate
      antidiuretic hormone
SICD   serum isocitric dehydrogen-
      ase
SID   sudden infant death
SIDS   sudden infant death syn-
      drome
sig   let it be labeled (*signetur*)
    significant
SIJ   sacroiliac joint
simul   at the same time
sing   of each (*singuli*)
SISI   short-increment sensitivity
      index
SIW   self-inflicted wound
SJR   Shinawora-Jones-Reinhart
      (units)
SK   streptokinase
SKSD   streptokinase-streptodor-
      nase
SL   sensation level
    streptolysin
sl   according to law (*secundum
    legem*)
    slight
SLA   sacrolaeva anterior
SLD or
SLDH   serum lactic dehydrogenase
SLE   St. Louis encephalitis
    systemic lupus erythematosus
SLEV   St. Louis encephalitis virus

SLI   splenic localization index
SLKC   superior limbic keratocon-
      junctivitis
SLN   superior laryngeal nerve
SLO   streptolysin-O
SLP   sacrolaeva posterior
SLR   straight leg raising
    Streptococcus lactis R
SLT   sacrolaeva transversa
SM   simple mastectomy
    skim milk
    streptomycin
    submucous
    suction method
    symptoms
    systolic mean
    systolic murmur
sm   small
SMA   superior mesenteric artery
SMC   special monthly compensa-
      tion
SMO   slip made out
SMON   subacute myelo-optical
      neuropathy
SMP   slow-moving protease
    special monthly pension
SMR   somnolent metabolic rate
    standard mortality ratio
    submucous resection
SMRR   submucous resection and
      rhinoplasty
SN   serum-neutralizing
    suprasternal notch
sn   according to nature (*secundum
    naturam*)
SNB   scalene node biopsy
SO   salpingo-oophorectomy
SOA-MCA   superficial occipital
      artery to middle
      cerebral artery
SOB   short(ness) of breath
SOC   sequential-type oral contra-
      ceptive
SOL or

Sol solution
      space-occupying lesion
sol or
soln solution
solv dissolve (*solve*)
SOM secretory otitis media
      serous otitis media
SOP standing operating procedure
s op s if necessary (*si opus sit*)
sos if it is necessary (*si opus sit*)
SOTT synthetic medium old
      tuberculin trichloracetic
      acid precipitated
SP shunt procedure
    skin potential
    status post
    steady potential
    summating potential
    suprapubic
    symphysis pubis
    systolic pressure
sp species
    spirit (*spiritus*)
sp gr specific gravity
SPA suprapubic aspiration
SPAI steroid protein activity
      index
SPBI serum protein-bound iodine
SPCA serum prothrombin conver-
      sion accelerator
SPE serum protein electrophoresis
SPF specific pathogen-free
    split products of fibrin
SPH secondary pulmonary hemo-
      siderosis
sph spherical
    spherical lens
SPI serum precipitable iodine
spir spirit (*spiritus*)
SPL sound pressure level
    spontaneous lesion
spont spontaneous (delivery)
SPP suprapubic prostatectomy
spt spirit
SQ social quotient
    subcutaneous

sq square
SR sarcoplasmic reticulum
    secretion rate
    sedimentation rate
    sensitization response
    service record
    sigma reaction
    sinus rhythm
    skin resistance
    superior rectus
    system review
    systemic resistance
    systems research
SRBC sheep red blood cells
SRC sedimented red cells
    sheep red cells
SRF somatotropin-releasing factor
    split renal function
    subretinal fluid
SRFS split renal function study
SRNA soluble ribonucleic acid
SRR slow rotation room
SRS slow-reacting substance
SRSA slow-reacting substance of
      anaphylaxis
SRT speech reception test
    speech reception threshold
SS saturated solution
    side-to-side
    signs and symptoms
    soapsuds
    statistically significant
    subaortic stenosis
    sum of squares
    supersaturated
ss one-half (*semis*)
SSA salicylsalicylic acid
    skin-sensitizing antibody
    sulfosalicylic acid (test)
SSD source to skin distance
    sum of square deviations
SSE soapsuds enema
SSKI saturated solution of potas-
      sium iodide
SSN severely subnormal

SSP Sanarelli-Shwartzman phenomenon
     subacute sclerosing panencephalitis
SSPE subacute sclerosing panencephalitis
SSS layer upon layer (*stratum super stratum*)
     specific soluble substance
SSU sterile supply unit
SSV under a poison label (*sub signo veneni*)
ST esotropia
    sternothyroid
    subtalar
    subtotal
    surface tension
st let it stand (*stet*)
    stage (of disease)
    straight
STA serum thrombotic accelerator
STA-MCA superficial temporal artery to middle cerebral artery
stab stabnuclear neutrophil
staph staphylococcus
stat German unit of radium emanation
     immediately (*statim*)
STC soft tissue calcification
STD skin test dose
     skin to tumor distance
std saturated
STH somatotropic hormone
STK streptokinase
STM streptomycin
STP scientifically treated petroleum
     standard temperature and pressure
STPD standard temperature and pressure, dry (0°C, 760 mm Hg)
str or
strep streptococcus

STS serologic test for syphilis
     standard test for syphilis
STSG split thickness skin graft
STT serial thrombin time
STU skin test unit
STVA subtotal villose atrophy
SU sensation unit
su let the person take (*sumat*)
SUA serum uric acid
     single umbilical artery
subcu,
subcut or
subq subcutaneous
SUD sudden unexpected death
     sudden unexplained death
SUID sudden unexplained infant death
sum let the person take (*sumat*)
SUN serum urea nitrogen
sup superficial
    superior
surg surgery
SUS stained urinary sediment
SUUD sudden unexpected, unexplained death
SV severe
    simian virus
    snake venom
    stroke volume
    subclavian vein
    supravital
sv alcoholic spirit (*spiritus vini*)
SVAS supravalvular aortic stenosis
SVC slow vital capacity
     superior vena cava
SVCG spatial vectorcardiogram
SVD spontaneous vaginal delivery
     spontaneous vertex delivery
SVI stroke volume index
SVM syncytiovascular membrane
SVR systemic vascular resistance
svr rectified spirit of wine (*spiritus vini rectificatus*)
svt proof spirit (*spiritus vini tenuis*)

SW   spiral wound
    stroke work
SWI   stroke work index
Sx   signs
    symptoms
sym   symmetrical
    symptoms
symp   symptoms
syr   syrup
Sz   schizophrenia
T   temperature
    tension (intraocular)
    thoracic
    thorax
    time
    tumor
T.   *Taenia*
    Treponema
    Trichophyton
    Trypanosoma
t   temporal
    three times (*ter*)
    tertiary
    test of significance
T+   increased tension
T−   decreased tension
$T_{1/2}$ half-life
T_3 triiodothyronine
T_4 thyroxine
TA   alkaline tuberculin
    therapeutic abortion
    titratable acid
    toxin-antitoxin
T & A   tonsillectomy & adenoidec-
    tomy
tab   tablet
TAB   typhoid, paratyphoid A, and
    paratyphoid B
TACE   chlorotrianisene
TAD   thoracic asphyxiant dys-
    trophy
TADAC   therapeutic abortion,
    dilation, aspiration,
    curettage
TAF   albumose-free tuberculin

TAF (*continued*)
    toxoid-antitoxin floccules
    trypsin-aldehyde-fuchsin
TAH   total abdominal hysterec-
    tomy
tal   of such (*talis*)
TAL   tendo Achillis lengthening
    thymic alymphoplasia
TAM   toxoid-antitoxin mixture
TAME   toluene-sulpho-trypsin
    arginine methyl ester
TAO   thromboangiitis obliterans
    triacetyloleandomycin
TAPVD   total anomalous pulmo-
    nary venous drainage
TAR   thrombocytopenia with
    absence of the radius
TAT   tetanus antitoxin
    thematic apperception test
    thromboplastin activation
    test
    total antitryptic activity
    toxin-antitoxin
    turn-around time
    tyrosine aminotransferase
TB   toluidine blue
    total base
    total body
    tracheobronchitis
    tubercle bacillus
    tuberculosis
TBA   tertiary butylacetate
    testosterone-binding affinity
    thiobarbituric acid
TBC   tuberculosis
TBD   total body density
TBF   total body fat
TBG   thyroxine-binding globulin
TBGP   total blood granulocyte
    pool
TBI   thyroxine-binding index
    total body irradiation
TBK   total body potassium
TBM   tuberculous meningitis
TBN   bacillus emulsions

TBP thyroxine-binding protein
TBPA thyroxine-binding pre-
    albumin
TB-RD tuberculosis-respiratory
    disease
TBS total body solute
    tribromosalicylanilide
    triethanolamine-buffered
    saline
tbsp tablespoonful
TBT tolbutamide test
    tracheobronchial toilet
TBV total blood volume
TBW total body water
    total body weight
TBX whole body irradiation
TC taurocholate
    temperature compensation
    tetracycline
    tissue culture
    to contain
    total capacity
    total cholesterol
    tubocurarine
Tc technetium
TCA tricarboxylic acid
    trichloroacetate
    trichloroacetic acid
TCAP trimethylcetylammonium
    pentachlorophenate
TCC trichlorocarbanilide
TCD tissue culture dose
TCD_{50} median tissue culture dose
TCE trichloroethylene
TCF total coronary flow
TCH total circulating hemoglobin
TCI to come in
    transient cerebral ischemia
TCID tissue culture infective dose
$TCID_{50}$ median tissue culture in-
    fective dose
TCIE transient cerebral ischemic
    episode
TCM tissue culture medium
TCP therapeutic continuous peni-
    cillin

TCSA tetrachlorosalicylanilide
TCT thrombin-clotting time
    thyrocalcitonin
TD tetanus-diphtheria
    therapy discontinued
    thoracic duct
    three times a day
    threshold of discomfort
    thymus-dependent
    time disintegration
    to deliver
    tone decay
    torsion dystonia
    total disability
    transverse diameter
    treatment discontinued
TDF thoracic duct fistula
    thoracic duct flow
TDI toluene-diisocyanate
    total-dose infusion
TDL thoracic duct lymph
TDP thoracic duct pressure
    thymidine diphosphate
tds or
TDS three times a day (*ter*
    die sumendum)
TDT tone decay test
TE threshold energy
    tissue-equivalent
    tooth extracted
    total estrogen (excretion)
    tracheo-esophageal
Te tetanus
TEA tetraethylammonium
TEAC tetraethylammonium
    chloride
TED threshold erythema dose
    thromboembolic disease
TEE tyrosine ethyl ester
TEF tracheoesophageal fistula
TEIB triethyleneiminobenzoquin-
    one
TEL tetraethyl lead
TEM transmission electron micros-
    copy
    triethylenemelamine

TEN   toxic epidermal necrolysis
tenac   tenaculum
TEP   thromboendophlebectomy
TEPP   tetraethyl pyrophosphate
TER   three times
    threefold
TES   trimethylaminoethane-
    sulfonic acid
Tet   tetanus
    tetralogy of Fallot
tet   tetanus
TETD   tetraethylthiuram disulfide
TF   tactile fremitus
    tetralogy of Fallot
    thymol flocculation
    tissue-damaging factor
    to follow
    total flow
    transfer factor
    tuberculin filtrate
    tubular fluid
TFA   total fatty acids
TFE   tetrafluoroethylene
TFS   testicular feminization syn-
    drome
TG   thioguanine
    thyroglobulin
    toxic goiter
    triglyceride
TGA   transposition of the great
    arteries
TGAR   total graft area rejected
TGFA   triglyceride fatty acid
TGL   triglyceride
    triglyceride lipase
TGT   thromboplastin generation
    test
    thromboplastin generation
    time
TGV   thoracic gas volume
    transposition of the great
    vessels
TH   thyrohyoid
th   thoracic
THA   total hydroxyapatite

THAM   trihydroxymethylamino-
    methane
THC   tetrahydrocannabinol
THDOC   tetrahydrodeoxycortico-
    sterone
THE   tetrahydrocortisone
ther   therapy
THF   humoral thymic factor
    tetrahydrocortisol
    tetrahydrofolic acid
THFA   tetrahydrofolic acid
THO   titrated water
THP   total hydroxyproline
TI   thoracic index
    time interval
    transverse inlet
    tricuspid incompetence
    tricuspid insufficiency
TIA   transient ischemic attack
TIBC   total iron-binding capacity
TIC   trypsin-inhibitory capacity
TID   titrated initial dose
tid   three times a day (*ter in die*)
TIE   transient ischemic episode
tin   three times a night (*ter in
    nocte*)
tinct   tincture
TIS   tumor in situ
TIT   triiodothyronine
TIVC   thoracic inferior vena cava
TKA   transketolase activity
TKD   tokodynamometer
TKG   tokodynagraph
TL   time lapse
    time-limited
    total lipids
    tubal ligation
TLA   translumbar aortogram
TLC   tender loving care
    thin-layer chromatography
    total L-chain concentration
    total lung capacity
    total lung compliance
TLD   thermoluminescent dosim-
    eter

TLD (*continued*)
    tumor lethal dose
T/LD_{100} minimum dose causing death or malformation of 100 per cent of fetuses
TLE thin-layer electrophoresis
TLQ total living quotient
TLV threshold limit value
TM temporomandibular
    time motion
    trademark
    transmetatarsal
    tympanic membrane
T_m maximal tubular excretory capacity of the kidneys
TMAS Taylor Manifest Anxiety Scale
T_{mG} or
TmG maximal tubular reabsorption of glucose
TMJ temporomandibular joint
TML tetramethyl lead
TMP thymidine monophosphate
    trimethoprim
TMTD tetramethylthiuram disulfide
TMV tobacco mosaic virus
TN total negatives
    true negative
Tn normal intraocular tension
TND term normal delivery
TNI total nodal irradiation
TNM (primary) tumor, (regional lymph) nodes, (remote) metastases—cancer grading system
TNT trinitrotoluene
TNTC too numerous to count
TO original tuberculin
    telephone order
    tincture of opium
TOA tubo-ovarian abscess
TOCP triorthocresyl phosphate
tonoc tonight

TOPS Take Off Pounds Sensibly
TOPV trivalent oral poliovirus vaccine
TORP total ossicular replacement prosthesis
tot prot total protein
TP temperature and pressure
    thrombocytopenic purpura
    total positives
    total protein
    true positive
    tryptophan
    tube precipitin
    tuberculin precipitation
TPA *Treponema pallidum* agglutination
TPBF total pulmonary blood flow
TPCF *Treponema pallidum* complement-fixation
TPG transplacental gradient
TPH transplacental hemorrhage
TPI *Treponema pallidum* immobilization
    treponemal immobilization test (cardiolipin)
    triose phosphate isomerase
TPIA *Treponema pallidum* immobilization (immune) adherence
TPM triphenylmethane
TPN triphosphopyridine nucleotide
TPNH reduced triphosphopyridine nucleotide
TPP thiamine pyrophosphate
TPR temperature, pulse, and respiration
    testosterone production rate
    total peripheral resistance
    total pulmonary resistance
TPS tumor polysaccharide substance
TPT typhoid-paratyphoid (vaccine)
TPTZ tripyridyltriazine

TPVR   total pulmonary vascular resistance
TQ   tourniquet
TR   tetrazolium reduction
    therapeutic radiology
    time released
    total resistance
    total response
    tuberculin R (new tuberculin)
tr   tincture
    trace
TRA   transaldolase
TRAM   Treatment Rating Assessment Matrix
    Treatment Response Assessment Method
TRBF   total renal blood flow
TRC   tanned red cell
    total ridge-count
TRF   thyrotropin-releasing factor
TRH   thyrotropin-releasing hormone
TRI   tetrazolium reduction inhibition
TRIC   trachoma-inclusion conjunctivitis
trit   triturate
TRK   transketolase
TRMC   tetramethylrhodamino-isothiocyanate
tRNA   transfer RNA
troch   troche (*trochiscus*)
TRP   tubular reabsorption of phosphate
TRPT   theoretical renal phosphorus threshold
TRU   turbidity-reducing unit
TS   test solution
    thoracic surgery
    total solids
    triple strength
    tropical sprue
TSA   technical surgical assistance
    trypticase soy agar
T$_4$SA   thyroxine-specific activity

TSB   trypticase soy broth
TSC   technetium sulfur colloid
    thiosemicarbizide
TSD   target skin distance
    Tay-Sachs disease
    theory of signal detectability
TSE   trisodium edetate
TSF   tissue-coding factor
TSH   thyroid-stimulating hormone
TSI   triple sugar iron (agar)
TSP   total serum protein
tsp   teaspoonful
TSPAP   total serum prostatic acid phosphatase
TSR   thyroid-to-serum ratio
TSS   tropical splenomegaly syndrome
TST   tumor skin test
TSTA   tumor-specific transplantation antigen
TSY   trypticase soy yeast
TT   tetrazol
    thrombin time
    thymol turbidity
    tooth, treatment of
    total thyroxine
    total time
    transit time
    transthoracic
TTC   triphenyltetrazolium chloride
TTD   tissue tolerance dose
TTH   thyrotropic hormone
    tritiated thymidine
TTI   time-tension index
    tension-time index
TTP   thrombotic thrombocytopenic purpura
    thymidine triphosphate
TTS   temporary threshold shift
TTT   tolbutamide tolerance test
TU   thiouracil
    toxic unit
    tuberculin unit
tuberc   tuberculosis
TUG   total urinary gonadotropin

TUR   transurethral resection
TURB   transurethral resection of
the bladder
TURP   transurethral resection of
the prostate
tus   cough (*tussis*)
TV   tidal volume
trial visit
tuberculin volutin
TVC   timed vital capacity
total volume capacity
transvaginal cone
TVH   total vaginal hysterectomy
TW   tap water
TWL   transepidermal water loss
Tx   traction
treatment
Ty   type
typhoid
TZ   tuberculin zymoplastiche
U   unit
unknown
upper
urology
UA   umbilical artery
unaggregated
uric acid
urine analysis
uterine aspiration
UB   ultimobranchial body
UBBC   unsaturated vitamin B_{12}-
binding capacity
UBF   uterine blood flow
UBI   ultraviolet blood irradiation
UC   ulcerative colitis
ultracentrifugal
unchanged
unclassifiable
unit clerk
urea clearance
urethral catheterization
uterine contractions
U & C   usual and customary
UCD   usual childhood diseases
UCG   urinary chorionic gonadotropin

UCHD   usual childhood diseases
UCO   urethral catheter out
UCP   urinary coproporphyrin
UCS   unconditioned stimulus
unconscious
UD   urethral discharge
uroporphyrinogen decarboxy-
lase
UDP   uridine diphosphate
UDPG   uridine diphosphoglucose
UDPGA   uridine diphosphoglu-
curonic acid
UDPGT   uridine diphosphogly-
cyronyl transferase
UE   upper extremity
UFA   unesterified fatty acid
UG   urogenital
UGI   upper gastrointestinal
UH   upper half
UI   uroporphyrin isomerase
UIBC   unsaturated iron-binding
capacity
UIF   undegraded insulin factor
UIQ   upper inner quadrant
UK   unknown
urokinase
UL   upper lobe
U & L   upper and lower
ULN   upper limits of normal
ULQ   upper left quadrant
UM   uracil mustard
umb   umbilicus
UMP   uridine monophosphate
UN   urea nitrogen
ung   ointment (*unguentum*)
uni-   one (prefix)
unk or
unkn   unknown
UOQ   upper outer quadrant
UP   upright posture
ureteropelvic
uroporphyrin
U/P   urine-plasma ratio
UPG   uroporphyrinogen
UPI   uteroplacental insufficiency
UPJ   ureteropelvic junction

UPOR usual place of residence
UR upper respiratory
    utilization review
ur urine
URD upper respiratory disease
URI upper respiratory infection
urol urology
URQ upper right quadrant
URTI upper respiratory tract in-
    fection
US ultrasonic
USN ultrasonic nebulizer
USO unilateral salpingo-oophorec-
    tomy
USR unheated serum reagin (test)
ut dict as directed (*ut dictum*)
UTBG unbound thyroxine-binding
    globulin
utend to be used (*utendus*)
UTI urinary tract infection
UTP uridine triphosphate
UU urine urobilinogen
UUN urine urea nitrogen
UV ultraviolet
    umbilical vein
    urinary volume
UVJ ureterovesical junction
UVL ultraviolet light
V vein
    vision
    visual acuity
    voice
    volume
V. *Vibrio*
v see (*vide*)
    very
    volt
VA vacuum aspiration
    ventriculoatrial
    vertebral artery
    visual acuity
Va alveolar ventilation
    visual acuity
vag vagina
    vaginal
VALE visual acuity, left eye

VAMP vincristine, amethopterine,
    6-mercaptopurine, and
    prednisone
var variation
VARE visual acuity, right eye
VASC Verbal Auditory Screen for
    Children
vasc vascular
VB viable birth
    vinblastine
VBL vinblastine
VBS veronal-buffered saline
VBS:FBS veronal-buffered saline–
    fetal bovine serum
VC acuity of color vision
    vena cava
    ventilatory capacity
    vincristine
    vital capacity
VCG vectorcardiogram
VCR vincristine
VCU voiding cystourethrogram
VD vapor density
    venereal disease
VDA visual discriminatory acuity
VDBR volume of distribution of
    bilirubin
VDG venereal disease – gonorrhea
vdg voiding
VDH valvular disease of the heart
VDL visual detection level
VDM vasodepressor material
VDP vincristine, daunorubicin,
    prednisone
VDRL Venereal Disease Research
    Laboratory
VDRS Verdun Depression Rating
    Scale
VDS venereal disease – syphilis
VE visual efficiency
    volumic ejection
V & E Vinethene and ether
VEE Venezuelan equine enceph-
    alomyelitis (virus)
VEM vasoexcitor material
vent ventricular

VEP   visual evoked potential
VER   visual evoked response
ves   bladder (*vesica*)
     vesicular
vesic   blister (*vesicula*)
VF   left leg (electrode)
     ventricular fibrillation
     ventricular fluid
     visual field
     vocal fremitus
VFP   ventricular fluid pressure
VG   ventricular gallop
VH   vaginal hysterectomy
     venous hematocrit
     viral hepatitis
VHD   viral hematodepressive
     disease
VHF   visual half-field
VI   volume index
VIA   virus-inactivating agent
vib   vibration
VIG   vaccinia-immune globulin
vin   wine (*vinum*)
VIP   vasoactive intestinal polypep-
     tide
     very important patient
     voluntary interruption of
     pregnancy
VIS   vaginal irrigation smear
vit   vitamin
     yolk (*vitellus*)
vit cap   vital capacity
VL   left arm (electrode)
VLDL or
VLDLP   very low density lipopro-
     tein
VM   viomycin
     voltmeter
VMA   vanillylmandelic acid
VMR   vasomotor rhinitis
VN   virus-neutralizing
VO   verbal order
VOD   vision, right eye (*visio
     oculus dextra*)
vol   volume

vos   dissolved in yolk of egg
     (*vitello ovi solutus*)
     vision, left eye (*visio oculus
     sinister*)
VOU   vision, each eye (*visio oculus
     uterque*)
voxel   volume element
VP   vasopressin
     venipuncture
     venous pressure
     Voges-Proskauer (reaction)
     volume-pressure
     vulnerable period
V & P   vagotomy and pyloroplasty
VBP   ventricular premature beat
VPC   ventricular premature con-
     traction
     volume per cent
VPRC   volume of packed red cells
V/Q   ventilation-perfusion
VR   right arm (electrode)
     valve replacement
     vascular resistance
     venous return
     ventilation ratio
     vocal resonance
     vocational rehabilitation
VRBC   red blood cell volume
VR & E   vocational rehabilitation
     and education
VRI   viral respiratory infection
VRP   very reliable product (writ-
     ten on prescription)
VS   vaccination scar
     venisection
     verbal scale (IQ)
     vital signs
     volumetric solution
     without glasses
vs   against (*versus*)
     vibration seconds
     voids
VsB   bleeding in the arm (*venae-
     sectio brachii*)
VSD   ventricular septal defect

VSOK vital signs normal
VSS vital signs stable
VSULA vaccination scar upper
    left arm
VSV vesicular stomatitis virus
VSW ventricular stroke work
VT tidal volume
    vacuum tuberculin
    ventricular tachycardia
V & T volume and tension
V_T tidal volume
VTSRS Verdun Target Symptom
    Rating Scale
VV viper venom
vv veins
v/v volume for volume
V/VI grade 5 on a 6-grade basis
VW vessel wall
    von Willebrand's disease
VZ varicella-zoster
W water
    Weber (test)
    week
    wehnelt (unit of roentgen ray
    penetrating ability)
    weight
    widowed
    wife
W+ weakly positive
w watt
    with
WAIS Wechsler's Adult Intelli-
    gence Scale
WB weight bearing
    Willowbrook (virus)
    whole blood
    whole body
WBC white blood cell
    white blood count
WBF whole-blood folate
WBH whole-blood hematocrit
WBR whole-body radiation
WC water closet
    white cell
    white cell casts
    whooping cough

WC (*continued*)
    work capacity
WC' whole complement
WCC white cell count
WD wallerian degeneration
    well-developed
    well-differentiated
    with disease
WDWN well-developed, well-
    nourished
WE Western encephalitis
    Western encephalomyelitis
WEE Western equine encephalo-
    myelitis (virus)
WF Weil-Felix (reaction)
    white female
WFR Weil-Felix reaction
WG water gauge
WH well-healed
WIA wounded in action
WISC Wechsler's Intelligence Scale
    for Children
WK Wernicke-Korsakoff (syn-
    drome)
wk weak
    week
WL waiting list
    wavelength
    work load
WM white male
    whole milk
WMF white middle-aged female
WMM white middle-aged male
WMR work metabolic rate
WN well-nourished
WNF well-nourished female
WNL within normal limits
WNM well-nourished male
wo without
W/O water in oil
WP weakly positive
    working point
WPRS Wittenborn Psychiatric
    Rating Scale
WPW Wolff-Parkinson-White
    (syndrome)

WR   Wassermann reaction
    weakly reactive
wr   wrist
WRC   washed red cells
WRE   whole ragweed extract
WS   water swallow
ws   watts-second
wt   weight
    white
WV   whispered voice
w/v   weight per volume
X   homeopathic symbol for the
    decimal scale of potencies
    Kienbock's unit of x-ray dosage
    magnification
    removal of
    respirations (anesthesia chart)
    start of anesthesia
    times
XC   excretory cystogram
XDP   xeroderma pigmentosum
XM   crossmatch
XP   xeroderma pigmentosum
XR   x-ray

XS   excess
    xiphisternum
XT   exotropia
XU   excretory urogram
Xu   x-unit
Y   year
yd   yard
YF   yellow fever
YO   year old
YOB   year of birth
yr   year
YS   yellow spot (of the retina)
    yolk sac
Z   atomic number
    zero
    Zuckung (contraction)
Z/D   zero defects
ZE   Zollinger-Ellison (syndrome)
Z/G or
ZIG   zoster immune globulin
Zz   ginger (*zingiber*)
Z, Z', Z''   increasing degrees of
    contraction

SYMBOLS

Ⓛ	left	○	female
Ⓜ	murmur	♂	male
Ⓡ	right trademark	♀	female
⊙	start of operation	*	birth
⊗	end of operation	†	death
□	male	τ	life (time)

$\tau\frac{1}{2}$	half-life (time)	Δt	time interval
$\bar{p}$	after	$3 = D$	delayed double diffusion (test)
$\bar{a}$	before		
$\bar{c}$	with	606	arsphenamine
$\bar{s}$	without	914	neoarsphenamine
?	question of questionable possible	R	take
		6-MP	6-mercaptopurine
$\sim$	approximate	^3HT	H_3T, tritiated thymidine
$\pm$	not definite	2d	second
$\downarrow$	decreased depression	$2°$	secondary
		2ndry	secondary
$\uparrow$	elevation increased	$2\times$	twice
$\Uparrow$	up	$\times 2$	twice
$\rightarrow$	causes transfer to	$1\times$	once
		$°$	degree
$\leftarrow$	is due to	$'$	foot
$\ominus$	normal	$''$	inch
$\sqrt{c}$	check with	$\ddot{\overline{ii}}$	two
φ	none	$/$	of per
$\vee$	systolic blood pressure		
$\wedge$	diastolic blood pressure	$:$	ratio (is to)
#	gauge number weight	$+$	positive present
$24°$	24 hours	$-$	absent negative

$\overline{X}$	average of all X's	$\mu\mu$g	micromicrogram (picogram)
α	alpha particle is proportional to	μM	micromolar
$\neq$	does not equal	μr	microroentgen
$>$	greater than	μsec	microsecond
$<$	less than	μu	microunit
χ^2	chi square (test)	μv	microvolt
σ	1/100 of a second standard deviation	μw	microwatt
		$\mu\gamma$	milligamma (nanogram)
℈	scruple	mμc	millimicrocurie (nanocurie)
℥	ounce		
f ℥	fluid ounce	mμg	millimicrogram (nanogram)
μ	micron		
$\mu\mu$	micromicron	mμ	millimicron
μc	microcurie	ℨ	drachm dram
μEq	microequivalent	f ℨ	fluidrachm fluidram
μf	microfarad		
μg	microgram	$\triangle$	prism diopter
μl	microliter	∞	infinity
$\mu\mu$c	micromicrocurie (picocurie)	$\frown$	combined with

TABLE OF ELEMENTS

NAME	SYMBOL	AT. NO.	AT. WT.*
Actinium	Ac	89	(227)
Aluminum	Al	13	26.982
Americium	Am	95	(243)
Antimony	Sb	51	121.75
Argon	Ar	18	39.948
Arsenic	As	33	74.922
Astatine	At	85	(210)
Barium	Ba	56	137.34
Berkelium	Bk	97	(247)
Beryllium	Be	4	9.012
Bismuth	Bi	83	208.980
Boron	B	5	10.811
Bromine	Br	35	79.909
Cadmium	Cd	48	112.40
Calcium	Ca	20	40.08
Californium	Cf	98	(249)
Carbon	C	6	12.011
Cerium	Ce	58	140.12
Cesium	Cs	55	132.905
Chlorine	Cl	17	35.453
Chromium	Cr	24	51.996
Cobalt	Co	27	58.933
Copper	Cu	29	63.54
Curium	Cm	96	(247)
Dysprosium	Dy	66	162.50
Einsteinium	Es	99	(254)
Erbium	Er	68	167.26
Europium	Eu	63	151.96
Fermium	Fm	100	(253)
Fluorine	F	9	18.998
Francium	Fr	87	(223)
Gadolinium	Gd	64	157.25
Gallium	Ga	31	69.72
Germanium	Ge	32	72.59
Gold	Au	79	196.967
Hafnium	Hf	72	178.49
Hahnium	Ha	105	(260)
Helium	He	2	4.003
Holmium	Ho	67	164.930
Hydrogen	H	1	1.008
Indium	In	49	114.82
Iodine	I	53	126.904
Iridium	Ir	77	192.2
Iron	Fe	26	55.847
Krypton	Kr	36	83.80
Lanthanum	La	57	138.91
Lawrencium	Lw	103	(257)
Lead	Pb	82	207.19
Lithium	Li	3	6.939
Lutetium	Lu	71	174.97
Magnesium	Mg	12	24.312

*Atomic weights are corrected to conform with the 1961 values of the Commission on Atomic Weights, expressed to the fourth decimal point, rounded off to the nearest thousandth. The numbers in parentheses are the mass numbers of the most stable or most common isotopes.

NAME	SYMBOL	AT. NO.	AT. WT.*
Manganese	Mn	25	54.938
Mendelevium	Md	101	(256)
Mercury	Hg	80	200.59
Molybdenum	Mo	42	95.94
Neodymium	Nd	60	144.24
Neon	Ne	10	20.183
Neptunium	Np	93	(237)
Nickel	Ni	28	58.71
Niobium	Nb	41	92.906
Nitrogen	N	7	14.007
Nobelium	No	102	(253)
Osmium	Os	76	190.2
Oxygen	O	8	15.999
Palladium	Pd	46	106.4
Phosphorus	P	15	30.974
Platinum	Pt	78	195.09
Plutonium	Pu	94	(242)
Polonium	Po	84	(210)
Potassium	K	19	39.102
Praseodymium	Pr	59	140.907
Promethium	Pm	61	(147)
Protactinium	Pa	91	(231)
Radium	Ra	88	(226)
Radon	Rn	86	(222)
Rhenium	Re	75	186.2
Rhodium	Rh	45	102.905
Rubidium	Rb	37	85.47
Ruthenium	Ru	44	101.07
Rutherfordium	Rf	104	(261)
Samarium	Sm	62	150.35
Scandium	Sc	21	44.956
Selenium	Se	34	78.96
Silicon	Si	14	28.086
Silver	Ag	47	107.870
Sodium	Na	11	22.990
Strontium	Sr	38	87.62
Sulfur	S	16	32.064
Tantalum	Ta	73	180.948
Technetium	Tc	43	(99)
Tellurium	Te	52	127.60
Terbium	Tb	65	158.924
Thallium	Tl	81	204.37
Thorium	Th	90	232.038
Thulium	Tm	69	168.934
Tin	Sn	50	118.69
Titanium	Ti	22	47.90
Tungsten	W	74	183.85
Uranium	U	92	238.03
Vanadium	V	23	50.942
Xenon	Xe	54	131.30
Ytterbium	Yb	70	173.04
Yttrium	Y	39	88.905
Zinc	Zn	30	65.37
Zirconium	Zr	40	91.22

*Atomic weights are corrected to conform with the 1961 values of the Commission on Atomic Weights, expressed to the fourth decimal point, rounded off to the nearest thousandth. The numbers in parentheses are the mass numbers of the most stable or most common isotopes.

(Courtesy of Dorland's Illustrated Medical Dictionary, 26th ed. P. 429. Philadelphia, W.B. Saunders Company, 1981.)

TABLES OF WEIGHTS AND MEASURES*

Measures of Mass

AVOIRDUPOIS WEIGHT

GRAINS	DRAMS	OUNCES	POUNDS	METRIC EQUIVALENTS, GRAMS
1	0.0366	0.0023	0.00014	0.0647989
27.34	1	0.0625	0.0039	1.772
437.5	16	1	0.0625	28.350
7000	256	16	1	453.5924277

APOTHECARIES' WEIGHT

GRAINS	SCRUPLES (℈)	DRAMS (ʒ)	OUNCES (℥)	POUNDS (lb.)	METRIC EQUIVALENTS, GRAMS
1	0.05	0.0167	0.0021	0.00017	0.0647989
20	1	0.333	0.042	0.0035	1.296
60	3	1	0.125	0.0104	3.888
480	24	8	1	0.0833	31.103
5760	288	96	12	1	373.24177

*Courtesy of Miller, B. F., and Keane, C. B.: Encyclopedia and Dictionary of Medicine, Nursing, and Allied Health, 2nd ed. Philadelphia, W. B. Saunders Company, 1978.

TROY WEIGHT

GRAINS	PENNYWEIGHTS	OUNCES	POUNDS	METRIC EQUIVALENTS, GRAMS
1	0.042	0.002	0.00017	0.0647989
24	1	0.05	0.0042	1.555
480	20	1	0.083	31.103
5760	240	12	1	373.24177

METRIC WEIGHT

MICROGRAM	MILLIGRAM	CENTIGRAM	DECIGRAM	GRAM	DECAGRAM	HECTOGRAM	KILOGRAM	EQUIVALENTS	
								AVOIRDUPOIS	APOTHECARIES'
1	...	...	...	...	...	...	...	0.000015 grains	
10^3	1	...	...	...	...	...	...	0.015432 grains	
10^4	10	1	...	...	...	...	...	0.154323 grains	
10^5	10^2	10	1	...	...	...	...	1.543235 grains	
10^6	10^3	10^2	10	1	...	...	...	15.432356 grains	
10^7	10^4	10^3	10^2	10	1	...	...	5.6438 dr.	7.7162 scr.
10^8	10^5	10^4	10^3	10^2	10	1	...	3.527 oz.	3.215 oz.
10^9	10^6	10^5	10^4	10^3	10^2	10	1	2.2046 lb.	2.6792 lb.
10^{12}	10^9	10^8	10^7	10^6	10^5	10^4	10^3	2204.6223 lb.	2679.2285 lb.

TABLES OF WEIGHTS AND MEASURES – *Continued*

Measures of Capacity

APOTHECARIES' (WINE) MEASURE

MINIMS	FLUID DRAMS	FLUID OUNCES	GILLS	PINTS	QUARTS	GALLONS	EQUIVALENTS		
							CUBIC INCHES	MILLI-LITERS	CUBIC CENTIMETERS
1	0.0166	0.002	0.0005	0.00013	...	...	0.00376	0.06161	0.06161
60	1	0.125	0.0312	0.0078	0.0039	...	0.22558	3.6967	3.6967
480	8	1	0.25	0.0625	0.0312	0.0078	1.80468	29.5737	29.5737
1920	32	4	1	0.25	0.125	0.0312	7.21875	118.2948	118.2948
7680	128	16	4	1	0.5	0.125	28.875	473.179	473.179
15360	256	32	8	2	1	0.25	57.75	946.358	946.358
61440	1024	128	32	8	4	1	231	3785.434	3785.434

METRIC MEASURE

MICROLITER	MILLILITER	CENTILITER	DECILITER	LITER	DEKALITER	HECTOLITER	KILOLITER	MYRIALITER	EQUIVALENTS (APOTHECARIES' FLUID)
1	...	...	...	...	...	...	...	...	0.01623108 min.
10^3	1	...	...	...	...	...	...	...	16.23 min.
10^4	10	1	...	...	...	...	...	...	2.7 fl. dr.
10^5	10^2	10	1	...	...	...	...	...	3.38 fl. oz.
10^6	10^3	10^2	10	1	...	...	...	...	2.11 pts.
10^7	10^4	10^3	10^2	10	1	...	...	...	2.64 gal.
10^8	10^5	10^4	10^3	10^2	10	1	...	...	26.418 gal.
10^9	10^6	10^5	10^4	10^3	10^2	10	1	...	264.18 gal.
10^{10}	10^7	10^6	10^5	10^4	10^3	10^2	10	1	2641.8 gal.

1 liter = 2.113363738 pints (Apothecaries').

TABLES OF WEIGHTS AND MEASURES—*Continued*

Measures of Length

METRIC MEASURE

MICRON	MILLI-METER	CENTI-METER	DECI-METER	METER	DEKA-METER	HEKTO-METER	KILO-METER	MYRIA-METER	MEGA-METER	EQUIVALENTS	
1	0.001	10^{-4}	…	…	…	…	…	…	…	0.000039	inch
10^3	1	10^{-1}	…	…	…	…	…	…	…	0.03937	inch
10^4	10	1	…	…	…	…	…	…	…	0.3937	inch
10^5	10^2	10	1	…	…	…	…	…	…	3.937	inch
10^6	10^3	10^2	10	1	…	…	…	…	…	39.37	inch
10^7	10^4	10^3	10^2	10	1	…	…	…	…	10.9361	yards
10^8	10^5	10^4	10^3	10^2	10	1	…	…	…	109.3612	yards
10^9	10^6	10^5	10^4	10^3	10^2	10	1	…	…	1093.6121	yards
10^{10}	10^7	10^6	10^5	10^4	10^3	10^2	10	1	…	6.2137	miles
10^{11}	10^8	10^7	10^6	10^5	10^4	10^3	10^2	10	1	62.1370	miles

Conversion Tables

AVOIRDUPOIS — METRIC WEIGHT

Ounces	Grams
1/16	1.772
1/8	3.544
1/4	7.088
1/2	14.175
1	28.350
2	56.699
3	85.049
4	113.398
5	141.748
6	170.097
7	198.447
8	226.796
9	255.146
10	283.495
11	311.845
12	340.194
13	368.544
14	396.893
15	425.243
16 (1 lb.)	453.59

Pounds	
1 (16 oz.)	453.59
2	907.18
3	1360.78 (1.36 kg.)
4	1814.37 (1.81 ")
5	2267.96 (2.27 ")
6	2721.55 (2.72 ")
7	3175.15 (3.18 ")
8	3628.74 (3.63 ")
9	4082.33 (4.08 ")
10	4535.92 (4.54 ")

METRIC — AVOIRDUPOIS WEIGHT

GRAMS	OUNCES
0.001 (1 mg.)	0.000035274
1	0.035274
1000 (1 kg.)	35.274 (2.2046 lb.)

APOTHECARIES' — METRIC LIQUID MEASURE

Minims	Milliliters
1	0.06
2	0.12
3	0.19
4	0.25
5	0.31
10	0.62
15	0.92
20	1.23
25	1.54
30	1.85
35	2.16
40	2.46
45	2.77
50	3.08
55	3.39
60 (1 fl.dr.)	3.70

Fluid drams	
1	3.70
2	7.39
3	11.09
4	14.79
5	18.48
6	22.18
7	25.88
8 (1 fl.oz.)	29.57

Fluid ounces	
1	29.57
2	59.15
3	88.72
4	118.29
5	147.87
6	177.44
7	207.01
8	236.58
9	266.16
10	295.73
11	325.30
12	354.88
13	384.45
14	414.02
15	443.59
16 (1 pt.)	473.18
32 (1 qt.)	946.36
128 (1 gal.)	3785.43

METRIC — APOTHECARIES' LIQUID MEASURE

MILLILITERS	MINIMS	MILLILITERS	FLUID DRAMS	MILLILITERS	FLUID OUNCES
1	16.231	5	1.35	30	1.01
2	32.5	10	2.71	40	1.35
3	48.7	15	4.06	50	1.69
4	64.9	20	5.4	500	16.91
5	81.1	25	6.76	1000 (1 L.)	33.815
		30	7.1		

TABLES OF WEIGHTS AND MEASURES – *Continued*

CONVERSION TABLES

APOTHECARIES' – METRIC WEIGHT		METRIC – APOTHECARIES' WEIGHT	
Grains	Grams	Milligrams	Grains
1/150	0.0004	1	0.015432
1/120	0.0005	2	0.030864
1/100	0.0006	3	0.046296
1/80	0.0008	4	0.061728
1/64	0.001	5	0.077160
1/50	0.0013	6	0.092592
1/48	0.0014	7	0.108024
1/30	0.0022	8	0.123456
1/25	0.0026	9	0.138888
1/16	0.004	10	0.154320
1/12	0.005	15	0.231480
1/10	0.006	20	0.308640
1/9	0.007	25	0.385800
1/8	0.008	30	0.462960
1/7	0.009	35	0.540120
1/6	0.01	40	0.617280
1/5	0.013	45	0.694440
1/4	0.016	50	0.771600
1/3	0.02	100	1.543240
1/2	0.032		
1	0.065	Grams	
1 1/2	0.097 (0.1)	0.1	1.5432
2	0.12	0.2	3.0864
3	0.20	0.3	4.6296
4	0.24	0.4	6.1728
5	0.30	0.5	7.7160
6	0.40	0.6	9.2592
7	0.45	0.7	10.8024
8	0.50	0.8	12.3456
9	0.60	0.9	13.8888
10	0.65	1.0	15.4320
15	1.00	1.5	23.1480
20 (1.3)	1.30	2.0	30.8640
30	2.00	2.5	38.5800
Scruples		3.0	46.2960
1	1.296 (1.3)	3.5	54.0120
2	2.592 (2.6)	4.0	61.728
3 (1 5)	3.888 (3.9)	4.5	69.444
Drams		5.0	77.162
1	3.888	10.0	154.324
2	7.776		
3	11.664		Equivalents
4	15.552	10	2.572 drams
5	19.440	15	3.858 "
6	23.328	20	5.144 "
7	27.216	25	6.430 "
8 (1 5)	31.103	30	7.716 "
Ounces		40	1.286 oz.
1	31.103	45	1.447 "
2	62.207	50	1.607 "
3	93.310	100	3.215 "
4	124.414	200	6.430 "
5	155.517	300	9.644 "
6	186.621	400	12.859 "
7	217.724	500	1.34 lb.
8	248.828	600	1.61 "
9	279.931	700	1.88 "
10	311.035	800	2.14 "
11	342.138	900	2.41 "
12 (1 lb.)	373.242	1000	2.68 "

TABLES OF WEIGHTS AND MEASURES — *Concluded*

Metric Doses With Approximate Apothecary Equivalents*

These *approximate* dose equivalents represent the quantities usually prescribed, under identical conditions, by physicians trained, respectively, in the metric or in the apothecary system of weights and measures. In labeling dosage forms in both the metric and the apothecary systems, if one is the approximate equivalent of the other, the approximate figure shall be enclosed in parentheses.

When prepared dosage forms such as tablets, capsules, pills, etc., are prescribed in the metric system, the pharmacist may dispense the corresponding *approximate* equivalent in the apothecary system, and vice versa, as indicated in the following table.

Caution — For the conversion of specific quantities in a prescription which requires compounding, or in converting a pharmaceutical formula from one system of weights or measures to the other, *exact* equivalents must be used.

LIQUID MEASURE		LIQUID MEASURE	
METRIC	APPROX. APOTHECARY EQUIVALENTS	METRIC	APPROX. APOTHECARY EQUIVALENTS
1000 ml.	1 quart	3 ml.	45 minims
750 ml.	1 1/2 pints	2 ml.	30 minims
500 ml.	1 pint	1 ml.	15 minims
250 ml.	8 fluid ounces	0.75 ml.	12 minims
200 ml.	7 fluid ounces	0.6 ml.	10 minims
100 ml.	3 1/2 fluid ounces	0.5 ml.	8 minims
50 ml.	1 3/4 fluid ounces	0.3 ml.	5 minims
30 ml.	1 fluid ounce	0.25 ml.	4 minims
15 ml.	4 fluid drams	0.2 ml.	3 minims
10 ml.	2 1/2 fluid drams	0.1 ml.	1 1/2 minims
8 ml.	2 fluid drams	0.06 ml.	1 minim
5 ml.	1 1/4 fluid drams	0.05 ml.	3/4 minim
4 ml.	1 fluid dram	0.03 ml.	1/2 minim

WEIGHT		WEIGHT	
METRIC	APPROX. APOTHECARY EQUIVALENTS	METRIC	APPROX. APOTHECARY EQUIVALENTS
30 Gm.	1 ounce	30 mg.	1/2 grain
15 Gm.	4 drams	25 mg.	3/8 grain
10 Gm.	2 1/2 drams	20 mg.	1/3 grain
7.5 Gm.	2 drams	15 mg.	1/4 grain
6 Gm.	90 grains	12 mg.	1/5 grain
5 Gm.	75 grains	10 mg.	1/6 grain
4 Gm.	60 grains (1 dram)	8 mg.	1/8 grain
3 Gm.	45 grains	6 mg.	1/10 grain
2 Gm.	30 grains (1/2 dram)	5 mg.	1/12 grain
1.5 Gm.	22 grains	4 mg.	1/15 grain
1 Gm.	15 grains	3 mg.	1/20 grain
0.75 Gm.	12 grains	2 mg.	1/30 grain
0.6 Gm.	10 grains	1.5 mg.	1/40 grain
0.5 Gm.	7 1/2 grains	1.2 mg.	1/50 grain
0.4 Gm.	6 grains	1 mg.	1/60 grain
0.3 Gm.	5 grains	0.8 mg.	1/80 grain
0.25 Gm.	4 grains	0.6 mg.	1/100 grain
0.2 Gm.	3 grains	0.5 mg.	1/120 grain
0.15 Gm.	2 1/2 grains	0.4 mg.	1/150 grain
0.12 Gm.	2 grains	0.3 mg.	1/200 grain
0.1 Gm.	1 1/2 grains	0.25 mg.	1/250 grain
75 mg.	1 1/4 grains	0.2 mg.	1/300 grain
60 mg.	1 grain	0.15 mg.	1/400 grain
50 mg.	3/4 grain	0.12 mg.	1/500 grain
40 mg.	2/3 grain	0.1 mg.	1/600 grain

Note — A milliliter (ml.) is the approximate equivalent of a cubic centimeter (cc.).

* Adopted by the latest Pharmacopeia, National Formulary, and New and Nonofficial Remedies, and approved by the Federal Food and Drug Administration.

COMBINING FORMS
IN MEDICAL TERMINOLOGY*

The following is a list of combining forms encountered frequently in the vocabulary of medicine. A dash or dashes are appended to indicate whether the form usually precedes (as ante-) or follows (as -agra) the other elements of the compound or usually appears between the other elements (as -em-). Following each combining form, the first item of information is the Greek or Latin word, or both a Greek and a Latin word, from which it is derived. Those words that are not printed in Greek characters are Latin. Information necessary to an understanding of the form appears next in parentheses. Then the meaning or meanings of the word are given, followed where appropriate by reference to a synonymous combining form. Finally, an example is given to illustrate the use of the combining form in a compound English derivative.

a-	a- (n is added before words beginning with a vowel) negative prefix. Cf. in-³. ametria	alve-	alveus trough, channel, cavity. alveolar
ab-	ab away from. Cf. apo-. abducent	amph-	See amphi-. ampheclexis
abdomin-	abdomen, abdominis. abdominoscopy	amphi-	ἀμφί (i is dropped before words beginning with a vowel) both, doubly. amphicelous
ac-	See ad-. accretion	amyl-	ἄμυλον starch. amylosynthesis
acet-	acetum vinegar. acetometer	an-¹	See ana-. anagogic
acid-	acidus sour. aciduric	an-²	See a-. anomalous
acou-	ἀκούω hear. acouesthesia. (Also spelled acu-)	ana-	ἀνά (final a is dropped before words beginning with a vowel) up, positive. anaphoresis
acr-	ἄκρον extremity, peak. acromegaly		
act-	ago, actus do, drive, act. reaction	ancyl-	See ankyl-. ancylostomiasis
		andr-	ἀνήρ, ἀνδρός man. gynandroid
actin-	ἀκτίς, ἀκτῖνος ray, radius. Cf. radi-. actinogenesis	angi-	ἀγγεῖον vessel. Cf. vas-. angiemphraxis
acu-	See acou-. osteoacusis	ankyl-	ἀγκύλος crooked, looped. ankylodactylia. (Also spelled ancyl-)
ad-	ad (d changes to c, f, g, p, s, or t before words beginning with those consonants) to. adrenal	ant-	See anti-. antophthalmic
		ante-	ante before. anteflexion
aden-	ἀδήν gland. Cf. gland-. adenoma	anti-	ἀντί (i is dropped before words beginning with a vowel) against, counter. Cf. contra-. antipyogenic
adip-	adeps, adipis fat. Cf. lip- and stear-. adipocellular		
aer-	ἀήρ air. anaerobiosis	antr-	ἄντρον cavern. antrodynia
aesthe-	See esthe-. aesthesioneurosis	ap-¹	See apo-. apheter
af-	See ad-. afferent	ap-²	See ad-. append
ag-	See ad-. agglutinant	-aph-	ἅπτω, ἀφ- touch. dysaphia. (See also hapt-)
-agogue	ἀγωγός leading, inducing. galactagogue		
		apo-	ἀπό (o is dropped before words beginning with a vowel) away from, detached. Cf. ab-. apophysis
-agra	ἄγρα catching, seizure. podagra		
alb-	albus white. Cf. leuk-. albocinereous		
		arachn-	ἀράχνη spider. arachnodactyly
alg-	ἄλγος pain. neuralgia	arch-	ἀρχή beginning, origin. archenteron
all-	ἄλλος other, different. allergy		

*Compiled by Lloyd W. Daly. A.M., Ph.D., Litt. D., Allen Memorial Professor of Greek, University of Pennsylvania.

arter(i)-   ἀρτηρία elevator (?), artery. arteriosclerosis, periarteritis

arthr-   ἄρθρον joint. Cf. articul-. synarthrosis

articul-   articulus joint. Cf. arthr-. disarticulation

as-   See ad-. assimilation

at-   See ad-. attrition

aur-   auris ear. Cf. ot-. aurinasal

aux-   αὔξω increase. enterauxe

ax-   ἄξων or axis axis. axofugal

axon-   ἄξων axis. axonometer

ba-   βαίνω, βα- go, walk, stand. hypnobatia

bacill-   bacillus small staff, rod. Cf. bacter-. actinobacillosis

bacter-   βακτήριον small staff, rod. Cf. bacill-. bacteriophage

ball-   βάλλω, βολ- throw. ballistics. (See also bol-)

bar-   βάρος weight. pedobarometer

bi-¹   βίος life. Cf. vit-. aerobic

bi-²   bi- two (see also di-¹). bilobate

bil-   bilis bile. Cf. chol-. biliary

blast-   βλαστός bud, child, a growing thing in its early stages. Cf. germ-. blastoma, zygotoblast.

blep-   βλέπω look, see. hemiablepsia

blephar-   βλέφαρον (from βλέπω; see blep-) eyelid. Cf. cili-. blepharoncus

bol-   See ball-. embolism

brachi-   βραχίων arm. brachiocephalic

brachy-   βραχύς short. brachycephalic

brady-   βραδύς slow. bradycardia

brom-   βρῶμος stench. podobromidrosis

bronch-   βρόγχος windpipe. bronchoscopy

bry-   βρύω be full of life. embryonic

bucc-   bucca cheek. distobuccal

cac-   κακός bad, abnormal. Cf. mal-. cacodontia, arthrocace. (See also dys-)

calc-¹   calx, calcis stone (cf. lith-), limestone, lime. calcipexy

calc-²   calx, calcis heel. calcaneotibial

calor-   calor heat. Cf. therm-. calorimeter

cancr-   cancer, cancri crab, cancer. Cf. carcin-. cancrology. (Also spelled chancr-)

capit-   caput, capitis head. Cf. cephal-. decapitator

caps-   capsa (from capio; see cept-) container. encapsulation

carbo(n)-   carbo, carbonis coal, charcoal. carbohydrate, carbonuria

carcin-   καρκίνος crab, cancer. Cf. cancr-. carcinoma

cardi-   καρδία heart. lipocardiac

cary-   See kary-. caryokinesis

cat-   See cata-. cathode

cata-   κατά (final a is dropped before words beginning with a vowel) down, negative. catabatic

caud-   cauda tail. caudad

cav-   cavus hollow. Cf. coel-. concave

cec-   caecus blind. Cf. typhl-. cecopexy

cel-¹   See coel-. amphicelous

cel-²   See -cele. celectome

-cele   κήλη tumor, hernia. gastrocele

cell-   cella room, cell. Cf. cyt-. celliferous

cen-   κοινός common. cenesthesia

cent-   centum hundred. Cf. hect-. Indicates fraction in metric system. [This exemplifies the custom in the metric system of identifying fractions of units by stems from the Latin, as centimeter, decimeter, millimeter, and multiples of units by the similar stems from the Greek, as hectometer, decameter, and kilometer.] centimeter, centipede

cente-   κεντέω puncture. Cf. punct-. enterocentesis

centr-   κέντρον or centrum point, center. neurocentral

cephal-   κεφαλή head. Cf. capit-. encephalitis

cept-   capio, -cipientis, -ceptus take, receive. receptor

cer-   κηρός or cera wax. ceroplasty, ceromel

cerat-   See kerat-. aceratosis

cerebr-   cerebrum. cerebrospinal

cervic-   cervix, cervicis neck. Cf. trachel-. cervicitis

chancr-   See cancr-. chancriform

cheil-   χεῖλος lip. Cf. labi-. cheiloschisis

cheir-   χείρ hand. Cf. man-. macrocheiria. (Also spelled chir-)

chir-   See cheir-. chiromegaly

chlor-   χλωρός green. achloropsia

chol-   χολή bile. Cf. bil-. hepatocholangeitis

chondr-   χόνδρος cartilage. chondromalacia

chord-   χορδή string, cord. perichordal

chori-   χόριον protective fetal membrane. endochorion

chro-   χρώς color. polychromatic

chron-   χρόνος time. synchronous

chy-   χέω, χυ- pour. ecchymosis

-cid(e)   caedo, -cisus cut, kill. infanticide, germicidal

cili-   cilium eyelid. Cf. blephar-. superciliary

cine-   See kine-. autocinesis

-cipient   See cept-. incipient

circum-   circum around. Cf. peri-. circumferential

-cis-   caedo, -cisus cut, kill. excision

clas-   κλάω, κλασ- break. cranioclast

clin-   κλίνω bend, incline, make lie down. clinometer

clus-   claudo, -clusus shut. Malocclusion

co-   See con-. cohesion

cocc-   κόκκος seed, pill. gonococcus

coel-   κοῖλος hollow. Cf. cav-. coelenteron. (Also spelled cel-)

col-¹   See colon-. colic

col-²   See con-. collapse

colon- κόλον lower intestine. *colon*ic

colp- κόλπος hollow, vagina. Cf. sin-. endo*colp*itis

com- See con-. *com*masculation

con- con- (becomes co- before vowels or *h*; col- before *l*; com- before *b*, *m*, or *p*; cor- before *r*) with, together. Cf. syn-. *con*traction

contra- *contra* against, counter. Cf. anti-. *contra*indication

copr- κόπρος dung. Cf. sterco-. *copr*oma

cor-¹ κόρη doll, little image, pupil. iso*cor*ia

cor-² See con-. *cor*rugator

corpor- *corpus*, *corporis* body. Cf. somat-. intra*corpor*al

cortic- *cortex*, *corticis* bark, rind. *cortic*osterone

cost- *costa* rib. Cf. pleur-. inter*cost*al

crani- κρανίον or *cranium* skull. peri*crani*um

creat- κρέας, κρεατ- meat, flesh. *creat*orrhea

-crescent *cresco*, *crescentis*, *cretus* grow. ex*crescent*

cret-¹ *cerno*, *cretus* distinguish, separate off. Cf. crin-. dis*crete*

cret-² See -crescent. ac*cret*ion

crin- κρίνω distinguish, separate off. Cf. cret-¹. endo*crin*ology

crur- *crus*, *cruris* shin, leg. brachio*crur*al

cry- κρύος cold. *cry*esthesia

crypt- κρύπτω hide, conceal. *crypt*orchism

cult- *colo*, *cultus* tend, cultivate. *cult*ure

cune- *cuneus* wedge. Cf. sphen-. *cune*iform

cut- *cutis* skin. Cf. derm(at)-. sub*cut*aneous

cyan- κύανος blue. antho*cyan*in

cycl- κύκλος circle, cycle. *cycl*ophoria

cyst- κύστις bladder. Cf. vesic-. nephro*cyst*itis

cyt- κύτος cell. Cf. cell-. plasmo*cyt*oma

dacry- δάκρυ tear. *dacry*ocyst

dactyl- δάκτυλος finger, toe. Cf. digit-. hexa*dactyl*ism

de- *de* down from. *de*composition

dec-¹ δέκα ten. Indicates multiple in metric system. Cf. dec-². *deca*gram

dec-² *decem* ten. Indicates fraction in metric system. Cf. dec-¹. *deci*para, *deci*meter

dendr- δένδρον tree. neuro*dendr*ite

dent- *dens*, *dentis* tooth. Cf. odont-. inter*dent*al

derm(at)- δέρμα, δέρματος skin. Cf. cut-. endo*derm*, *derm*atitis

desm- δεσμός band, ligament. syn*desm*opexy

dextr- *dexter*, *dextr*- right-hand. ambi*dextr*ous

di-¹ *di*- two. *di*morphic. (See also bi-²)

di-² See dia-. *di*uresis.

di-³ See dis-. *di*vergent.

dia- διά (*a* is dropped before words beginning with a vowel) through, apart. Cf. per-. *dia*gnosis

didym- δίδυμος twin. Cf. gemin-. epi*didym*al

digit- *digitus* finger, toe. Cf. dactyl-. *digit*igrade

diplo- διπλόος double. *diplo*myelia

dis- *dis*- (*s* may be dropped before a word beginning with a consonant) apart, away from. *dis*location

disc- δίσκος or *discus* disk. *disc*oplacenta

dors- *dorsum* back. ventro*dors*al

drom- δρόμος course. hemo*drom*ometer

-ducent See duct-. ad*ducent*

duct- *duco*, *ducentis*, *ductus* lead, conduct. ovi*duct*

dur- *durus* hard. Cf. scler-. in*dur*ation

dynam(i)- δύναμις power. *dynam*oneure, neuro*dynam*ic

dys- δυσ- bad, improper. Cf. mal-. *dys*trophic. (See also cac-)

e- *e* out from. Cf. ec- and ex-. *e*mission

ec- ἐκ out of. Cf. e- *ec*centric

-ech- ἔχω have, hold, be. syn*ech*otomy

ect- ἐκτός outside. Cf. extra-. *ect*oplasm

ede- οἰδέω swell. *ede*matous

ef- See ex-. *ef*florescent

-elc- ἕλκος sore, ulcer. ent*elc*osis. (See also helc-)

electr- ἤλεκτρον amber. *electr*otherapy

em- See en-. *em*bolism, *em*pathy, *em*phlysis

-em- αἷμα blood. an*em*ia. (See also hem(at)-)

en- ἐν (*n* changes to *m* before *b*, *p*, or *ph*) in, on. Cf. in-². *en*celitis

end- ἔνδον inside. Cf. intra-. *end*angium

enter- ἔντερον intestine. dys*enter*y

ep- See epi-. *ep*axial

epi- ἐπί (*i* is dropped before words beginning with a vowel) upon, after, in addition. *epi*glottis

erg- ἔργον work, deed. en*erg*y

erythr- ἐρυθρός red. Cf. rub(r)-. *erythr*ochromia

eso- ἔσω inside. Cf. intra-. *eso*phylactic

esthe- αἰσθάνομαι, αἰσθη- perceive, feel. Cf. sens-. an*esthe*sia

eu- εὖ good, normal. *eu*pepsia

ex- ἐξ or *ex* out of. Cf. e-. *ex*cretion

exo- ἔξω outside. Cf. extra-. *exo*pathic

extra- *extra* outside of, beyond. Cf. ect- and exo-. *extra*cellular

faci- *facies* face. Cf. prosop-. brachio*faci*olingual

-facient	*facio, facientis, factus, -fectus* make. Cf. poie-. cale*facient*
-fact-	See facient-. arte*fact*
fasci-	*fascia* band. *fasci*orrhaphy
febr-	*febris* fever. Cf. pyr-. *febr*icide
-fect-	See -facient. de*fect*ive
-ferent	*fero, ferentis, latus* bear, carry. Cf. phor-. ef*ferent*
ferr-	*ferrum* iron. *ferr*oprotein
fibr-	*fibra* fibre. Cf. in-¹. chondro*fibr*oma
fil-	*filum* thread. *fil*iform
fiss-	*findo, fissus* split. Cf. schis-. *fiss*ion
flagell-	*flagellum* whip. *flagell*ation
flav-	*flavus* yellow. Cf. xanth-. ribo*flav*in
-flect-	*flecto, flexus* bend, divert. de*flect*ion
-flex-	See -flect-. re*flex*ometer
flu-	*fluo, fluxus* flow. Cf. rhe-. *flu*id
flux-	See flu-. af*flux*ion
for-	*foris* door, opening. per*for*ated
-form	*forma* shape. Cf. -oid. ossi*form*
fract-	*frango, fractus* break. re*fract*ive
front-	*frons, frontis* forehead, front. naso*front*al
-fug(e)	*fugio* flee, avoid. vermi*fuge*, centri*fug*al
funct-	*fungor, functus* perform, serve, function. mal*funct*ion
fund-	*fundo, fusus* pour. in*fund*ibulum
fus-	See fund-. dif*fus*ible
galact-	γάλα, γάλακτος milk. Cf. lact-. dys*galact*ia
gam-	γάμος marriage, reproductive union. a*gam*ont
gangli-	γάγγλιον swelling, plexus. neuro*gangli*itis
gastr-	γαστήρ, γαστρός stomach. cholangio*gastr*ostomy
gelat-	*gelo, gelatus* freeze, congeal. *gelat*in
gemin-	*geminus* twin, double. Cf. didym-. quadri*gemin*al
gen-	γίγνομαι, γεν-, γον- become, be produced, originate, or γεννάω produce, originate. cyto*gen*ic
germ-	*germen, germinis* bud, a growing thing in its early stages. Cf. blast-. *germ*inal, ovi*germ*
gest-	*gero, gerentis, gestus* bear, carry. con*gest*ion
gland-	*glans, glandis* acorn. Cf. aden-. intra*gland*ular
-glia	γλία glue. neuro*glia*
gloss-	γλῶσσα tongue. Cf. lingu-. tricho*gloss*ia
glott-	γλῶττα tongue, language. *glott*ic
gluc-	See glyc(y)-. *gluc*ophenetidin
glutin-	*gluten, glutinis* glue. ag*glutin*ation
glyc(y)-	γλυκύς sweet. *glyc*emia, *glycyr*rhizin. (Also spelled gluc-)
gnath-	γνάθος jaw. ortho*gnath*ous
gno-	γιγνώσκω, γνω- know, discern. dia*gno*sis
gon-	See gen-. amphi*gon*y
grad-	*gradior* walk, take steps. retro*grad*e
-gram	γράφω, γραφ- + -μα scratch, write, record. cardio*gram*
gran-	*granum* grain, particle. lipo*gran*uloma
graph-	γράφω scratch, write, record. histo*graph*y
grav-	*gravis* heavy. multi*grav*ida
gyn(ec)-	γυνή, γυναικός woman, wife. andro*gyn*y, *gyn*ecologic
gyr-	γῦρος ring, circle. *gyr*ospasm
haem(at)-	See hem(at)-. *haem*orrhagia, *haemat*oxylon
hapt-	ἅπτω touch. *hapt*ometer
hect-	ἑκτ- hundred. Cf. cent-. Indicates multiple in metric system. *hect*ometer
helc-	ἕλκος sore, ulcer. *helc*osis
hem(at)-	αἷμα, αἵματος blood. Cf. sanguin-. *hem*angioma, *hemat*ocyturia. (See also -em-)
hemi-	ἡμι- half. Cf. semi-. *hemi*ageusia
hen-	εἷς, ἑνός one. Cf. un-. *hen*ogenesis
hepat-	ἧπαρ, ἥπατος liver. gastro*hepat*ic
hept(a)-	ἑπτά seven. Cf. sept-¹. *hept*atomic, *hepta*valent
hered-	*heres, heredis* heir. *hered*oimmunity
hex-¹	ἕξ six. Cf. sex-. *hex*yl-. An *a* is added in some combinations.
hex-²	ἔχω, ἑχ- (added to σ becomes ἑξ-) have, hold, be. ca*hex*y
hexa-	See hex-¹. *hexa*chromic
hidr-	ἱδρώς sweat. hyper*hidr*osis
hist-	ἱστός web, tissue. *hist*odialysis
hod-	ὁδός road, path. *hod*oneuromere. (See also od- and -ode¹)
hom-	ὁμός common, same. *hom*omorphic
horm-	ὁρμή impetus, impulse. *horm*one
hydat-	ὕδωρ, ὕδατος water. *hydat*ism
hydr-	ὕδωρ, ὑδρ- water. Cf. lymph-. achlor*hydr*ia
hyp-	See hypo-. *hyp*axial
hyper-	ὑπέρ above, beyond, extreme. Cf. super-. *hyper*trophy
hypn-	ὕπνος sleep. *hypn*otic
hypo-	ὑπό (ο is dropped before words beginning with a vowel) under, below. Cf. sub-. *hypo*metabolism
hyster-	ὑστέρα womb. colpo*hyster*opexy
iatr-	ἱατρός physician. ped*iatr*ics
idi-	ἴδιος peculiar, separate, distinct. *idi*osyncrasy
il-	See in-². ³. *il*linition (in, on), *il*legible (negative prefix)
ile-	See ili-. [ile- is commonly used to refer to the portion of the

intestines known as the ileum]. *ile*ostomy

ili-   *ilium (ileum)* lower abdomen, intestines [ili- is commonly used to refer to the flaring part of the hip bone known as the ilium]. *ilio*sacral

im-   See in-². ³. *im*mersion (in, on), *im*perforation (negative prefix)

in-¹   ἴς, ἰνός fiber. Cf. fibr-. *in*osteatoma

in-²   *in* (n changes to l, m, or r before words beginning with those consonants) in, on. Cf. en-. *in*sertion

in-³   *in-* (n changes to l, m, or r before words beginning with those consonants) negative prefix. Cf. a-. *in*valid

infra-   *infra* beneath. *infra*orbital
insul-   *insula* island. *insul*in
inter-   *inter* among, between. *inter*carpal
intra-   *intra* inside. Cf. end- and eso-. *intra*venous

ir-   See in-². ³. *ir*radiation (in, on), *ir*reducible (negative prefix)
irid-   ἶρις, ἴριδος rainbow, colored circle. *kerato*irido*cyclitis
is-   ἴσος equal. *iso*tope
ischi-   ἰσχίον hip, haunch. *ischio*pubic
jact-   *iacio, iactus* throw. *jact*itation
ject-   *iacio, -iectus* throw. *in*jection
jejun-   *ieiunus* hungry, not partaking of food. gastro*jejun*ostomy
jug-   *iugum* yoke. con*jug*ation
junct-   *iungo, iunctus* yoke, join. con*junct*iva
kary-   κάρυον nut, kernel, nucleus. Cf. nucle-. mega*kary*ocyte. (Also spelled cary-)
kerat-   κέρας, κέρατος horn. *kerat*olysis. (Also spelled cerat-)
kil-   χίλιοι one thousand. Cf. mill-. Indicates multiple in metric system. *kil*ogram
kine-   κινέω move. *kine*matograph. (Also spelled cine-)
labi-   *labium* lip. Cf. cheil-. gingivo*labi*al
lact-   *lac, lactis* milk. Cf. galact-. gluco*lact*one
lal-   λαλέω talk, babble. glosso*lal*ia
lapar-   λαπάρα flank. *lapar*otomy
laryng-   λάρυγξ, λάρυγγος windpipe. *laryng*endoscope
lat-   *fero, latus* bear, carry. See -ferent. trans*lat*ion
later-   *latus, lateris* side. ventro*later*al
lent-   *lens, lentis* lentil. Cf. phac-. *lent*iconus
lep-   λαμβάνω, ληπ- take, seize. cata*lep*tic
leuc-   See leuk-. *leuc*inuria
leuk-   λευκός white. Cf. alb-. *leuk*orrhea. (Also spelled leuc-)

lien-   *lien* spleen. Cf. splen-. *lieno*cele
lig-   *ligo* tie, bind. *lig*ate
lingu-   *lingua* tongue. Cf. gloss-. sub*lingual*
lip-   λίπος fat. Cf. adip-. glyco*lip*in
lith-   λίθος stone. Cf. calc-¹. nephro*lith*otomy
loc-   *locus* place. Cf. top-. *loc*omotion
log-   λέγω, λογ- speak, give an account. *logo*rrhea, embry*ology*
lumb-   *lumbus* loin. dorso*lumb*ar
lute-   *luteus* yellow. Cf xanth-. *lute*oma
ly-   λύω loose, dissolve. Cf. solut-. *kerato*lysis
lymph-   *lympha* water. Cf. hydr-. *lymph*adenosis
macr-   μακρός long, large. *macr*omyeloblast
mal-   *malus* bad, abnormal. Cf. cac- and dys-. *mal*function
malac-   μαλακός soft. osteo*malac*ia
mamm-   *mamma* breast. Cf. mast-. sub*mamm*ary
man-   *manus* hand. Cf. cheir-. *man*iphalanx
mani-   μανία mental aberration. *ma*nigraphy, klepto*mani*a
mast-   μαστός breast. Cf. mamm-. hyper*mast*ia
medi-   *medius* middle. Cf. mes-. *medi*frontal
mega-   μέγας great, large. Also indicates multiple (1,000,000) in metric system. *mega*colon, *mega*dyne. (See also megal-)
megal-   μέγας, μεγάλου great, large. acro*megal*y
mel-   μέλος limb, member. sym*mel*ia
melan-   μέλας, μέλανος black. hippo*melan*in
men-   μήν month. dys*men*orrhea
mening-   μῆνιγξ, μήνιγγος membrane. encephalo*mening*itis
ment-   *mens, mentis* mind. Cf. phren-, psych- and thym-. de*ment*ia
mer-   μέρος part. poly*mer*ic
mes-   μέσος middle. Cf. medi-. *meso*derm
met   See meta-. *met*allergy
meta-   μετά (a is dropped before words beginning with a vowel) after, beyond, accompanying. *meta*carpal
metr-¹   μέτρον measure. stereo*metr*y
metr-²   μήτρα womb. endo*metr*itis
micr-   μικρός small. photo*micr*ograph
mill-   *mille* one thousand. Cf. kil-. Indicates fraction in metric system. *milli*gram, *milli*pede
miss-   See -mittent. intro*miss*ion
-mittent   *mitto, mittentis, missus* send. inter*mittent*

mne-	μιμνήσκω, μνη- remember pseudomnesia
mon-	μόνος only, sole. monoplegia
morph-	μορφή form, shape. polymorphonuclear
mot-	moveo, motus move. vasomotor
my-	μῦς, μυός muscle. inoleiomyoma
-myces	μύκης, μύκητος fungus. myelomyces
myc(et)-	See -myces. ascomycetes, streptomycin
myel-	μυελός marrow. poliomyelitis
myx-	μύξα mucus. myxedema
narc-	νάρκη numbness. toponarcosis
nas-	nasus nose. Cf. rhin-. palatonasal
ne-	νέος new, young. neocyte
necr-	νεκρός corpse. necrocytosis
nephr-	νεφρός kidney. Cf. ren-. paranephric
neur-	νεῦρον nerve. esthesioneure
nod-	nodus knot. nodosity
nom-	νόμος (from νέμω deal out, distribute) law, custom. taxonomy
non-	nona nine. nonacosane
nos-	νόσος disease. nosology
nucle-	nucleus (from nux, nucis nut) kernel. Cf. kary-. nucleide
nutri-	nutrio nourish. malnutrition
ob-	ob (b changes to c before words beginning with that consonant) against, toward, etc. obtuse
oc-	See ob-. occlude.
ocul-	oculus eye. Cf. ophthalm-. oculomotor
-od-	See -ode¹. periodic
-ode¹	ὁδός road, path. cathode. (See also hod-)
-ode²	See -oid. nematode
odont-	ὁδούς, ὁδόντος tooth. Cf. dent-. orthodontia
-odyn-	ὀδύνη pain, distress. gastrodynia
-oid	εἶδος form. Cf. -form. hyoid
-ol	See ole-. cholesterol
ole-	oleum oil. oleoresin
olig-	ὀλίγος few, small. oligospermia
omphal-	ὀμφαλός navel. periomphalic
onc-	ὄγκος bulk, mass. hematoncometry
onych-	ὄνυξ, ὄνυχος claw, nail. anonychia
oo-	ὠόν egg. Cf. ov-. perioothecitis
op-	ὁράω, ὀπ- see. erythropsia
ophthalm-	ὀφθαλμός eye. Cf. ocul-. exophthalmic
or-	os, oris mouth. Cf. stom(at)-. intraoral
orb-	orbis circle. suborbital
orchi-	ὄρχις testicle. Cf. test-. orchiopathy
organ-	ὄργανον implement, instrument. organoleptic
orth-	ὀρθός straight, right, normal. orthopedics
oss-	os, ossis bone. Cf. ost(e)-. ossiphone
ost(e)-	ὀστέον bone. Cf. oss-. enostosis, osteanaphysis
ot-	οὖς, ὠτός ear. Cf. aur-. parotid
ov-	ovum egg. Cf. oo-. synovia
oxy-	ὀξύς sharp. oxycephalic
pachy(n)-	παχύνω thicken. pachyderma, myopachynsis
pag-	πήγνυμι, παγ- fix, make fast. thoracopagus
par-¹	pario bear, give birth to. primiparous
par-²	See para-. parepigastric
para-	παρά (final a is dropped before words beginning with a vowel) beside, beyond. paramastoid
part-	pario, partus bear, give birth to. parturition
path-	πάθος that which one undergoes, sickness. psychopathic
pec-	πήγνυμι, πηγ- (πηκ- before τ) fix, make fast. sympectothiene. (See also pex-)
ped-	παῖς, παιδός child. orthopedic
pell-	pellis skin, hide. pellagra
-pellent	pello, pellentis, pulsus drive. repellent
pen-	πένομαι need, lack. erythrocytopenia
pend-	pendeo hang down. appendix
pent(a)-	πέντε five. Cf. quinque-. pentose, pentaploid
peps-	πέπτω, πεψ- (before σ) digest bradypepsia
pept-	πέπτω digest. dyspeptic
per-	per through. Cf. dia-. pernasal
peri-	περί around. Cf. circum-. periphery
pet-	peto seek, tend toward. centripetal
pex-	πήγνυμι, πηγ- (added to σ becomes πηξ-) fix, make fast. hepatopexy
pha-	φημί, φα- say, speak. dysphasia
phac-	φακός lentil, lens. Cf. lent-. phacosclerosis. (Also spelled phak-)
phag-	φαγεῖν eat. lipophagic
phak-	See phac-. phakitis
phan-	See phen-. diaphanoscopy
pharmac-	φάρμακον drug. pharmacognosy
pharyng-	φάρυγξ, φαρυγγ- throat. glossopharyngeal
phen-	φαίνω, φαν- show, be seen. phosphene
pher-	φέρω, φορ- bear, support. periphery
phil-	φιλέω like, have affinity for. eosinophilia
phleb-	φλέψ, φλεβός vein. periphlebitis
phleg-	φλέγω, φλογ- burn, inflame. adenophlegmon
phlog-	See phleg-. antiphlogistic
phob-	φόβος fear, dread. claustrophobia
phon-	φωνή sound. echophony

phor- See pher-. Cf. -ferent. exo*phoria*

phos- See phot-. phosphorus

phot- φῶς, φωτός light. *phot*erythrous

phrag- φράσσω, φραγ- fence, wall off, stop up. Cf. sept-[1]. dia*phrag*m

phrax- φράσσω, φραγ- (added to σ becomes φραξ-) fence, wall off, stop up. emp*hrax*is

phren- φρήν mind, midriff. Cf. ment-. meta*phren*ia, meta*phren*on

phthi- φθίνω decay, waste away. ophthalmo*phthis*is

phy- φύω beget, bring forth, produce, be by nature. noso*phyte*

phyl- φῦλον tribe, kind. *phyl*ogeny

-phyll φύλλον leaf. xantho*phyll*

phylac- φύλαξ guard. *prophylac*tic

phys(a)- φυσάω blow, inflate. *phys*ocele, *phys*alis

physe- φυσάω, φυση- blow, inflate. em*physe*ma

pil- pilus hair. epi*pil*ation

pituit- pituita phlegm, rheum. *pituit*ous

placent- placenta (from πλακοῦς) cake. extra*placent*al

plas- πλάσσω mold, shape. cine*plas*ty

platy- πλατύς broad, flat. *platy*rrhine

pleg- πλήσσω, πληγ- strike. di*pleg*ia

plet- pleo, -pletus fill. de*plet*ion

pleur- πλευρά rib, side. Cf. cost-. peri*pleur*al

plex- πλήσσω, πληγ- (added to σ becomes πληξ-) strike. apo*plex*y

plic- plico fold. com*plic*ation

pne- πνοιά breathing. trauma*topne*a

pneum(at)- πνεῦμα, πνεύματος breath, air. *pneum*odynamics, *pneum*atothorax

pneumo(n)- πνεύμων lung. Cf. pulmo(n)-. *pneumo*centesis, *pneumo*notomy

pod- πούς, ποδός foot. *pod*iatry

poie- ποιέω make, produce. Cf. -facient. sarco*poie*tic

pol- πόλος axis of a sphere. peri*pol*ar

poly- πολύς much, many. *poly*spermia

pont- pons, pontis bridge. *ponto*cerebellar

por-[1] πόρος passage. myelo*por*e

por-[2] πῶρος callus. *por*ocele

posit- pono, positus put, place. re*posit*or

post- post after, behind in time or place. *post*natal, *post*oral

pre- prae before in time or place. *pre*natal, *pre*vesical

press- premo, pressus press. *press*oreceptive

pro- πρό or pro before in time or place. *pro*gamous, *pro*cheilon, *pro*lapse

proct- πρωκτός anus. entero*proct*ia

prosop- πρόσωπον face. Cf. faci-. di*prosop*us

pseud- ψευδής false. *pseud*oparaplegia

psych- ψυχή soul, mind. Cf. ment-. *psych*osomatic

pto- πίπτω, πτω- fall. nephro*ptos*is

pub- pubes & puber, puberis adult. ischio*pub*ic. (See also puber-)

puber- puber adult. *puber*ty

pulmo(n)- pulmo, pulmonis lung. Cf. pneumo(n)-. *pulmo*lith, cardio*pulmo*nary

puls- pello, pellentis, pulsus drive. pro*puls*ion

punct- pungo, punctus prick, pierce. Cf. cente-. *punct*iform

pur- pus, puris pus. Cf. py-. sup*pur*ation

py- πύον pus. Cf. pur-. nephro*py*osis

pyel- πύελος trough, basin, pelvis. nephro*pyel*itis

pyl- πύλη door, orifice. *pyl*ephlebitis

pyr- πῦρ fire. Cf. febr-. galacto*pyr*a

quadr- quadr- four. Cf. tetra-. *quadr*igeminal

quinque- quinque five. Cf. pent(a)-. *quinque*cuspid

rachi- ῥαχίς spine. Cf. spin-. encephalo*rachi*dian

radi- radius ray. Cf. actin-. ir*radi*ation

re- re- back, again. *re*traction

ren- renes kidneys. Cf. nephr-. ad*ren*al

ret- rete net. *ret*othelium

retro- retro backwards. *retro*deviation

rhag- ῥήγνυμι, ῥαγ- break, burst. hemor*rhag*ic

rhaph- ῥαφή suture. gastror*rhaph*y

rhe- ῥέω flow. Cf. flu-. diar*rhe*al

rhex- ῥήγνυμι, ῥηγ- (added to σ becomes ῥηξ-) break, burst. metror*rhex*is

rhin- ῥίς, ῥινός nose. Cf. nas-. basi*rhin*al

rot- rota wheel. *rot*ator

rub(r)- ruber, rubri red. Cf. erythr-. bili*rub*in, *rub*rospinal

salping- σάλπιγξ, σάλπιγγος tube, trumpet. *salping*itis

sanguin- sanguis, sanguinis blood. Cf. hem(at)-. *sanguin*eous

sarc- σάρξ, σαρκός flesh. *sarc*oma

schis- σχίζω, σχιδ- (before τ or added to σ becomes σχισ-) split. Cf. fiss-. *schis*torachis, rachi*schis*is

scler- σκληρός hard. Cf. dur-. *scler*osis

scop- σκοπέω look at, observe. endo*scope*

sect- seco, sectus cut. Cf. tom-. *sect*ile

semi- semi- half. Cf. hemi-. *semi*flexion

sens- sentio, sensus perceive, feel. Cf. esthe-. *sens*ory